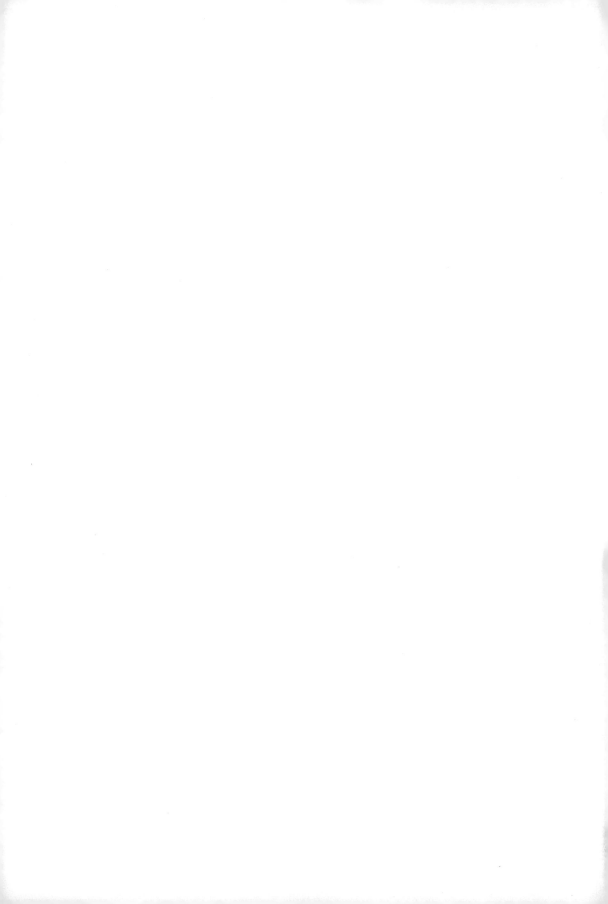

CLINICS IN DEVELOPMENTAL MEDICINE NOS. 113/114
PROBLEMS OF INTRACRANIAL PRESSURE IN CHILDHOOD

Clinics in Developmental Medicine Nos. 113/114

PROBLEMS OF
INTRACRANIAL PRESSURE
IN CHILDHOOD

Edited by
R. A. MINNS

1991
Mac Keith Press

Distributed by:
OXFORD: Blackwell Scientific Publications Ltd.
NEW YORK: Cambridge University Press.

©1991 Mac Keith Press
5a Netherhall Gardens, London NW3 5RN

First published 1991

British Library Cataloguing in Publication Data

Problems of intracranial pressure in childhood.
 1. Children. Brain. Intracranial pressure
 I. Minns, R. A. II. Series
 618.928

ISBN (UK) 0 901260 82 7
    (USA) 0 521 41272 2

Printed in Great Britain at The Lavenham Press Ltd., Lavenham, Suffolk
Mac Keith Press is supported by **The Spastics Society, London, England**

To Dr T. T. S. Ingram

CONTENTS

CONTRIBUTORS

ROGER BAYSTON — Senior Lecturer in Bacteriology, Department of Paediatric Surgery, Institute of Child Health, Guilford Street, London, and Honorary Bacteriologist, National Hospital for Nervous Diseases.

P. S. BAXTER — Lecturer in Paediatrics, University of Sheffield, Department of Paediatrics, Children's Hospital, Sheffield.

NEVILLE R. BELTON — Senior Lecturer, Department of Child Life and Health, University of Edinburgh.

J. K. BROWN — Consultant Paediatric Neurologist, Royal Hospital for Sick Children, Edinburgh.

CONCEZIO DI ROCCO — Associate Professor of Paediatric Neurosurgery, Institute of Neurosurgery, Section of Paediatric Neurosurgery, Catholic University Medical School, Rome.

A. H. HAMILTON — Senior Registrar in Paediatrics, St Luke's Hospital, Paediatric Unit, Little Horton Lane, Bradford.

F. J. KIRKHAM — Senior Registrar in Paediatrics, Newcomen Centre, Guy's Hospitals, St Thomas Street, London.

J. R. S. LEGGATE — Consultant Neurosurgeon, North Manchester General and Booth Hall Children's Hospitals, Manchester.

MALCOLM I. LEVENE — Professor of Paediatrics and Child Health, Honorary Consultant Paediatrician, Clarendon Wing, General Infirmary at Leeds.

NEIL McINTOSH — Professor of Child Life and Health, University of Edinburgh.

M. V. MERRICK — Consultant Radiologist, Medical Radioisotope Department, Western General Hospital, Edinburgh.

J. DOUGLAS MILLER — Professor of Surgical Neurology, Department of Clinical Neurosciences, University of Edinburgh.

R. A. MINNS   Senior Lecturer, University of Edinburgh Department of Child Life and Health, and Consultant Paediatric Neurologist, Royal Hospital for Sick Children, Edinburgh.

A. J. W. STEERS   Consultant Neurosurgeon, Western General Hospital and Royal Hospital for Sick Children, Edinburgh.

FOREWORD

The understanding of intracranial dynamics, and in particular the mechanism and treatment of raised intracranial pressure, is of increasing importance in the management of many disorders where there is a component of disordered cerebral function. Such disorders may result from primary cerebral problems, such as meningitis and encephalitis, or from more widespread problems—the metabolic encephalopathy associated with Reye's syndrome being a particularly well recognised example.

The measurement of intracranial pressure has been routine for many years in the Edinburgh Child Neurology Unit, where infants and children with a wide range of neurological problems have been studied. More recently the measurement of cerebral blood flow in conjunction with intracranial pressure has led to further understanding of these complex neurological problems. While this volume does not aim to be a comprehensive dissertation on all aspects of cerebral blood flow and intracranial pressure, it does provide the most up-to-date overview of the management of these children. The considerable advances in clinical and experimental research, particularly with regard to the monitoring techniques and the therapeutic possibilities, have made this volume necessary.

It discusses the basic physiological mechanisms of cerebral blood flow and intracranial pressure and the changes brought about by raised intracranial pressure. The measurement of intracranial pressure and the management of raised intracranial pressure and abnormal intracranial dynamics do not just concern specialised paediatric neurology units: they involve any paediatrician who may encounter the problem, as early and correct management at this stage is important for an over-all successful outcome. The neonatologist may be particularly involved because of the high incidence of congenital and acquired problems in the neonate. This Clinic considers these problems, and gives a detailed discussion of mortality, morbidity and the postnatal and metabolic encephalopathies.

As a general paediatrician with a neonatal bias, I read the volume with great interest. Its combination of basic science and clinical issues brings together material of great importance for the development of neurology and the critical care of young children in the future. The presentation is clear and comprehensive, and I believe this book will have a widespread appeal.

NEIL McINTOSH

ABBREVIATIONS

ACTH	adrenocorticotrophic hormone
ADH	antidiuretic hormone
ADP	adenosine diphosphate
AF	anterior fontanelle
AFB	acid fast bacilli
ATNR	asymmetrical tonic neck reflex
ATP	adenosine triphosphate
$AVDO_2$	arteriovenous oxygen difference
AVP	arginine vasopressin
BCG	bacille Calmette-Guérin
BIHT	benign intracranial hypertension
BP	blood pressure
BSEP	brainstem evoked potentials
cAMP	cyclic adenosine monophosphate
CBF	cerebral bloodflow
CBV	cerebral blood volume
CCS	children's coma score
CFAM	cerebral function analysing monitor
CK	creatine kinase
CMRGl	cerebral metabolic rate for glucose
$CMRO_2$	cerebral metabolic rate for oxygen
CNS	central nervous system
CPAP	continuous positive airway pressure
CPM	central pontine myelinolysis
CPP	cerebral perfusion pressure
CPR	cardio-pulmonary resuscitation
CPS	carbamyl phosphate synthetase
CRA	cardio respiratory arrest
CRP	C-reactive protein
CSF	cerebrospinal fluid
CT	computed x-ray tomography
CVP	central venous pressure
DIC	diffuse intravascular coagulation
DFI	direction of flow index
DOPA	dihydroxyphenylalanine
DQ	developmental quotient
ECD	ethyl cysteinate dimer
ECF	extracellular fluid
ECG	electrocardiogram
EEG	electroencephalogram
EM	electron microscopy
EOM	external ocular movements
EVD	external ventricular drain
FFT	fast Fourier transformation

GABA	gamma-aminobutyric acid
GCS	Glasgow coma scale
GHB	gamma-hydroxybutyric acid
GI	gastrointestinal
HC	head circumference
HI	head injury
5-HIAA	5-hydroxyindoleacetic acid
HMPAO	hexamethyl propylene amine oxide
HSV	herpes simplex virus
HVA	homovanillic acid
ICP	intracranial pressure
ICU	intensive care unit
IMP	I paraiodo-amphetamine
IPPV	intermittent positive pressure ventilation
IQ	intelligence quotient
IVH	intraventricular haemorrhage
JVO	jugular venous oxygen
JVP	jugular venous pressure
kPa	kilopascals
lCBF	local cerebral bloodflow
LDH	lactic dehydrogenase
LP	lumbar puncture
MAP	mean arterial pressure
MBP	myelin basic protein
MBq	megabecquerels
MCA	middle cerebral artery
MHPG	methoxy-4-hydroxyphenyl glycol
MR	mental retardation
MRI	magnetic resonance imaging
MTT	mean transit time
NADH/	nicotinamide adenine dinucleotide, reduced
NAD+	and oxidised forms
NAI	non-accidental injury
NMRS	nuclear magnetic resonance spectroscopy
OFR	oxygen free radical
OTC	ornithine transcarbamylase
$PaCO_2$	partial pressure of arterial carbon dioxide
PAE	post-asphyxial encephalopathy
PCO_2	partial pressure of carbon dioxide
PET	positron emission tomography
PI	pulsatility index
PHVD	post-haemorrhagic ventricular dilatation
PLEDS	periodic lateralising epileptic discharges
PO_2	partial pressure of oxygen
PaO_2	partial pressure of arterial oxygen

PRI	Pourcelot resistance index
P_{SAS}	pressure in subarachnoid space
P_{SSS}	superior sagittal sinus pressure
PTAH	phosphotungstic acid hematoxylin
PTR	prothrombin ratio
PVH	periventricular haemorrhage
PVI	pressure-volume index
PVL	periventricular leukomalacia
PVS	persistent vegetative state
RAV	resistance across arachnoid villi
rCBF	regional cerebral bloodflow
REM	rapid eye movement
RI	resistance index
RICP	raised intracranial pressure
RNA	ribonucleic acid
S/A	subarachnoid
SAP	systemic arterial pressure
SAS	subarachnoid space
S/D	subdural
SIADH	syndrome of inappropriate ADH secretion
SPECT	single photon emission computed tomography
SSP	sagittal sinus pressure
SVC	superior vena cava
TBM	tuberculous meningitis
TCD	transcranial Doppler
TM	tympanic membrane
TP	theco-peritoneal
VDU	video display unit
VEP	visual evoked potentials
VFP	ventricular fluid pressure
VMA	vanillylmandelic acid
VP	venous pressure
VPR	volume-pressure response
WBC	white blood cell

PREFACE

Paediatric neurologists are interested in all conditions of children which involve the brain and peripheral nervous system, from abnormalities of higher cortical function to the neuropathic bladder. While paediatric neurology certainly encompasses the important study of neurodegenerative disease, it also includes conventional neurology (neuromuscular diseases, epilepsy and brain tumours) and neonatal neurology. In addition to making a contribution to community paediatrics (development, learning disorders, and neurological handicap), the paediatric neurologist is also involved in acute neurological emergencies (encephalopathies, status epilepticus and CNS trauma). This area of neuro-intensive care constitutes one of the most recent paediatric sub-specialities, and one in which there is increasing interest.

Neuro-intensive care is one of the most complex areas of paediatrics. It differentiates between the primary brain insult and the 'secondary injury' due to fits, pressure, infection and homeostatic derangements, and it also guides the manipulation of cerebral bloodflow (CBF) to meet the brain's metabolic needs based on a knowledge of the cerebral perfusion, cerebrovascular autoregulation, and cerebral metabolism. This area of paediatric neurology is exclusively hospital-based. The sick child presents to a children's hospital and the paediatrician is the first in attendance. This emergency treatment is often a major determinant of the outcome. The paediatric neuro-intensive care and monitoring unit should be sited in a children's hospital with on-site expertise and co-operation between paediatric intensivists, anaesthetists, neurosurgeons, and neurologists.

Neuro-intensive care requires a combination of knowledge, skills and technology: knowledge of the pathophysiology, procedural and assessment skills of both medical and nursing personnel, and the technology involved in the various forms of monitoring together with laboratory and imaging back-up.

This book does not aspire to be a comprehensive treatise on all aspects of neuro-intensive care, nor is it a monograph on the underlying neurosciences, about which the reader would be advised to consult such standard works as Davson, Milhorat and Klatzo. We hope, however, that it will give a better understanding of the pathophysiology and therapeutic options available in practice for managing the child with an encephalopathy or hydrocephalus. In preparing this text I have focused particularly on practical issues relating to abnormal intracranial dynamic problems seen commonly in children.

The book is designed as a series of lectures or essays and the multispeciality nature of the conditions is reflected in the choice of contributors: among them paediatric neurologists, paediatric neurosurgeons, a neonatologist, a nuclear medicine specialist, a bacteriologist and a biochemist. The contributions are biased towards the personal therapeutic preferences of the authors, and the justification for this is that it offers a decisive viewpoint in areas that have been successful in practice.

Many colleagues have helped with advice and comments in the preparation of this text, including members of the Department of Child Life and Health in the University of Edinburgh and my medical, surgical, and anaesthetic colleagues at the Royal Hospital for Sick Children, as well as the Department of Clinical Neurosciences in Edinburgh. Apart from the contributors who wrote and revised their text with much patience, I must mention a number of people to whom I am especially grateful: Professor Neil McIntosh, Emeritus Professor J. O. Forfar, Dr T. T. S. Ingram, Mr John Shaw, Dr Chris Steer, Dr Guy Besley, Professor Douglas Miller and Dr Mike Hendry.

My thanks are particularly due to Their Royal Highnesses The Duke and Duchess of York and Action Research for the Crippled Child, Dr John Ward and his colleagues in the Department of Neurosciences at Medical College Virginia, Richmond, USA, Mrs Midge Clark and the Neurophysiology Staff at the Royal Hospital for Sick Children (RHSC) Edinburgh, Miss Anne Caldow and the nursing staff of the Ingram Neurology Ward, RHSC Edinburgh, Miss Lesley Skeates and Mr Len Cumming for the graphics and photography, the Earl of Elgin and Mr Charles MacGregor from the TSB Foundation, and Mr Donald McLaughlan with Gaeltec Research Limited. Mrs Kaye Kaufmann worked for many months to prepare much of this text and I am greatly indebted to her; and to Dr Martin Bax, Dr Pamela Davies and Mr Edward Fenton, who looked after the in-house editing.

ROBERT A. MINNS
MARCH 1990

1
BASIC INTRACRANIAL DYNAMICS

J. Douglas Miller

A number of brain disorders of infancy and childhood result ultimately in secondary ischaemic brain damage that is often disabling and sometimes fatal. The process common to such damage is a critical reduction in the vascular perfusion pressure to the brain, produced most often by an increase in the intracranial pressure (ICP). Understanding of the mechanisms that govern the regulation of CBF and ICP is therefore central to the development of strategies of management of many neurological and neurosurgical disorders of childhood. These include head injury, hydrocephalus, brain tumours, encephalopathies, craniospinal infection and intracranial haemorrhage.

Intracranial pressure
If a needle is inserted into the lumbar subarachnoid space, and the cerebrospinal fluid (CSF) allowed to run up a glass manometer, the fluid meniscus attains a certain positive pressure measured in centimetres of water (or more properly of CSF), and it exhibits two forms of pulsation, one rapid and synchronous with the pulsebeat, the other slower and synchronous with respiration. This is a display of the CSF pressure. If the needle or catheter is inserted into the lateral ventricle, cerebral subarachnoid space or cisterna magna of a normal recumbent subject, using the same pressure reference point, an identical pressure recording would be obtained. Under these circumstances the CSF pressure is synonymous with the ICP. Such conditions no longer hold when the CSF pathways are occluded or obstructed because of intracranial mass lesions or the swelling of brain tissue, and measurements of ICP made from below the tentorium are likely to underestimate the true intracranial pressure (Langfitt *et al.* 1964).

Because of the need to compare the ICP with the arterial pressure, it is customary to express ICP in the same units of measurement. In most countries this is mmHg (1mmHg = 1.36cmH$_2$O), but SI units are also used; ICP is then expressed as kilopascals (1kPa = 7.5mmHg). Because of the pulsatile nature of the pressure, it is necessary to follow an agreed convention in calculating mean ICP. This is calculated as for arterial pressure with respect to the rapid pulsation (mean pressure = systolic + 2.diastolic / 3). When there is also a sizeable respiratory component, this is usually sinusoidal and the mean is derived from the 'diastolic' pressure plus half of the 'pulse pressure'. The normal ICP is usually given in the adult as the range 0 to 15mmHg (0 to 2kPa), but negative pressures can be recorded. In children, the upper limit of normal ICP is lower, at 5mmHg below two years of age and 10mmHg below five years (Welch 1980).

ICP rises briefly, for seconds at a time, during coughing, straining, crying and

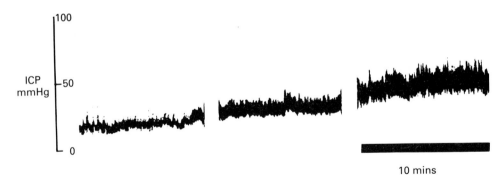

Fig. 1.1. Chart recording of three 10-minute recordings of ICP showing the increase in pulse amplitude that accompanies rising ICP.

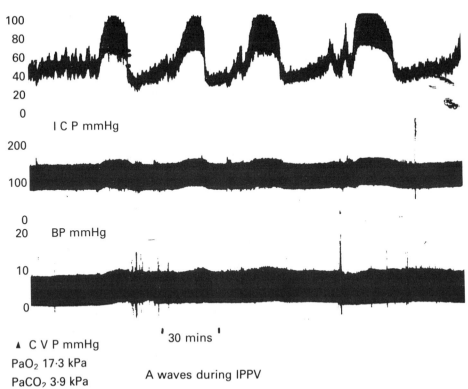

Fig. 1.2. Chart recording of ICP, arterial pressure (BP) and cerebral venous pressure (CVP) in a head-injured patient exhibiting plateau or A waves. Note the accompanying rise in BP.

other activities that increase central venous pressure. Sustained rises in ICP are generally considered pathological when mean ICP exceeds 20mmHg for more than a minute. Elevations in ICP may be in the form of steady, sustained rises in pressure, or intermittent, in the form of pressure waves. As mean ICP increases, there is usually an increase in the pulse pressure or amplitude of the ICP wave (Fig. 1.1).

In his classic study, Lundberg (1960) defined three principal types of intracranial pressure wave . The first were 'A' waves or plateau waves. These consist of an abrupt rise in ICP from levels just above normal to 50mmHg or more; ICP remains at this level for between five and 20 minutes, accompanied at times by complaints of headache or fullness of the head, facial flushing or transient worsening of neurological dysfunction, then returns spontaneously to normal or near-normal levels (Fig. 1.2). The second basic type of pressure pattern—the 'B' wave—consists of a series of sharply peaked waves, occurring at intervals of between 30 seconds and two minutes. Both A and B waves are thought to result from cerebral vasodilatation; A waves occur against a background of reduced craniospinal compliance, in which small increments of volume result in large increases of pressure. In some instances of B wave activity, the timing of the pressure peaks coincides with periodic respiration, and it has been proposed that the B waves result from fluctuations in cerebral vascular calibre due to corresponding alterations in arterial carbon dioxide tension. It is also recognised, however, that B wave activity can be seen in patients during periods of artificial ventilation, when arterial PCO_2 is constant. The third type of ICP wave is the 'C' wave: rapid sinusoidal fluctuations occurring about six times per minute, and corresponding to Traube-Hering-Mayer fluctuations in arterial pressure.

The clinical correlates of raised ICP, headache, vomiting and papilloedema, have a traditional place in the neurological literature. They remain valuable signs when present, but their absence cannot be construed as indicating that ICP is normal (Selhorst *et al.* 1985). Accumulated experience of ICP monitoring in a wide range of conditions has shown that ICP can be high in the absence of all three signs. The later signs of impairment of consciousness, pupillary dilatation and changes in heart rate and blood pressure are really indications of brain shift or brainstem ischaemia; they may therefore appear at different levels of ICP, depending upon the cause of the intracranial hypertension (Langfitt 1969, Miller and Adams 1984).

Causes of raised intracranial pressure (RICP)
The basis for understanding the causes of RICP is the Monro-Kellie doctrine. In its original form, this stated that because the brain and the blood within it were both largely liquid and therefore incompressible, any addition to the bulk of the brain must either be accompanied by an equivalent reduction in the blood volume or an increase in ICP. This theory had to be modified by Burrows to take account of the presence of CSF in the cranial cavity, and its important role in the process of compensating for intracranial mass lesions (Langfitt 1969). This much was established by the middle of the last century, then slightly modified by Weed early in this century to allow for the participation by the spinal dural sac in the process of spatial compensation for intracranial masses.

3

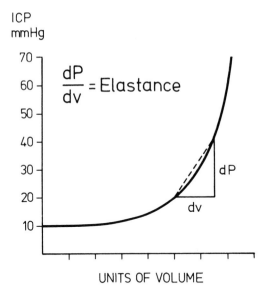

ICP
mmHg

$$\frac{dP}{dv} = Elastance$$

UNITS OF VOLUME

Fig. 1.3. Theoretical diagram of the ICP–volume relationship.

Experimental and clinical observations at the turn of the century (by Duret, von Bergmann, Kocher and Cushing) established the concept of brain compression being comprised of an initial phase of spatial compensation, during which an equivalent volume of CSF and venous blood was expressed from the cranial cavity and ICP remained normal, followed by a phase in which ICP rose slowly at first, then increasingly steeply as decompensation became total; the final stage was reached when the ICP reached the level of the blood pressure and the cerebral circulation arrested. Between 1964 and 1968, there was a series of studies of experimental brain compression from the University of Pennsylvania, defining the ICP volume curve under controlled circumstances, and introducing the important concept of cerebral vasomotor paralysis (Langfitt *et al.* 1965*a,b*). In this state, cerebral blood vessels lost their normal capacity to react to changes in arterial pressure and arterial PCO_2, and the recording of ICP showed a high-amplitude trace that varied directly with the arterial pressure waveform. Vasomotor paralysis occurred at a late stage in progressive brain compression, even when that compression had been abruptly relieved.

The causes of RICP can be an addition to the cranial contents (an extradural haematoma or a metastatic brain tumour, for example) or it may result from an increase in the volume of one or more of the normal constituents: an increase in brain-tissue water content constitutes brain oedema; an increase in cerebral blood volume may result from active cerebral vasodilatation or because of venous obstruction; if the CSF pathways become obstructed, hydrocephalus may follow and be a cause of RICP.

The actual increase in ICP that results from a given increment in volume depends on the ICP-volume status at that point. Thus a patient with a slowly expanding mass lesion may have entirely normal ICP under resting conditions, yet

4

when he goes to sleep and cerebral vasodilatation occurs during the rapid eye movement (REM) sleep phase, ICP may increase suddenly and dramatically (Miller 1975a). The factors that cause increased ICP may be additive, as for example hydrocephalus or brain oedema complicating a brain tumour.

Langfitt showed that the relationship between ICP and the volume of a progressively expanding intracranial mass was exponential, with little rise in ICP at first, then progressive steepening of the curve as compensatory volumes of CSF and blood became exhausted (Fig. 1.3). Marmarou and Shulman (1975) showed that the relationship between ICP and the volume of bolus additions to CSF volume was also exponential. This meant that by adding small volumes of fluid to the cranial CSF space it was possible to extrapolate information about lumped craniospinal compliance—the volume-pressure relationship (Miller 1975a).

Miller also described the volume-pressure response (VPR) as the increase in ICP in mmHg per ml of CSF volume added, or withdrawn, in one second. Normal values were 0 to 2mmHg/ml; values of 3mmHg/ml or more at baseline ICP levels of 30mmHg or less indicated reduced craniospinal compliance (or more correctly, increased elastance) (Miller and Leech 1975).

Marmarou defined the pressure-volume index (PVI) as the notional volume which, if added to the CSF, would produce a tenfold rise in ICP. It is an extrapolation from the results of injecting a much smaller bolus, derived from:

$$\text{PVI} = \Delta v / \log_{10} [\text{Pp}/\text{Po}] \ (\text{ml})$$

where Po = baseline CSF pressure and Pp the peak ICP after injection of a fluid bolus (Δv).

The normal range of PVI in an adult is 25 to 30ml; in a child it is lower, from 12 to 25ml. Marmarou and colleagues (1975, 1987) also developed equations to measure CSF formation and absorption rates based upon controlled bolus additions and withdrawals of CSF.

Interactions between intracranial pressure and brain shift
When a mass expands in the supratentorial space, brain adjacent to the mass tends to flow away from it, providing that there is adequate time. Because the brain tissue is virtually incompressible it displaces, to usurp space normally occupied by the CSF. Thus the third ventricle and the supratentorial subarachnoid space over the surface of the hemisphere, in the cisterns round the midbrain and at the base, almost disappear; this can be recognised on CT (Teasdale *et al.* 1984). The lateral ventricle on the same side of the brain as the mass also becomes smaller. The cingulate gyrus begins to herniate under the lower margin of the falx cerebri, as the midline of the brain is displaced to the opposite side (Miller and Adams 1984). When supratentorial midline shift is pronounced, there may be dilatation of the lateral ventricle contralateral to the mass as a result of obstruction of the foramen of Monro; when identified on CT this is also a reliable indication that ICP is increased. The medial part of the temporal lobe also herniates, through the tentorial hiatus between the free edge of the tentorium and the mid-brain. This process further obliterates the normal CSF pathway, progressively cutting off the supratentorial

5

cavity from the posterior fossa and spinal canal. At the same time the entire brainstem is shifted axially downward toward the foramen magnum; this process tends to distract the brainstem from its blood supply via the central perforating branches of the basilar artery. This combination of shift, distortion and ischaemia in the medulla is considered to be the explanation for the changes in blood pressure embodied in the well known Cushing Response.

Corresponding with the process of brain shift and herniation, a pressure differential or gradient develops in which the CSF pressure above the tentorium becomes progressively greater than the CSF pressure below the tentorium, in the cisterna magna or in the lumbar subarachnoid space. This pressure gradient serves to increase the driving force propelling the herniating brain; furthermore, applying a stimulus that would normally cause a uniform increase in ICP (for example a vasodilating anaesthetic or an increase in arterial PCO_2), may produce the classical signs of tentorial herniation (dilatation of the pupil and decerebrate motor response) (Fitch and McDowall 1971, Miller 1975b).

When the mass lesion expands in the posterior cranial fossa, the effects of brainstem embarrassment are seen at an earlier stage because of direct distortion of the medulla or herniation of the cerebellar tonsils through the foramen magnum. If ICP becomes elevated, it is usually because of obstruction of the CSF pathway. On CT this is signalled by enlargement of the lateral ventricles.

Intractranial pressure, cerebral venous pressure and cerebral perfusion pressure
When ICP is increased, there is a corresponding increase in the pressure within the thin-walled veins in the cerebral subarachnoid space. This rise in venous pressure has been shown to occur experimentally to pressure levels over 100mmHg (Johnston and Rowan 1974). The cerebral venous pressure remains about 3mmHg above the mean ICP. This is necessary, because if ICP were to exceed the venous pressure the veins would collapse and the cerebral circulation would cease. Strictly speaking, the cerebral perfusion pressure (CPP) should be defined as the difference between the arterial and the venous exit pressure; it is easier and more practical to define it as the difference between arterial and intracranial pressure.

The relationship between ICP, CPP and CBF is a complex one, since RICP can both be caused by an increase in CBF and be a limiting factor producing a reduction in CBF (see below).

Cerebral bloodflow and brain energy metabolism
The brain depends continuously and almost entirely upon the oxidative metabolism of glucose in large quantities. Under resting conditions the bloodflow to the brain accounts for one fifth of the cardiac output, and its oxygen consumption is one sixth of that of the entire body. There is no energy reserve; if the supply of blood, oxygen and glucose is abruptly cut off, the electrical activity of the brain ceases within 15 seconds, and if the supply is not resumed within 15 minutes, structural and permanent damage to neurons begins to occur (Siesjo 1978, Astrup 1982). If the blood supply is progressively reduced, electrical activity can be maintained until flow falls to 40 per cent of normal. Beyond that point there is slowing then loss of

electro-encephalographic and evoked potential activity. As flow goes below the 20 per cent threshold there is leakage of potassium from the neuronal cell body, followed by ingress of water and calcium ions as the cell membrane pump and ion channel systems begin to fail. Thereafter, triggered by the calcium, a cascade of damaging events ensues, involving lipolysis, formation of eicosanoids from arachidonic acid and, as by-products, of free oxygen radicals. In this way, a process that began as neuronal dysfunction proceeds to ischaemic neuronal necrosis, and a reversible state becomes irreversible.

The key issue for maintenance of the structural integrity of the brain is therefore to secure and preserve a steady and adequate supply of blood, oxygen and glucose to all parts of the brain, and a run-off of bloodflow sufficient to clear the products of metabolism from the tissue. For preservation of the capacity of the brain to receive, process and transmit electrochemical information, the regional blood supply should be able to increase to meet the local metabolic demand as specific groups of neurons begin firing and increasing their energy requirement.

The content of oxygen in the blood is determined by the quantity of haemoglobin and its degree of saturation by oxygen which depends in turn upon blood oxygen tension, pH and temperature. The volume flow of blood is determined by the perfusion pressure and a number of factors that together comprise the conductance, including vascular calibre, length of the vascular bed, and the viscosity of the blood. The perfusion pressure of the brain is the difference between the arterial (inflow) pressure and the cerebral venous (outflow) pressure. The latter is difficult to measure, and a reasonable approximation is provided by ICP. Thus CPP is most commonly calculated from the difference between arterial and intracranial pressure. The cerebrovascular resistance is calculated as CPP divided by the CBF, and expressed as mmHg per ml per 100g brain per minute.

The carriage of oxygen or glucose to the brain is calculated as the product of CBF and the content of oxygen or glucose in the blood. The rate of cerebral oxygen or glucose uptake, utilisation or metabolism (interchangeable terms) is derived from the product of CBF and the cerebral arteriovenous content difference for oxygen or glucose, and expressed as ml (oxygen) per 100g brain per minute. In a similar way the cerebral lactate production rate can be estimated from the product of bloodflow and the venous-arterial difference for lactate. To obtain cerebral venous blood, a catheter is passed up the internal jugular vein as far as the jugular bulb and its position verified radiographically. The corresponding measurements of bloodflow should ideally use the same source of cerebral venous blood as part of the calculation, or they should at least be measures of total CBF.

Measurements of cerebral bloodflow
The major advance in the measurement of CBF in man was the application of the Fick Principle to obtain an estimate of the volume of blood flowing through a given weight of brain tissue per minute (Kety and Schmidt 1945). The method involved inhalation of a metabolically inert gas that diffused freely into brain tissue from the blood-stream and then diffused out again when the arterial supply to the brain no longer contained the tracer gas. By giving the gas over a prolonged time, until the

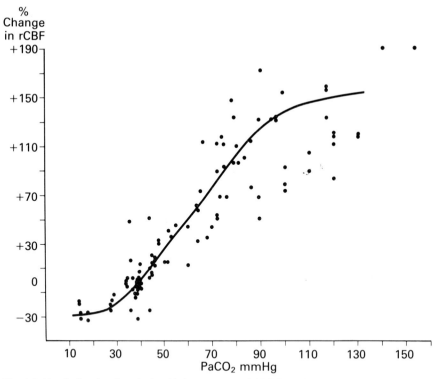

Fig. 1.4. Graph showing the relationship between arterial PCO_2 and percentage change in regional CBF measured by thermal clearance. (From Miller *et al.* 1969, reproduced by permission).

brain was saturated with tracer, the cerebral venous blood was able to be used as an index of brain content of tracer at saturation, and CBF could be calculated from the cerebral tissue (venous) level of tracer divided by the integrated arteriovenous difference for the tracer during its administration. This yielded a measure of bloodflow in ml blood per 100g brain per minute. The normal value in man is 50ml/100g/min. Since the normal cerebral arteriovenous oxygen content difference is 6ml/100ml blood, the normal cerebral oxygen uptake rate is the product of the two: 3ml/100g/min.

Such figures referring to total averaged brain bloodflow are of limited value, and quite fail to reveal the considerable changes in regional CBF that can occur during the activation of specific parts of the brain. Thus bloodflow in the lateral geniculate nuclei can increase to more than 200ml/100g/min with light stimulation, while neighbouring parts of the brain show no change in flow. Newer methods of bloodflow measurement involving the use of radio-isotopes, and the new imaging systems—single photon emission tomography (SPECT) and positron emission tomography (PET)—now permit display of regional CBF in specific regions of the brain, including structures deep in the hemisphere and brainstem (Phelps *et al.* 1982).

Despite the limitations of the earlier methods of measuring CBF, most of our

8

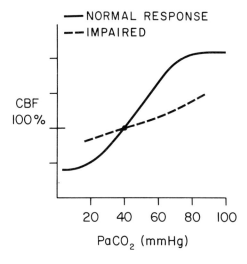

NORMAL RESPONSE
IMPAIRED

CBF
100%

20 40 60 80 100

PaCO₂ (mmHg)

Fig. 1.5. Diagram showing the normal and impaired response of CBF to altered arterial PCO₂.

knowledge of how the cerebral circulation responds to normal physiological stimuli and to pathological insults was gathered at that time.

There is coupling between CBF and brain metabolism. When consciousness is lost, the cerebral metabolic rate for oxygen falls from 3 to below 2ml/100g/min and mean CBF falls from 50 to 30ml/100g/min or less.

Cerebrovascular response to carbon dioxide and oxygen

Normal values for CBF in man are referenced to arterial PCO_2 levels of 5.5kPa. As soon as arterial PCO_2 rises above this normal level, CBF increases; it doubles when arterial PCO_2 rises from 5.3 to 10.6kPa (Fig. 1.4). Above this level there is less of an increase in flow (Harper and Glass 1965). Conversely, when arterial PCO_2 falls, CBF decreases due to cerebral vasoconstriction; CBF halves as arterial PCO_2 falls from 5.3 to 2.7kPa. Below that level there is less decrease in flow, but the electro-encephalogram (EEG) shows slow-wave activity and lactate begins to accumulate in the CSF. If the hypocapnia is accompanied by administration of hyperbaric oxygen, the CSF lactic acidosis does not occur and bloodflow falls further. These changes suggest that mild hypoxia is reversing the hypocapnic cerebral vasoconstriction by causing an opposing cerebral vasodilatation (Miller and Ledingham 1971). The changes in CBF that are produced by changes in arterial PCO_2 also cause changes in cerebral blood volume (CBV), and these in turn cause changes in ICP. The magnitude of the ICP changes depends upon the ICP-volume status at the time. Under the right circumstances, induction of hypocapnia by hyperventilation can be a useful means of reducing RICP, particularly when this has largely been related to cerebral vasodilatation. The danger is the worsening of brain ischaemia if hyperventilation is applied when CBF is already low (Miller 1975).

The mechanism by which carbon dioxide produces changes in the calibre of cerebral resistance vessels is not fully understood, but it has been known for some time that this form of vascular responsiveness can be attenuated or even lost altogether (Fig. 1.5). The loss may be global or regional; in the latter case, the

9

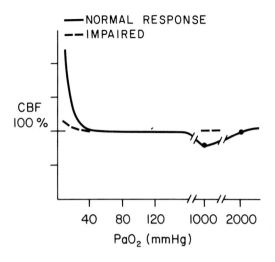

CBF
100 %

40 80 120 1000 2000

PaO₂ (mmHg)

Fig. 1.6. Diagram showing normal and impaired response of CBF to altered arterial PO₂.

concepts of 'steal' and 'inverse steal' arise. When arterial PCO_2 rises, bloodflow in the normal brain increases, but in the unresponsive zone the vessels cannot dilate and flow may actually fall; conversely, when arterial PCO_2 is reduced, bloodflow falls only in the normal brain areas, while in the unresponsive zone the vessels fail to constrict and flow may actually increase (the so-called 'inverse steal'). This mechanism has been cited as supporting the use of hyperventilation in patients with focal brain damage. Localised loss of vascular responsiveness has been seen in stroke, intracerebral haematoma, tumour and brain contusion (Lewelt *et al.* 1982).

When arterial oxygen tension changes, CBF does not alter until oxygen desaturation begins to occur, at PO_2 levels of about 7.0kPa; at this point CBF increases, and by the time arterial PO_2 has fallen to 4kPa, CBF has tripled (Fig. 1.6). The effects of hyperoxia are much less impressive; a rise in arterial PO_2 to 133.3kPa, obtained under hyperbaric conditions, produces a 20 per cent reduction in CBF. When the response to carbon dioxide is lost, so also is the response to hypoxia and hyperoxia (Miller *et al.* 1970).

Pressure regulation in the cerebral circulation

Cerebral bloodflow usually remains virtually constant over a range of arterial pressure levels, from 60 to 140mmHg (8 to 18.7kPa) in normal individuals. This autoregulation is accomplished by progressive dilatation of small cerebral vessels during falling pressure; it appears that vessels of different calibre respond to different pressure thresholds (Kontos *et al.* 1978). Below 60mmHg (8kPa) the vascular dilatation is no longer adequate to maintain flow at a constant level, and flow falls progressively to zero at the critical closing pressure of the cerebral circulation. When blood pressure rises above 140mmHg (18.7kPa), the point of 'breakthrough of autoregulation' is reached and CBF increases, accompanied usually by progressive formation of cerebral oedema. In cases of chronic arterial hypertension, the upper and lower thresholds of autoregulation are reset at a higher level; and blood pressure levels that seem adequate may in fact be

10

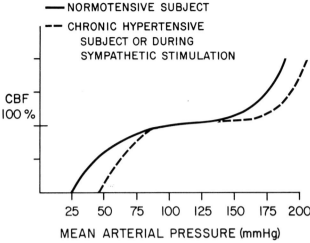

— NORMOTENSIVE SUBJECT

-- CHRONIC HYPERTENSIVE
   SUBJECT OR DURING
   SYMPATHETIC STIMULATION

CBF
100 %

25   50   75   100   125   150   175   200

MEAN ARTERIAL PRESSURE (mmHg)

Fig. 1.7. Diagram showing the relationship between arterial pressure and CBF in the normal subject and the 'resetting' of the curve that occurs with chronic arterial hypertension.

inadequate to sustain a normal flow level (Strandgaard *et al.* 1974).

Autoregulation may be impaired or lost on a global or a regional basis. This can be seen in cases of post-hypoxic insult, trauma, intracranial haemorrhage, brain tumour, meningitis, and encephalitis. In addition, in head injury and other conditions in which CBF is already reduced and cerebrovascular resistance increased, the levels of arterial and CPP required to provide an adequate flow level may be 30 or 40mmHg higher than 'normal' (Fig. 1.7).

When ICP is increased, CBF often remains normal until CPP falls to 40 or 50mmHg (5.3 or 6.7kPa) (Miller *et al.* 1972). This maintenance of flow is also accompanied by dilatation of the small resistance vessels, and appears to be mediated by the same autoregulatory mechanism as the response to changes in blood pressure. Thus, when autoregulation is impaired, CBF tends to fall as soon as ICP rises above normal. Unfortunately many of the conditions in which autoregulation is lost are also frequently associated with increased ICP. It can also be appreciated that the relationship between ICP and CBF is complex, since an increase in CBF may bring about a rise in ICP and an increase in ICP may be responsible for a decrease in CBF.

Conclusion

Understanding of the intricate interplay between CBF, brain metabolism and the perfusion pressure of the brain is crucial to the development of strategies for the urgent and effective treatment of a number of serious disorders of the child's brain.

REFERENCES

Astrup, J. (1982) 'Energy-requiring cell functions in the ischaemic brain.' *Journal of Neurosurgery*, **56**, 482–497.
Fitch, W., McDowall, D. G. (1971) 'Effect of halothane on intracranial pressure gradients in the presence of intracranial space-occupying lesions.' *British Journal of Anaesthesia.* **43**, 904–912.
Harper, A. M., Glass, H. I. (1965) 'Effect of alterations in the arterial carbon dioxide tension on the

blood flow through the cerebral cortex at normal and low arterial blood pressures.' *Journal of Neurology, Neurosurgery and Psychiatry*, **28**, 449–452.

Johnston, I. H., Rowan, J. O. (1974) 'Raised intracranial pressure and cerebral blood flow. 3: Venous outflow tract pressures and vascular resistances in experimental intracranial hypertension.' *Journal of Neurology, Neurosurgery and Psychiatry*, **37**, 392–402.

Kety, S. S., Schmidt, C. F. (1945) 'Determination of cerebral blood flow in man by the use of nitrous oxide in low concentrations.' *American Journal of Physiology*, **143**, 53–66.

Kontos, H. A., Wei, E. P., Navari, R. M., Levasseur, J. E., Rosenblum, W. I., Patterson, J. L. (1978) 'Responses of cerebral arteries and arterioles to acute hypotension and hypertension.' *American Journal of Physiology*, **234**, H371–H383.

Langfitt, T. W. (1969) 'Increased intracranial pressure.' *Clinical Neurosurgery*, **16**, 436–471.

—— Weinstein, J. D., Kassell, N. F., Simeone, F. A. (1964) 'Transmission of increased intracranial pressure. I. Within the craniospinal axis.' *Journal of Neurosurgery*, **21**, 989–997.

—— Kassell, N. F., Weinstein, J. D. (1965) 'Cerebral blood flow with intracranial hypertension.' *Neurology*, **15**, 761–773.

—— Weinstein, J. D., Kassell, N. F. (1965) 'Cerebral vasomotor paralysis produced by intracranial hypertension.' *Neurology*, **15**, 622–641.

Lewelt, W., Jenkins, L. W., Miller, J. D. (1982) 'Effects of experimental fluid percussion injury of the brain on cerebrovascular reactivity to hypoxia and hypercapnia.' *Journal of Neurosurgery*, **56**, 332–338.

Lundberg, N. (1960) 'Contusions recording and control of ventricular fluid pressure in neurosurgical practice.' *Acta Psychiatrica Scandinavica*, **36**, Suppl. 149. pp. 1–193.

Marmarou, A., Shulman, K. (1975) 'Pressure-volume relationships—basic aspects.' *In* McLaurin, R. L. (Ed.) *Head Injuries. Proceedings of the Second Chicago Symposium on Neural Trauma.* New York: Grune & Stratton. pp. 233–236.

—— —— Lamorgese, J. (1975) 'Compartmental analysis of compliance and outflow resistance of the cerebrospinal fluid system.' *Journal of Neurosurgery*, **43**, 523–534.

—— Maset, A. L., Ward, J. D., Ohpi, S., Brooks, D., Lutz, H. A., Moulton, R. J., Muizelaar, J. P., Desalles, A., Young, H. F. (1987) 'Contribution of CSF and vascular factors to elevation of ICP in severely head-injured patients.' *Journal of Neurosurgery*, **66**, 883–890.

Miller, J. D. (1975a) 'Volume and pressure in the craniospinal axis.' *Clinical Neurosurgery*, **22**, 76–105.

—— (1975b) 'Effects of hypercapnia on pupillary size, ICP and cerebral venous PO$_2$ during experimental brain compression.' *In* Lundberg, N., Ponten, U., Brock, M. (Eds.) *Intracranial Pressure. Vol. II.* Berlin: Springer. pp. 444–446.

—— Fitch, W., Cameron, B. D. (1969) 'Measurement of cerebral blood flow in the presence of raised intracranial pressure.' *Journal of Surgical Research*, **9**, 399–407.

—— Ledingham, I. McA., Jennett, W. B. (1970) 'The effect of hyperbaric oxygen on intracranial pressure and cerebral blood flow in experimental cerebral oedema.' *Journal of Neurology, Neurosurgery and Psychiatry*, **33**, 745–755.

—— —— (1971) 'Reduction of increased intracranial pressure: comparison between hyperbaric oxygen and hyperventilation.' *Archives of Neurology*, **24**, 210–216.

—— Stanek A. E., Langfitt, T. W. (1972) 'Concepts of cerebral perfusion pressure and vascular compression during intracranial hypertension.' *Progress in Brain Research*, **35**, 411–432.

—— Leech, P. J. (1975) 'Effects of mannitol and steroid therapy on intracranial volume-pressure relationships in patients.' *Journal of Neurosurgery*, **45**, 274–281.

—— Adams, J. H. (1984) 'The pathophysiology of raised intracranial pressure.' *In* Adams, J. H., Corsellis, J. A. N., Duchen, L. W. (Eds.) *Greenfield's Neuropathology, 4th Edn.* London: Arnold. pp. 53–84.

Phelps, M., Mazziotta, J. C., Huang, S.-C. (1982) 'Study of cerebral function with positron computed tomography.' *Journal of Cerebral Blood Flow and Metabolism*, **2**, 113–162.

Selhorst, J. B., Gudeman, S. K., Butterworth, J. F., Harbison, J. W., Miller, J. D., Becker, D. P. (1985) 'Papilledema after acute head injury.' *Neurosurgery*, **66**, 357–363.

Siesjö, B. K. (1978) *Brain Energy Metabolism.* New York: Wiley.

Strandgaard, S., MacKenzie, E. T., Sengupta, D., Rowan, J. O., Lassen, N. A., Harper, A. M. (1974) 'Upper limit of autoregulation of cerebral blood flow in the baboon.' *Circulation Research*, **34**, 435–440.

Teasdale, E., Cardoso, E., Galbraith, S., Teasdale, G. (1984) 'A new CT scan appearance with raised intracranial pressure in severe diffuse head injury.' *Journal of Neurology, Neurosurgery and Psychiatry*, **46**, 600–603.

Welch, K. (1980) 'The intracranial pressure in infants.' *Journal of Neurosurgery*, **52**, 693–699.

12

2
MECHANISMS OF PRODUCTION OF RAISED INTRACRANIAL PRESSURE

J. K. Brown

Many different diseases can produce a rise in intracranial pressure, and in clinical practice each disease may cause a rise in ICP by several different mechanisms. This rise in pressure may then produce new symptoms and signs, but can also result in new 'secondary' pathological changes in the brain. Those secondary pathological changes may themselves result in death or long-term handicap (Brown *et al.* 1973); they are characteristic of RICP but are not specific to the cause.

In cases of head injury, prolonged status epilepticus, perinatal asphyxia, drowning and poisoning, the primary injury is usually well established by the time the child is first seen by a paediatrician. The main reason for intensive care is to prevent secondary hypoxic/ischaemic injury from RICP, fits, or defects in homeostasis (Brown and Habel 1975).

The symptoms and signs of RICP will be discussed in the next chapter: but many of the symptoms and signs thought to be typical of meningitis, for example (drowsiness, irritability, vomiting and neck stiffness), are in fact due not to the disease itself but to the RICP (Nugent *et al.* 1979) and may dramatically disappear after treatment of the increased ICP before the bacterial infection itself has been treated (Minns *et al.* 1989).

Mechanisms of production of RICP

The mechanisms whereby a rise in ICP is produced are summarised in Table 2.I.

Space occupation as a cause of RICP

A pathological process (usually tumour, blood clot, cyst or abscess) causes further volume to be added to the normal volume of blood, brain and CSF in a skull of fixed volume. There can also be metabolic material stored within cells, causing a true increase in brain volume (*i.e.* megalencephaly). In cases of cerebral oedema and hydrocephalus, the rise in ICP is really also due to space occupation by water: and in cerebral congestion the increase in CBV acts as a space-occupying lesion.

In the small infant with unfused skull bones, gradual increase in the volume of the intracranial contents (due to hydrocephalus, chronic subdural haematoma or a slow-growing tumour) results in accommodation of the extra volume by an increase in the size of the head (macrocephaly). This can be due to a true increase in the size of the skull, due to bony growth at the suture lines (which may show marked interdigitation), or by stretching of them (producing splaying or diastasis of the suture lines). Splaying is more likely to occur when the addition of extra volume is relatively rapid. In chronic cases there may be demineralisation of the skull bones

13

TABLE 2.I

Causes of RICP

Space occupation	Tumour
	Abscess
	Cyst
	Blood clot
Hydrocephalus	Excess production of CSF
	Obstruction to CSF pathways
	Failure of absorption of CSF
Brain swelling	Cerebral congestion
	Cerebral oedema—intracellular
	extracellular
	myelin
Craniocerebral disproportion	

at the suture margins, giving a false impression of even greater splaying. The inner table of the skull may also be eroded, resulting in craniolacunae and craniotabes. The ultimate limiting factor which decides whether ICP rises quickly, or macrocephaly alone occurs, is the elasticity of the dura.

In older children in whom the sutures have fused, so that intracranial volume is fixed, any additional volume must be accommodated by displacement of one of the other intracranial contents: brain, CBV, blood in venous sinuses or CSF. In the normal situation the brain occupies 70 per cent of the skull volume, CBV 10 per cent and CSF 10 per cent. There is therefore only 10 per cent normally available for physiological variations without causing a rise in ICP (Boyle's law [P] [V] is a constant).

Brain itself is for all practical purposes incompressible (needing a pressure of 10,000 tons to reduce it to half volume) even though it shows elastic properties and is readily deformable (*e.g.* by a finger at operation or into any oddly shaped skull, as seen in moulding at birth or some of the odd craniostenoses). This elastic deformability also allows the brain to be displaced as a shift or cone (see Chapter 3). Brain volume is not fixed, however, and can be varied by changes in brain water, as seen after the long-term use of steroids when apparent cerebral atrophy results. The accommodation of slow-growing tumours such as meningiomas causes indentation of the brain with marked space-occupying effect and apparently little effect on cerebral function.

If one blows up a balloon inside the head of an experimental animal, at first there is accommodation of the extra volume as venous sinuses are compressed and CSF is reabsorbed or displaced into the spinal theca. Once these compensatory mechanisms are exhausted—the ventricles are empty of CSF and compressed—any additional increase in volume results in a very rapid rise in ICP as there is poor compliance. At this stage even the increase in blood in the head during one cardiac systole may be sufficient to give a large pulse-wave artifact on the ICP recording (Fig. 2.1). The marked rise in CBF which normally occurs during REM sleep will also cause a rise in ICP.

The balloon experiment for compliance is used in a modified way in clinical practice by injecting a bolus of fluid and observing the rise in pressure; or

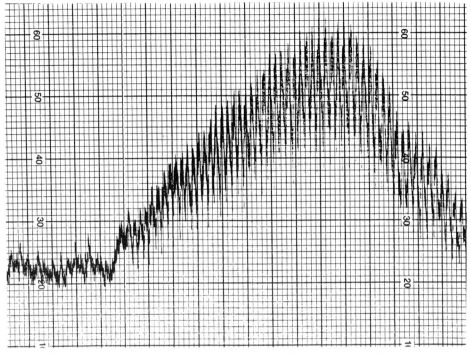

Fig. 2.1. ICP monitoring trace. The amplitude of the p-wave artifact rises as well as the baseline pressure when compliance becomes poorer.

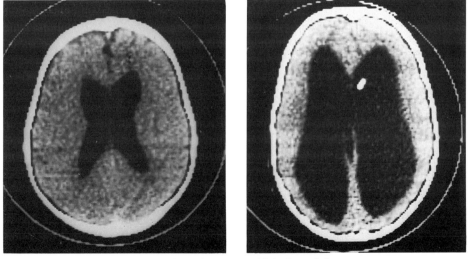

Fig. 2.2. Generalised lateral ventricular enlargement with hydrocephalus.

conversely, if the pressure is high, removing a known volume and observing the fall in pressure.

Hydrocephalus as a cause of RICP

This signifies an increase in the total volume of CSF within the head with a secondary increase in the CSF spaces (Fig. 2.2). There may be a true hydrocephalus from an increase in CSF production, obstruction to its circulation or impaired absorption. This can be hypertensive or normotensive. Alternatively it may be a 'false' or '*ex vacuo*' hydrocephalus due to a shrinkage of the brain from cerebral atrophy. The remaining volume (vacuum) within the skull is passively filled by an expansion of the CSF pathways. This latter is really a form of cranio-cerebral disproportion.

CSF production by the choroid plexus is regulated in a similar manner to the production of urine by the kidney (Rubin *et al.* 1966) in that an ultrafiltrate from the plasma accumulates in the choroid interstitial space, similar to glomerular filtrate by the kidney (McComb 1983). The capillaries in the choroid plexus differ from brain capillaries in that they have fenestrated rather than tight endothelial junctions allowing protein molecules, sucrose and inulin into the choroidal extracellular space (Cutler *et al.* 1968, Davson *et al.* 1987). This is then modified in the choroid epithelium, not simply by further ultrafiltration but by active transport systems which are selective, again similar to the renal tubule. The sodium, protein, bicarbonate, magnesium content and pH of CSF are different from plasma, and changes in plasma are not necessarily reflected by similar changes in CSF. A marked hydrogen ion or osmolar gap can exist between the two. Even small molecules such as glucose do not show parallel changes (*e.g.* during a glucose tolerance test). CSF secreted by the choroid plexus has a different chemical composition from lymph and brain extracellular fluid. The latter is mixed with choroidal secretion to form CSF, which is therefore modified in chemical composition from each source.

The perfusing pressure and reactivity of the choroid capillaries are the main controlling factors for filtration. Selective secretion depends upon biochemical factors such as an active sodium transport system which appears to depend upon the enzyme carbonic anhydrase and can be blocked by the use of acetazolamide. The choroid epithelium is also rich in beta 2 adrenergic receptors, and it is thought that beta-blocking drugs such as propanolol can reduce CSF production rate (Rubin *et al.* 1960, Juncos *et al.* 1982). There are also receptors in the choroid plexus for vasoactive intestinal peptide, whose function is unknown. It is not known which are the most important physiological mechanisms for control of CSF production, nor by what afferent feedback control system the normal volume of CSF and the ICP is determined (Lorenzo *et al.* 1970).

It is thought that increased back pressure, such as a raised intraventricular pressure, will also decrease CSF production rates by decreasing choroidal perfusion (Hochwald and Sahar 1971, Sklar *et al.* 1980). CSF is not secreted at a constant rate but appears to cycle with bursts of production as though it had a biological rhythm (Bering 1958, Minns *et al.* 1988). The normal CSF production rates can vary from 0.3ml to 0.5ml per minute. A low intraventricular pressure such as when the child is placed on open ventricular drainage, without a hydrostatic head of pressure, causes increased volumes to be produced, often several hundred ml per 24 hours (Cutler *et al.* 1968).

The function of CSF is mechanical, chemical, protective and excretory. The mechanical properties are that it suspends the brain, decreases brain weight and prevents different tissue inertias, causing brain and skull to move at different speeds when the head moves. If the CSF is removed then venous tears and subdural haematomas are more common from relatively trivial injury. CSF allows macrophages to remove and clear up debris. It functions as brain lymph, allowing removal of fluid and large molecules which escape the closed capillaries (tight junctions) and cannot get back into the bloodstream. The blood CSF barrier, along with the blood brain barrier, is protective against entry of drugs, antibodies and large molecules which may damage the brain. Since normal brain function is very dependent on ionic shift, the concentration of sodium, potassium, magnesium, calcium and pH is vital: otherwise any change in blood level might cause 'cerebral short-circuits'. The brain is therefore encased in its own protective *milieu intérieur*. This means that substances which act as neurotransmitters in the brain do not all leak out into the circulation, and conversely circulating neuropeptides and transmitters cannot gain ready access with undesirable results.

Causes of hydrocephalus
CSF PRODUCTION

Hydrocephalus is known to occur with an increased rate of production of CSF in choroid papillomas. Hydrocephalus can be treated by choroid plexectomy. CSF production rates may fail to keep pace with drainage rates in the use of open ventricular drainage or low-pressure shunts so that ventricular collapse with the slit ventricle syndrome can result. Again it is not known how much CSF production rate plays a part in the continued progression or sudden deterioration of children with obstructive hydrocephalus (McComb 1983). Deterioration often appears to follow a virus infection, and this can be due either to an effect on choroidal CSF secretion or the volume of production of brain lymph secondary to an action on the endothelial cells of brain capillaries. The CSF production rate is thought to increase with any increase in body temperature and decrease with hypothermia. Ventriculitis is associated with a choroid plexitis with vasodilatation of the choroidal capillaries and an increase in CSF production so that a partially functioning shunt may be unable to cope.

CSF OBSTRUCTION

Obstruction to CSF flow can occur at any level; at the level of the foramen of Monro (usually from tumour but occasionally in children after a subependymal haemorrhage or severe ventriculitis) a unilateral hydrocephalus results. Obstruction to the third ventricle may arise from a colloid cyst or due to hypothalamic tumours such as craniopharyngioma, glioma, meningioma or cyst.

The aqueduct is thought to be the site of obstruction in many of the cases of isolated congenital hydrocephalus. It may be genetic (either sex-linked recessive or autosomal) and may be associated with clasp thumbs or chromosome abnormali-

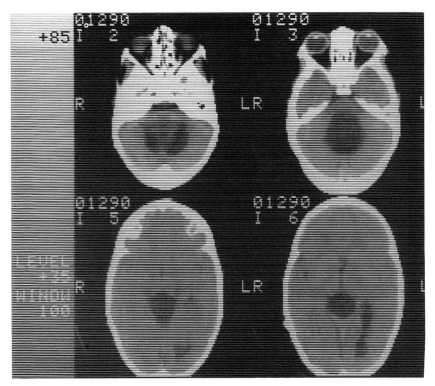

Fig. 2.3. Isolated fourth ventricular hydrocephalus.

ties. The aqueduct may show partial or total atresia or forking and reduplication. Chronic RICP in children results not only in a cone at the level of the tentorium but in downward displacement (shift) of the midbrain, so that secondary distortion and kinking of the aqueduct may convert a communicating into a non-communicating hydrocephalus. If contrast such as myodil is placed into the posterior end of the third ventricle it does not pass down the aqueduct. The myodil passes freely if ICP is lowered by tapping the lateral ventricle, but the aqueduct is tented like the hind leg of a dog. The aqueduct can also be obstructed from gliosis as a result of peri-aqueductal inflammation as a result of infection with toxoplasmosis, mumps or torulosis. In neonates surviving a subependymal haemorrhage, the secondary aqueductal inflammation following infection with toxoplasmosis, mumps or Luschka by organised blood clot—results in isolation of the fourth ventricle, which can develop hydrocephalus even though the lateral ventricles are well controlled. (Fig. 2.3). A similar situation arises as a congenital malformation in the Dandy-Walker syndrome.

The outlet to the fourth ventricle can be obstructed, causing a fourth ventricle hydrocephalus, due to organising haemorrhage or secondary to meningitis. The foramina may be absent in Dandy-Walker or obstructed in Arnold-Chiari malformation, platybasia or basilar impression. The latter may occur in achondroplasia, Klippel-Feil syndrome or metabolic bone diseases.

Other posterior fossa abnormalities such as occipital encephaloceles, Meckel-Gruber syndrome and Joubert's syndrome are often associated with hydrocephalus. The commonest cause of hydrocephalus after the neonatal period is obstruction to the CSF pathway by tumour, and since the commonest tumours in children are posterior fossa tumours (*e.g.* medulloblastoma, ependymoma, haemangioblastoma, primitive neuroectodermal tumour, glioblastoma, and cerebellar astrocytoma), the signs of RICP due to hydrocephalus are the common presenting features. The pontine glioma is unusual in that it can be very large and yet does not cause hydrocephalus as an early feature.

The CSF is thought to be propelled from the posterior fossa over the surface of the brain by the pulsatility of the brain and blood vessels against the inner surface of the skull. If there is loss of contact as after removal of a cerebellar tumour or a hemispherectomy the 'hole' may cause failure of CSF propulsion and so forms a space-occupying cyst which can itself cause RICP. A deep subarachnoid space will tend to maintain itself after any arachnoid obstruction has resolved for the same reason. Arachnoid adhesions may cause a pouch with a valve-like entrance so that CSF is pumped into it but cannot escape, resulting in an arachnoid cyst which causes RICP due to space occupation. The subarachnoid space may be obstructed or obliterated by fibrin deposition and adhesions due to arachnoiditis in meningitis, post-subarachnoid haemorrhage and in the idiopathic arachnoiditis associated with very high CSF protein.

CSF ABSORPTION

The problem of absorption of CSF remains as much if not more of a mystery than the control of secretion of CSF. There is no doubt that there are pressure-controlled valves which allow CSF to gain direct access to the bloodstream in the sagittal sinus via the arachnoid granulations (Welch and Friedman 1960). These can be blocked by blood in cases of subarachnoid haemorrhage, inflammatory matter in meningitis or by clot in cases of venous sinus thrombosis. Back pressure from venous obstruction has become a contender for the mechanism of production of hydrocephalus in some conditions such as achondroplasia as well as the so-called lateral sinus syndrome or otitic hydrocephalus and is also thought to play a part in some cases of benign intracranial hypertension.

Studies with 'heavy water', however, suggest that the arachnoid mater itself plays a part in water regulation. This regulation may be under the control of antidiuretic hormone (ADH), since arginine vasopressin (AVP) is present in the CSF in man and is thought to regulate brain water permeability. AVP levels rise when ICP rises, and if one infuses AVP, ICP will rise. The effect could be on brain extracellular fluid (ECF) volume or CSF absorption (see below). It is however thought that the amount of tritiated water found in the jugular vein increases after AVP administration (Raichle and Grubb 1978). Even in the case of subdural haematoma, the free passage of water and albumin from bloodstream into the collection suggests that there must be a controlling mechanism. It could be that inappropriate ADH secretion may be inappropriate for the brain in its action on the

19

kidney, as it causes water intoxication, but very appropriate for the brain if it decreases CSF production and increases absorption of water from the CSF—possibly through a direct effect on arachnoid permeability.

Hydrocephalus is often spoken of as external or internal, or communicating and non-communicating, but one cannot always make this clear distinction in clinical practice. Nowadays one tends to count the number of ventricles involved.

Craniocerebral disproportion
This occurs when there is a discrepancy between the size of the skull (which may be too large or too small in volume for the size of brain), together with the normal intracranial volumes of blood and CSF. RICP is likely to occur when there is craniostenosis. An over-enlarged ventricular system or subarachnoid spaces can give a false impression of external hydrocephalus or subdural haematoma when the cranial cavity is too large for the size of the brain (*e.g.* Sotos syndrome).

The brain weighs about 340g at birth and about 1340g at four years. This continued brain growth requires a gradual increase in intracranial volume, and normally the maintained stretch on the suture lines causes the bony (cranial) growth to keep pace with cerebral growth. If the brain is small (microencephaly) then the skull is small (microcephaly). If the brain ceases to grow as a result of perinatal asphyxial damage, then the skull also stops growing (secondary microcephaly). If the brain is larger than normal (*e.g.* in primary familial megalencephaly or a megalencephaly secondary to some form of storage disease) the skull grows correspondingly large (macrocephaly). If the skull cannot accommodate this normal brain growth (craniostenosis) from premature fusion or absence of sutures (*e.g.* in Crouzon's disease, Apert's syndrome, turricephaly or scaphocephaly) then there can be a rise in ICP with brain damage and blindness.

Certain metabolic diseases of the cranial bones themselves, such as hypophosphatasia, can also result in failure of skull bones to accommodate continuing brain growth, and in the past this was aggravated by treatment with calcitonin.

If a child suffering from congenital hydrocephalus is shunted with a low-pressure valve (especially one without an anti-syphon device), then CSF production may not keep pace with removal and the ventricles become collapsed and slit-like on CT scan. This allows brain growth to continue into the existing skull volume but removes the continued stretch on the suture lines, which may then fuse prematurely. A paradox subsequently arises: brain growth continues until there is no further room, when the child returns with symptoms of severe RICP but without hydrocephalus (the ventricles will be slits on the CT scan). Unless the suture line is split and the craniocerebral disproportion relieved, severe intracranial hypertension will result.

The reverse can also be seen, when a child with a chronic or subacute subdural haematoma presents with macrocephaly. If the subdural haematoma is successfully treated but there is no decrease in intracranial volume, the volume of CSF in the subarachnoid space will have to increase to fill the increased space. Unless this is appreciated one may continue to perform unnecessary 'subdural' (*i.e.* subarachnoid) taps. Failure of the subarachnoid pump means that these cases of *ex vacuo* or

TABLE 2.II

Brain swelling

Expanded intravascular volume
Expanded extracellular volume
Increased intracellular water
Increased cell volume—metabolic storage
Myelin oedema (not same as white-matter oedema)

external hydrocephalus may develop pressure and require to be shunted—decision on treatment depends upon measurement of the pressure in the collection.

The slit ventricle (as seen on CT scan) can therefore be due to several mechanisms: (i) inability of the ventricle to expand due to stiffness, at the subependyma, *e.g.* due to ventriculitis, toxoplasmosis or cytomegalovirus infection, (ii) chronic low pressure from overdrainage or syphoning from a shunt, or (iii) restriction of expansion caused by too small a skull volume from craniostenosis, *i.e.* craniocerebral disproportion. Slit ventricles can therefore be associated with a low, normal or high ICP (Engel *et al.* 1979).

Brain swelling as a cause of RICP
The brain may swell as a result of an increase in the CBV (cerebral congestion) or due to an increase in the total water content of the brain (cerebral oedema). There are in turn several types of cerebral oedema, since the increase in water content may be intracellular (cytotoxic oedema), in the extracellular extravascular space (vasogenic oedema), or due to oedema of myelin (myelinoclastic oedema) (Brown and Steer 1986) (see Table 2.II).

The brain may also swell due to an increase in number or size of the cells. We have discussed increase in size of the cells causing macrocephaly in storage disorders such as some of the gangliosidoses. Diffuse astrocyte proliferation can occasionally be seen in diseases such as neurofibromatosis or tuberose sclerosis.

Cerebral congestion
The control of the cerebral circulation is discussed in more detail in Chapter 3. The CBV depends upon the size of the vascular bed, which in turn depends upon (i) the degree of arteriolar vasoconstriction (autoregulation), (ii) the size of the capillary bed (which in turn is influenced by local metabolic demand, pH, lactate and PCO_2) (Bruce 1984), and (iii) the capacity of the venous system. Certain physiological functions, such as REM sleep, increase CSF and CBV. The local bloodflow to a part of the brain increases as that part of the brain is active.

The bloodflow and volume increases markedly under certain pathological situations. Epileptic activity has a marked effect on CBF. Asphyxia in the neonate can lead to paralysed autoregulation and massive dilatation of bloodvessels with cerebral congestion. Head injury in children may differ from that in adults, as a massive increase in white-matter bloodflow means that cerebral congestion may sometimes be more important as a cause of RICP than cerebral oedema. Carbon dioxide is a very potent vasodilator or inhibitor of autoregulation so that cerebral

TABLE 2.III

Types of cerebral oedema

Extracellular oedema
        Vasogenic
        Hydrostatic
        Hydrocephalic
        Osmotic
        Necrotic
Intracellular oedema
        Osmotic
        Failure of cell to excrete H_2O
Myelinoclastic oedema
        Metabolic
        Toxic

---

congestion is often seen at its most florid in the hot vasodilated chronic bronchitic with papilloedema and massive retinal vasodilatation. In children suffering from cyanotic congenital heart disease or congestive cardiac failure (or any cause of a high central venous pressure) there is cerebral congestion, with associated scalp vein dilatation, retinal vein dilatation and sometimes a pulsatile fontanelle with an intracranial bruit.

The use of certain drugs and anaesthetic agents can paralyse autoregulation, thus allowing systolic blood pressure to reach the microcirculation and increasing the risk of hydrostatic cerebral oedema (Johansson 1974). Nitroprusside, nitrites, halothane and chlorpromazine can do this to varying degrees (Cottrell *et al.* 1978). The headache associated with the use of nitrites (*e.g.* inhaled amyl nitrite) shows how rapid this effect can be.

Apart from paralysis of autoregulation and pooling in the microcirculation we need also to consider the third arm of the circulation, *i.e.* the venous system. Any venous obstruction can cause a rapid increase in CBV and a secondary rise in ICP; this is the basis of the Queckenstedt test and should never be performed in the presence of suspected RICP. A severe rise in ICP may result from any venous thrombosis, obstruction from glomus jugulare tumours or tumours of the base of the skull, or high intrathoracic pressure from chest injury or poor ventilator technique.

Cerebral oedema
Cerebral oedema has already been defined as an increase in volume in the whole or part of the brain due to an increase in the water content (Pappius and Feindel 1976). The increase in water may be in one or several compartments: (i) intracellular, especially within astrocytes (cytotoxic), (ii) extracellular/extra vascular (vasogenic), or (iii) in myelin sheaths (myelinoclastic) (Table 2.III).

The term cerebral oedema is still often used loosely as if it were interchangeable with cerebral congestion or brain swelling. It also used to be fashionable to divide it into wet or dry oedema, depending on whether the cut surface wept at post-mortem examination, and into grey- or white-matter oedema. Vasogenic oedema is more likely to be wet and to affect white matter, while

22

cytotoxic oedema is more likely to be dry and affect grey matter (Feigin and Popoff 1962).

Pathophysiology of cerebral oedema
The brain differs from other tissues of the body in several respects: it does not possess a system of lymphatic channels, the capillary endothelial cells are tightly bound together and not fenestrated, there is no fat within the brain, it has its own reticulo-endothelial scavenger tissue in the microglia, and there are no lymph follicles or lymphoid tissue within the dura.

The absence of lymphatic channels and lymph nodes does not mean that brain extracellular fluid cannot be removed. Fifty years ago Harvey Cushing postulated that the CSF circulation was in fact a lymphatic system for the brain with a circulating force provided by the secretion of CSF from the choroid plexus. The extracellular fluid emerges from the brain via pores in the ependyma, and is diluted by the CSF from the choroid plexus and circulated through the lateral third and fourth ventricle to be propelled over the surface of the brain by vascular pulsation as well as the 'vis a tergo' from the choroid production. It is then absorbed into the arachnoid granulations, the surface arachnoid and the spinal theca (Milhorat *et al.* 1971, Milhorat 1987). Brain extracellular fluid can also emerge from the surface of the brain into the subarachnoid space. The pia mater is lined by a layer of glial cells and there are pores in this pial/glial membrane similar to those in the ependyma. These are separate from the blind pial pockets, which penetrate quite deep into the brain conveying bloodvessels (*i.e.* the Virchow-Robin spaces).

Further evidence for a lymphatic system is that drainage of CSF from the anterior part of the skull does pass via the ethmoid lymphatics into the cervical glands and so into the systemic lymphatic system.

It is thought that about 60 per cent of CSF comes from the choroid plexus and about 40 per cent from brain extracellular fluid. In children with obstructive hydrocephalus (*e.g.* from aqueduct stenosis) there may be a reverse transcephalic flow of CSF from ventricle through brain extracellular space and out over the surface to be absorbed. This can be seen dramatically as a type of extracellular cerebral oedema on CT scan. Dyes injected into the CSF such as trypan blue will also penetrate into the brain to give *in vivo* cellular staining.

In pathological states of subependymal scarring (gliosis, as in toxoplasmosis, post ventriculitis or scarring following a subependymal bleed) there is a kind of lymphatic obstruction, necessitating reverse flow of brain ECF to the surface.

The blood brain barrier
For many years debate continued as to whether there was an actual extracellular space in the brain. With the advent of electron microscopy it was settled that the brain possesses extracellular space like other tissues.

The brain capillaries differ from those in extracerebral tissues due to their tighter junctions between cells, so less extracellular fluid should form as a passive transudate. The endothelial cells in brain capillaries are in close contact with each other and are cemented or 'welded' together by a five-layer plasma membrane so that no gap exists between adjacent cells (*i.e.* there are tight endothelial junctions). Unlike the extracerebral tissues, there are no fenestrations in the capillary wall, meaning that they are more watertight. The capillary wall itself is also surrounded by small cells known as pericytes, and it is thought that these are contractile. A further protection of the capillary surface area from the extracellular space is by the close application of the astrocytic foot processes which cover over 80 per cent of the capillary surface. It should be remembered that neurons are not in direct contact with their blood supply but require an intermediary in the form of the astrocyte which acts as a 'mother cell' or 'food-taster'. The blood brain barrier is formed by the composite of tight endothelial junctions together with the pericytes and astrocytic foot processes. This forms a barrier to drugs, amino acids, neurotransmitters and antibodies: even movement of water, sodium and chloride must be controlled.

The endothelial cells possess masses of mitochondria, up to 10 per cent by volume. This is five times more than in endothelial cells of extracerebral tissue and emphasises the metabolic activity of the cerebral endothelial cell. They also contain large amounts of GABA transaminase and DOPA transaminase to detoxicate any circulating neurotransmitters which would seriously upset brain function if they penetrated. The astrocytic foot processes can be seen to swell on electron-microscopic examination with any disruption of the blood brain barrier (Nag *et al.* 1976). The astrocytes contain abundant carbonic anhydrase and may influence hydrogen ion transfer, but also are thought to regulate the extracellular potassium concentration and control the brain ammonia by connecting it to glutamine.

Large molecules such as proteins can if necessary be transported across the endothelial cell by pinocytosis. This process may allow albumin transport in certain pathological states (*e.g.* hypoxic/ischaemic or cold injury), causing vasogenic oed-ema. Damage to the endothelial cells, pericytes or loosening of the junctions would cause the same leakage of protein into brain ECF (Murphy and Johansson 1985).

Vasoactive substances (such as histamine, serotonin, prostaglandins, angioten-sin 2, vasoactive intestinal peptide, vasopressin, free fatty acids, kinins and liperoxides as well as free radicles) could all theoretically influence transport across the microcirculation, but we are still ignorant of their relative importance. Bradykinin causes the release of vasodilator prostaglandins, PGE$_2$ and PG$_{12}$, which have different effects between the internal and external carotid circulation.

Once fluid has escaped from the vessels into the ECF it is thought to move towards the ependyma by passing along the nerve tracts or along the vessels themselves to the pial surface.

Classification of brain oedema
We will consider the various types of brain oedema under the following headings: (i) vasogenic oedema, (ii) hydrostatic oedema, (iii) hydrocephalic oedema, (iv) intracellular oedema, (v) osmotic oedema, (vi) necrotic oedema, and (vii) myelinoclastic oedema (Table 2.III). These are not clear-cut single entities; several may coexist in the same patient, and in clinical practice one may not be able to differentiate one from another, but the pathophysiological background is different and separation makes discussion easier.

TABLE 2.IV

Causes of vasogenic oedema

Capillary damage
    Trauma, shaking injury
    Hypertensive encephalopathy
    Vasculitis (meningococcal and *Haemophilus influenzae* cerebritis)
    Hypoxic / ischaemic damage
    Herxheimer reaction
    Cerebral malaria
    Status epilepticus
    Radiation vasculitis
    Endothelial failure—mitochondriopathies
Biochemical factors
    Necrotic tissue, infarct or abscess, with release vasoactive peptides
    Tumour
    5 OH tryptamine, histamine, prostaglandins
    Steroid withdrawal
Increased pinocytosis
    Ischaemia
Opening tight junctions
    Hydrostatic oedema
    Osmotic agents
Lymphatic obstruction
    Hydrocephalic oedema
Venous obstruction

Extracellullar oedema

This can be due to vasogenic oedema, hydrostatic oedema, hydrocephalic oedema, osmotic oedema or necrotic oedema.

VASOGENIC OEDEMA

Damage to the endothelial cells or their junctions can result in breakdown of the blood brain barrier (Reulen 1976). Alternatively, as happens in hydrostatic oedema, a very high perfusion pressure blows sodium and water through the existing pores. Vasogenic oedema can be produced experimentally in several ways by the use of 5-hydroxy tryptamine, localised cold injury or injection of a hyperosmolar bolus (Beks and Kerckhoffs 1972).

In clinical practice capillary damage can result from many causes (Table 2.IV) such as asphyxia, head injury (especially in non-accidental shaking injuries when vascular damage is easily seen in the fundus—Caffey 1972), and in vasculitis associated with serum sickness, Herxheimer reactions or infective vasculitis as is seen in meningococcal septicaemia and *Haemophilus influenzae* cerebritis (Raimondi and Di Rocco 1979, Conner and Minielly 1980, Horwitz *et al.* 1980).

Anoxic ischaemic damage paralyses local autoregulation; lactate, acidosis and hypercarbia also affect vessel permeability. It is also thought that active transport of albumin molecules from bloodstream to extracellular space, across the endothelial cell, can occur by pinocytosis. Opening of the endothelial junctions by the pericytes also allows leakage of osmotically active molecules. The large number of mitochondria in the endothelial cells suggests that they are oxygen-dependent (Brierley 1977), and could become 'leaky' in hypoxia, and metabolic diseases (*e.g.*

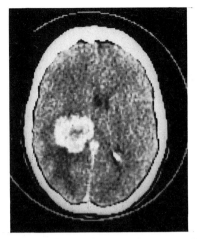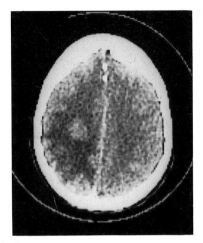

Fig. 2.4. Oedema around a focal area of brain damage.

Reye's syndrome). The same mechanisms are seen dramatically in the focal oedema which surrounds a persistently discharging epileptic focus.

Tumours or necrotic brain appear to secrete vasoactive substances which cause breakdown of focal areas of the blood brain barrier (Fig. 2.4). This can be demonstrated in the experimental animal by fluorescein staining of an infarct following carotid ligation. A similar 'natural experiment' occurs if a jaundiced patient sustains a stroke, when the infarct is the only part of the brain to show yellow staining. Kernicteric staining of the brain in perinatal asphyxia also occurs in the periventricular regions. Brain oedema occurs in humans following focal brain infarction, and if this results in a rise in ICP above 15mmHg the prognosis is poor (Ropper and Shafran 1984). If mannitol is given therapeutically, however, because of breakdown of the blood brain barrier in the infarct, the mannitol penetrates the infarct. When subsequently the plasma osmolality falls, it can cause rebound oedema of the infarct. Damage to the vascular endothelium with loss of the local blood brain barrier is also seen as a late complication of radiotherapy, when the onset of the focal oedema can be quite acute.

The loss of protein from the vascular to the extravascular space will result in a loss of oncotic pressure gradients to hold fluid in the capillaries. Albumin may also selectively bind water molecules in addition to the osmotic effect. If the albumin is broken down into peptides this can increase the osmotic effect more than a hundredfold. The elegant experiments of Klatzo's laboratory show that escape of albumin molecules is important in vasogenic oedema through the opened blood brain barrier, and that other small molecules may continue to escape for some time even after the oedema has resolved.

The breakdown of the blood brain barrier can be demonstrated clinically by the injection of sucrose intravenously. This normally stays within the vascular compartment but it can be measured in the CSF (lymph) if there is a leaky blood brain barrier. Experimentally radioactive-labelled sucrose, transferrin, I 131-

26

labelled albumin, Evans blue, horseradish peroxidase or fluorescein are all used (Pappenheimer 1962, Klatzo and Seitelberger 1967, Bryar *et al.* 1969, Nag *et al.* 1976).

In the presence of a severe vasogenic leak the proteins in the CSF should resemble a plasma protein profile rather than the very selective protein pattern from choroid plexus CSF. Occasionally there is continued vascular leak of protein and fluid, which flows through the brain and into the CSF without any impedance so that there is 'bulk extracellular flow'.

HYDROSTATIC OEDEMA

Hydrostatic oedema implies that the fluid content of the brain is increased as a result of fluid being forced under pressure from one compartment to another.

We have already discussed the mechanism of hydrocephalic oedema, when obstruction to the ventricular outflow causes a rise in pressure and reversed transcephalic flow across the brain with an increase in extracellular fluid easily visible on CT scan.

If the blood pressure is steadily increased, there comes a point of maximum protective vasoconstriction: autoregulation is overcome and a vastly increased perfusion pressure is transmitted to the microcirculation (Van Vught *et al.* 1976). This not only damages the vessels, but allows filtration under pressure to force open the blood brain barrier so that water and sodium are pumped into the extracellular space. This is seen at its most florid in hypertensive encephalopathy. Klatzo and Seitelberger (1967) used this as an experimental model using pressures as high as 350 to 400mmHg in experimental animals. Pressures as low as 120mmHg will open up the blood brain barrier in infant experimental animals, compared to 150mmHg in the adult animal (Robinson 1985).

If the normal protective autoregulation is lost (due to paralysis from hypoxia/ischaemia, prolonged seizures, trauma, severe hypercarbia or the use of drugs such as nitroprusside or papaverine) then even a normal blood pressure will be transmitted in full to the microcirculation and can result in oedema (Johansson 1974).

In the case of back pressure from venous obstruction the pressure is transmitted 'vis a fronte' instead of 'vis a tergo', and the pressure in the venous capillaries is increased without any protective autoregulation. Oedema will coexist with cerebral congestion, and the increase in CBV in these cases may be just as important as the oedema.

INTRACELLULAR OEDEMA

Accumulation of water within the cells of the brain usually denotes astrocytic rather than neuronal oedema. The oligodendroglia may also swell. Hypoxia results in swelling of the mitochondria and accumulation of glycogen within the cell, which is seen as an early sign on electron microscopy. Glucose is broken down to produce energy in the form of adenosine triphosphate (ATP), which is necessary to energise the membrane pumps in order to pump sodium out of the cell. The end result of complete aerobic glycolysis is carbon dioxide and water. The cell has to excrete this water, so as not to develop severe hydrops. Interference with energy supply will therefore cause water retention in several ways, *i.e.* failure to exclude sodium or to excrete water. If the cell is damaged, intracellular proteolysis releases idiogenic osmols, which will then also encourage water to be drawn into the cell by osmosis.

Intracellular oedema is likely in hypoxic ischaemic states, but also in disorders of energy metabolism such as mitochondrial disorders, for instance the congenital mitochondrial metabolic diseases (especially those likely to produce Reye's syndrome such as medium-chain acyl coenzyme A dehydrogenase deficiency) or the acquired mitochondriopathies (*i.e.* acquired parainfectious and toxic causes of Reye's syndrome). The free fatty acids liberated into the bloodstream in Reye's syndrome will add vasogenic oedema from toxic effect on the endothelium to the primary mitochondrial disorder. The experimental model used in the laboratory for cytotoxic oedema is poisoning with triethyl tin.

OSMOTIC OEDEMA

There are several compartments within the brain across which an osmotic gradient can develop, encouraging fluid shifts from one to the other:
(1) across the endothelium between blood and extracellular fluid
(2) across the cell membranes between extracellular and intracellular fluid
(3) across the arachnoid between blood and CSF, and
(4) across the ependyma between brain ECF and CSF.
We have already described the osmotic gradient between blood and brain extracellular fluid (*i.e.* across the blood brain barrier). The albumin binds water and exerts colloid osmotic pressure, but may also be broken down into much more osmotically active fragments.

The osmotic forces play a part in intracellular oedema, and the ionic exchange of sodium and potassium across the cell membranes need not balance each other. After an hypoxic/ischaemic episode there may be a marked leakage of potassium into the ECF within five minutes, while sodium may not change dramatically for 30 minutes. This will dehydrate the cells and may cause fits if the astrocytes cannot mop up the potassium.

An osmotic gradient as high as 50 milliosmols can exist across the very thin arachnoid membrane between blood and CSF (see below). There is a marked time-lag of up to six hours for equilibration between blood and CSF (Habel and Simpson 1976).

There are specific clinical situations in which osmotic oedema is likely to arise:
Hyperosmolar plasma to brain. Water is drawn from brain into plasma if the osmolality of the blood is higher than that of brain (as in hypernatraemic dehydration, diabetic ketoacidosis, uraemia or after the administration of mannitol, glycerol, sorbitol, urea or sucrose). The brain shrinks, with the risk of intracranial bleeding; plasma water expands and may be associated with hypertension or pulmonary oedema (Finberg *et al.* 1959, Bruck *et al.* 1968, Metzger and Rubenstein 1970).
Hyperosmolar brain to plasma. Water intoxication may result if the osmolality of the plasma is suddenly reduced, as in the over-use of electrolyte-free intravenous

fluids (when dextrose is mopped up by the liver into glycogen, leaving osmotically 'free' water). The ability to excrete a water load depends not only upon antidiuretic hormone but also glucocorticoids. The ability to excrete a given percentage of a water load was part of the old Kepler test of adrenal function. Glucocorticoid function is intricately related to the stress reaction, and children who are ill will not excrete the theoretical fluid load if given intravenously and may become water-intoxicated. They will develop hyponatraemia and hypo-osmolality. The results of careless fluid-balance regimes are often wrongly attributed to inappropriate ADH secretion. Infusion of normal saline and glucose does not change ICP, and infusion of 5 per cent glucose raises the ICP (Fishman 1953, Bakay *et al.* 1954). This is because the lag in equilibration leaves the brain relatively hyperosmolar and causes cerebral oedema by drawing water into it. As already discussed, if mannitol or urea has been used and there is a breakdown in blood brain barrier, the hyperosmolar agent penetrates the lesion but does not fall immediately; but the plasma levels fall and so there is a reversed osmotic gradient. A similar situation arises in hyper-natraemic dehydration. At first plasma volume is preserved with tissue dehyd-ration. Some of the increase in plasma sodium penetrates the brain and CSF. If the treatment now suddenly reduces plasma osmolality, *e.g.* by using non-electrolyte dextrose solutions, sudden rebound and often fatal cerebral oedema results.

A sudden increase in plasma water can also occur in true inappropriate ADH secretion, which often complicates meningitis, asphyxia, encephalitis, head injury, status epilepticus or acute encephalopathies (Friedman and Segar 1979). The failure to excrete water by the kidney results in 'strong' hyperosmolar urine and diluted hypo-osmolar plasma. There is oedema (of eyelids, dorsum of hands, pre-tibia and ankles), dilutional hyponatraemia, weight gain from water intoxication and severe brain swelling from cerebral oedema. A fall in serum sodium below 120mmol/l results in fits no matter whether the sodium is low due to salt loss or dilution. An osmolality below 255mosmol is again nearly always associated with severe cerebral oedema. Fits, coma and decerebration in meningitis may therefore be due to the electrolyte upset rather than the infection.

Dysequilibrium occurs if one reduces plasma osmolality more quickly than 1.0mosmol per hour *i.e.* 25mosmol in 24 hours. The osmolality of plasma depends mainly on sodium, glucose, urea concentrations and the presence of idiogenic osmols. Elevation of these parameters in hypernatraemic dehydration, diabetic ketoacidosis, uraemia or shock syndromes usually causes the clinician to want to reduce them quickly. Hypernatraemic dehydration should be treated by restoring plasma volume with plasma, colloid, albumin or normal saline and then the sodium should be gradually reduced over the next 72 hours.

Excessive haste results in cerebral oedema; mannitol simply restores the hyperosmolar state so that one can start again. Mannitol causes controlled hyperosmolar dehydration and so the control of maintenance fluid to prevent rebound is vital (Becker and Vries 1972). The use of dialysis to reduce high blood urea or sudden reduction of hyperglycaemia (even the type without ketoacidosis) can result in fatal cerebral oedema (Duck and Wyatt 1988). CT scan shows many children with diabetic ketoacidosis to have cerebral oedema, even if not severe enough to cause a cone and reduced consciousness. Activation of the NA/H+ exchange system in plasma membranes, due to the effects of weak organic acids in diabetic ketoacidosis, could also be a possible mechanism in the genesis of cerebral oedema (Van der Meulen *et al.* 1987). Just as important as the partition of osmolar active substances is the partition of hydrogen ions, and there may be a marked difference between plasma and CSF pH or between intracellular and extracellular pH. If there is a marked CSF hydrogen ion gap, an encephalopathy may result independent of the causal disease (Posner *et al.* 1965, Posner and Plum 1967).

OEDEMA OF MYELIN

Myelinoclastic (myelinogenic) oedema is not the same as white-matter oedema: as already discussed, vasogenic oedema causes an increase in extracellular fluid which tracks along the bundles of fibres in the white matter to reach the ependymal pores.

Myelinogenic oedema is less common and is usually due to swelling of the myelin sheaths themselves, often with vacuolation of the white matter on histological examination. The experimental animal model involves the use of toxins such as triethyl tin. In humans, metabolic diseases (such as galactosaemia) or toxins (such as the antiseptic hexachlorophane and the drug vigabatrine) have been incriminated. However, it is not common as a cause of RICP in the common acute encephalopathies of childhood.

NECROTIC OEDEMA

There is widespread infarction of brain in children with a serious impairment of CPP either secondary to RICP or due to a drop in systemic arterial pressure (Bruce *et al.* 1981). Cells die and lysosomes burst, releasing enzymes and peptides which are osmotically active and cause local oedema (idiogenic osmols). The endothelium is also damaged and autoregulation to the area is lost. Thromboplastin is rich in brain, and liberation from the damaged tissue causes thrombosis in the microcirculation and veins draining the tissue, thus further impairing blood supply and increasing the swelling due to an increase in blood volume in the infarct. The loss of autoregulation means that the ICP will follow systemic blood pressure. There may be a rise in ICP which is totally resistant to hyperventilation (as there is no autoregulation) and to mannitol (as the bloodvessels and cell walls are all disrupted).

If the blood pressure falls or rises, the ICP may follow passively by the same amount. This situation represents a stage of brain death and the oedema is in essence brain liquefaction (what Courville crudely but aptly called 'a bag of mush brain'). A fatal outcome is usually to be expected; survival is usually with severe mental and physical disability (Bannister 1983).

Clinical diagnosis of cerebral oedema

In clinical practice the diagnosis of cerebral oedema can be made with varying degrees of certainty, dependent on the urgency of the situation and the ready availability of imaging and neurophysiological tests.

Situational

In certain clinical situations, if a child develops symptoms and signs such as those of tentorial herniation, suggesting RICP, it is reasonable to assume cerebral oedema is the cause and to institute treatment without any further investigation (Batzdorf 1976, Bruce 1983, Brown and Steer 1986).

Cerebral oedema can be assumed in a child admitted with prolonged status epilepticus who does not recover consciousness after the fits are controlled. The administration of mannitol is then often very dramatic, with the child recovering full consciousness and being neurologically intact as rapidly as if one gives glucose in hypoglycaemia. This, along with the use of mannitol in the young infant with meningitis, is among the most dramatic responses which convince the clinician of the need to be constantly aware of the problem of RICP.

A similar situation arises in the child with scalds encephalopathy. The scald begins to swell and blister as the child becomes jittery and febrile with fits and loss of consciousness. Untreated s/he may die; s/he can be assumed to have cerebral oedema, and again will awaken as soon as the diuresis from mannitol occurs. Just as impressive in these cases is the visible reduction in swelling of the scald itself.

Another clinical situation can arise during the treatment of hyperosmolar dehydration, whether from hypernatraemia, diabetes or hyperosmolar-hyperglycaemic coma or dysequilibrium syndrome in renal failure, when the onset of fits, decerebration, and further decrease in conscious level can be assumed to be due to cerebral oedema. The RICP in cases of Reye's syndrome is usually due to cerebral oedema, and treatment is empirical in many centres where routine ICP monitoring is not performed. The correct management of RICP influences outcome, and treatment should really only be undertaken in centres able to monitor ICP (Shaywitz *et al.* 1980).

There are other situations when, although cerebral oedema may be present, the symptoms may be due to other factors. Extensor hypertonus following asphyxia may be due to oedema, but is more often a dystonia due to basal ganglia involvement—so-called post-asphyxial rigidity. This is not influenced by treatment to reduce ICP which is often normal or due to necrotic oedema (Seshia *et al.* 1979). In the case of head injury, RICP may be due to a mass lesion (space occupation) or cerebral congestion rather than oedema. Treatment of presumed oedema without imaging could then result in a dangerous delay in removing a mass lesion.

Clinical signs of RICP

If during the course of an acute illness such as meningitis, encephalitis (especially due to herpes simplex virus), metabolic disease or Reye's syndrome there are sudden signs of midbrain compression with tentorial herniation, it is usual to assume that these are due to RICP from cerebral oedema and to treat with mannitol and frusemide, while making arrangements for CT scanning and ICP monitoring (see Chapter 3).

CT scan in cerebral oedema

All children with an acute encephalopathy should have an emergency CT scan,

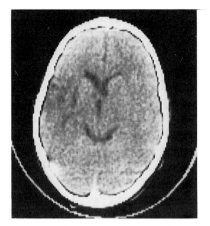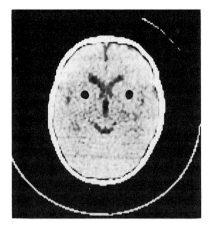

Fig. 2.5. *Left:* lateral ventricles, third ventricle and cisterna ambiens on a normal CT scan. *Right:* eyes placed artifactually to demonstrate why it is called the 'happy smiling face' sign.

especially if there is any reduction in conscious level. It may show swelling of one hemisphere with a shift, or the white matter may be focally or generally of reduced density and expanded. The cause may be obvious, as with an intracerebral haemorrhage or abscess. The lateral ventricles are compressed as pressure rises; the third ventricle becomes compressed and then the periaqueductal cisterns become obliterated (*i.e.* the 'happy smiling face' disappears, see Fig. 2.5). These CT scan appearances are thought to mirror the ICP (*e.g.* compressed lateral ventricles signify pressure, third ventricle compression 20mmHg, and cisterna ambiens obliteration 35mmHg). However, severely raised ICP can occur with a normal scan. The CT scan is an anatomical test. If one needs to understand the physiology (*i.e.* the ICP), the only sure way is to measure it rather than guessing from CT scan appearances.

The ventricles can be enlarged with a degree of hydrocephalus, and this can coexist with cerebral oedema. A fatal rise in ICP may occur before any of the above appearances are seen. Although in cases of active hydrocephalus the ventricles appear rounded and smooth-edged, the CT must not be used as a guide to the presence or absence of raised pressure or blindness may result.

Measurement of ICP
There may be no reliable clinical signs of RICP until a tentorial cone has occurred: and by this time there is imminent danger of secondary brainstem infarction with progressive and possibly irreversible brainstem failure. Papilloedema is unreliable and is usually absent in acute encephalopathy. CT scan is not a fail-safe diagnostic tool for RICP, which must be measured when there is any doubt. All children with impaired consciousness level (except in cases of obvious poisoning), should be considered for ICP monitoring, as should all children with impaired consciousness associated with trauma, Reye's syndrome, status epilepticus, acute encephalitis (especially due to herpes simplex virus), and meningitis (especially *Haemophilus influenzae* cerebritis). The most difficult decisions are in relation to acute anoxic

TABLE 2.V

Methods of monitoring ICP

Lumbar puncture (transducer attached to needle)
Cisternal puncture
Subarachnoid puncture (neonatal via angle of fontanelle)
Direct ventricular puncture via fontanelle
Burrhole and ventricular puncture
Burrhole and ventricular catheter
Perforation skull with sternal marrow needle and catheter,
    into ventricle
Insertion of ventriculostomy reservoir
Surface catheter via burrhole
Surface transducer via burrhole
Insertion Leeds screw or Philadelphia bolt

ischaemic insults such as perinatal asphyxia, near-miss cot-death, post-cardiac bypass or post-cardiac arrest resuscitation, as the relationship of raised pressure and its treatment to outcome in these cases is still in doubt.

In a normal person, lying horizontal, the pressure is the same in the subarachnoid space, ventricles and lumbar theca. If the foramen of Monro is blocked or the aqueduct is obstructed or a lumbar puncture has been performed, pressure may vary within different compartments, and this is what causes shifts and cones.

The basic equipment required is a pressure transducer, amplifier and pen recorder. A busy unit may need more sophisticated equipment, with digitisation of the signal to allow for computer storage and long-term analysis of the waveforms: but the basic equipment required is available in most hospitals.

The modern non-displacement miniature transducers allow measurement through a needle, cannula or screw with Luer fitting (Table 2.V). The pressure may therefore be measured through: (i) a needle at lumbar puncture, (ii) an intravenous catheter placed via the lateral angle of the fontanelle into the subarachnoid space in the neonate, (iii) direct ventricular tap in infants with hydrocephalus, (iv) cisterna magna puncture, or even (v), when the fontanelle is closed, by a catheter passed through a sternal marrow needle after perforation of the relatively thin skull bones (Minns 1977, McWilliam and Stephenson 1984, Brown and Steer 1986).

In most clinical situations the favourite methods are either a catheter placed by a neurosurgeon into the subdural/subarachnoid space for surface measurement, or some means of cannulating the ventricle: either using an infant feeding tube for direct puncture and exteriorisation (with risk of infection) or, ideally, a subcutaneous ventriculostomy reservoir such as those designed by Rickham or Ommaya. The Leeds bolt or Philadelphia screw was favoured for young children who might be restless, as it was fixed firmly by screwing into a reamed burrhole. Unfortunately at high pressures it did not show good linearity with direct ventricular pressure recording, which is generally accepted as the ideal.

Surface transducers inserted through a burrhole are expensive, and they are difficult to zero. The earlier ones were also very dependent upon the position of the child, and occipital pressure sores from immobilisation were common. At present they do not appear to have any advantage over a cordis catheter attached to a standard miniature transducer.

Non-invasive surface monitoring, such as applanation tonometry through the fontanelle, is of limited value and is not usually reliable in children with acute encephalopathies. A direct method of measurement is to be preferred because, although invasive, its risks are outweighed by the worsened prognosis of uncontrolled ICP.

A single pressure measurement may suffice when performing a lumbar puncture on a child with suspected meningitis. In most cases (80 per cent of cases of proven meningitis), the pressure will be found to be high and the needle will need to be left *in situ* for 30 minutes during administration of mannitol and frusemide. With ICP monitoring the procedure needs to be continued for several days, as baseline pressure may be normal but unpredictable pathological plateaus can cause serious clinical deterioration. The same applies to the effects of sleep, fits, ventilation techniques and the use of drugs (Lundberg 1960, Langfitt 1973, Miller 1978) (see Chapter 3).

Neurosurgical diagnosis
The brain may be very tight and flattened against the skull with flattening of the gyri and compression of the veins when the dura is opened at craniotomy. One must differentiate a 'tight brain' due to oedema from that due to cerebral congestion as a result of faulty anaesthetic technique. In severe cases the brain oozes out through the burrholes like toothpaste. The brain may swell so much that any attempt to re-close the dura is impossible. In fulminant cases the brain may then herniate out through the wound as a 'brain fungus'.

Magnetic resonance imaging
This is the most accurate way of assessing brain water in a living person, and the method allows estimation of CSF production rates and CSF volume as well as brain water content. The tl value gives the value for brain water content.

Neuropathological confirmation
Before modern imaging techniques, a retrospective diagnosis of cerebral oedema was often the only proof available. Some clinicians were suspicious of a diagnosis of brain swelling and never treated children with acute encephalopathies for RICP. The use of ICP monitoring and imaging has shown that the findings of generations of pathologists do apply at the bedside. The swollen, infarcted, necrotic and liquefied brain is the undesirable end result of total infarction from raised pressure. Shifts and cones described at post-mortem examination can now be diagnosed in life by clinical symptoms and imaging.

Biochemical estimation
Brain water can be measured at post-mortem examination or on brain biopsy and compared to sodium:potassium ratios as a measure of cerebral oedema in childhood.

Cerebral metabolism can be measured at the cotside using near infrared spectrophotometry (Wyatt *et al.* 1986). Regional cerebral metabolism for oxygen and glucose can be measured using PET scanning. Biochemical markers in CSF (*e.g.* lactate, pH, hypoxanthine and creatine phosphokinase) give some idea of impaired cerebral metabolism secondary to RICP or impaired perfusion (see Chapter 14). MRI and spectroscopy now allow estimations to be made in life (Cruckard *et al.* 1987).

Summary

The mechanisms of production of RICP are complex and multifactorial. Many different mechanisms may be acting in the same child. For example in the newborn infant suffering from hypoxic/ischaemic encephalopathy, (i) the mother may have been given excess intravenous dextrose in labour, causing water intoxication in the baby, (ii) the infant may be being continued on intravenous fluids and cannot excrete a water load, (iii) s/he may have excess ADH secretion, (iv) s/he may have renal damage from the hypoxia, (v) there may be loss of autoregulation for several days after the insult, (vi) there may be cerebral congestion with increase in white-matter blood volume, (vii) there may be vascular damage with vasogenic oedema, (viii) there may be artificial ventilation, pneumothorax and suction, which raises central venous pressure, (ix) there may be intracellular oedema which results from the hypoxia, (x) there may be necrotic oedema arising from infarcted brain, (xi) s/he may haemorrhage into infarcted areas causing space occupation, and (xii) subarachnoid bleeding may give rise to secondary hydrocephalus. Although at present one cannot measure each parameter at the bedside, and one may not even be able to say in a specific clinical situation whether oedema is present or not, a knowledge of pathophysiology is necessary to understand the rationale of treatment and the timing of clinical deterioration or improvement.

REFERENCES

Bakay, L., Crawford, J. D., White, J. C. (1954) 'The effects of intravenous fluids on cerebrospinal fluid pressure.' *Surgery, Gynaecology and Obstetrics*, **99**, 48–52.
Bannister, R. (1983) 'Reappraising death.' *British Medical Journal*, **286**, 710.
Batzdorf, U. (1976) 'The management of cerebral oedema in pediatric practice.' *Pediatrics*, **58**, 78–87.
Becker, D. P., Vries, J. K. (1972) 'The alleviation of increased ICP by the chronic administration of osmotic agents.' *In* Brock, M., Dietz, H. *Intracranial Pressure. Vol. I.* Berlin: Springer. pp. 309–315.
Beks, J. W. F., Kerckhoffs, H. P. H. (1972) 'Studies on the water content of cerebral tissues and intracranial pressure in vasogenic brain oedema.' *In* Brock, M., Dietz, H. *Intracranial Pressure. Vol. I.* Berlin: Springer. pp. 119–126.
Bering, E. A. Jr (1958) 'Problems of the dynamics of the cerebrospinal fluid with particular reference to the formation of cerebrospinal fluid and its relationship to cerebral metabolism.' *Clinical Neurosurgery*, **5**, 77–96.
Brierley, J. B. (1977) 'Experimental hypoxic brain damage.' *Journal of Clinical Pathology*, **30**, Suppl., 181–187.
Brown, J. K., Ingram, T. T. S., Seshia, S. S. (1973) 'Patterns of decerebration in infants and children: defects in homeostasis and sequelae.' *Journal of Neurology and Neurosurgery*, **36**, 431–434.
—— Habel, A. H. (1975) 'Toxic encephalopathy and acute brain swelling in children.' *Developmental Medicine and Child Neurology*, **17**, 659–679.
—— Steer, C. R. S. (1986) 'Strategies in the management of acute encephalopathies.' *In* Gordon, N., McKinlay, I. *Children with Neurological Disorders II: Neurologically Sick Children. Treatment and Management.* Oxford: Blackwell. pp. 219–294.

Bruce, D. A. (1983) 'Management of cerebral oedema.' *Pediatrics in Review*, **4**, 217–224.

—— (1984) 'Effects of hyperventilation on cerebral blood flow and metabolism.' *Clinics in Perinatology*, **11**, 673–680.

—— Alavi, A., Bilaniuk, L., Dolinskas, C., Obrist, W., Uzzell, B. (1981) 'Diffuse cerebral swelling following head injuries in children. The syndrome of malignant brain oedema.' *Journal of Neurosurgery*, **54**, 170–178.

Bruck, E., Abal, G., Aceto, T. (1968) 'Pathogenesis and pathophysiology of hypertonic dehydration with diarrhoea.' *American Journal of Diseases of Children*, **115**, 122–144.

Bryar, G. E., Goldstein, N. P., Svien, H. J., Sayre, G. P., Jones, J. D. (1969) 'Experimental cerebral edema—vital staining with Evans Blue during the developmental and regressive phases.' *Journal of Neurosurgery*, **30**, 391–397.

Caffey, J. (1972) 'On the theory and practice of shaking infants.' *American Journal of Diseases of Children*, **124**, 161–169.

Conner, W. T., Minielly, J. A. (1980) 'Cerebral oedema in fatal meningococcaemia.' *Lancet*, **2**, 967–969.

Cottrell, J. E., Patel, K., Turndorf, H., Ransohoff, J. (1978) 'Intracranial pressure changes induced by sodium nitroprusside in patients with intracranial mass lesions.' *Journal of Neurosurgery*, **48**, 329–331.

Cruckard, H. A., Gadan, D. G., Frackowiack, R. S. J., Proctor, E., Allen, K., Williams, S. R., Ross Russell, R. W. (1987) 'Acute cerebral ischaemia: concurrent changes in cerebral blood flow, energy metabolites, pH and lactate measured with hydrogen clearance 31p and 1H nuclear magnetic resonance spectroscopy. II: Changes during ischaemia.' *Journal of Cerebral Blood Flow and Metabolism*, **7**, 394–402.

Cutler, R. W. P., Page, L., Galwich, F., Waters, G. V. (1968) 'Formation and absorption of cerebrospinal fluid in man.' *Brain*, **91**, 707–720.

Davson, H., Welch, K., Segal., M. B. (1987) *The Physiology and Pathophysiology of the Cerebrospinal Fluid*. Edinburgh: Churchill Livingstone. pp. 445–451.

Duck, S. C., Wyatt, D. T. (1988) 'Factors associated with brain herniation in the treatment of diabetic ketoacidosis.' *Journal of Pediatrics*, **113**, 10–14..

Engel, M., Carmel, P. W., Chutorian, A. M. (1979) 'Increased ventriculomegaly in children with shunts; "normal volume" hydrocephalus.' *Neurosurgery*, **5**, 549.

Feigin, I., Popoff, N. (1962) 'Neuropathological observations on cerebral edema.' *Archives of Neurology*, **6**, 151–160.

Finberg, L., Luttrell, C., Redd, H. (1959) 'Pathogenesis of lesions in the nervous system in hypernatremic states. II: Experimental studies of gross anatomic changes and alterations of chemical composition of the tissues.' *Pediatrics*, **23**, 46–53.

Fishman, R. A. (1953) 'Effects of isotonic intravenous solutions on normal and increased intracranial pressure.' *Archives of Neurology and Psychiatry*, **70**, 350–360.

Friedman, A. L., Segar, W. E. (1979) 'Antidiuretic hormone excess.' *Journal of Pediatrics*, **94**, 521–526.

Habel, A. H., Simpson, H. (1976) 'Osmolar relation between cerebrospinal fluid and serum in hyperosmolar hypernatraemic dehydration.' *Archives of Disease in Childhood*, **51**, 660–666.

Hochwald, G. M., Sahar, A. (1971) 'Effect of spinal fluid pressure on cerebrospinal fluid formation.' *Experimental Neurology*, **32**, 30–40.

Horwitz, S. J., Boxerbaum, B., O'Bell, J. (1980) 'Cerebral herniation in bacterial meningitis in childhood.' *Annals of Neurology*, **7**, 525–528.

Johansson, B. (1974) 'Blood brain barrier dysfunction in acute arterial hypertension after papaverine-induced vasodilation.' *Acta Neurologica Scandinavica*, **50**, 573–580.

Juncos, J., Epstein, F., Hunnicutt, E., Nathanson, J. (1982) 'Human choroid plexus: pharmacologic characterization of hormone receptors in vitro.' (Abstract) *Neurology*, **32**, A70.

Klatzo, I., Seitelberger, F. (1967) 'Brain edema.' *Proceedings of the Vienna Symposium*. Berlin: Springer.

Langfitt, T. W. (1973) 'Increased intracranial pressure.' *In* Youmans, J. R. (Ed.) *Neurological Surgery*, Vol. I. Philadelphia: W. B. Saunders. p. 443.

Lorenzo, A. V., Page, L. K., Watters, G. V. (1970) 'Relationship between cerebrospinal fluid formation, absorption, and pressure in human "hydrocephalus".' *Brain*, **93**, 679–692.

Lundberg, N. (1960) 'Continuous recording and control of ventricular fluid pressure in neurosurgical practice.' *Acta Psychologica et Neurologica Scandinavica*, **36**, Suppl. 149, 1–193.

McComb, J. G. (1983) 'Recent research into the nature of cerebrospinal fluid formation and absorption.' *Journal of Neurosurgery*, **59**, 369–383.

McWilliam, R. C., Stephenson, J. B. P. (1984) 'Rapid bedside technique for intracranial pressure monitoring.' *Lancet*, **2**, 73–75.

Metzger, A. L., Rubenstein, A. H. (1970) 'Reversible cerebral oedema complicating diabetic ketoacidosis.' *British Medical Journal*, **3**, 746–747.

Milhorat, T. H. (1987) *Cerebrospinal Fluid and the Brain Edemas*, New York: Neuroscience Society.

—— Hammock, M. K., Fenstor-Macher, J. D., Rall, D. P., Levin, V. A. (1971) 'Cerebrospinal fluid production by the choroid plexus and brain.' *Science*, **173**, 330–332.

Miller, J. D. (1978) 'Intracranial pressure monitoring.' *British Journal of Hospital Medicine*, **19**, 497–503.

Minns, R. A. (1977) 'Clinical application of ventricular pressure monitoring in children.' *Zeitschrift für Kinderheilkunde und Grenzgebiete*, **224**, 430–443.

—— Brown, J. K., Engelman, H. M. (1988) 'CSF production rate, "realtime" estimation.' *Zeitschrift für Kinderchirurgie*, **42**, Suppl. 1, 36–40.

—— Engelman, H. M., Stirling, H. (1989) 'Cerebrospinal fluid pressure in pyogenic meningitis.' *Archives of Disease in Childhood*, **64**, 814–820.

Murphy, V. A., Johansson, C. E. (1985) 'Adrenergic-induced enhancement of brain barrier system permeability to small nonelectrolytes: choroid plexus versus cerebral capillaries.' *Journal of Cerebral Blood Flow and Metabolism*, **5**, 401–412.

Nag, S., Robertson, D. M., Dinsdale, H. B., Haas, R. A. (1976) 'Determination of cerebral edema by quantitative morphometry.' *In* Pappius, H. M., Feindel, W. (Eds.) *Dynamics of Brain Edema*. Berlin: Springer. p. 32.

Nugent, S. K., Bausher, J. A., Moxon, E. R., Rogers, M. C. (1979) 'Raised intracranial pressure. Its management in *Neisseria meningitidis* meningoencephalitis.' *American Journal of Diseases in Children*, **133**, 260–262.

Pappenheimer, J. R. (1962) 'Bulk flow and diffusion in the cerebrospinal fluid system of the goat.' *American Journal of Physiology*, **203**, 775–781.

Pappius, H. M., Feindel, W. (1976) *Dynamics of Brain Edema*. Berlin: Springer.

Posner, J. B., Swanson, A. G., Plum, F. (1965) 'Acid-base balance in cerebrospinal fluid.' *Archives of Neurology*, **12**, 479–496.

—— Plum, F. (1967) 'Spinal fluid pH and neurologic symptoms in systemic acidosis.' *New England Journal of Medicine*, **227**, 605–613.

Raichle, M. E., Grubb, R. L. (1978) 'Regulation of brain water permeability by centrally released vasopressin.' *Brain Research*, **143**, 191–194.

Raimondi, A. J., Di Rocco, C. (1979) 'The physiopathogenic basis for the angiographic diagnosis of bacterial infections of the brain and its coverings in children. I: Leptomeningitis; II: Cerebritis and brain abscess.' *Child's Brain*, **5**, 1–13, 398–407.

Reulen, H. J. (1976) 'Vasogenic brain oedema—new aspects in its formation, resolution and therapy.' *British Journal of Anaesthesia*, **48**, 741–752.

Robinson, J. S. (1985) 'Opening of the blood-brain barrier by framine-induced hypertension in adult and immature rats.' *Journal of Pediatric Neurosciences*, **1**, 203–209.

Ropper, A. H., Shafran, B. (1984) 'Brain edema after stroke. Clinical syndrome and intracranial pressure.' *Archives of Neurology*, **41**, 26–29.

Rubin, R. C., Henderson, E. S., Ommaya, A. K., Walker, M. D., Rall, D. P. (1966) 'The production of cerebrospinal fluid in man and its modification by acetazolamide.' *Journal of Neurosurgery*, **25**, 430–436.

Seshia, S. S., Chow, P. N., Sankaran, K. (1979) 'Coma following cardio-respiratory arrest in childhood.' *Developmental Medicine and Child Neurology*, **21**, 143–153.

Shaywitz, B. A., Rothstein, P., Venes, J. L. (1980) 'Monitoring and the management of increased intracranial pressure in Reye syndrome: results in 29 children.' *Pediatrics*, **66**, 198–204.

Sklar, F. H., Reisch, J., Elashvilli, T., Smith, T., Long, D. M. (1980) 'Effects of pressure of cerebrospinal fluid formation: non-steady state management in dogs.' *American Journal of Physiology*, **239**, R277–R284.

Van der Meulen, J. A., Klip, A., Grinstein, S. (1987) 'Possible mechanism for cerebral oedema in diabetic ketoacidosis.' *Lancet*, **2**, 306–308.

Van Vught, A. J., Troost, J., Willemse, J. (1976) 'Hypertensive encephalopathy in childhood.' *Neuropädiatrie*, **7**, 92–100.

Welch, K., Friedman, V. (1960) 'The cerebrospinal fluid values.' *Brain*, **83**, 454–469.

Wyatt, J. S., Cope, M., Delpy, D. T., Wray, S., Reynolds, E. O. R. (1986) 'Quantifications of cerebral oxygenation and haemodynamics in sick newborn infants by near infra red spectophotometry.' *Lancet*, **2**, 1063–1065.

37

3
THE PATHOLOGICAL EFFECTS OF RAISED INTRACRANIAL PRESSURE

J. K. Brown

Raised intracranial pressure causes two distinct pathological processes: a reduction of CBF, or shifts and cones. These secondary pathological processes may cause further brain damage, additional to the primary process, and are responsible for many of the clinical symptoms and signs which are the basis of neurological observations and ICU monitoring (Brown and Steer 1986, Minns *et al.* 1989).

RICP and the cerebral circulation
Anatomy of the cerebral circulation
All major vessels (*i.e.* carotid, vertebral and their major divisions) are anatomically distinct by seven weeks of gestation. The most preterm infant possesses the major anatomical vessels, but not a mature pattern of circulation (Roach and Riela 1988). The cerebral circulation develops from mesoderm when solid cords of primitive endothelial cells (angioblasts) bud off existing mature capillaries and penetrate the developing neuro-ectodermal cerebral vesicle. In anencephaly, there is no penetration of the telencephalon and one sees masses of aberrant vessels in a haemangiomatous-looking mass instead of the normal cerebral hemisphere.

The new vessels develop in order to keep pace with the increasing metabolic demands of the developing tissues which can no longer be met by simple diffusion from a vascular plexus which encases the developing nervous system. It is thought that this corresponds in time with the differentiation of astroglia and the formation of dendrites (Jacobson 1978).

The capillaries are not static once they have formed, as changes in the whole vasculature of the brain occur between the second and third trimester, and thousands of capillaries already formed have to undergo a process of involution. In the preterm infant before 28 weeks' gestation all the cell division and massive metabolic activity is in the subependymal germinal plate which is supplied from the basal circulation by Heubner's artery and the choroidal vessels. The cerebral cortex is supplied by short penetrating spiral arteries (Pape and Wigglesworth 1989). After 28 weeks' gestation the cell division in the germinal plate stops, and all the germinal cells undergo dissolution and absorption. The basal circulation is now less dominant, the cerebral cortex is developing and also the oligodendroglia now require a rich nutrition in order to sustain the rapid phase of myelination. Long penetrating cortical vessels therefore need to develop. The short spiral arteries also increase in calibre and become less spiralled.

In the early stages of development, the carotid artery supplies all the

38

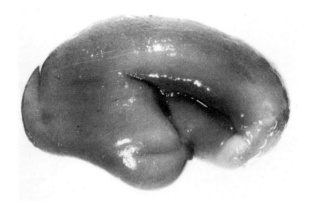

Fig. 3.1. Brain at 20 weeks when the cerebral cortex is rudimentary and supplied by only small surface vessels. The main blood supply is from the basal circulation.

developing cerebral hemisphere and divides into cranial (rostral) and caudal portions. The cranial portion develops into the anterior and middle cerebral artery and continues to supply the anterior two-thirds of the hemisphere. The caudal portion (posterior cerebral and posterior communicating arteries) supplies occipital cortex, posterior temporal lobe and midbrain. This portion becomes more dependent upon vertebral flow as the posterior communicating artery becomes functionally less significant than the basilar. The occipital lobe (calcarine visual area) is thought to remain dependent on carotid rather than basilar blood supply in 25 per cent of people (Roach and Riela 1988). The vertebral arteries may show marked variation between individuals.

These anatomical changes are important, as consumptive asphyxia is more of a threat in the most metabolically active parts of the brain. In impaired CBF, the watershed zones between adjacent vascular territories are most susceptible. It can be appreciated that this may shift with age, from between centrifugal and centripetal arteries (causing periventricular leucomalacia in the newborn) to between middle and posterior cerebral arteries, causing infarcts in the pericentral white matter of the optic radiation and posterior temporal lobe (see below). The venous system also changes as the Galenic system (draining the basal parts of the brain) becomes less dominant, and the cortical veins (draining into the sagittal sinus) become more conspicuous. Connections across the skull bones allow intracranial venous blood to drain into the extracranial venous circulation (*i.e.* blood from the brain into the external jugular vein). There is also a significant flow into the vertebral veins, which increases if the internal jugular vein is obstructed. Blood from the face and eye may pass in the opposite direction, into the cavernous sinus, and so drain into the internal jugular vein. Apart from its importance in the spread of infection it means that sampling of blood from the jugular bulb is not sampling blood solely from the brain (Kirsch *et al.* 1985). About 20 per cent of tracer or dye injected into the internal carotid artery will appear in the external jugular vein. The purpose of this brief review is to show that in paediatric practice one must always remember that one is dealing with a developing nervous system, and that even anatomy is not static (Figs. 3.1, 3.2).

39

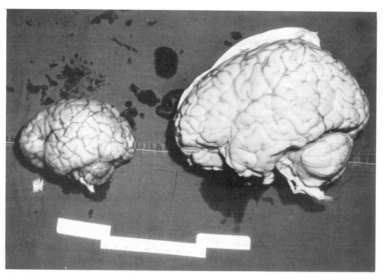

Fig. 3.2. Brain at three months and at four years, demonstrating the tremendous amount of brain growth that occurs in the first few years of life.

Normal control of the cerebral circulation

The control of CBF is governed by similar principles as other organs (Meyer *et al.* 1971) (Fig. 3.3, Table 3.I). The brain cannnot withstand periods of ischaemia without permanent damage, and in the upright position gravitational forces mean that the brain would be the first to be deprived of blood supply; so a very precise control of cerebral circulation is necessary in order to stop us fainting or being unable to think every time we stand up. The head is also balanced on a very mobile neck. Turning one's head completely occludes one vertebral artery, and tilting it may cause kinking of the carotids. Four vessels feeding into an equilibration system (as seen in the circle of Willis) ensure flow regardless of head position.

CBF depends upon CPP (which is not the same as aortic blood pressure) and

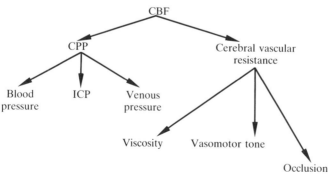

Fig. 3.3. Major factors controlling CBF.

TABLE 3.I

Factors affecting cerebral autoregulation

Changes in systemic blood pressure
Use of part of brain
Drugs—halothane, nitroprusside, nitrites, ketamine
Sleep
Lactic acid
Carbon dioxide
Seizures
Anoxic ischaemic damage
Brainstem bloodflow

inversely on cerebral vascular resistance (radius of vessel, length of vessel and viscosity of fluid). A general rule is that arteries change resistance and veins change capacitance. The arteries, even in the preterm infant, all possess a well developed tunica media of smooth muscle and in normal circumstances are maintained in a state of partial contraction—vasomotor tone, which is the basis of cerebrovascular autoregulation. If fully dilated, as in vasoparalytic shock or with loss of autoregulation, then the volume of the cerebral circulation (CBV) is vastly increased. With intense vasoconstriction (cerebral vasospasm), the opposite is the case. The bloodflow in any vessel can be fast or slow and still deliver the same volume of blood per minute, depending upon perfusion pressure and diameter of the vessel. In other words, one can increase flow through a vessel of fixed diameter by increasing pressure, or in spite of a fixed perfusion pressure by increasing vessel diameter. This must be remembered when interpreting Doppler velocity of flow as synonymous with volume of flow.

One can increase CBV and yet decrease flow by producing stasis within the system as with vasoparalysis.

Autoregulation

If one makes a window in the skull in an experimental animal, so that one can observe the blood vessels of the pia mater, one can see that the vessels constrict when the blood pressure rises and dilate when it falls. This maintains the CBF constant in spite of widely varying blood pressure (*i.e.* CPP). This is what is meant by cerebral autoregulation (Meyer *et al.* 1971). Flow is thought to be regulated by the small arteries and arterioles, and not the major vessels. The relative constancy of the major vessels is helpful from the point of view of Doppler velocitometry. They are however capable of intense vasospasm such as to cause infarction as seen in the intense vasospasm following subarachnoid bleeding, migraine or trauma. Human CBF is maintained between blood pressures of 60 to 160mmHg in the adult. Raising ICP reduces the effective CPP, and again the vessels dilate to maintain the flow at the lower perfusion pressure. This is what is meant by cerebral autoregulation. Postural hypotension causes blood pressure to fall if the person stands suddenly, so there must be an increase in peripheral sympathetic discharge to reduce the size of the vascular bed to accommodate the fixed blood volume and so maintain blood pressure. At the same time the cerebral vessels must do the opposite and dilate. If the brainstem reflexes are disrupted (see below) then severe postural hypertension, may result due to excess swings in sympathetic tone. In autonomic neuropathy, as in diabetes or with sympathetic ganglion-blocking drugs, this compensation is lost and postural hypotension and syncope result.

At blood pressures below 60mmHg no further compensation is possible, and the CBF falls in parallel with any further drop in systemic perfusion pressure.

Blood pressure may rise to a point of maximum vasoconstriction, when any further rise is transmitted to the brain microcirculation. This will also damage small bloodvessels, resulting in hypertensive encephalopathy and retinopathy, with the risk of intracerebral haemorrhage.

If cerebral vasomotor tone is abolished—due either to brainstem damage, for example because of asphyxia (Friis-Hansen 1985), or drugs (Johansson 1974)—then the perfusing pressure will be transmitted to the microcirculation at normal blood pressure, which can be seen on the ICP trace as a marked increase in amplitude of the pulse-wave artefact. This also encourages the development of hydrostatic oedema which may be the start of an often fatal vicious circle.

The most potent override of vasomotor tone is by carbon dioxide which causes cerebral vasodilatation and a massive increase in CBF (Harper and Glass 1965, Harper *et al.* 1972). Kinins and atrial natriuretic peptide are also thought to promote cerebral vasodilatation, as are drugs such as halothane, nitrites and nitroprusside. Peripheral vasoconstrictors such as noradrenaline, vasopressin, neuropeptide, and angiotensin II do not have a profound effect on cerebral vasomotor tone. This is probably because they do not pass the blood brain barrier.

The neurogenic control of cerebral vasomotor tone (*i.e.* autoregulation) is thought in the case of extraparenchymal vessels to be mediated by noradrenergic fibres from the superior cervical ganglion, which in turn are thought to originate in the locus ceruleus in the medulla. It is thought that there is a direct pathway from brainstem to intraparenchymal vessels (Raichle *et al.* 1976). The extracerebral vessels can be shown to be rich in noradrenergic endings (Rennels and Nelson 1973). Intraparenchymal nerve-endings on the smaller bloodvessels are rich in dopamine hydroxylase, and these nerves may also influence tight junctions and water permeability. It is thought that autoregulation is achieved by a varied tonic constriction rather than by an active dilator nerve supply.

The brain is able to monitor its own blood supply by a centre in the medulla, possibly the locus ceruleus. If perfusion is reduced, CBF is preserved by a built-in compensatory mechanism: systemic hypertension (*i.e.* the Cushing effect). Sympathetic discharge to the heart increases cardiac output and cerebral vasodilatation. Stimulation of the brainstem in experimental animals can be shown to cause cerebral vasodilatation (Molnar and Szanto 1964, Langfitt and Kassell 1968).

CBF is not usually influenced by beta-blockers such as propanolol or anticholinesterases such as atropine. Intravenous bradykinin, which is a powerful vasodilator, causes a drop in systemic blood pressure and a rise in ICP, presumably secondary to a rise in CBV from cerebral vasodilatation.

Physiology of autoregulation

The control of the circulation is basically a series of feedback systems. The baroreceptors respond to stretch and monitor the systemic blood pressure in the aortic arch and carotid sinus. Those baroreceptors in the carotid sinus resemble the Golgi tendon organs in muscle, which measure the degree of muscle tension. This information is transmitted back to the brain via the ninth cranial nerve from the carotid sinus and vagal afferents from the aortic arch. It is first relayed to the nucleus of the tractus solitarius. There is then a simple reflex to the nucleus ambiguus allowing modification of vagotonia to the heart, *i.e.* slowing the heart and decreasing output to lower the blood pressure. Alternatively, if blood pressure falls, a decrease in vagotonia causes a rise in heart-rate (since the heart is controlled mainly by changes in vagal tone rather than sympathetic activity, which is reserved for emergency stress reactions). The vagus affects the heart-rate and is chronotropic, whereas the sympathetic affects force of contraction and is inotropic.

The nucleus of the tractus solitarius also sends messages from the baroreceptors to the vasomotor centre. Peripheral vasomotor tone depends upon sympathetic tonic activity, and this can be modified independently of heart-rate to decrease or increase vasomotor tone, according to whether one wants to increase or decrease the volume of the systemic circulation (*i.e.* the tightness with which the particular blood volume is held and so determine the systemic blood pressure).

The respiratory centre is closely linked with these other brainstem nuclei and is sensitive to carbon dioxide as well as pH. In the brainstem, the area postrema—like the hypothalamus—contains no blood brain barrier, having fenestrated capillaries so that the PCO_2, PO_2 and pH can be monitored here just as osmolarity, glucose and temperature are monitored at the hypothalamic receptor system. The carotid body also monitors acid-base status.

We can regard the brainstem as an intensive-care computer system with an afferent information service coming from the lungs by the Hering Breuer reflex, acid base from carotid body and area postrema, carbon dioxide and oxygen from the area postrema and carotid body, blood pressure from aortic and carotid sinus baroreceptors, and central venous pressure from right atrial receptors. This information is computed to adjust heart-rate, blood pressure, and rate and depth of respiration in order to maintain the internal milieu at preset levels.

The locus ceruleus also has connections to all these inputs and can override the other reflex systems in order to maintain cerebral perfusion. Massive hypertension, tachycardia over 200 per minute, hyperventilation, hyperglycaemia and cerebral vasodilatation can all occur if the feedback system is disrupted.

Paralysis of all these functions, as in brainstem failure, produces the reverse clinical picture of apnoea unresponsive to PCO_2, vasoparalytic shock, a fixed heart-rate and total loss of cerebral autoregulation.

Isolation of individual reflexes means that severe postural hypertension can occur every time the patient is put in a standing position. Individual patients may have hyperventilation to the point of tetany, Ondine's curse with loss of automatic respiration in sleep, repeated cardiac arrest from vagotonia without brainstem compression, cerebral diabetes or the pseudo-phaeochromocytoma syndrome.

Lassen (1968) has been the main protagonist for a local biochemical control of the cerebral circulation as being more important than neurogenic control. He demonstrated local bloodflow changes in response to vision, speech, music or even anticipation of an act; total bloodflow is a gross concept therefore, and possibly the most dynamic control of bloodflow is the fine tuning of changes in CBF to discrete but active parts of the brain. It is more likely that local changes in pH and lactate will override neurogenic control to enable flow to follow metabolism. Carbon dioxide and drugs such as nitrites or nitroprusside will also override neurogenic control (Huff *et al.* 1972, Paul *et al.* 1972). The same applies to the extraparenchymal vessels when breakdown products of blood in the CSF override the 'correct tone' imposed by the medulla and cause intense, maybe fatal, vasospasm. CBF is therefore regulated basically by two systems: a monitoring system for total flow and a fine-tuned system linking local metabolism and its blood supply.

Cerebral perfusion pressure
This depends basically upon the blood pressure, and although in the adult one can talk of a normal blood pressure, this is more difficult in children. Systolic blood pressure at birth may be only 40mmHg, rising to systolic/diastolic averages of 80/55mmHg in the first year, 85/60mmHg in the preschool years and 90/60mmHg during the school years, meaning that perfusion pressure is more easily encroached upon than in adults. Theoretically the perfusion pressure is blood pressure minus venous pressure. A rise in venous pressure is a very effective way of decreasing perfusion pressure and so flow (Miller *et al.* 1972). In practice ICP is usually very similar (slightly less) to venous pressure and so is used to measure CPP (which is said to equal systemic arterial pressure minus ICP). Pressure at the cerebral arterioles is the true CPP and the above equation does not always hold true. Arteriolar pressure is about one-third aortic pressure, *i.e.* 15mmHg in the newborn and 40mmHg in the adult. Clinical experience shows that these are the absolute ICPs at which brain ischaemia begins to appear. In adults with head injuries an ICP over 40mmHg carries a very poor prognosis (death, or survival in a persistent vegetative state). Focal oedema can act as a local space-occupying lesion and causes a decrease in regional flow in spite of adequate perfusion pressure. Sludging of the microcirculation from hyperviscosity or the local liberation of thromboplastic substances means that regional perfusion and total bloodflow are not absolutely linked.

Perfusion pressures of less than 50mmHg cause concern in the older child; pressures of less than 40mmHg make the risk of infarction high, and of less than 20mmHg mean that survival is unlikely (Lou *et al.* 1977, Raju *et al.* 1981). One does see exceptions, however, such as children with basal vessel damage following meningitis or some cases of craniocerebral disproportion, when the very low CPP which can occur in sleep would normally make one very anxious about continuing brain damage. Otherwise the children appear very well (Fig. 3.4).

Systemic hypotension with peripheral circulatory failure (*i.e.* shock) may occur in children with head injuries, the septic shock of meningococcal septicaemia, and in neonates with intracranial haemorrhage (intraventricular, subgaleal and extradural). The fall in systemic blood pressure may then be the principal cause of

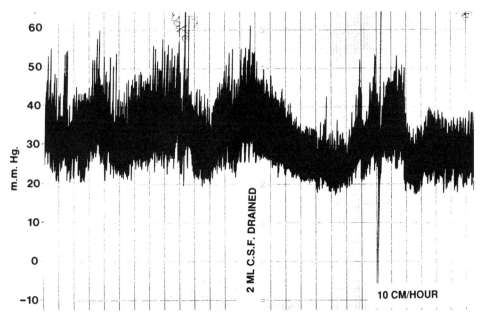

Fig. 3.4. RICP associated with craniocerebral disproportion. This is not responsive to hyperventilation and removal of CSF, or mannitol.

cerebral circulatory failure and infarction. With progressive brainstem failure there is a loss of the normal vasomotor tone to the systemic circulation which is normally adjusted for a given volume to maintain a predetermined blood pressure at the aortic receptor, carotid body and medulla. If this fails, the capacity of the circulation is too great for the blood volume. Relative hypovolaemia and severe hypotension ensue (*i.e.* vasoparalytic shock or cerebral shock). This will cause further cerebral ischaemia and usually death.

The effects of even a modest rise in ICP can be seen in the infant by the use of transcranial Doppler. Complete cessation of diastolic flow may occur at ICP around 10 to 15mmHg, which would not be considered significant in the older child and adult. Removal of CSF with reduction in ICPs to normal rapidly restores the flow. Because of the low blood pressure, failure of cerebral circulation with brain infarction is often more prominent in the neonate than shifts or cones, which require a higher pressure than the expansile head usually allows to develop. ICPs over 30mmHg are required in the older child to seriously impair cerebral perfusion.

Severe intracranial hypertension will stop all CBF, as seen in the so-called 'carotid stop' on angiography.

Normal CBF
The normal CBF is around 50ml per 100g of brain tissue per minute (Lassen and Christensen 1976). In the adult with a brain weight of 1500g this means that 750ml of a total cardiac output of 3500ml goes to the brain each minute. The percentage of cardiac output which goes to the brain is much higher in the small infant.

Bloodflow varies from region to region and is normally five times higher in grey (100ml per 100g) than white matter (20ml per 100g). The order of flow, from highest to lowest, can be placed in a league table: (i) inferior colliculus, (ii) sensory cerebral cortex, (iii) motor cerebral cortex, (iv) geniculate bodies, (v) superior colliculus (vi) caudate nucleus, (vii) thalamus, (viii) cerebellum and (ix) cerebral white matter.

When the subject is awake and vigilant, the frontal lobes normally maintain an increase in flow which is thought to relate to constant forward planning. This disappears in sleep, anaesthesia or dementia (Lassen 1968). REM sleep is associated with a 40 per cent increase in CBF, and this can be used as a physiological test of compliance. When part of the brain is planning or executing a cognitive ability, a motor skill or an emotional task, the corresponding part of the brain can be shown to have an increase in flow (Obrist *et al.* 1975, Ingvar and Philipson 1977). The limbic system can be shown to do the same in anxiety states.

Measurement of CBF

Measurement of CBF has been attempted for over 50 years (Ferris 1941), yet there are still great technical difficulties in the measurement of bloodflow at the bedside in the intensive-care unit.

RADIO-ISOTOPE METHODS

In the CBF laboratory, the use of radioactive xenon has stood the test of time and tends to be used as the gold standard against which other methods are compared (Obrist *et al.* 1975, Matsuda *et al.* 1984). Krypton, xenon and nitrous oxide have all been used as inert gases on the basis of the so-called Kety-Schmidt (1945) principle (*i.e.* brain uptake equals arterial content minus venous content multiplied by CBF). An inert gas is not metabolised in the brain and so the total amount is constant. The technique requires an arterial sample and a venous sample from the jugular bulb. This is invasive and technically difficult, and allows total rather than regional flow, with errors due to venous admixture already described.

The use of isotopes of these inert gases is therefore an advantage in that gamma cameras can be used outside the head, without the need for jugular bulb venous sampling. Xenon 133 is a gamma-emitter with a half-life of five days. It is eliminated in the breath mostly with a single pass through the lungs (Kirsch *et al.* 1985). It is given by inhalation, intravenous or intra-arterial injection. The advent of portable gamma cameras and computerisation means that portable equipment like the Encephalotec are available for bedside intensive-care unit measurements.

There are still several disadvantages because of the radiation. Costeloe and Rolfe (1989) estimated that this is equivalent to eight chest x-rays in the newborn. One cannot get repeat measurements to see trends with changing ICP and CPP. Partition of the gas is different between grey and white matter, but particularly between normal and infarcted brain. One also has the problem of easy access to isotope when it is needed unpredictably in an emergency situation. In many of the studies of CBF in children the effects of ICP were not measured; different methods of administering the gas, different pathological conditions and widely different ages of

46

patients mean that very few studies are comparable (Lou *et al.* 1977, Greisen 1984, Ment *et al.* 1984).

Other isotope methods include iodine-labelled amphetamine (n-isopropyl-p-I 123 iodo amphetamine), but this is a research tool at present (Kuhl *et al.* 1982).

The use of isotope encephalography with the measurement of mean transit time is a method which most nuclear medicine departments could carry out on a routine basis (see Chapter 4).

NITROUS OXIDE METHOD

The use of the old nitrous oxide method of Kety and Schmidt is used occasionally during anaesthesia with neurosurgery or cardiac surgery (McHenry 1966, Kirsch 1985). It still requires someone able to perform jugular bulb sampling. Eyre (1988) is investigating this technique to see if it can be developed into a useful bedside test for children.

MERCURY STRAIN GAUGE PLETHYSMOGRAPHY

Non-invasive techniques, such as mercury strain gauge plethysmography, were restricted to very young infants (Cross *et al.* 1979, Milligan 1979). In this technique the change in head size in the infant with unfused skull sutures is measured using a mercury strain gauge around the head. The change in CBV with each systolic pulse and the cumulative effect of venous compression, can be measured. This method did give physiological data on carbon dioxide responsiveness of very small infants, and could give sequential data not available from the xenon method which would have been unethical in these infants. However, one was never sure how much blood was simply shunted into the vertebral veins, and it has now been replaced by Doppler velocitometry.

IMPEDANCE PLETHYSMOGRAPHY

Rheoencephalography or impedance plethysmography had a limited vogue for a short while in paediatrics, and it may still prove to be a useful technique. Four electrodes are placed around the head: two act as transmitters and emit a small current of 2 to 4 milliamps at high frequency (100kHz), the other two receive electrodes and allow the impedance of the head to the current to be measured. This produces a pulsatile waveform which is thought to follow stroke volume rather than the CBF or velocity (Costeloe and Rolfe 1989). Impedance falls as the blood in the head increases. It is not now used as a measure of CBF, although it does allow continuous monitoring in a non-invasive way. It warrants further comparison with the ICP trace to see if it correlates with pulse-wave artifact and can be used as a continuous non-invasive method of measuring changes in autoregulation.

DOPPLER VELOCITOMETRY

This is a method currently undergoing intense clinical assessment. It depends upon the well known Doppler principle of a change in sound-frequency from a moving object as perceived by a stationary observer. The moving object which reflects the sound is the red blood corpuscle. The change in frequency is given by twice the

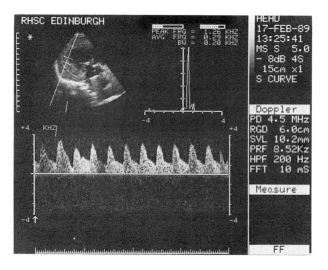

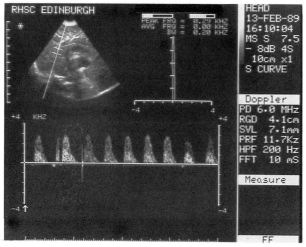

Fig. 3.5. Doppler flow studies along with Doppler imaging which allow the vessel to be identified.

transmitter frequency, multiplied by the cosine velocity of flow divided by the speed of sound. It assumes that the red cells all move at the same speed, which is not the case, as those in the centre move faster than at the edges. One also needs to know the angle of the beam to the direction of flow in the bloodvessel, as this significantly reduces the measured velocity as the probe moves away from a right-angle. One cannot measure flow without knowing the diameter of the vessel and one must be wary of equating CBF velocity directly with CBF. The correlation with xenon estimates of CBF is disappointing. Greisen (1984) compared Doppler and xenon and found a correlation of 0.56; in dogs and pigs, using the Pourcelot index, the correlation to CBF was 0.424 (Bishop *et al.* 1986). Several hardware improvements and changes in technique and measurement calculation have been introduced.

One can use two crystals in the probe: one for transmission and the other as a receiver so that continuous Doppler measurements of frequency change only are possible. If one crystal is used with a pulsed soundwave, then by measuring time delay as well as frequency change, the distance can be measured and so the depth of the vessel being monitored. In the case of large vessels, the diameter of the vessel can also be measured. Combining Doppler with ultrasound imaging allows greater accuracy in determining which particular vessel is being measured (Fig. 3.5). The display can be made on a colorscan, and the use of sonic contrast injections may help.

Some form of fixation is desirable so that one always hits the same vessel from the same angle in order to enable sequential studies (*e.g.* when removing CSF, reducing carbon dioxide, using mannitol, or changing systemic blood pressure). The greatest difficulty is in knowing how to analyse and measure the waveform. There are several possibilities: (i) maximum systolic or diastolic velocity, (ii) peak systolic velocity—peak diastolic velocity/systolic, (iii) the Pourcelot index, *i.e.* peak systolic frequency—diastolic frequency/mean, or (iv) the area under the curve. There are specific abnormalities which are very helpful such as cessation of diastolic flow or reversal of diastolic flow (Perlman *et al.* 1981). Reversal of flow during diastole is more often seen when there is a low diastolic pressure associated with a wide pulse pressure due to an 'aortic run-off' from a patent ductus arteriosus, aortic incompetence or peripheral vasodilatation. It also occurs when cerebral vascular resistance is very high as in sludging of the microcirculation in necrotic brain. Cessation of diastolic flow is likely when ICP rises to near diastolic blood pressure in the cerebral arterioles, and it may be the first indication of impaired CBF even if one cannot measure an absolute flow. It can therefore help in deciding when one should proceed to the more invasive measurement of ICP. There appears to be a good correlation between Doppler velocitometry and CO_2 response, *i.e.* vascular reactivity. The use of Doppler through the fontanelle in the newborn, pulsed Doppler through the squamous temporal in older children and large neck-vessel studies in stroke have established Doppler as a useful method of looking at the cerebral circulation (Kirkham *et al.* 1986, Rennie *et al.* 1987). It is safe, repeatable and without radiation risk, and is likely to remain the only practical bedside tool for studying the cerebral circulation for the foreseeable future (Batton *et al.* 1983, Hansen *et al.* 1983, Bode and Wais 1988, Levene *et al.* 1988, Costeloe and Rolfe 1989).

MISCELLANEOUS METHODS

PET scans allow regional metabolism and bloodflow to be studied. This has shown that in epilepsy there may be an increase in bloodflow during the fit but a cold underperfused area between fits. Even seizures thought to be due to diffuse brain disease such as infantile spasms can be shown to have regional cold areas which are amenable to surgery and result in an improvement in seizure control. PET scanning is certainly the most dramatic way of demonstrating infarction and the local results of cerebral ischaemia. Since proximity to a cyclotron is needed it is likely that it will remain a research tool to enable us to understand pathology and pathophysiology.

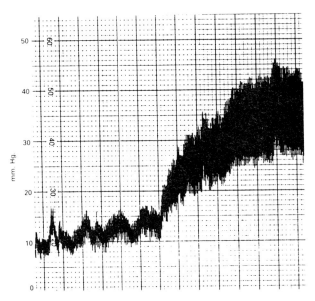

Fig. 3.6. Plateau wave. Note the tremendous increase in the size of the pulse-wave artifact as the pressure rises so that it is difficult to work out a mean.

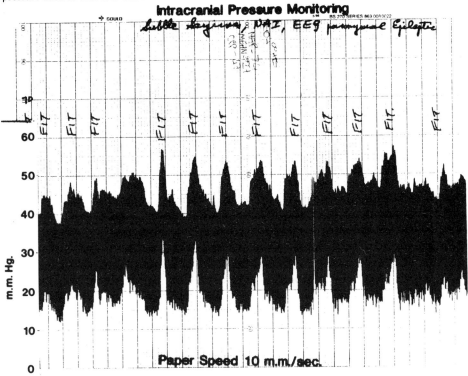

Fig. 3.7. Very wide pulse amplitude due to failure of autoregulation together with a saw-tooth effect as the child has changes in CBF associated with a fit.

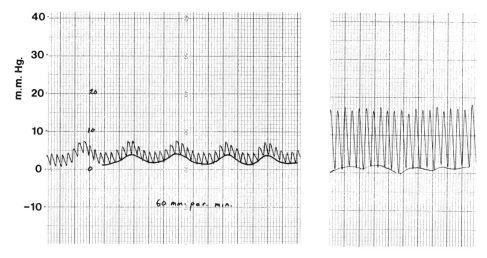

PAPER SPEED 60 MM./MIN.

Fig. 3.8. Pulse-wave artifact and respiratory artifact on a normal ICP trace at normal ICP, run at a fast paper speed of 60mm/minute. The second part of the trace shows the pulse-wave artifact grossly increased to 15mmHg.

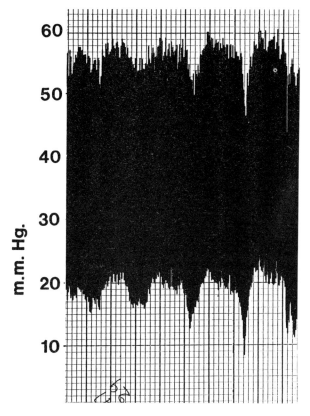

Fig. 3.9. Total loss of autoregulation with pulse-wave artifact of 35mmHg.

The advent of 'the poor man's PET' (*i.e.* SPECT) is more likely to become available for routine clinical use.

SPECT using I^{123} amphetamine shows good regional bloodflow, including increase in flow with epileptic foci as shown on EEG (Hill *et al.* 1982). Nuclear magnetic resonance (NMR) imaging is another method which is being investigated to study bloodflow; at present it seems likely to be more useful for observing water molecules within the brain in cerebral oedema, hydrocephalus and CSF production (Singer and Crooks 1983).

ICP WAVEFORM ANALYSIS

Analysis of the waveforms on the ICP trace is widely used (Lundberg 1960, Bruce *et al.* 1977). The normal ICP trace is discussed in Chapter 7. It can be regarded as showing three main groups of waveforms: baseline pressure, physiological waves and pathological waveforms.

The baseline pressure is usually easy to see when the pressure is low and the pulse pressure wave of low amplitude (Fig. 3.6). If the pulse amplitude is high, even though the pressure may be normal, it is difficult to work out the mean pressure simply by inspecting the trace (Fig. 3.7) and a computerised system is then essential.

The physiological waveforms are those associated with either a change in arterial pressure or a change in central venous pressure. The change in arterial pressure between systolic and diastolic shows as the pulse-wave artifact (Fig. 3.8). Because of autoregulation this is damped to represent normally a swing in ICP of only about 2 or 3mmHg. If autoregulation is lost, the normal brain pulsation increases as felt through the fontanelle; and the pulse-wave pressure on the ICP trace gets bigger and eventually may be the same as the systolic/diastolic pressure difference, *i.e.* more than 40mmHg (Fig. 3.9). The same type of increase in amplitude in pulse waveform is seen when there is severely reduced compliance so that a small increase in intracranial blood volume makes a large difference to the pressure. It may be difficult to know if an increase in amplitude of the pulse waveform is due to reduced compliance or loss of autoregulation. Technically one can test compliance by changing intracranial volume either by injecting fluid into the ventricle or removing a known amount in aliquots and observing the pressure change. In the same way raising or lowering the blood pressure and observing the difference in ICP and pulse-wave amplitude would tell us about autoregulation. These techniques can be used occasionally, for instance with hydrocephalus with a ventriculostomy reservoir or for the child on blood-pressure support with dopamine. If the amplitude of the pulse waveform is reduced or there is a smooth line with no pulse-wave artifact, the first consideration must be to exclude a mechanical fault with the catheter or the transducer causing a dampening of the signal. It is however of very low amplitude in the preterm infant or in severe hydrocephalus, as well as in brains with a low flow as in severe atrophy in a persistent vegetative state.

Respiration causes changes in central venous pressure and these are also reflected on the normal trace as a slower and lower amplitude fluctuation of the baseline than the pulse-wave artifact. In pathological states the venous swings may

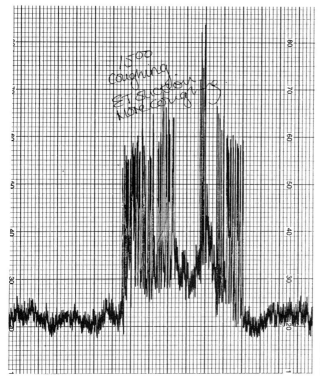

Fig. 3.10. Effect of coughing and suction on the endotracheal tube upon ICP.

lessen and the arterial increase so that the p / r ratio increases (Miller 1988). Other physiological waves are usually also due to rises in venous pressure such as coughing, straining at stool, crying and Valsalva manoeuvres (Fig. 3.10). Crying or nasopharyngeal suction may cause very high plateaus of ICP (around 88mmHg), with only a slow return to baseline if the child has poor compliance.

A particularly useful physiological variable is the increase in CBF that occurs in REM sleep, as this is a natural model for increasing CBF and CBV in order to examine the compliance. If there is adequate reserve the extra CBV can be accommodated without a rise in pressure. If compliance is compromised a very high rise in ICP can then occur with each phase of REM sleep (Rahilly 1980). It is for this reason that we usually monitor ICP in children through at least two phases of REM sleep. The situation can be mimicked by a ketamine compliance test when the effects of a small dose of intravenous ketamine on ICP is monitored. This should only be used if immediate measures to relieve ICP are available (*e.g.* by aspiration of CSF from a ventriculostomy reservoir) since otherwise the rise in ICP is uncontrollable and may reach very high levels.

The pathological waveforms are of two types: either abnormalities of the physiological waveforms, or additional waves or plateaus known as A waves, B waves (ramp and sinusoidal), C waves and tonic D waves.

The pathological ICP waves are not seen in the normal child. A waves are

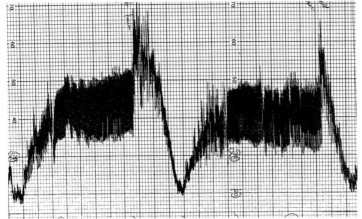

Fig. 3.11. Plateau wave of over 40mmHg.

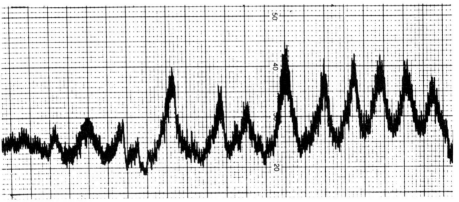

Fig. 3.12. *Above:* typical saw-tooth B waves. *Below:* small B waves superimposed on the trace which gradually increase in amplitude to produce a plateau of longer duration due to poor compliance in a child with hydrocephalus.

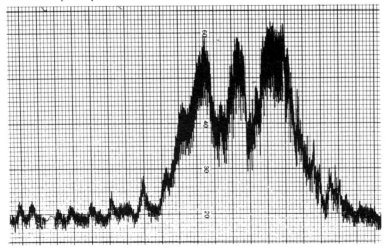

54

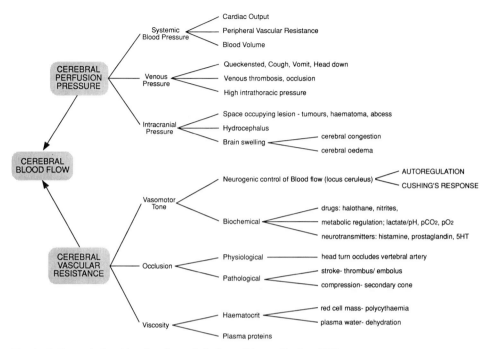

Fig. 3.13. Interrelationship of various clinical conditions affecting CBF.

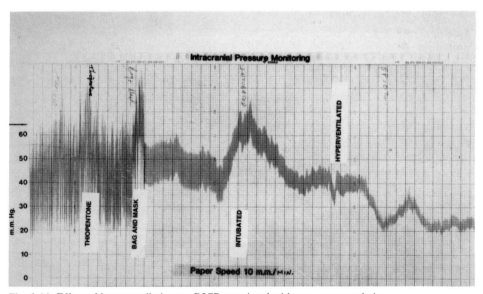

Fig. 3.14. Effect of hyperventilation on RICP associated with poor autoregulation.

synonymous with plateau waves of Lundberg plateaus: they are of high amplitude (50 to 100mmHg) and of long duration (between five and 20 minutes). They represent autoregulation failure with an increase in CBV (*i.e.* cerebral congestion). The excessive rise in pressure encourages further coning, and a vicious circle of progressive deterioration (Fig. 3.11).

B waves are of shorter duration (0.5 to two per minute) and from the normal pressure range to 50mmHg (*i.e.* of lower amplitude than A waves). They relate to brainstem failure and periodic respiration, and are abolished by paralysis and artificial ventilation but do not correlate directly with a rise in the carbon dioxide level in plasma. They appear as the common saw-tooth waves (Fig. 3.12).

C waves are faster waves occurring about six per minute (range four to eight) and to not more than 20mmHg in amplitude. They are thought to represent an exaggeration of a normal cycling of systemic blood pressure (the so-called Traub–Herring–Meyer waves). They can be very marked in the raised pressure associated with meningitis.

EEG and evoked-response studies only demonstrate damage once it has occurred and are too indirect for routine use when monitoring is aimed at identifying impaired cerebral perfusion whilst it is still treatable and before the vicious cycle outlined above is entered (Goitein *et al.* 1983).

Abnormal CBF
The pathological factors which can cause a reduction in CBF are shown diagrammatically in Figure 3.13.

CARBON DIOXIDE
The single most potent effect on CBF is a rise in the plasma carbon dioxide level (Shalit *et al.* 1967), when it stimulates marked hyperventilation not only in the normal brain; for every rise in PCO_2 of 1 kilopascal the CBF rises by 15ml per 100g tissue. Hypercapnia interferes with the normal autoregulation in response to a change in systemic blood pressure and so makes the situation worse by overriding the compensatory mechanism (Miller 1975). Respiratory failure with a rise in PCO_2 will therefore increase CBF, increase CBV, cause cerebral congestion and raise ICP. Any rise in ICP will also cause central neurogenic hyperventilation to lower the PCO_2 and by an inborn compensatory mechanism bring down the ICP. In many children with acute encephalopathies the PCO_2 is already less than 4.0kPa when first seen, *i.e.* the correct level (3.5 to 4.0kPa) when initiating intermittent positive pressure ventilation (IPPV) (Fig. 3.14). There is still debate as to whether megaventilation in order to reduce the PCO_2 to 2.0kPa or less reduces CBF sufficiently to cause ischaemia, so defeating the purpose for trying to reduce ICP pressure using hyperventilation (Bruce 1984). It is in this area where most clinical difficulty arises: a rise in PCO_2 may cause a rise in ICP, but lowering it may reduce CBF. We need to adjust ICP and CO_2 to achieve optimal bloodflow for the brain's immediate metabolic needs, and so it is here that bedside methods of measuring sequential or continuous CBF are most needed.

If the PCO_2 is lowered too rapidly, wide swings in CSF pH may cause a Posner encephalopathy and precipitate severe inappropriate ADH secretion. The Cushing response, inappropriate ADH and hyperventilation are compensatory mechanisms the brain possesses to try and maintain its perfusion and lessen ICP.

HYPOXIA

Severe hypoxia causes a serious fall in CBF with loss of autoregulation and the risk of hydrostatic and vasogenic oedema as well as intracellular oedema (see Chapter 2) (Lou *et al*. 1977). Moderate hypoxia does not have the same marked effect on CBF as hypercapnia, so a fall in PO_2 from 12.7 to 8kPa results in little change in CBF, while severe hypoxia (*e.g.* a drop from 8 to 4kPa) will double CBF, probably due to tissue hypoxia and liberation of lactate rather than a chemoreceptor effect on the locus ceruleus (Lassen 1968). Severe hypoxic/ischaemic encephalopathy is seen in children from 'extrinsic' cerebral causes in perinatal asphyxia, prolonged status epilepticus, near-miss cot-death, drowning, poisoning, cardiac arrest or post-cardiac bypass surgery. Pathological evidence of hypoxic ischaemic damage is found as the predominant finding in most children dying of head injury, Reye's syndrome, meningitis or other metabolic encephalopathies due to 'intrinsic' failure of cerebral perfusion (most commonly the result of RICP). Following an extrinsic or extracerebral hypoxic/ischaemic cause there is loss of autoregulation which may last several days, with a fall in cerebral perfusion which can last much longer than the acute episode. In cases of severe systemic hypotension, such as cardiac arrest, cerebral oedema is probably not as important a cause of secondary brain damage as autoregulatory failure and direct neuronal death, and ICP is very often normal. Post-asphyxial rigidity is often thought wrongly to be decerebration due to a midbrain herniation from pressure. CBF may increase in the early stages as the vessels open from loss of autoregulation, especially in white matter. Perinatal asphyxia has been much more thoroughly studied than other types of hypoxic ischaemic encephalopathy and demonstrates the loss of autoregulation, loss of carbon dioxide reactivity, lowered CBF, initial raised white-matter flow, decreased white-matter flow in periventricular leukomalacia, and extensive ischaemic infarction in subependymal haemorrhage (Hill and Volpe 1982; Volpe *et al*. 1982, 1983; Levene *et al*. 1988; Costeloe and Rolfe 1989).

FITS

CBF is markedly increased in children during seizures, often by several hundred per cent. As already described, in the interictal period there may be cold areas of hypometabolism and hypoperfusion. Changes in bloodflow during seizures can be shown by xenon, Doppler, and PET scan (Shimizu *et al*. 1983). There is again a need for sequential studies in children with status epilepticus to see if the brain damage causing mesial temporal sclerosis or hemiplegia is related to a mismatch between bloodflow and metabolism.

HEAD INJURY

RICP due to an intracranial haematoma or cerebral oedema may impair cerebral perfusion causing secondary cerebral infarction, *i.e.* the so-called secondary injury.

The management of head injury in intensive care can do little to diminish the effects of the primary injury, but children may show a good recovery if secondary anoxic ischaemic damage can be prevented (Graham *et al.* 1989). In children with head injuries, however, a different mechanism also occurs: an increase in bloodflow through the cerebral white matter causing cerebral congestion. This may be associated initially with a 50 per cent rise in CBF (Obrist *et al.* 1983). The CBF may therefore be increased, normal or seriously diminished in children with head injuries, and the management will vary with the pattern, so again a bedside method of sequential bloodflow measurement would be invaluable. At present a single reading from the Encephalotec or Doppler flow studies are all most centres can use.

DRUGS

Drugs such as ketamine also increase CBF by some 60 per cent. If compliance is critical then both natural and induced sleep may be associated with a dramatic rise in ICP which can cause apnoea or a serious deterioration in the patient's condition. Ketamine should not be used as an anaesthetic agent for medical procedures if there is any possibility of RICP.

Anaesthetic agents such as halothane will also cause cerebral vasodilatation and an increase in CBF, which can be a great nuisance to the neurosurgeon by causing a tight swollen brain. It can also decompensate a child with critical compliance (*e.g.* having a shunt changed for hydrocephalus) when, if CSF has not been removed from a ventriculostomy reservoir prior to surgery, the use of wrong anaesthetic technique may result in a blind child post-operatively. Halothane should not be used in order to view the fundi of a difficult child.

If nitroprusside is used to 'open' the peripheral circulation and allow volume expansion (*e.g.* in septic shock)it may also cause paralysis of cerebral autoregulation and the rise in systemic blood pressure can be associated with a marked rise in ICP. Unless one can measure CBF, one does not know whether the impairment of CPP from the rise in ICP is more than offset by improved perfusion. In most situations it is a fall in CBF which is the main concern as a cause of death or disability from brain infarction. Even if cerebral perfusion is maintained, a rise in ICP may still cause shifts and cones with progressive brainstem failure, secondary ischaemia from compression of vessels, and death.

Most children who die of an acute encephalopathy do so because of the brain infarction, and hypoxic ischaemic damage overshadows the initial pathology.

Cerebral infarction from impaired perfusion

There may be infarction as a result of interference with CBF from RICP, due to vessel compression from shifts and cones, due to vessel occlusion (arterial or venous) or secondary to systemic hypotension. In experimental animals and humans, infarction has been shown to occur when the CPP falls below 20mmHg (Jones *et al.* 1981, Raju *et al.* 1981). Ischaemia is divided into phases by neuropathologists:

In *phase 1*, the mitochondria in neurons swell, the brain swells as astrocytes and neurons swell from water retention (cystostatic oedema). The anoxic neurons rapidly release potassium which is mopped up by the astrocytes. This may also alter the osmolality of the cytoplasm, causing swelling (Fujimoto *et al.* 1976).

In *phase 2*, the endothelial cells leak and allow protein to escape into the extracellular space and in severe cases allow blood into the tissues (*i.e.* a haemorrhagic infarct). In these cases the plasma escapes as extracellular brain lymph and the red cells become packed, crenated and break down causing iron and bilirubin to be formed in the tissues. This ferruginisation is used to date the infarct. The leakage of protein into the infarct can last 10 days so that radioactive technetium is taken up by a relatively old infarct.

Phase 3 is characterised by death of cells in the infarcted area with lysosomal rupture: resulting in breakdown of tissue proteins with swelling of the infarct, breakdown of blood brain barrier, loss of autoregulation, sludging of the microcirculation and liquefaction of tissues. The swelling of astrocytes and endothelial cells compresses the capillaries, and electron microscopy shows the erythrocytes to be stuck. In experimental head injury, haemodilution to prevent microcirculatory sludging lessens the degree of brain damage. It is thought that mannitol may also act in this way. A further cause of sludging is due to release of thromboplastic substances (which can be measured in the CSF). The resulting necrotic tissue may then be absorbed by macrophages to leave a cyst, as in periventricular cystic leukomalacia, or one large porencephalic cyst. In other cases an astrocyte reaction gradually replaces the dead tissue with a glial scar. Capillaries proliferate and new ones grow into the damaged area.

The actual site of infarction is determined by several factors, since a fall in blood pressure does not result in uniform infarction of the whole brain (Bruce *et al.* 1973). Basal ganglia may catch the brunt on one side and cortical grey matter on the other; leg area may be more affected than arm. The circle of Willis, with a supply system of four arteries, means that there must be areas where the pressures even out, or there would be retrograde flow. These areas of no flow mean that one may see a pattern of predominant middle cerebral artery infarction from a general drop in perfusion pressure. The difference between centrifugal and centripetal flow in the neonate has been discussed as the basis for periventricular leukomalacia. The same applies to the separation of the carotid circulation by the posterior cerebral becoming more basilar-artery dependent. The area between major vascular territories is very susceptible, since the cerebral arterioles are end arteries and do not anastomose; therefore the area between anterior and middle (*i.e.* the leg area of the motor strip) can be selectively infarcted, as may be the parietal watershed, or alternatively selective infarction of the basilar territory. This is in addition to the selective vascular occlusion due to a cone (discussed in the next section).

Certain parts of the brain are more susceptible than others to anoxia such as the hippocampus, basal ganglia and cerebellar Purkinje cells and can be selectively damaged. Jennett and Teasdale (1981) showed that in head injuries there was hypoxic ischaemic damage to these selective areas as well as watershed zone infarction *e.g.* hippocampus 81 per cent, basal ganglia 79 per cent, cerebral cortex 46 per cent and cerebellum 44 per cent.

There is much interest in the actual cellular mechanisms whereby ischaemia causes cell damage and death (Table 3.II), *i.e.* whether due to free radicles (Fong *et*

TABLE 3.II

Mechanisms of anoxic brain damage

Consumptive asphyxia (demand outstrips supply energy)
Excitotoxicity (glutamate stimulation of cell beyond energy supply)
Substrate failure (hypoglycaemia, failure of ketone production)
Intracellular acidosis (aggravated by excess substrate supply *e.g.* glucose)
ATP depletion
Rupture of lysosomes (cell suicide)
Calcium invasion with cytotoxicity
Release of S-S/S-H groups
Free radical toxicity (*e.g.* epoxides)
Failure of microcirculation from thromboplastin release
Osmotic disruption—release of idiogenic osmols and failure to excrete metabolic water

al. 1973), entry of calcium ions into the cell, lysosomal rupture or simply loss of energy (*i.e.* ATP). Nuclear magnetic spectroscopy shows that creatine phosphate falls and inorganic phosphate rises, but the cells appear to retain some ATP to the end (Cady *et al.* 1983). This has led to the use of calcium antagonists and free radicle scavengers (mannitol, vitamin E and vitamin C) in order to try and limit the extent of the ischaemic damage. It is also the logic of using haemodilution and aspirin to prevent sludging or phenobarbitone to lessen the cells' energy needs.

Another cause of cell disruption could be severe intracellular acidosis (Rehncrona *et al.* 1980). It used to be thought that the intracellular enzymes could not function at pH below 6.7, and that metabolism would grind to a halt. The use of nuclear magnetic spectroscopy of muscle suggests that degrees of intracellular acidosis may be much more severe than thought possible. The argument as to the use of THAM to correct intracellular acidosis is not answered.

s-s or disulphide groups are thought to damage cell membrane whilst s-H (*i.e.* sulphydryl groups) stabilise—hence the theoretical use of glutathione to stabilise the cell membranes. It is also thought that certain neurotransmitters such as glutamate could stimulate the cell beyond the point that it can sustain increased electrical activity by increased metabolism, *i.e.* excitotoxicity (Meldrum 1985, Rothman and Olney 1986).

RICP with shifts and cones

The rise in pressure as a result of oedema, congestion, space occupation or hydrocephalus need not be generalised but may occur in one intracranial compartment more than another. This is obvious with a tumour, clot or abscess: an infarct will be focal, oedema may be around a tumour or infarct, one ventricle may be involved in hydrocephalus so that pressure gradients develop:

(1) between right and left supratentorial compartments across the falx
(2) between both supratentorial compartments and the posterior fossa
(3) between the posterior fossa and the supratentorial compartments (upward shift and cone), or
(4) between posterior fossa and spinal cord across the foramen magnum.

The pressure gradient need only be a few mmHg to cause a shift and cone. In

TABLE 3.III

Signs of tentorial herniation

Sunset sign, loss of upward conjugate deviation
Sixth-nerve weakness
Dilatation ipsilateral pupil
Coma
Tonic fits
Doggy paddling arms, cycling legs
Decerebrate rigidity
Hypertension
Bradycardia
Central neurogenic hyperventilation
Ipsilateral hemiplegia
Calcarine infarction—blindness
Hemianopia
Fixed dilated pupils—bilateral

chronic conditions such as chronic subdural haematoma one can have marked but gradual shifts to accommodate the extra volume without the need for severe intracranial hypertension. If the ICP rises acutely and to a high level then impaction is likely, with resultant necrosis (*i.e.* impaction of the brain either under the free edge of the falx or into the tentorial orifice or foramen magnum). The impaction causes local ischaemia and necrosis, but also vascular compression with the possibility of more distant infarction (Meyer 1920).

Supratentorial shift
If the pressure is different between the right and left supratentorial compartments, then one hemisphere tries to migrate to the other side under the free edge of the falx. This causes impaction of the cingulate gyrus which is infarcted (supracallosal hernia), but also may entrap one of the branches of the anterior cerebral, causing infarction in the corresponding leg area. The inferior sagittal sinus is also involved in the compression. The increase in pressure bows the falx, and is seen as a shift of the midline on scan or ultrasound.

Tentorial herniation
A rise in supratentorial pressure more often causes a tentorial herniation (Johnson and Yates 1956*a,b*). The diencephalon moves backwards, stretching and twisting the gyrus rectus, and putting traction on the optic nerves with descent downwards of the brainstem. The cerebral hemispheres move back along the tentorial shelf impacting against the dorsal midbrain and compressing the superior colliculus. The medial temporal lobe is squashed down through the tentorial orifice which causes a deep notch on the parahippocampal gyrus, often with necrosis (Kernohan and Woltman 1929). The brainstem is compressed from side to side and distorted, as well as having its vascular supply impaired. This causes ischaemia of the brainstem with secondary haemorrhagic infarction. Nerves such as the sixth and third are compressed, as are vessels such as the posterior cerebral which passes through the tentorial orifice.

TABLE 3.IV

Eye signs in RICP

Sunset sign
Loss of upward conjugate deviation
Sixth-nerve weakness
Ptosis
Third-nerve palsy
Hippus (unilateral optic nerve traction)
Hemianopia (unilateral calcarine ischaemia)
Papilloedema or venous distension
Optic atrophy
Pinpoint pupils
Hutchinson's pupils
Blindness from calcarine ischaemia
Bitemporal hemianopia, hernia of third ventricle
Watershed of optic radiation
Balint's syndrome
Nystagmus

Many of the signs which we see in RICP are the result of tentorial herniation and most of the monitoring and observation in acute encephalopathy is aimed at detecting these at an early stage in order to relieve ICP (Table 3.III) (Horwitz *et al.* 1980, Minns *et al.* 1989).

EYE SIGNS

The various eye signs are listed in Table 3.IV. As the pressure causes local compression of the superior colliculus, there is loss of upward conjugate deviation (a well known sign of pressure in this area in Parinaud's syndrome from a pinealoma but also in chronic subdural haematoma). The common sunsetting sign—downward deviation of the eyes—is really paralysis of conjugate upward gaze.

Compression of the sixth nerve causes a squint with loss of abduction of the eye. Third-nerve palsies may be partial, with the child simply presenting with a ptosis. Compression of the third nerve may involve its peripheral part or the oculomotor centre in the periaqueductal grey matter, in which case it is a sign of impending fatal brainstem compression. Isolated third-nerve palsies may occur after recovery from head injury due to compression of the nerve in its extracerebral course. Pupil changes, apart from the dilatation of the ipsilateral pupil as part of the classical Hutchinson's pupil signs of pressure, may also consist of hippus or—as brainstem failure progresses—pinpoint pupils of pontine failure and the cadaveric denervated pupil of severe brainstem failure (midpoint and unreactive to light, accommodation or pain).

Blindness may arise secondary to papilloedema. Papilloedema is a late sign in acute encephalopathies and absent more often than present. Normal fundi do not exclude very severe intracranial hypertension. Blindness can also arise due to optic-nerve traction, infarction of the optic radiation in periventricular leukomalacia. Balint's syndrome of visual agnosia arises if there is infarction of the watershed area

TABLE 3.V

TABLE 3.V

Acute motor signs in RICP

Ipsilateral hemiplegia
Doggy paddling arms, cycling legs
Tonic fits (intermittent decerebration)
Decerebrate rigidity
Decorticate postures
Midbrain flexor rigidity
Hypotonia
Erb's palsy
Spinal flexion with uninhibited flexor withdrawal
Return of primitive reflexes (such as ATNR)

between middle and posterior cerebral artery territories. A hemianopia results if one posterior cerebral artery is compressed, but more often it is bilateral with severe calcarine infarction. This is the most feared complication in children with acute pressure, as total and irrecoverable blindness may result. Optic atrophy may be seen in children who survive episodes of severe RICP, even if they have never exhibited any papilloedema. Distension of the retinal veins due to the draining of intracranial blood into extracranial veins, together with pulsation of the veins which ceases when ICP reaches 15mmHg, are more common signs in children with RICP as papilloedema is often absent in the acute situation. Absence of papilloedema does not mean that it is safe to perform a lumbar puncture. The visual-evoked response is distorted or disappears in RICP, returning to normal after reduction of the pressure.

MOTOR SIGNS (Table 3.V)
Compression of the cerebral peduncle causes a hemiplegia and since this is prior to decussation of the pyramids in the medulla it can be ipsilateral or contralateral to the mass lesion in one hemisphere. If it is ipsilateral, as is often the case, then it can act as a false localising sign by making one think that the lesion is in the opposite hemisphere. The sixth nerve winds around the peduncle, and so a corresponding loss of abduction of the eye may also act as a false localising sign.

As the midbrain is compressed the child begins to show extensor hypertonus at first in the legs; the arms start to 'doggy paddle' and the legs to cycle (Fig. 3.15). This causes a true localising sign (*e.g.* a hemplegia in a child with an extradural haematoma) to disappear and be replaced by doggy paddling. Adult-orientated neurosurgeons may feel that these are now normal movements and indicate no focal mass lesion.

As midbrain compression continues there are episodes of sudden opisthotonus, often thought to be epileptic fits: but these 'tonic fits', 'brainstem fits' or 'cerebellar fits' are due not to a cerebral arrhythmia, but to release of the medullary reticular nuclei, and lead eventually to true decerebrate rigidity (more correctly decerebrate spasticity). Table 3.VI shows the spectrum of diseases which can present as decerebration in children.

There may be unilateral decerebrate postures with a hemiplegic (decorticate)

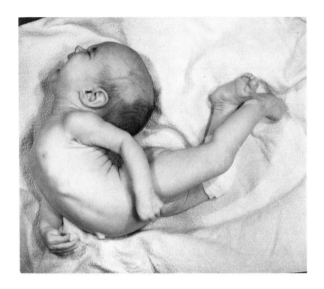

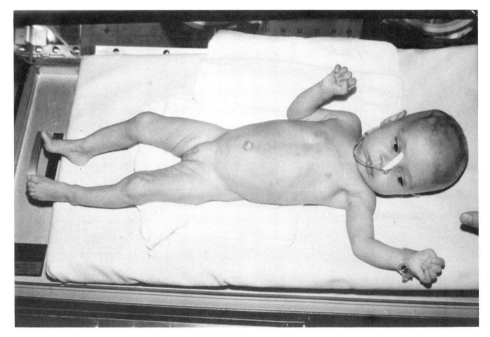

Fig. 3.15. *Left:* gross neck retraction associated with RICP. *Below:* child is immobile extended with return of the asymmetrical tonic neck reflex and some doggy paddling of the upper limbs.

posture on the opposite side. Should brainstem compression and failure progress then sudden hypotonia, spinal flexion or even an Erb's palsy may develop.

CONSCIOUS LEVEL

Consciousness depends upon the reticular system arousing the cerebral cortex and is what we mean by level of arousal, vigilance or awareness. Only the person

TABLE 3.VI
Aetiology of decerebrate rigidity in 64 children

	Cases (N)
Intracranial haemorrhage (30%)	
Subdural haemorrhage—battered baby	5
—other causes	5
Intraventricular haemorrhage	6
Arteriovenous malformation	1
Other	2
Infection (30%)	
Meningitis	8
Encephalitis	6
Abscess	1
Cortical thrombophlebitis	1*
Septicaemia (with intravascular coagulation)	2
Fatty liver encephalopathy	1
Hypoxia (18%)	
Cardiac arrest (anaesthetic)	3
Neonatal hypoxia	6
Drowning	1
Post convulsion	2
Metabolic (14%)	
Hypernatraemic dehydration (gastro-enteritis)	3
Alkalotic tetany	2
Kernicterus	1
Burns encephalopathy	2
Water intoxication (transfusion)	1
Other (8%)	
Birth trauma	3
Congenital malformation	1
Sagittal sinus injury	1

*Plus two in meningitic group.
(After Brown *et al.* 1973.)

involved knows if s/he is conscious. To an observer the response to a verbal command or visual or tactile stimulus is interpreted as showing conscious behaviour. If we paralyse all behavioural responses as with a muscle relaxant, one does not know if the patient is conscious or not—as shown by the increasing number of people claiming to be awake during surgical operations.

It may be that the neonate has no stored memories, or that they have been destroyed by extensive cortical damage, so that there is no content to consciousness (*i.e.* no thought or understanding—a persistent vegetative state). Loss of behavioural response to a stimulus (*e.g.* eye opening, tactile localisation and speech) also occurs in akinetic mutism. One may wrongly assume a person to be still in coma when in reality he is fully conscious and aware.

The child will lose consciousness as midbrain compression progresses, reducing reticular arousal of the cerebral cortex. If this is lost permanently we say that the person is brain-dead. The child becomes irritable and drowsy, able to be aroused but not recognising where s/he is, gradually responding to pain by purposeful movements and subsequently only by decerebrate movements. This is

TABLE 3.VII

Glasgow coma scale

	N
Eye opening	
Spontaneous	4
To speech	3
To pain	2
Nil	1
Best motor response	
Obeys	6
Localises	5
Withdraws	4
Abnormal flexion	3
Extensor response	2
Nil	1
Verbal response	
Orientated	5
Confused speech	4
Inappropriate words	3
Inappropriate sounds	2
Nil	1

Score is 3 to 15.
(After Teasdale and Jennett 1974.)

TABLE 3.VIII

Glasgow coma scale—modified children's coma scale

Eye opening	
Spontaneous	4
Reaction to speech	3
Reaction to pain	2
No response	1
Best motor response	
Obeys verbal command	6
Localises painful stimulus	5
Withdraws from pain	4
Abnormal flexion (decorticate response)	3
Extensor response (decerebrate response)	2
No response to painful stimulus	1
Verbal response	
Orientated, smiles, interacts	5
Consolable if crying, interacts inappropriately	4
Inconsistently consolable, moaning only interaction	3
Inconsolable, irritable, restless	2
No crying, no interaction	1

Score is 3 to 15.
(After Hahn *et al.* 1988.)

TABLE 3.IX

Aetiology of coma in 75 children

Aetiology	N	%
Intracranial infection	26	34.7
Meningitis 14		
Encephalitis 12		
Septicaemia	3	4.0
Gram-negative 2		
Pneumococcal 1		
Anoxia diffuse ischaemia	18	24.0
Cardiorespiratory arrest 15		
Operative, postoperative hypotension 3		
Primary epilepsy	11	14.7
'Metabolic'	11	14.7
Gastro-enteritis 4		
Poisoning 4		
Hepatic 3		
Intracranial vascular lesions	3	4.0
Middle cerebral artery occulsion 1		
Cortical venous thrombophlebitis 1		
Intraventricular haemorrhage 1		
Non-accidental injury	2	2.6
Histiocytosis	1	1.3
Totals	75	100.0

(From Seshia *et al.* 1977.)

the basis of the Glasgow coma scale (Table 3.VII). It does not measure coma as defined in terms of conscious awareness, but is a very useful clinical tool to assess deterioration or improvement by a limited standardised examination which is not too dependent on observer error, as occurred with the previous terminology ('drowsy', 'stupor' and 'coma'). It cannot be used in small children when the modified score (Table 3.VIII) is used.

Children with midbrain herniation often become mute and may even become mute in cerebellar disease. The differentiation of brainstem mutism from a cortical aphasia is often impossible. Recovery of speech may be extremely rapid from nothing to normal in a few days in mutism. The child with an aphasia is likely to remain with speech, reading and writing disorders in the long term.

The reappearance of sleep-wake cycles is the best guide as to when a child emerges from coma into akinetic mutism, decorticate mute (aphasic) or persistent vegetative state. Presentation of acute encephalopathies with coma shows the same disease spectrum as those presenting with decrebrate rigidity (Table 3.IX).

Coma due to RICP will nearly always be accompanied by other signs, especially ocular, of midbrain compression. The child who presents in coma with normal reacting pupils and eye movements should be suspected of poisoning or metabolic disease.

Coma due to anoxic ischaemic encephalopathy does not show any correlation between level of consciousness and ICP, nor does the outcome bear any relationship to ICP as the damage is parenchymatous and not just a result of ICP. The level of ICP is important, however, in determining the prognosis in cases of Reye's syndrome, hydrocephalus and head injury, and to a large extent in meningitis and possibly status epilepticus.

It is important to differentiate coma due to ICP from that due to toxic or anoxic causes (Seshia *et al.* 1983).

DISORDERS OF HOMEOSTASIS
Midbrain compression is usually accompanied by hypertension and bradycardia with a respiratory arrhythmia of tachypnoea or periodic (Cheyne–Stokes) respiration type (see below).

Foramen magnum impaction
Pressure exerted on the midbrain causes secondary compression of vessels supplying the central portions of the pons. The descent of the brainstem and pressure on the cerebellum transmits the pressure to the foramen magnum (Fig. 3.15). If an injudicious lumbar puncture (LP) is performed (Brown 1976, Addy 1987), then although only a few drops are removed, a large quantity of CSF continues to leak into the epidural space (Slack 1980). If contrast medium is placed in the theca at LP it can be shown to leak extradurally and along the course of the intercostal nerves. The puncture therefore not only lowers pressure, and so produces a pressure gradient between posterior fossa and spinal theca, but by removing CSF creates space for further downward herniation of intracranial contents. The cerebellar tonsils herniate posteriorly as far as c6 or 7, they become

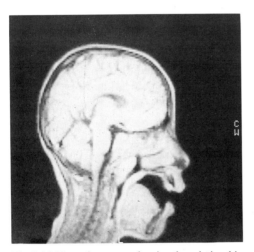

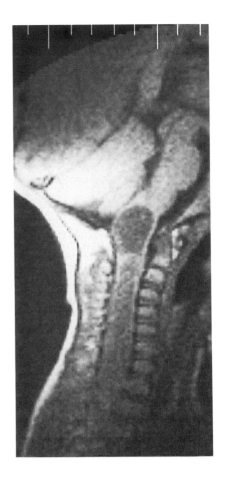

Fig. 3.16. Normal anatomy showing the relationship between the medulla and the cerebellar tonsil; the MRI scan on the right shows expansion of the cervical medullary junction with space occupation at the foramen magnum.

impacted in the foramen magnum, they become necrotic and break off, and may descend into the lumbar theca so that Purkinje cells can be seen in lumbar CSF and pieces of cerebellum seen through the meninges in the lumbar region at post-mortem examination. The descent pulls down the vertebral arteries and may cause spinal ischaemia, resulting in an acute Erb's palsy. The posterior inferior cerebellar arteries are compressed with resultant cerebellar infarction. The medulla descends and is compressed. It is not surprising, therefore, that after establishment of RICP with unrelieved tentorial herniation, the picture becomes dominated by progressive brainstem failure leading eventually to the brain-death syndrome.

Prior to considering progressive brainstem failure, it is useful to summarise how shifts and cones have added to the pathology of infarction and hypoxia:

Loss of cerebral perfusion
1. Total brain ischaemia
2. Centrifugal/centripetal failure (periventricular leukomalacia)

TABLE 3.X

Brainstem failure (vegetative failure)

Hypertension—Cushing response
Hypertension—pseudo-phaeochromocytoma syndrome
Hypotension—vasoparalytic shock
Sinus arrhythmia
Sinus tachycardia
Sinus bradycardia
ECG changes
Nodal rhythm
Fixed heart-rate (pain, fits, anxiety, suction)
Central neurogenic hyperventilation
Cheyne–Stokes respiration
Bradypnoea
Apnoeic attacks
Pulmonary oedema
Laryngeal stridor
Hyperglycaemia (cerebral diabetes)
Hypoglycaemia
Hypothermia
Severe hyperthermia (poikilothermia)
Loss sodium/osmolality control

3. Circle of Willis 'no flow' areas leading to specific vascular territory infarction *e.g.* middle cerebral artery
4. Watershed between anterior and middle cerebral arteries *i.e.* leg area
5. Watershed between middle and posterior cerebral territories causing Balint's syndrome.

Specific vascular compression
1. Anterior cerebral artery by transcallosal or cingulate hernia
2. Posterior cerebral arteries with calcarine infarction in tentorial herniation
3. Posterior inferior cerebellar arteries in foramen magnum cone
4. Anterior spinal artery in foramen magnum descent and impaction
5. Central midbrain and pontine vessels with secondary brainstem haemorrhagic infarction in tentorial herniation.

Local pressure necrosis
1. Cingulate gyrus
2. Uncus and parahippocampal gyrus
3. Cerebellar tonsils
4. Orbital part of frontal lobe.

This list of secondary pathological effects of RICP should leave no one in any doubt about the importance of suspecting and treating RICP, which can complicate practically any acute neurological disease. A disease with a good prospect of cure may then result in death or severe residual neurological disability.

Progressive brainstem failure
If the pressure effects continue, the decerebrate postures of tentorial herniation

69

TABLE 3.XI

Signs of foramen magnum cone

Bradypnoea
Apnoea
Stridor
Tongue fasciculation
Erb's palsy
Decerebration replaced by atonia
Return of spinal flexion
Vasoparalytic shock
Hyperglycaemia
Bradycardia replaced by fixed heart-rate
Cardiac arrest
Absent caloric responses
Doll's eyes response returns then disappears
Loss of sodium? osmolality control
Loss of temperature control
Cerebellar infarction (pica compressed)

may suddenly disappear as the child becomes profoundly hypotonic; the only signs of neurological activity are a flexor withdrawal reflex in the legs (Table 3.X). In the very young infant with non-myelinated pyramidal tracts, and in whom spinal shock does not develop, there may be a return to spinal flexion with brisk flexor withdrawal and dermatome to myotome contractions. This is easily misdiagnosed as an improvement. Occasionally the picture of fasiculation of the tongue, bulbar palsy and an Erb's palsy may be predominant and confusing.

Pupils may be small and pinpoint. More often the external ophthalmoplegia becomes complete so that there is loss not only of doll's eye but also caloric responses: in other words, even vestibular input to the stem does not elicit any eye movements. At the same time the pupils assume the mid-range or cadaveric position being completely unresponsive to light. A widely dilated pupil still has some innervation. Coma is deep with no responses apart from reflex withdrawal. There is no gag reflex, cough, sneeze or vomit— *i.e.* even the protective reflexes are lost.

However brainstem failure is dominated by loss of homeostasis (Table 3.XI) —respiratory, cardiovascular, glucose, temperature, osmolality and autonomic control.

With tentorial herniation there is a tachypnoea with rates often over 100 per minute and a low PCO_2 (*i.e.* central neurogenic hyperventilation). This may be replaced by periodic breathing with periods of apnoea (known as Cheyne–Stokes when the periods of apnoea are regular). As pressure to the medullary respiratory centres increases, a gradual reduction in rate is the hallmark. Sudden apnoea does not usually come unannounced provided careful monitoring of respiratory rate has been performed (Table 3.XII). The result is collapse, with respiratory arrest and total apnoea. The bradypnoea persists below 10 per minute and is usually interpolated with sighs, which continue as gasping after regular respiration has ceased. It is thought that respiratory rate may normally be controlled by the beat between two oscillators, and these become disconnected and independent.

TABLE 3.XII

Defects in homeostasis: respiratory

Respiratory arrhythmias
 Tachypnoea—central neurogenic hyperventilation
 Bradypnoea—central neurogenic hypoventilation
 Atactic irregular respiration
 Ictal respiratory arrhythmias
 Apnoeic attacks
 Gasping/sighing
 Periodic breathing—Cheyne–Stokes respiration

Respiratory failure
 Ventilation perfusion defect (PO_2 reduced)
 Central ventilatory failure — (PCO_2 raised)
 Tonic muscle spasm restricting ventilation

Laryngeal
 Loss of cough, gag, sneeze, *i.e.* protective reflexes,
   with laryngeal incompetence and aspiration

TABLE 3.XIII

Defects in homeostasis: gut

Vomit
Increased acid output
Cushing's ulcers
Aspiration coffee grounds or haematemesis
Oesophageal reflux
Reflex pharyngeal apnoea
Aspiration gastric contents
Borborygmi +++
Defaecation

Respiratory arrhythmias may occur with erratic respiration tachyrhythmias, bradyrhythmias and apnoeic periods together with varying depths of inspiration and expiration, sometimes called ataxic respiration. We feel that one should consider respiratory arrhythmias as seriously as one considers cardiac arrhythmias. Some are reversed with xanthines such as aminophylline, and some appear to have an epileptic basis and may be reversed with intravenous diazepam (which can also cause apnoea so must only be given in an ICU situation). Episodes may be bizarre, such as when the child develops a tachycardia of 200 per minute, yawns with sudden reduction to 60 per minute and goes apnoeic at the same time; this pattern may be repeated dozens of times a day and can only be regarded as a type of brainstem seizure. Epileptic apnoea is rare in older children, but well documented in the neonate. Failure of automatic ventilation is seen in some cases of poisoning with phenothiazine-type drugs when the child will voluntarily breathe in and out to command, but remains apnoeic when not instructed. Occasionally this will respond to naloxone. Failure of the vocal cords to open at inspiration reflexly may cause severe laryngeal stridor. If there is also cerebral pulmonary oedema then croup and wet lungs may not immediately suggest a cerebral cause.

Pulmonary oedema appears to be due to a massive sympathetic discharge

TABLE 3.XIV

Defects in homeostasis: cardiovascular

Blood pressure
   Hypertension—Cushing response
   Hypertension—pseudo-phaeochromocytoma
   Postural hypertension
   Hypotension—vasoparalytic shock (ischaemic
     sympathectomy)

Cardiac rhythm
   Bradycardia
   Tachycardia
   Asystole
   Exaggerated sinus arrhythmia
   Fixed heart-rate

ECG changes
   Absent p wave, nodal escape
   Deep Q waves
   Broadened QRS

(Ducker *et al*. 1969). This may also cause severe hypertension and hyperglycaemia.

One must constantly beware of the secondary respiratory problems such as severe pulmonary oedema as part of Mendelsohn's syndrome due to aspiration of acid gastric contents, especially as excess acid secretion with acute erosions and gastro-intestinal haemorrhage can be severe. Massive haematemesis can result from these 'Cushing's ulcers'. This is why the use of alkali prophylactically and cimetidine forms an integral part of management of the unconscious child should there be any aspirated blood from the nasogastric tube (Table 3.XIII).

The cardiovascular system is affected both peripherally and centrally (Table 3.XIV). The heart is normally under a controlling vagotonia; if this is lost a tachycardia results. Increase in vagal tone occurs at first with tentorial herniation and this may progress to vagal cardiac arrest. Tachycardia occurs in pontine lesions and at surgery one can show tachycardia when the pons is stimulated and bradycardia with the upper stem. This also produces marked ECG changes so that p-waves may disappear with nodal escape or pattern resembling myocardial infarction well described after subarachnoid haemorrhage. Ischaemic vagotomy often results in a fixed heart-rate between 130 and 150 per minute.

Preservation of sinus arrhythmia is a good guide to intact vagal innervation. The rate normally rises with anxiety and pain as when the endotracheal tube is aspirated. A fixed heart-rate unresponsive to stimulation means ischaemic brainstem vagotomy and is a very bad sign. The peripheral circulation is under sympathetic control and so there may again be excess or diminished activity. The Cushing response of hypertension, often with hyperglycaemia and tachycardia, has been described as a possible compensatory mechanism of the brain when its perfusion is threatened (Cushing 1902). If the reflexes are damaged, there can be severe postural hypertension or the cerebral pseudo-phaeochromocytoma picture of very severe hypertension, tachycardia, sweating, pallor and hyperglycaemia (Eden *et al*. 1977). This picture need not be associated with RICP but can cause

TABLE 3.XV

Defects in homeostasis: biochemical endocrine

Hypoglycaemia
Hyperglycaemia (cerebral diabetes)
Diabetes insipidus
Inappropriate antidiuretic hormone secretion
Essential hypernatraemia
Natriuretic hyponatraemia
Hyperprolactinaemia
Hypocalcaemia
Hypothermia, hyperthermia, poikilothermia

retinal haemorrhages, fits and signs of hypertensive encephalopathy. The blood pressures are extremely high for young children (*e.g.* 260/150mmHg).

Serum potassium concentrations are often low, whilst sodium concentrations —which may have been low initially as part of the water intoxication due to inappropriate ADH secretion—may now range from 60 to 300mmol/l as compared to the usual very narrow range of 135 to 145mmol/l. Glucose may be high with cerebral diabetes, or low with persistent hypoglycaemia. Fever, sometimes with hyperthermia, may give way to hypothermia or poikilothermia (Table 3.XV). The hypothalamic monitoring of temperature, glucose and osmolality is either destroyed or the regulatory system cut off from the sensors. The same applies to the brainstem sensors for respiration, heart-rate and blood pressure. The expected picture is apnoea, a fixed heart-rate and vasoparalytic shock with total loss of vasomotor tone due in effect to an ischaemic sympathectomy. Blood pressure drops, core to skin temperature is in keeping with peripheral circulatory failure, and there are cold extremities with poor capillary return. The blood volume is inadequate to fill the vastly increased volume of the circulatory bed without vasomotor tone. Plasma expansion and pharmacological vasoconstriction with dopamine may restore some CPP, but the prognosis by this stage is usually hopeless.

The end stage of apnoea unresponsive to CO_2, vasoparalytic dopamine-dependent shock, coma, fixed heart-rate, unresponsive cadaveric pupils, absent 'doll's eye' and caloric responses, absent protective gag and cough reflexes, constitutes brainstem death. The patterns by which this is arrived at will vary from child to child, depending upon the areas of pons and medulla which are compressed and infarcted.

REFERENCES

Addy, D. P. (1987) 'When not to do a lumbar puncture.' *Archives of Disease in Childhood*, **62**, 873–875.
Batton, D. G., Hellmann, J., Hernandez, M. J., Makels, M. J. (1983) 'Regional cerebral blood flow, cerebral blood velocity, and pulsatility index in newborn dogs.' *Pediatric Research*, **19**, 67–70.
Bishop, C. C. R., Powell, S., Rutt, D., Browse, N. L. (1986) 'Transcranial Doppler measurement of middle cerebral artery blood flow velocity: a validation study.' *Stroke*, **17**, 913–915.
Bode, H., Wais, U. (1988) 'Age dependence of flow velocities in basal cerebral arteries.' *Archives of Disease in Childhood*, **63**, 606–611.
Brown, J. K. (1976) 'Lumbar puncture and its hazards.' *Developmental Medicine and Child Neurology*, **18**, 803–816.

—— Ingram, T. T. S., Seshia, S. S. (1973) 'Patterns of decerebration in infants and children.' *Journal of Neurology and Neurosurgery*, **36**, 431–434.

—— Steer, C. R. S. (1986) 'Strategies in the management of acute encephalopathies.' *In* Gordon, N., McKinlay, I. *Children with Neurological Disorders. II: Neurologically Sick Children. Treatment and Management.* Oxford: Blackwell. pp. 219–294.

Bruce, D. A. (1984) 'Effects of hyperventilation on cerebral blood flow and metabolism.' *Clinics in Perinatology*, **II**, 673–680.

—— Langfitt, T. W., Miller, J. D. (1973) 'Regional cerebral blood flow, intracranial pressure and brain metabolism in comatose patients.' *Journal of Neurosurgery*, **38**, 131.

—— Berman, W. A., Schut, L. (1977) 'Cerebrospinal fluid monitoring in children. Physiology, pathology and clinical usefulness.' *Advances in Paediatrics*, **24**, 233.

Cady, E. B., Dawson, M. J., Hope, P. L., Tofts, P. S., Costello, A. M., Delpy, D. T., Reynolds, E. O. R., Wilkie, D. R. (1983) 'Non-invasive investigation of cerebral metabolism in newborn infants by phosphorus nuclear magnetic resonance spectroscopy.' *Lancet*, **2**, 1059–1062.

Costeloe, K., Rolfe, P. (1989) 'Techniques for studying cerebral perfusion in the newborn.' *In* Pape, K. E., Wigglesworth, J. S. (Eds.) *Perinatal Brain Lesions.* Oxford: Blackwell. pp. 135–190.

Cross, K. W., Dear, P. R. F., Hathorn, M. K. S., Hyams, A., Kerslake, D. McK., Milligan, D. W. A., Rahilly, P. M., Stothers J. K. (1979) 'An estimation of intracranial blood flow in the newborn infants.' *Journal of Physiology*, **289**, 329–345.

Cushing, H. (1902) 'Some experimental and clinical observations concerning states of increased intracranial tension.' *American Journal of the Medical Sciences*, **124**, 375.

Ducker, T. B., Simmons, R. L., Martin, A. M. (1969) 'Pulmonary edema as a complication of intracranial disease.' *American Journal of Diseases of Children*, **118**, 638–641.

Eden, O. B., Sills, J. A., Brown, J. K. (1977) 'Hypertension in acute neurological diseases of childhood.' *Developmental Medicine and Child Neurology*, **19**, 437–445.

Eyre, J. (1988) *Paper presented to British Paediatric Neurology Association Meeting.*

Ferris, E. B. (1941) 'Objective measurement of relative intracranial blood flow in man with observations concerning hydrodynamics of the craniovertebral system.' *Archives of Neurology and Psychiatry*, **46**, 377–401.

Fong, K. L., McCay, P. R., Poyer, J. L. (1973) 'Evidence that peroxidation of lysosomal membranes is initiated by hydroxyl free radicals produced during flavin enzyme activity.' *Journal of Biology and Chemistry*, **248**, 77–92.

Friis-Hansen, B. (1985) 'Perinatal brain injury and cerebral blood flow in newborn infants.' *Acta Paediatrica Scandinavica*, **74**, 323–331.

Fujimoto, T., Walker, J. T. Jr., Spatz, M., Klatzo, I. (1976) 'Pathophysioloical aspects of ischaemic edema.' *In* Pappius, H. M., Feindel, W. (Eds.) *Dynamics of Brain Edema.* Berlin: Springer. pp. 171–180.

Goitein, K. J., Fainmesser, P., Sohmer, H. (1983) 'Cerebral perfusion pressure and auditory brain-stem responses in childhood CNS diseases.' *American Journal of Diseases of Children*, **137**, 777–781.

Graham, D. I., Ford, I., Adams, J. H., Doyle, D., Teasdale, G. M., Lawrence, A. E., McLellan, D. R. (1989) 'Ischaemic brain damage is still common in fatal non-missilehead injury.' *Journal of Neurology, Neurosurgery and Psychiatry*, **52**, 346–350.

Greisen, G. (1984) 'CBF in the newborn infant: issues and methods with special reference to the intravenous [133]xenon clearance technique.' *CBF Bulletin*, **7**, 134–143.

—— Johansen, K., Ellison, P. H., Fredriksen, P. S., Mali, N., Friis-Hansen, B. (1984) 'Cerebral blood flow in the newborn infant: comparison of Doppler ultrasound and [133] xenon clearance.' *Journal of Pediatrics*, **104**, 411–418.

Hahn, Y. S., Chyung, C., Barthel, M. J., Bailes, J., Flannery, A. M., McLone, D. G. (1988) 'Head injuries in children under 36 months age.' *Child's Nervous System*, **4**, 34–40.

Hansen, N. B., Stonestreet, B. S., Rosenkrantz, T. S., Oh, W. (1983) 'Validity of Doppler measurements of anterior cerebral artery blood flow velocity correlation with brain blood flow in pig labs.' *Pediatrics*, **72**, 526–531.

Harper, A. M., Deshmukh, V. D., Rowan, J. O., Jennett, W. B. (1972) 'The influence of sympathetic nervous activity on cerebral blood flow.' *Archives of Neurology*, **27**, 1–6.

—— Glass, H. J. (1965) 'Effect of alterations in the arterial carbon dioxide tension on the blood through the cerebral cortex at normal and low arterial blood pressures.' *Journal of Neurology, Neurosurgery and Psychiatry*, **28**, 449–452.

Hill, A., Volpe, J. J. (1982) 'Decrease in pulsatile flow in the anterior cerebral arteries in infantile hydrocephalus.' *Pediatrics*, **69**, 4–7.

Hill, T. C., Holman, B. L., Lovett, R., O'Leary, D. H., Front, D., Magistretti, P., Zimmerman, R. E.,

Moire, S., Slouse, M. E., Wu, J. L., Lin, T. D., Baldwin, R. H. (1982) 'Initial experience with SPECT (Single-photon computerized tomography) of the brain using N-isopropyl I 123. p-iodoamphetamine concise communication.' *Journal of Nuclear Medicine*, **23**, 191–195.

Horwitz, S. J., Boxerbaum, B., O'Bell, J. (1980) 'Cerebral herniation in bacterial meningitis in childhood.' *Annals of Neurology*, **7**, 525–528.

Huff, J. T., Harper, M., Sengupta, D., Jennett, B. (1972) 'Effect of alpha-adrenergic blockade on response of cerebral circulation to hypocapnia in the baboon.' *Lancet*, **2**, 1337–1339.

Ingvar, D. H., Philipson, L. (1977) 'Distribution of cerebral blood flow in the dominant hemisphere during motor icleation and motor performance.' *Annals of Neurology*, **2**, 230–237.

Jacobson, M. (1978) *Developmental Neurobiology*. New York: Plenum.

Jennett, B., Teasdale, G. (1981) *Management of Head Injuries*. Philadelphia: F. A. Davis. pp. 19–43.

Johansson, B. (1974) 'Blood brain barrier dysfunction in acute arterial hypertension after papaverine induced vaso dilation.' *Acta Neurologica Scandinavica*, **50**, 573–580.

Johnson, R. T., Yates, P. O. (1956a) 'Brain stem haemorrhages in expanding supratentorial conditions.' *Acta Radiologica (Stockholm)*, **46**, 250–256.

—— —— (1956b) 'Clinico pathological aspects of pressure changes at the tentorium.' *Acta Radiologica (Stockholm)*, **46**, 242–249.

Jones, T. H., Morametz, P. B., Growell, R. M., Marcoux, F. W., Fitzgibbon, S. J., De Girola, M. I., Vojemann, R. E. (1981) 'Thresholds of focal cerebral ischaemia in awake monkeys.' *Journal of Neurosurgery*, **54**, 773–782.

Kernohan, J. W., Woltman, H. W. (1929) 'Incisura of the crus due to contralateral brain tumour.' *Archives of Neurology and Psychiatry*, **21**, 274–287.

Kety, S. S., Schmidt, C. F. (1945) 'The determination of cerebral blood flow in man by the use of nitrous oxide in low concentration.' *American Journal of Physiology*, **143**, 53–66.

Kirkham, F. J., Padayachee, T. S., Parsons, S., Seargeant, L. S., Howe, F. R., Gosling, R. G. (1986) 'Transcranial measurements of blood velocity in the basal cerebral arteries using pulsed Doppler ultrasound = velocity as an index of flow.' *Ultrasound in Medicine and Biology*, **12**, 15–21.

Kirsch, J. R., Traystman, R. J., Rogers, M. C. (1985) 'Cerebral blood flow measurement techniques in infants and children.' *Pediatrics*, **75**, 887–895.

Kuhl, D. E., Barrio, J. R., Huang, S. C., Selin, C., Ackerman, R. F., Lear, J. L., Wu, J. L., Lin, T. H., Phelps, M. E. (1982) 'Quantifying local cerebral blood flow by N-isopropyl-p- [123I] iodoamphetamine (IMP) tomography.' *Journal of Nuclear Medicine*, **23**, 196–203.

Langfitt, T. W., Kassell, N. F. (1968) 'Cerebral vasodilatation produced by brain-stem stimulation: neurogenic US autoregulation.' *American Journal of Physiology*, **215**, 90–97.

Lassen, N. A., (1968) 'Brain extracellular pH the main factor controlling cerebral blood flow.' *Scandinavian Journal of Clinical and Laboratory Investigation*, **22**, 247–251.

—— Christensen, M. S. (1976) 'Physiology of cerebral blood flow.' *British Journal of Anaesthesia*, **48**, 719–734.

Levene, M. I., Bennett, J. J., Punt, J. (1988) *Fetal and Neonatal Neurology and Neurosurgery*. Edinburgh: Churchill Livingstone. pp. 312–325.

Lou, H. C., Lassen, A., Friis-Hansen, B. (1977) 'Cerebral blood flow determination in newborns.' *Neuropädiatrie*, **8** (Suppl.), 533–535.

Lundberg, N. (1960) 'Continuous recording and control of ventricular fluid pressure in neurosurgical practice.' *Acta Psychiatrica Scandinavica*, **149**, 1–193.

Matsuda, H., Maeda, T., Yamada, M., Gui, L., Tonami, N., Hisada, K. (1984) 'Age-matched normal values and topographic maps for regional cerebral blood flow measurements by Xe–133 inhalation.' *Stroke*, **15**, 336–342.

McHenry, L. C. Jr. (1966) 'Cerebral blood flow.' *New England Journal of Medicine*, **274**, 82–90.

Meldrum, B. (1985) 'Possible therapeutic applications of antagonists of excitatory amino acid neurotransmitters.' *Clinical Science*, **68**, 113–122.

Ment, L. R., Duncan, C. C., Ehrenkranz, R. A. (1984) 'Intraventricular hemorrhage in the preterm neonate: timing and cerebral blood flow changes.' *Journal of Pediatrics*, **104**, 419–425.

Meyer, A. (1920) 'Herniation of the brain.' *Acta Neurologica et Psychiatrica*, **4**, 387–400.

Meyer, J. S., Teraura, T., Sakamoto, K., Kondo, A. (1971) 'Central neurogenic control of cerebral blood flow.' *Neurology*, **24**, 247–262.

Molnar, I., Szanto, J. (1964) 'The effect of electrical stimulation of the bulbar vasomotor centre on the cerebral blood flow.' *Quarterly Journal of Experimental Physiology*, **49**, 184–193.

Miller, J. D. (1975) 'Effects of hypercapnia on pupillary size, intracranial pressure and cerebral venous PO_2 during experimental brain compression.' *In* Lundberg, N., Ponten, U., Brock, M. (Eds.)

Intracranial Pressure, II. Berlin: Springer. p. 444.

—— (1988) *Personal communication.*

—— Stanck, A., Langfitt, T. W. (1972) 'Concept of cerebral perfusion pressure and vascular compression during intracranial hypertension.' *Progress in Brain Research*, **35**, 411–432.

Milligan, D. W. A. (1979) 'Cerebral blood flow and sleep state in the normal newborn infant.' *Early Human Development*, **3/4**, 321–328.

Minns, R. A., Engelman, H. M., Stirling, H. (1989) 'Cerebrospinal fluid pressure in pyogenic meningitis.' *Archives of Disease in Childhood*, **64**, 814–820.

Obrist, W. D., Thompson, H. K., Wang, H. S., Wilkinson, W. E. (1975) 'Regional cerebral blood flow estimated by [133] xenon inhalation.' *Stroke*, **6**, 245–256.

—— Langfitt, T. W., Dolinskas, C. A., Jaggi, J. L., Segawa, H. (1983) 'Factors relating to intracranial hypertension in acute head injury.' *Intracranial Pressure, V.* Berlin: Springer. pp. 491–494.

Pape, K., Wigglesworth, J. S. (1989) *Perinatal Brain Lesions. 5. Contemporary Issues in Fetal and Neonatal Medicine.* Oxford: Blackwell.

Paul, R. L., Polanco, O., Turney, S. Z., McAslan, T. C., Cowley, R. A. (1972) 'Intracranial pressure responses to alterations in arterial carbon dioxide pressure in patients with head injuries.' *Journal of Neurosurgery*, **36**, 714–720.

Perlman, J. M., Hill, A., Volpe, J. J. (1981) 'The effect of patent ductus arteriosus on flow velocity in the anterior cerebral arteries: ductal steal in the premature newborn infant.' *Journal of Pediatrics*, **99**, 767–771.

Rahilly, P. M. (1980) 'Effects of sleep state and feeding on cranial blood flow of the human neonate.' *Archives of Disease in Childhood*, **55**, 265–270.

Raichle, M. E., Eichling, J. D., Grubb, P. L. Jr., Hartman, B. K. (1976) 'Central noradrenergic regulation of brain microcirculation.' *In* Pappius, H. M., Feinder, W. (Eds.) *Dynamics of Brain Edema* Berlin: Springer. p. 11.

Raju, T. N. K., Vidyasagar, D., Papazafiratou, C. (1981) 'Cerebral perfusion pressure and abnormal intracranial pressure wave forms: their relation to outcome in birth asphyxia.' *Critical Care Medicine*, **9**, 449–453.

Rehncrona, S., Rosen, I., Siesjo, B. K. (1980) 'Excessive cellular acidosis: an important mechanism of neuronal damage in the brain?' *Acta Physiologica Scandinavica*, **110**, 435–437.

Rennels, M. L., Nelson, E. (1973) 'Capillary innervation in the mammalian CNS.' *American Journal of Anatomy*, **144**, 233–241.

Rennie, J. M., South, M., Morley, C. T. (1987) 'Cerebral blood flow velocity variability in infants receiving assisted ventilation.' *Archives of Disease in Childhood*, **62**, 1247–1251.

Roach, E. S., Riela, A. R. (1988) *Pediatric Cerebrovascular Disorders.* New York: Futura.

Rothman, S. M., Olney, J. W. (1986) 'Glutamate and the pathophysiology of hypoxic-ischemic brain damage.' *Annals of Neurology*, **19**, 105–111.

Seshia, S. S., Seshia, M. M. K., Sachdeva, R. K. (1977) 'Coma in childhood.' *Developmental Medicine and Child Neurology*, **19**, 614–628.

—— Johnston, B., Kasian, G. (1983) 'Non-traumatic coma in childhood: clinical variables in prediction of outcome.' *Developmental Medicine and Child Neurology*, **25**, 493–501.

Shalit, M. N., Shimojya, S., Reinmuth, O. M. (1967) 'Carbon dioxide and cerebral circulatory control.' *Archives of Neurology*, **17**, 298–303.

Shimizu, H., Tagawa, T., Futagi, Y., Tawaka, J. (1983) 'Cerebral bloodflow in children with intractable epilepsy.' *Brain Development*, **5**, 36–40

Singer, S. R., Crooks, L. E (1983) 'Nuclear magnetic resonance blood flow measurements in the human brain.' *Science*, **221**, 654–656.

Slack, J. (1980) 'Coning and lumbar puncture.' *Lancet*, **2**, 474–475.

Teasdale, G., Jennett, B. (1974) 'Assessment of coma and impaired consciousness.' *Lancet*, **2**, 81–84.

Volpe, J. J., Perlman, J. M., Hill, A., McMenamin, J. B. (1982) 'Cerebral blood flow velocity in the human newborn. The value of its determination.' *Pediatrics*, **70**, 147–152.

—— Herscovitch, P., Perlman, J. M., Raichle, M. E. (1983) 'Positron emission tomography in the newborn: extensive impairment of regional cerebral blood flow with intraventricular hemorrhage and hemorrhagic intracerebral involvement.' *Pediatrics*, **72**, 589–601.

4
CEREBRAL BLOODFLOW

M. V. Merrick

An adequate blood supply is essential for all tissues. Any reduction in the supply of oxygen or substrates to, and the removal of the end-products of metabolism from an organ, impairs its efficiency. The effects of ischaemia are particularly rapid in the brain, which has no effective reserves of oxygen or glucose (despite its high rate of oxidative metabolism), and is therefore critically dependent on the maintenance of an adequate blood supply.

Many methods have been developed for measuring bloodflow (Table 4.I). Standard reference techniques, which give a direct or absolute measurement of bloodflow, are often not practical as clinical tools, but nevertheless any indirect method must be validated initially against one of them. Not all of the methods suggested in the literature have been confirmed in this way.

Before proceeding further it is important to define certain terms. In particular, the difference between bloodflow and perfusion must be appreciated. *Bloodflow* is expressed as the quantity (volume or weight) of blood entering or leaving the region under investigation per unit of time, typically millilitres of blood per minute. *Perfusion* is defined as the flow per unit weight of tissue, most commonly expressed in millilitres of blood per 100g of brain per minute. The practical difference can be appreciated by considering the example of a volume which includes only the superior sagittal sinus. The bloodflow may be quite high, perhaps 50 to 100ml/min; but as there is no brain within the sinus, the perfusion will be zero.

Another potential source of confusion is the way in which the term 'flow' is used. This is correctly defined as above, in units such as ml/min. However, it is sometimes employed when referring to the velocity with which blood is moving: this is measured in cm/min (or equivalent units) and is properly termed 'velocity of flow'.

Experimental or reference techniques of measuring bloodflow
Flow meters
The most direct method of measuring cerebral bloodflow in experimental animals is to place a flow meter in series with the internal carotid artery (Schmidt *et al.* 1945). The technique is valid in most species but not in homo sapiens (or femina sapientia) because of the presence of a functioning circle of Willis. There is considerable individual variation in the adequacy of this anastomotic pathway. Alternatively an electro-magnetic or ultrasonic flow meter, which measures the velocity of blood, may be positioned around the afferent artery. Flow can be determined if the cross-sectional area has been accurately measured. Inserting such a detector, in series with a vessel or around it, is an invasive operative procedure, impractical in clinical practice. Even in experimental animals, accurate positioning of the detector is

TABLE 4.I

Methods of measuring bloodflow, velocity or perfusion

Technique	Page	In vitro global	In vitro regional	Global or regional in vivo	Quantitative imaging in vivo	Qualitative imaging in vivo
Flow meter	77	X				
Electrical impedance	77	X		?		
Auto-radiography	80,97		X		X	
Wash-out	81,93	X	X	X	X	
Wash-in	93	X		X	X	
Microspheres	79	X	X		X	X
Ultrasound	82			X		X
MRI	86				X	X
SPECT	95					X
PET	97				X	
First pass	99			X	X	

technically demanding, and it can be difficult to determine the exact dimension where it passes through the probe. Variations in blood velocity (across the diameter of the vessel or between systole and diastole) may give rise to errors, depending on the length of time taken to make each measurement, the frequency of any variations and their amplitude. If recordings are made over a very short interval, the readings may not be representative of the mean unless a very large number of measurements are made at regular intervals. If each takes a long time, an average value is obtained which may not be truly representative.

It is also necessary to determine whether flow at the site of measurement is laminar or turbulent. When a small discrete quantity of tracer is added to fluid flowing through a tube, the volume in which the bolus is dispersed increases progressively. During streamlined flow, the velocity of tracer at the head of the bolus is double the mean velocity of the bolus as a whole (Taylor 1953). On the other hand when flow is turbulent, as it usually is in biological systems where the calibre of vessels varies and there are many branches, the relationship between peak flow and mean flow is more complex. It is therefore essential to determine whether the detecting system measures mean velocity of flow throughout the volume being interrogated, or if it is influenced by the peak velocity of flow and by turbulence, which can give rise to local reversals of flow. Such techniques are principally relevant to organs which have a single afferent artery such as the kidney, and are not readily applicable to measurement of total cerebral bloodflow.

Microspheres
Another method of measuring bloodflow employs the principle that, if a tracer is completely extracted from the blood on a single pass through an organ, the fraction of the amount originally administered which remains in that organ is in proportion to the fraction of cardiac output being supplied to it (Sapirstein 1956). This is true only if the tracer is completely extracted on a single pass, there is no recirculation, tracer is completely mixed in the output from the left ventricle and no streaming or unevenness of distribution occurs as it circulates.

Radioactive labelled microspheres correspond most closely to the ideal tracer for this purpose (Heyman *et al*. 1977). These are small insoluble particles which may be of albumin, of carbonised albumin or of plastic, large enough to be totally extracted by small arterioles or capillaries and which do not aggregate into larger collections or fragment into smaller ones. In principle, in order to obtain complete mixing with the blood leaving the left ventricle, it is desirable to inject into the left atrium. Intravenous injection results in complete extraction by the lungs unless there is a right-to-left shunt. The range of sizes present must be controlled within narrow limits; 'shimming' occurs if the variation is too great, the distribution across the diameter of larger vessels varying with particle size, with consequent preferential loss of larger particles into the proximal branches (Yipintsoi *et al*. 1973). As the quantity of radioactive tracer carried by each particle depends on its size, a small number of very large particles will spuriously alter the apparent distribution. Any particles too small to be trapped in capillaries are subsequently taken up by the reticulo-endothelial system, also affecting the distribution. The tracer must remain exclusively attached to the particles. Iron isotopes are usually unsuitable, as they are readily translocated from the microspheres onto circulating transferrin. In practice it is often adequate to inject into the aortic root. The distribution of the radioactivity is determined by counting excised organs of experimental animals and by PET (see p. 97) or suitably modified whole-body counting techniques in humans (Crean *et al*. 1986) and expressed as the fraction of the cardiac output in the whole organ or per unit weight.

This method by itself gives the relative or fractional distribution of the output from the left ventricle. In order to calculate absolute flow it is necessary to combine this with a measurement of cardiac output, most conveniently using a 'reference organ' consisting of a small cannula inserted into a suitable vessel (*e.g.* a limb artery) from which blood is withdrawn at a constant rate during the injection of the microspheres. The cardiac output can be calculated, provided there has been careful measurement of the total amount of activity injected (in the case of a bolus) or the rate of injection for a constant infusion, the rate of withdrawal through the cannula and the total quantity of tracer collected in the blood sample (Zierler 1962). By combining these two parameters the bloodflow to the brain (or any other organ which does not have a portal supply) can be calculated, from the ratio of activity in the 'reference organ' to that in the organ under investigation (Heikkila *et al.* 1983, Steinling *et al.* 1985). Unlike methods which measure the velocity of flow in arteries, this technique enables the distribution of flow to be measured into small vessels, by using quantitative autoradiography (see below and p. 97), even down to the capillary level. Although this is one of the best reference methods, as with so many techniques it is difficult to obtain accurate and reliable results, and it requires meticulous attention to detail. A number of clinically applicable methods are based on this technique (p. 95).

Autoradiography
This works on the principle that if a freely diffusable non-metabolised tracer is added to the arterial supply of any tissue or organ, the concentration (c_i) in any small volume (i) after a time T depends on the arterial concentration (c_a) during that time interval, the local perfusion (*i.e.* the flow to that region divided by its volume, F_i/v_i) and the effectiveness of the diffusion equilibrium between the capillary and tissue (m_1) (Kety *et al.* 1955).

$$c_i(T) = m_i F_i (v_i^{-1}) e^{-kT} \int_o^T c_a e^{kT} dt \qquad (1)$$

Trifluroiodomethane (CF_3I^{131}) was formerly employed, but being volatile, the arterial concentration reaches a plateau within two minutes. Subsequent administration is balanced by expiratory loss, reducing the sensitivity of the technique. With a non-volatile tracer such as ^{131}I antipyrine the arterial concentration rises almost linearly with time (Kety 1960).

To estimate the input, blood is drawn from an in-dwelling arterial catheter and passed through a suitable continuous-reading detector to obtain the arterial time/ concentration curve. Allowance must be made for distortion of the curve due to the dead-space in the tubing between the artery and the measuring device. It cannot be assumed that the shape of the arterial input curve to the brain is the same as that from a small peripheral artery, and this can lead to serious error (Iida *et al.* 1986).

After about a minute, the animal is decapitated and the head rapidly frozen in liquid nitrogen. It is then sectioned, and the slices are placed on autoradiographic film along with a number of gelatin discs containing a range of known concentrations of the isotope. After development, the concentration of isotope at each point is measured with a microdensitometer standardised using the gelatin discs. The partition coefficient is measured separately by maintaining a constant arterial concentration and making sequential measurements up to one hour, by which time there is complete equilibrium between blood and all structures in the brain. The solubility of CF_3I^{131} is very dependent upon the haematocrit and blood-lipid content, both of which vary appreciably from animal to animal. There is less variation with ^{131}I antipyrine. The diffusion coefficient (m) is usually assumed to be close to unity.

Inert tracer wash-out

The first practical method used a non-radioactive tracer, nitrous oxide (N_2O) (Kety and Schmidt 1945, 1948a,b). All subsequent clinical developments have used radioactive tracers, although non-radioactive ones still have a place in experimental animals. All the methods employ the same theoretical foundation, namely that if tracer is delivered at a measured rate, flow can be calculated from the total quantity of tracer removed from the blood divided by the nett mean concentration difference between the arterial and venous blood, provided that the system is in equilibrium and bloodflow is constant during the period of measurement (Fick 1870). In the original Kety-Schmidt method, the subject inhaled 15 per cent N_2O and the A-V concentration-difference was determined by measurement of consecutive samples of arterial and jugular venous blood over a timed period. The tracer content of the brain could not be measured directly but was derived from the total amount of N_2O removed from the blood—the indirect Fick principle. Flow (F) is then given by the equation:

$$F = \frac{Q_t}{_0\!\int^{\infty} (c_a - c_v)dt} \tag{2}$$

where Q_t is the quantity of N_2O taken up by the whole brain in time t, measured from the start of inhalation; c_a is the arterial concentration of nitrous oxide during any short time interval (dt), and c_v is the venous concentration of nitrous oxide during the same interval.

The tracer should be freely diffusible because its concentration in the venous outflow must be in equilibrium with the tracer content of the brain. Perfusion (P), by expressing flow in terms of a fixed weight of brain, facilitates intercomparison between subjects and species. This is obtained by dividing the flow by the weight (w) of the brain, thus giving concentration rather than total content; multiplying by 100 expresses the result in units of 100g rather than 1g of brain:

$$P = 100 \; F/w \tag{3}$$

substituting in (2)

$$P = \frac{100Q_t}{_0^w\!\int^t (c_a - c_v)dt} \tag{4}$$

The partition coefficient (λ) is the ratio of the quantity of tracer dissolved in brain to that in an equal weight of blood at the same time ($c_{v(t)}$):

$$\lambda = (Q_t/w)/c_{v(t)} \tag{5}$$

Substituting in equation 4:

$$P = \frac{100c_{v(T)}.\lambda}{_0\!\int^t (c_a - c_v)dt} \tag{6}$$

i.e. the perfusion is given by the venous concentration at time t, multiplied by a constant which takes account of differences in solubility, and divided by the quantity of tracer extracted from the blood up to that time.

81

If a freely diffusible tracer which does not become bound in any way is introduced as an instantaneous bolus (δ-function), provided that there is no recirculation and that—by the time blood has passed once through the region in question—the tracer concentration in brain is in equilibrium with that in blood, the rate at which tracer is subsequently washed out (dc_t/dt) is given by differentiating equation 6 and rearranging:

$$dc_t/dt = k(\lambda c_a - c_v) \tag{7}$$

Following bolus injection, the arterial concentration rapidly becomes negligible. Integrating gives:

$$c_t = c_o e^{-kt} \tag{8}$$

whilst in the case of a constant infusion, when the arterial concentration remains constant:

$$c_t = \lambda c_a (1 - e^{-kt}) \tag{9}$$

There are thus four related parameters which can be measured (Zierler 1965) and from which perfusion or flow can be derived:
1. Rate of wash-in
2. Rate of wash-out
3. Total quantity of tracer delivered
4. Variation of amount of tracer present with time.
Methods based on these principles have been used to measure regional cerebral bloodflow in experimental animals and in man. Xenon-enhanced CT uses the first of these (p. 93). The second has been employed in many guises (see below and pp. 87–94), in vitro with small beta particle detectors and low-energy beta-emitting tracers such as [85]Kr, which has a half-value thickness of 0.36mm in brain and thus effectively measures the clearance from a volume of cortex 1.5mm diameter around the detector (Ingvar and Lassen 1962, Lassen 1965). Hydrogen is an alternative non-radioactive biologically inert gas. The technology of measurement is different but the resultant curves are interpreted similarly (Aukland et al. 1964, Young 1980). The principle is that the oxidation of a substance at the surface of an electrode is associated with a current which reaches a plateau value unaffected by any further increase in voltage and proportional to the concentration gradient at the electrode surface. As biological systems contain only minimal amounts of substances which are oxidised or reduced at the voltage employed, the system is relatively specific for hydrogen in principle, but not in practice. A further technique, producing equivalent wash-out curves, measures the rate of removal of heat from the tip of a warmed probe (Betz et al. 1966). Autoradiography and microspheres use the third, while first-pass techniques use the last.

Clinical methods of bloodflow measurement
Ultrasound
The familiar Doppler effect is the basis of all current ultrasound methods of measuring blood velocity. This is based on the principle that the perceived

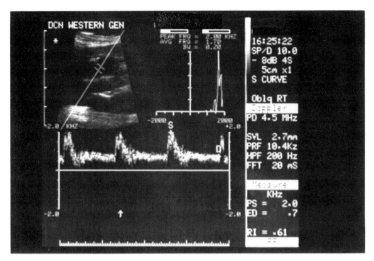

Fig. 4.1. Duplex ultrasound of carotid bifurcation. Cursor (*top left*) shows region from which the Doppler signal is being analysed. Doppler signal (*bottom panel*) shows blood velocity greatest in systole, with little movement in diastole (courtesy of Dr P. Sandercock).

wavelength of a waveform depends on the relative velocity of the source and the observer. The usual example cited is the apparent pitch of a train whistle, which rises as the train approaches the observer and falls as the train passes and moves into the distance.

To measure the velocity of flow in a bloodvessel, a beam of high-frequency sound, usually above the range of human hearing and therefore referred to as 'ultrasound', is directed towards the artery or vein in question. Some of the sound is reflected back to the transducer which has produced it, and which also acts as a detector. If the fluid is in motion, the wavelength will be altered depending on the fluid's velocity and whether it is moving towards or away from the probe. This method is therefore basically similar to the invasive use of ultrasonic flow meters, but the transducers are at some distance from the vessel. The depth of the vessel is determined by setting the time interval between emitting the pulse of sound and listening for the echo reflected back. This assumes that the velocity of sound in tissue is constant, an assumption which is sufficiently accurate for clinical purposes under most circumstances, but may be affected by pathological changes in the skull. Velocity is calculated from the difference in wavelength between the emitted pulse and the received echo. The wavelength of the echo is longer than that of the original pulse if the blood is moving away from the probe and shorter if the blood is flowing towards it. The angle of the vessel to the incident beam must also be measured if the true velocity is to be calculated. It must be remembered that the term 'velocity' implies direction as well as speed.

The movement of the blood in large superficial vessels (such as the femoral or carotid arteries) may be displayed as a 2D image in which the velocity at each point is represented by a shade of grey. This may be supplemented (Fig. 4.1) by

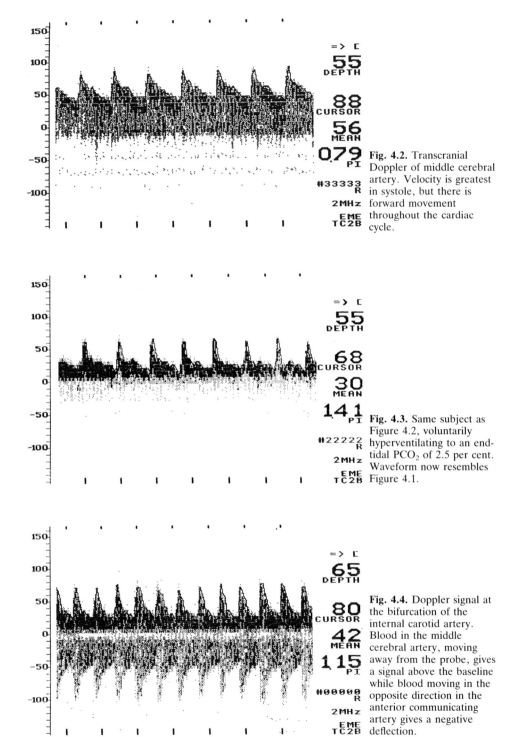

Fig. 4.2. Transcranial Doppler of middle cerebral artery. Velocity is greatest in systole, but there is forward movement throughout the cardiac cycle.

Fig. 4.3. Same subject as Figure 4.2, voluntarily hyperventilating to an end-tidal PCO_2 of 2.5 per cent. Waveform now resembles Figure 4.1.

Fig. 4.4. Doppler signal at the bifurcation of the internal carotid artery. Blood in the middle cerebral artery, moving away from the probe, gives a signal above the baseline while blood moving in the opposite direction in the anterior communicating artery gives a negative deflection.

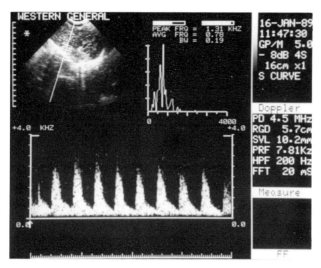

Fig. 4.5. The upper left quadrant is a sagittal section, slightly to one side of the midline, through the anterior fontanelle of a neonate. The two cross lines on the cursor indicate the region selected for analysis of the Doppler signal. The lower panel shows this Doppler signal. (PD = pulsed Doppler frequency 4.5Mh. RGD = range gate depth 5.7cm. SVC = sample volume length 10.2mm. PPF = pulse repetition frequency 7.81kH. HPF: high-pass filter 200Hz. FFT: fast Fournier transform at 20msecs (courtesy of Dr S. R. Wild).

conventional compound B mode ultrasound scanning which visualises the walls of the vessels with much better spatial resolution than can be achieved by Doppler alone (Spencer 1987). More sophisticated equipment employs colour to indicate the direction of flow. These techniques are not applicable to smaller and more deeply situated vessels such as the major intracranial arteries. A Doppler signal from these can however be recognised and the vessel from which it is originating inferred from the direction of the probe and the depth which has been selected. By making multiple measurements at regular intervals, variations in velocity throughout the cardiac cycle can be demonstrated. The pattern of velocity changes depends on the vessel under investigation and the state of the cerebral circulation. Figure 4.2 shows a typical tracing from the middle cerebral artery of a young adult. The height of the bars represents the velocity at that instant, and the horizontal displacement represents the time interval.

The maximum velocity occurs in systole and the minimum in end-diastole, but there is forward movement at all times. Hyperventilation produces a pattern similar to that in the aorta and common carotid at rest, with little or no movement in diastole (Fig. 4.3). At the bifurcation of a vessel, there is bidirectional flow as the blood moves towards the transducer in one branch, and away from it in the other (Fig. 4.4). What is measured is not absolute velocity, as the angle of the vessel to the probe cannot be determined, but the component of velocity towards or away from the transducer. Mean velocity (Aaslid *et al.* 1982) is not related to perfusion in any simple way, but is useful for assessing changes in an individual patient. The pulsatility index (PI)—a relationship between peak systolic velocity (v_a), end

85

diastolic velocity (v_d) and mean velocity (v_m)—has been suggested as an index of the peripheral resistance (Gosling *et al.* 1974).

$$PI = (v_s - v_d) / v_m \qquad (10)$$

Intracranial vessels are much more easily visualised in infants, through the fontanelles (Fig. 4.5).

Ultrasound is non-invasive, relatively quick, simple, safe and capable of very accurate measurements of velocity. Except in larger or superficial vessels it is not possible to estimate diameter accurately enough to calculate flow, so that in most cases velocity only can be measured. Like so many techniques in ultrasound, there is considerable dependence on the skill and expertise of the person performing the examination: it is nevertheless useful for obtaining sequential studies in the same individual. Disadvantages include the inability in most cases to measure flow (as distinct from velocity) and the absence of any indication of the more distal distribution of the blood. Thus velocity is increased proximal to an arteriovenous shunt, even though metabolically relevant flow to adjacent normal tissues may be reduced.

Other phenomena have also been employed. Changes in bloodflow are associated with alterations in electrical impedance (Jacquy *et al.* 1979). These have been used to detect pulsatile flow in neonates, having an advantage over ultrasound in that it remains practical even after closure of the fontanelles. Clinical experience is still restricted to a few centres, and the clinical place of this technique is unclear. The adult skull acts as a high impedance barrier, restricting the technique at present to babies.

Magnetic resonance
Magnetic resonance uses the radio signals given out when certain atoms (*in vivo* particularly hydrogen), having been aligned by a powerful magnetic field, emit radio waves when this field is disturbed. With the earlier MRI equipment blood-vessels appeared 'empty', *i.e.* as signal-free areas, as the time taken to make the measurement was long compared to the velocity of flow in the vessels, so that the blood which had initially been within the magnetic field was washed out before the signal from it could be measured. More recently a number of techniques have been developed for measuring the rate at which this signal is removed from the volume of interest or the way in which it is modified by the movement of the blood, and this has been applied to calculate the velocity of flow (Axel 1984, von Schulthess and Higgins 1985). The methods have the advantage that they can be used even at very low rates of flow, for example to measure the movement of CSF around the brainstem (Bradley *et al.* 1986, Ridgway *et al.* 1987), as well as for the measurement of the velocity of bloodflow. Velocity in capillary beds can also be measured, although the technique is subject to artefacts resulting from patient movement. It is also possible to produce a quantitative image showing the velocity of blood in the larger vessels by subtracting the 'stationary' from the 'moving' signal (Bogren *et al.* 1988). It is not clear whether the resolution is adequate for clinical purposes as a substitute for angiography.

These techniques are for the most part only applicable to fairly large vessels and, like ultrasound, give no indication of the subsequent distribution of bloodflow in the tissues supplied by them. The resolution of MRI equipment is inadequate for accurate measurement of vessel diameter, which is best estimated by ultrasound. The equipment required is seldom available, being much more expensive than that for any of the other techniques described, except PET (see below), nor is it portable. One virtue of the Doppler method is that it can be performed repeatedly in sick patients, using fairly compact equipment which can be taken to the bedside. Magnetic resonance requires the patient to be brought to the machine. Metallic equipment connected to the patient may cause problems because of the very high magnetic fields used.

Diffusible tracers

To calculate bloodflow *in vivo* it is necessary to measure both the volume of distribution and the mean transit time of the tracer. In many clinical situations the volume of distribution cannot be defined, and hence flow cannot be determined; it is nevertheless possible to derive perfusion from equation 14.

Tracers either (i) remain intravascular, are assayed during their first passage through the organ and are more useful for measurement of absolute flow (ml/min) (p. 99), or (ii) are diffusible, equilibrate with a volume larger than the blood volume, give perfusion and may be measured during wash-in or wash-out (ml/100g/min) (Bassingthwaighte and Holloway 1976). An important difference between Kety and Schmidt's original method using N_2O and subsequent modifications employing radioactive tracers is that the majority of the latter have been designed as far as possible to eliminate the need for arterial sampling. The more widely used methods which employ diffusible tracers will be described first.

Any suitable tracer, whether diffusible or non-diffusible, should be physiologically, chemically and metabolically inert—*i.e.* they should not undergo any chemical alteration whilst in the body, nor affect bloodflow or any other physiological variable, and should be detectable and accurately measurable by available gamma-counting techniques. At the concentration used by Kety and Schmidt (1945), N_2O has analgesic properties and thus does not comply with these criteria. The tracer must be fat-soluble in order to pass rapidly from blood into brain, so that extraction and equilibrium are faster than circulation. The most useful measure of lipophilicity is the octanol/water partition coefficient. This is the natural logarithm of the ratio of the solubility of the substance in octanol (a medium chain-length alcohol) to its solubility in water. If the solubility in octanol is too low, the extraction by brain on a single pass will be substantially less than 100 per cent. If the octanol solubility is too high, an excessive amount of the tracer will dissolve in the red cells and this also impairs the first pass extraction efficiency. The ln P_{oct} coefficient should optimally be between 0.9 and 2.5 (Dischino *et al.* 1983).

The amount of recirculation is determined by the route of administration, and by the efficiency of extracranial extraction and excretion. All tracers suitable for intravenous or inhalational use have appreciable recirculation. Unless appropriate corrections are made for this, the rate of wash-out will be underestimated.

Measurement of the uptake of a tracer such as ^{123}I-IMP or ^{99m}TC-HMPAO (p. xx) at equilibrium never gives an absolute measure of bloodflow because, no matter how high the extraction efficiency on the first pass, there is always some back-diffusion subsequently, so that the nett extraction efficiency on the second and subsequent passes is lower than on the first.

A large number of substances approximate sufficiently to the requirements for a diffusible tracer to be clinically useful, including isotopes of the noble gases xenon and krypton and many organo-halogen compounds, although none is ideal. ^{133}xe is the isotope most commonly used because it is readily available. Its gamma-ray energy of 80kev is rather low for *in vivo* measurements; in consequence the number of counts collected from a given quantity of radioactivity is strongly influenced by the depth of that radioactivity below the surface; a thickness of approximately 2cm halves the detected count-rate. Planar measurements are therefore disproportionately influenced by radioactivity in the scalp and more superficial parts of the cerebral cortex. Another xenon isotope, ^{127}xe, emits higher-energy gamma rays and is thus in principle a better isotope for this application, as the attenuation correction is proportionately very much smaller, although supplies are more restricted. Because of its higher energy, it requires thicker detectors surrounded by heavier shielding, making it more difficult to cluster several around the head in order to obtain information about the bloodflow to a number of regions simultaneously. Equipment designed for use with ^{133}xe is generally not suitable for use with ^{127}xe.

Krypton 77 has the disadvantage of a short half-life, so that it is available only close to the cyclotron which produces it. Moreover it emits positrons, which are detected as 511kev gamma rays. At this energy, very heavy shielding is necessary to collimate conventional detectors. It is best used in conjunction with a positron camera (Yamamoto *et al.* 1980). Other tracers which have been used include ^{79}kr, ^{18}F fluromethane, ^{18}F antipyrine, ^{131}I antipyrine, ^{11}c-labelled alcohols, ^{18}F-labelled ethanol, ^{15}o-labelled water or CO_2. Apart from the ^{131}I labels, the majority require PET. Although only ^{133}xe is commonly used in this class, the underlying principles are the same for all of these tracers.

Inert gas wash-out
Intra-arterial method

If an intra-arterial bolus of xenon (typically 100 MBq) or other suitable tracer dissolved in saline is given into a carotid artery, it will be largely taken up by the ipsilateral hemisphere during the first pass. The activity (quantity of radioactivity) necessary depends on the size and sensitivity of the detectors chosen and the duration of the measurement. Because only a small percentage of the original activity remains, larger initial activities are required to maintain adequate statistics towards the end of a 15-minute than a two-minute wash-out. The greater part of any activity which does reach the venous outflow is exhaled on traversing the lungs. Very little of the bolus thus recirculates or reaches the rest of the body. Transit time (τ) is defined as:

$$\tau = v_d/F \qquad (11)$$

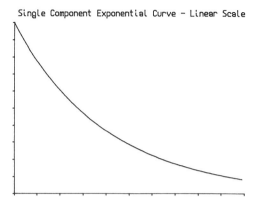

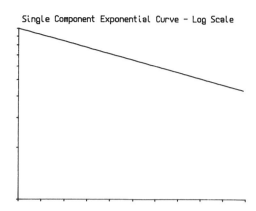

Fig. 4.6. Single exponential wash-out plotted on linear and semi-logarithmic scales.

where v_d is the volume of distribution (p. 100) and F is flow. Dividing both the numerator and denominator in equation 11 by the weight of tissue (w):

$$\tau = (v_d/w)/(F/w) \tag{12}$$

Substituting from (3) and rearranging:

$$P = 100v_d/\tau.w \tag{13}$$

By substituting from equations 4 and 6:

$$P = \lambda/\tau \tag{14}$$

Thus to determine perfusion it is not necessary to measure either the total quantity of tracer administered or the weight of tissue, only the rate of wash-out and the partition coefficient. Wash-out from the brain is usually measured for 15 minutes by one or more scintillation detectors positioned over the cranium (Lassen and Ingvar 1972). The extracranial concentration of tracer is extremely low and any removed from the head is almost entirely lost during its passage through the lungs, so that recirculation is negligible. There are three ways of calculating total, hemispheric or regional mean transit time (and hence perfusion), depending on the field of view of the detectors:

1. From the Kety-Schmidt equation (6), dividing the change in count-rate over a 10-minute period by the corresponding change in area under the wash-out curve.

2. If the wash-out curve (equation 7) is re-plotted as the natural logarithm of count-rate against time, the first two minutes correspond fairly closely to the theoretical prediction of a straight line (Fig. 4.6) (*i.e.* wash-out is approximately mono-exponential, equation 8), the slope of which is the wash-out rate from the regions having the higher bloodflow. The half-time ($t_{1/2}$) is the interval for the count-rate to fall from any value to half that value. The mean transit time is $0.693/t_{1/2}$. Perfusion (P_{init}), also known as initial slope index (ISI), approximates to that of grey matter:

$$P_{init} = 100.\lambda_g/\tau \tag{15}$$

with λ_g the partition coefficient for grey matter. Multiplying out the constants gives:

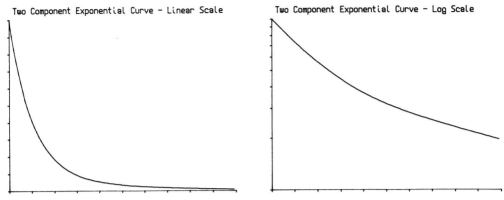

Two Component Exponential Curve – Linear Scale

Two Component Exponential Curve – Log Scale

Fig. 4.7. Sum of two exponential functions plotted on linear and semi-logarithmic scales.

$$P_{init} = 115.t_{1/2} \qquad (16)$$

The values obtained are slightly lower than those calculated using the bi-exponential fit described below, but the method is nevertheless clinically useful as the errors inherent in fitting a double exponential to clinical data often outweigh any improvement in accuracy theoretically attainable (Obrist and Wilkinson 1985).
3. The curve obtained over 15 minutes resembles Figure 4.7 (above left): it is not a single exponential, but corresponds rather better to the sum of two (Ingvar and Lassen 1962, Kety 1965), the suggestion being that the brain is not homogeneous, wash-out from grey and white matter occurring at different rates. A semi-logarithmic plot of this (above right) is not linear. Assuming that by the end of the study the faster compartment has effectively washed out, the counts in the later part of the curve must be due to the slower component. It is always possible to approximate a straight line to the last few points of any curve. Extrapolating backwards and subtracting the value at each point from the observed value at that point produces a new curve which may now give a straight line on semi-logarithmic graph paper. If it does not, repeating the process eventually gives a curve with so few counts that any deviation from linearity cannot be detected. If the values obtained do not agree with your preconceptions, they may be adjusted by fitting the initial line to a different set of points—*i.e.* earlier or later.

Virtually any curve can be fitted by the sum of a number of exponentials, and successfully fitting two or more to an experimental curve is not evidence that these correspond to any real physiological process. The slower is widely considered to be due to wash-out from extracranial structures and white matter (Häggendal *et al.* 1965) which, having a lower bloodflow than grey matter, are slower to lose any tracer which has been taken up. After subtracting this component, a second exponential function can be fitted to the residue, from which the half-time of the faster compartment is obtained. If the measurements are extended to 40 minutes, three exponentials can be fitted, ascribed to grey matter, white matter and extracranial structures (Obrist *et al.* 1967). Perfusion is calculated using equation 15. The results obtained yielded a poor correlation when compared with

TABLE 4.II

Absorbed radiation dose

Investigation	Effective dose equivalent (mSv)
[133]Xe planar counting (60MBq/L/15 min)	0.6
[133]Xe tomography (400MBq/L/90 sec)	0.6
[99m]Tc First Pass (750MBq)	7.5
[123]I IMP (150MBq)	5.8
[99m]Tc HMPAO (740MBq)	12.4
[18]F DG (175MBq)	3.8
Xe CT (5 points per curve)	17.5

(After Ell *et al.* 1987.)

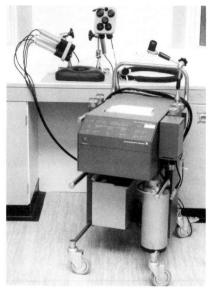

Fig. 4.8. Device to hold up to 10 detectors whilst measuring xenon wash-out.

simultaneous measurements using microspheres in dogs (Heikkila *et al.* 1983).

The average blood/whole-brain partition coefficient for xenon is 1.15 in subjects who are not anaemic; the coefficient for normal grey matter is 0.8 and for white matter 1.5 (Veall and Mallett 1965*a*). Different values should be employed in the presence of anaemia, depending on its severity, and in the presence of hyperlipidaemia. The larger the number of detectors employed, the better the information which can be obtained about regional differences in blood-flow, though at the cost of an increased absorbed radiation dose (Table 4.II), as each detector will be smaller and look at a smaller volume of brain; in order to obtain adequate statistics a larger quantity of tracer must therefore be administered.

This method may be performed using a pair of detectors with simple cylindrical collimators to give hemispheric information, a 'helmet' of detectors (Fig. 4.8) to give regional information (Lassen and Ingvar 1972) or a gamma-camera (Guldberg *et al.* 1977). There are a number of practical and theoretical disadvantages, in particular the requirement for an intra-arterial injection and the assumption that the partition coefficients are constant. This is approximately correct in normal brain, but is invalid in pathological areas (O'Brien and Veall 1974, van Duyl and Volkers 1980, Meyer *et al.* 1981). Moreover the separation of the experimental curve into fast and slow components does not yield a single unambiguous solution, but depends upon the section of the curve taken (Zierler 1965). The distinction is fairly straightforward in normal subjects, in whom flow through grey matter is much higher than through the other compartments. However, as grey-matter flow falls and the difference between the compartments decreases, 'curve stripping' becomes progressively more inaccurate (Herholz *et al.* 1983).

91

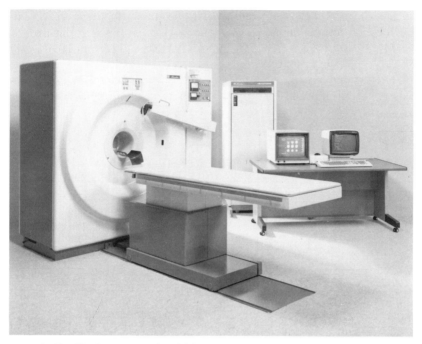

Fig. 4.9. The Headtome, a modern high resolution single photon tomographic scanner (courtesy of Shimatzu Corporation).

Inhalation or intravenous methods

An alternative method eliminating the need for intra-arterial injection was introduced by Mallett and Veall (1965) and further developed by Obrist *et al.* (1967). The subject inspires from a closed circuit containing a soda-lime absorber (to prevent accumulation of carbon dioxide) and a reservoir filled with sufficient oxygen to supply the patient's needs during the period. A suitable activity of ^{133}xe (20MBq/l) is introduced into the circuit; after rebreathing for three or four minutes, an equilibrium is obtained such that the concentration of xenon in brain is thereafter more or less constant. The closed circuit is then broken and the subject allowed to inhale room air while exhaled xenon is collected in a suitable trap or vented to the exterior. As in the intra-arterial method, two or more (up to 20) detectors positioned over the head record the rate of wash-out. The half-time of wash-out is calculated for each detector as in the intra-arterial method, but it is necessary to correct for two factors:

1. Radiation originating from the respiratory tract which is scattered into the field of view of the brain detectors, and
2. Recirculation of isotope.

The latter may be corrected by a detector sampling the expired air and measuring the end-tidal radioactivity, which originates from recirculating activity from all parts of the body and reflects the concentration in the arterial blood returning to the brain (Veall and Mallett 1965*b*). The former is minimised by discarding points on the head curves before the end-tidal radioactivity has fallen to 20 per cent of its initial peak level. This usually takes less than one minute. However as the greatest distinction between fast and slow components is in the early part of the curve, this reduces the accuracy, especially when the perfusion is low (Obrist *et al.* 1975).

The simplest equipment consists of a pair of detectors, one positioned to view each hemisphere. Devices which hold up to 10 per hemisphere are positioned in parallel planar jigs or in a helmet-shaped holder (Lassen and Ingvar 1972). An additional detector continuously samples air drawn from the mouthpiece in order to construct the recirculation correction curve (Veall and Mallett 1965*b*), as the end expiratory concentration is assumed to be in equilibrium with the arterial concentration. The end-tidal PCO$_2$ can be measured using the same sample.

More detailed anatomical information can be obtained by multi-detector systems encircling the head (Fig. 4.9) (Stokely *et al.* 1980, Kanno *et al.* 1981) or a gamma-camera (Podreka *et al.* 1983). The former oscillate or rotate, making repeated measurements of wash-out six times per minute, viewed from multiple positions around the head. Perfusion (P$_{init}$) is calculated for each point using equation 16, as when using stationary detectors; the same corrections are made, although there are fewer points to each curve. Tomographic cross-sections showing the distribution of perfusion, not only in the cortex but throughout the depth of the brain, are then reconstructed using standard filtered back-projection algorithms (Celsis *et al.* 1981). Because only the slope of the curve is required and not the absolute quantity, the lack of an accurate attenuation correction does not invalidate the result, although the relatively small number of counts originating from deeper structures limits the useful spatial resolution to regions greater than 3cm in diameter (Rezai *et al.* 1988). The highest count-rates originate from the grey matter because it has a higher bloodflow and a higher solvency for xenon.

Compton-scattered radiation, which results from the incomplete absorption of some of the emitted gamma-radiation originating within the brain, tends to affect the white-matter curves to a greater extent than those from grey matter, leading to an overestimate of white-matter perfusion (Lassen 1985). There is a good correlation between the planar and tomographic methods (Schroeder *et al.* 1986). Although the data thus obtained substantially improve the information content of the examination, they are of limited clinical applicability because of the high cost of such dedicated equipment, which has no other application. In order to obtain an adequate count-rate, much greater concentrations of radioactivity are required (700 to 800MBq/l) than with the static technique.

Stable xenon
An alternative approach has been to measure the wash-in of stable xenon using sequential transmission CT scans (Gur *et al.* 1981; Meyer *et al.* 1981, 1984). The patient breathes a mixture of 35 per cent xenon and 65 per cent oxygen for seven or eight minutes, after an initial period on 100 per cent oxygen to eliminate as much nitrogen as possible. Higher concentrations of xenon produce anaesthesia: there is some variation in the threshold at which effects are experienced. Sequential scans are made during the wash-in rather than the wash-out period, and end-tidal xenon

concentration is monitored as a measure of the arterial xenon concentration. Because of considerations of radiation dose (Table 4.II), the number of scans is limited and the wash-in curve may contain only five points. This technique gives better anatomical definition than any of the radio-isotopic techniques and permits regional estimation of partition coefficient, thus eliminating one of the major defects of xenon wash-out techniques; the disadvantages are the high radiation dose (especially to the lens of the eye, which is one of the most radiation-sensitive tissues), the need for the patient to remain absolutely immobile throughout the examination, and the changes in the cerebral perfusion rate induced by the abnormally high oxygen concentration both during the initial period of N_2O wash-out and during the xenon build-up. Moreover a great deal of CT scanner time is required.

Tomographic methods
Tomography is a technique for obtaining images of sections or slices through the body not obtainable by more direct means. In its original and simplest form, an x-ray tube and film are rotated about an axis. Objects in the plane of the axis remain stationary relative to the film and appear sharp while those in other planes move relative to the film and so are blurred. The more modern and sophisticated approach is to obtain a series of planar projections around the patient and from these to compute the distribution within the body. Emission computed tomography (ECT), which produces cross-sectional images of the distribution of administered radioactivity, must be distinguished from transmission CT, in which an external source of x-rays is used to produce an image of the distribution of substances such as fat, water, air and bone which differ in their relative opacity to x-rays. Although the technology of detection is totally different, the images produced by MRI are finally created by an exactly equivalent process.

There are two forms of ECT. Single photon ECT (SPECT) employs conventional gamma-ray emitting radio-isotopes such as ^{99m}Tc, ^{123}I or ^{133}Xe. The data are collected either by a conventional gamma camera, programmed to rotate around the patient and to collect multiple projections, or specially designed equipment employing a large number of detectors, each fitted with a separate collimator which limits its field of view to a predetermined volume (Fig. 4.9). These latter devices usually have a better resolution and sensitivity than a gamma camera when used for tomography, but are more expensive and less versatile. Few departments at present perform sufficient tomographic studies to justify such expensive dedicated equipment. SPECT studies are usually only semi-quantitative. Although uptake in large organs can be estimated to within ±10 per cent (Kirkos *et al.* 1987), it is not yet possible to make an accurate correction on a pixel-by-pixel basis for:
(1) attenuation of the gamma-ray flux as it leaves the patient, because the probability that any single gamma-ray will fail to be detected is a complex function of its site of origin within the patient,
(2) redistribution of the tracer during the tomographic acquisition.

PET employs radio-isotopes which emit positrons rather than gamma-rays. Positrons are beta-particles which differ from most other beta-particles and from orbiting electrons by carrying a positive rather than a negative charge. They behave initially like other beta-particles, interacting with molecules in their immediate neighbourhood, until they are travelling slowly enough to interact with a conventional orbiting electron. The two charges cancel out and the combined mass is converted into energy. This appears in the form of a pair of gamma-ray photons, each of 511kev, which move in opposite directions (to conserve momentum) at the speed of light. These may be detected by positioning a pair of detectors, one on either side of the patient (or source), and accepting only those gamma-rays which are seen simultaneously in both. This eliminates the need for the lead-grid collimator which must be used with all single-photon devices if positional information is required, but reduces their sensitivity one or two orders of magnitude.

Modern PET cameras surround the patient with several thousand pairs of detectors. In principle every event should be timed to within an accuracy of 5 picoseconds if accidental coincidences are to be eliminated and the source of the coincidence-pair determined uniquely. This is not yet possible, so the images still contain background or 'noise' due to these accidentals, reducing both the contrast in the images and the accuracy of uptake measurements. Nevertheless PET has a number of attractions.

Because a pair of gamma-rays is always detected, to perform an accurate attenuation correction it is only necessary to measure the total thickness of the patient at that point. True quantitation is therefore possible. The 'physiological' elements carbon, oxygen and nitrogen have no gamma-ray emitting isotopes but do have the positron emitters ^{11}C, ^{15}O and ^{13}N. Other useful positron-emitting isotopes include ^{77}Kr, ^{18}F, ^{82}Rb and ^{68}Ga. The disadvantage is that all but the last two have very short half-lives and therefore require a nearby cyclotron as a source of the isotopes.

Microsphere analogues and SPECT
Although direct intra-arterial injection of microspheres labelled with different tracers has been used to demonstrate functional changes in CBF (Etani *et al.* 1983), this technique has little practical application. A number of techniques have been proposed employing soluble tracers which can be injected intravenously, have almost 100 per cent extraction on their first pass through the brain and remain *in situ* long enough for their distribution to be measured by tomography. The only positron-emitting tracer suggested, ^{13}N-labelled ammonia, has an extraction efficiency of approximately 50 per cent (Phelps *et al.* 1982), which is too low and thus does not have a linear relationship between uptake and flow; because there are better methods of measuring CBF with PET, this one is not widely used.

However, the concept has found favour for SPECT. A number of compounds have been developed (Holman *et al.* 1982, Blau 1985, Nowotnik *et al.* 1985), the common feature being their high lipid solubility; the two to have been most widely used are N-isopropyl-^{123}I-paraiodo-amphetamine (IMP) and ^{99m}Tc (d,l) hexamethyl propylene amine oxime (HMPAO). The mechanism of fixation is not established for any of these compounds. The rate of wash-out of IMP varies in different parts of the

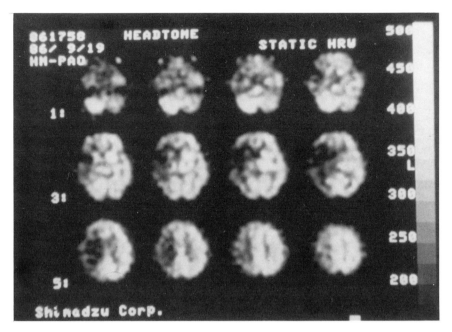

Fig. 4.10. Consecutive transaxial slices showing distribution of TcHMPAO in patient with right temporal cerebral infarction. (courtesy Shimatzu Corporation)

brain (Creutzig *et al.* 1986) and is slower than would be expected if diffusion were the only process involved. Uptake is non-saturable and is therefore not due to specific receptor binding (Winchell *et al.* 1980). It has been suggested that the difference in pH between the intracellular fluid (7.0) and blood (7.4) may be sufficient to allow IMP to polarise intracellularly and thus become lipophobic (Blau 1985), reducing the rate of egress. Thus although immediately after injection the distribution is largely a function of bloodflow and closely resembles the distribution of perfusion demonstrated by x-ray xenon-enhanced CT (Hellman *et al.* 1986), at later times the physiological significance of the distribution is ambiguous (Royal *et al.* 1985). Another disadvantage of IMP is the high cost of an adequate activity of [123]I.

HMPAO differs from IMP in a number of respects. There is now clear evidence that the distribution is not simply a function of bloodflow (Lucignani *et al.* 1990), although images obtained with the two compounds immediately after injection superficially appear similar (Leonard *et al.* 1986, Podreka *et al.* 1987) (Fig. 4.10). The labelled molecule is fairly unstable *in vitro* and must be administered within 15 minutes of preparation. *In vivo* as well as *in vitro*, the lipophilic form is fairly rapidly converted to an hydrophilic compound, but only the lipophilic species is taken up by brain (Ell *et al.* 1987). The actual uptake depends upon the fraction of the total administered technetium activity to reach the brain in lipophilic form. The relationship between HMPAO uptake and regional perfusion (rCBF) is not linear (Yonekura *et al.* 1988, Choksey *et al.* 1989).

96

Although the initial extraction by brain and fatty tissue is very high, the first-pass extraction by other tissues is lower and more variable: so there is a certain amount of recirculation. Because of the fairly rapid conversion of the lipophilic to the hydrophilic form, the cerebral distribution is (for 30 seconds or so after injection) principally a reflection of bloodflow, but other factors such as lipid mass and red-cell volume contribute. It has been suggested that retention is the consequence of intracellular conversion to a hydrophilic form which cannot diffuse out through the cell membrane. Glutathione may play an important part in this conversion, but as this is present in devitalised as well as viable tissues, HMPAO does not permit the distinction of viable from dead but perfused cerebral tissue. Unlike IMP, the distribution changes little with time. There is no satisfactory method of calculating the absolute perfusion, as there is no practical method of determining the amount of the active compound available to the brain for extraction or the local effective extraction efficiency. Nor is there an accurate method of making an attenuation correction for images obtained by SPECT. Various approximations adequate for imaging purposes have been proposed (Bailey *et al.* 1987), but they do not permit an accurate measurement of the absolute uptake. Indices such as the ratio of left-to-right or cortical-to-cerebellar count-rate have been employed (Lindegaard *et al.* 1986). The method is therefore only semi-quantitative, although it does give a useful pictorial representation which approximates to the regional distribution of perfusion to the grey matter.

A number of other technetium-labelled agents with a first-pass extraction efficiency close to 100 per cent, but more stable *in vitro* than HMPAO, such as ^{99m}Tc ethyl cysteinate dimer (ECD) have been described (Léveillé *et al.* 1988). Their role is not yet established, but they may be useful for autoradiography (see below). Constant infusion of the very short-lived gas ^{81m}Kr has also been employed (Fazio *et al.* 1980). The principle is identical to the continuous inhalation of $^{15}O_2$, but intra-arterial infusion is essential because there is negligible transpulmonary absorption of inhaled krypton.

Positron emission tomography
Three methods have been used to measure rCBF with PET. Inert gas wash-out using ^{77}Kr (Yamamoto *et al.* 1980), ^{11}c butanol or a variety of ^{18}F hydrocarbons makes use of the same principles as for single photon emitters (p. 94).

The continuous inhalation steady state method devised by Jones *et al.* (1976) for use with the older PET equipment, which was not capable of making images in rapid sequence, is a variant on this. ^{15}o-labelled water, which is assumed to be freely diffusible between blood and brain, is employed as the tracer. The patient inhales at a steady uniform rate air containing constant tracer quantities of carbon dioxide labelled with ^{15}O. PCO_2 must be maintained at a level which does not affect CBF. Because of the short half-life of ^{15}o (123 seconds), after a period of three to four half-lives (about 10 minutes) an equilibruim is reached such that the rate of arrival of labelled water at the brain is equal to the rate of loss by wash-out and radioactive decay. The concentration and distribution of radioactivity thereafter remain constant and a single image of the distribution at equilibrium may be

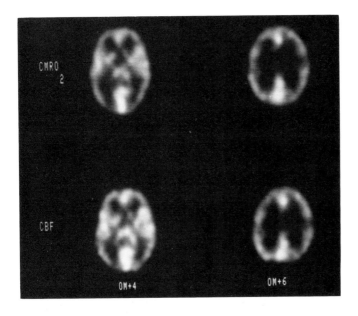

Fig. 4.11. Sections 4cm and 6cm above the orbito-meatal line: upper pair showing the regional metabolic rate for oxygen and the lower the rCBF (courtesy of Dr T. Jones).

obtained, taking as long as necessary to obtain adequate statistics (Fig. 4.11).

In the presence of carbonic anhydrase the conversion of carbon dioxide to carbonic acid is virtually instantaneous in the lungs; in consequence the oxygen in CO_2 is effectively in complete equilibrium with the oxygen in water. Perfusion is then given by the equation (Frakowiak *et al.* 1980).

$$P = \frac{D}{([H_2O]_a / [H_2O]_{brain}) - 1} \tag{17}$$

D is the radioactive decay constant for oxygen, $[H_2O]_a$ the arterial concentration of H_2O in an arterial blood sample, and $[H_2O]_{brain}$ the brain concentration measured by PET. Variations in the arterial input are not critical, provided they are correctly averaged over the entire period of the investigation (Meyer and Yamamoto 1984). Perfusion can therefore be estimated by measuring the concentration of ^{15}O-labelled water in a peripheral artery and the local amount of ^{15}O in the tissue. This technique gives lower values of rCBF than most other techniques because the assumption that water is freely diffusible is not wholly valid (Echling *et al.* 1974), and corrections must be made for residual intravascular radioactivity (Lammertsma *et al.* 1983), recirculation of water from other tissues and its rate of clearance from the body. Because of these effects the validity of this method for measuring brain bloodflow has been questioned (Bigler *et al.* 1981).

The relationship between flow and tissue-tracer concentration is linear only for a tracer with an infinitely short half-life, and falls off as the half-life of the radio-isotope increases. For oxygen the uptake is virtually flow-independent at flow-rates greater than approximately 100ml/min/100g (Huang *et al.* 1979). Nevertheless there is a good correlation between this method and intra-arterial microspheres in

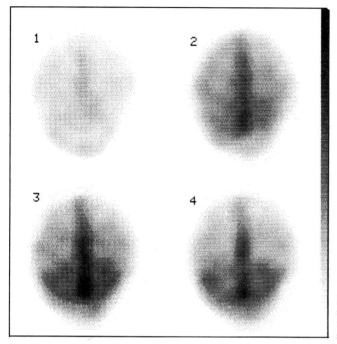

Fig. 4.12. Consecutive 0.5 second frames following rapid intravenous injection of sodium pertechnetate.

baboons for flows between 10 and 100ml/min/100g (Steinling *et al.* 1985). The method is therefore most useful for measuring low or normal flow rates with PET but may be misleading in those situations where the flow-rate is increased.

The third technique is an application of the principles of the original Kety/Schmidt quantitative autoradiographic method. ^{15}o water is usually employed as the tracer; ^{11}c-butanol is preferable because it is more freely diffusible, although any of the tracers used for inert gas wash-out would be suitable. PET provides the quantitative autoradiograph non-destructively (Herscovitch *et al.* 1983*a,b*; Raichle *et al.* 1983; Koeppe *et al.* 1985), but arterial blood sampling is still required and is a principal source of error (Iida *et al.* 1986), as the tracer content of small peripheral arteries differs appreciably in its time-course from that in the vessels supplying the brain. Further errors are due to variations in the time of arrival of the blood-borne radioactivity in different parts of the brain (Koeppe *et al.* 1987) and the finite time to obtain the tomographic image with even the fastest available PET scanners; some redistribution of the tracer occurs in this interval (Ter-Pogossian and Herscovitch 1985). Some modifications to this technique permit regional values of partition coefficient to be derived (Huang *et al.* 1982).

First-pass methods
Consecutive analogue images taken immediately after the intravenous injection of sodium pertechnetate reveal asymmetries of flow in almost two-thirds of patients with recent strokes, but also in up to a quarter of normal subjects (Rosenthall and Martin 1970, Moss *et al.* 1972). Digital recording (Fig. 4.12), combined with simple

indices such as an approximation to mean transit time (Oldendorf 1962), time of arrival, time to peak or modal transit time somewhat improves the sensitivity (Rowan *et al.* 1970, Bellina *et al.* 1980), as does measurement of interhemispheric differences in these parameters (Ahonen *et al.* 1981). Even so the overlap between normal and abnormal groups is such that these simple techniques are of limited clinical value. Only in patients with asymptomatic stenoses or transient ischaemic attacks is dynamic scintigraphy superior to CT (Buell *et al.* 1979).

More quantitative isotope methods derive ultimately from the concept of mean transit time (MTT) proposed by Stewart (1894) and subsequently refined by Hamilton *et al.* (1931). This is in effect a restatement of the definition of flow, which states that if a volume of blood (v) enters or leaves an organ or tissue in time (T), then flow (F) is given by:

$$F = v/T \tag{18}$$

When the tracer remains entirely intravascular, v is the blood volume. In the more general case, v_d is the volume of distribution of the particular tracer within the organ. This is the volume of blood containing the same amount of tracer as in the whole organ.

$$v_d = Q_t/C_{v(t)} \tag{19}$$

MTT (τ) is defined in equation 11 as the ratio of volume of distribution of the particular tracer in the organ or tissue to flow.

$$\tau = v_d/F \tag{11}$$

A formal proof of this relationship was subsequently provided by Meier and Zierler (1954). At the same flow, different tracers will have dissimilar transit times through an organ if their volumes of distribution differ, *e.g.* if they diffuse unequally out of the vascular bed or vary in protein binding. The physical meaning of MTT can be expressed in several ways which are exactly equivalent to each other and are equally valid. For a completely intravascular tracer the MTT may be considered either as the average time taken for a single particle or red cell to pass from the artery supplying an organ to the vein draining it; alternatively, it may be defined as the time in which the volume of blood entering or leaving the tissue under consideration is equal to the volume of blood actually in that tissue, *i.e.* the time required to replace the blood in the tissue once. For a tracer which does not remain intravascular, the equivalent volume (of distribution) rather than the actual blood volume is taken. The general equation for mean transit time (τ), which is true irrespective of the shape of the curve or the mathematical function which fits it, is

$$\tau = \Sigma_0^\infty c.t \, / \, \Sigma_0^\infty c \tag{20}$$

If the tracer remains wholly within the vascular bed, the transit time of blood can be calculated from the time-activity curve obtained from a region of interest following a rapid intravenous bolus. If the tracer has a larger volume of distribution, the transit time of that volume is obtained. These larger volumes of distribution are mathematical abstractions which do not correspond precisely to any anatomical region. It is therefore conceptually easier to use an intravascular tracer: though as the relationship between flow and transit time is valid for all tracers, different values of transit time will be obtained if tracers are employed which have different volumes of distribution.

It has been known for many years that if a small quantity of a tracer is added suddenly to a flowing stream of liquid, it becomes dispersed at a rate governed by a virtual coefficient of diffusivity into a progressively increasing volume, centred on a point which moves with the mean velocity of flow (Kinsman *et al.* 1929). Its concentration, measured in consecutive samples at any point downstream of the site of injection (Fig. 4.13), shows, after an interval which depends on the distance between the injection and sampling points, a rapid rise to a peak and then a rather slower fall which is terminated by a second slower and smaller rising phase due to recirculation. Cardiac output can be calculated from this curve; a correction for the recirculation (Fig. 4.14) is necessary because the tracer is usually not completely washed out of the region of interest before the leading edge of the returning bolus reappears. It is thus not possible to measure the complete first-pass curve directly. It was found empirically that the experimental curves could best be fitted by a complex power function known as a gamma variate (Thompson *et al.* 1964):

$$c(t) = \kappa(t-AT)^a\, e^{-(t-AT)/b} \tag{21}$$

κ is a simple constant of proportionality, a and b are other parameters. It should be noted that time, always measured from the same appearance time AT, appears twice: initially as a positive expression whose value increases to a fixed power function, and subsequently in a negative expression in which time is itself included in the power function. When the value of $(t-AT)$ is small the negative exponential which includes time is very small and the curve therefore rises. As $(t-AT)$ increases, the negative exponential component becomes the greater and the curve changes from a rising to a falling slope. Physiological changes can be correlated with alterations in the form of such curves (Klingensmith 1983).

To calculate MTT from equation 19 the entire first-pass curve is required, without any contribution from recirculation. In order to overcome this, for the first pass of a non-diffusible tracer, MTT can be approximated by the interval between the maximum rate of arrival, *i.e.* the maximum upslope, and the maximum rate of disappearance, *i.e.* the maximum downslope of this curve, identified from the first differential of the experimental curve (Oldendorf 1962). The former is the highest and the latter the lowest point of the differentiated curves. If this differential curve is differentiated a second time, the maxima and minima become the points at which this second differential curve crosses the zero line. Although Oldendorf did not do this, it is possible to solve the equation to find out the time interval represented by this difference.

In the case of the gamma-variate function this gives a value of 2b/a, while the true mean of this function is b(a + 1) (Newman *et al.* 1951, Thompson *et al.* 1964, Starmer and Clark 1970, Kuikka *et al.* 1974). This was subsequently applied to global and regional measurements of cerebral transit time (Kuikka *et al.* 1977, Szabo and Ritzl 1983). In practice, over the physiological range of transit times, the

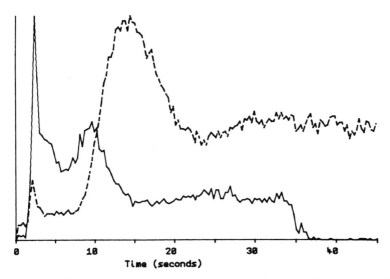

Fig. 4.13. Time/activity curves showing the first pass of a bolus of pertechnetate through the superior vena cava (*first peak*), aorta (*second peak*) and head (*dashed line*). The two curves are scaled individually.

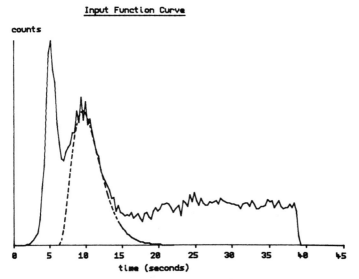

Fig. 4.14. Fitted aortic transit curve excluding both superior vena cava (SVC) activity and recirculation.

difference between 2b/a and b(a + 1) is usually small, although the former is consistently lower than the latter.

No physiological meaning was ascribed to the parameters a and b until Davenport (1983), using a model initially proposed by Kinsman *et al.* (1929) and elaborated by Newman *et al.* (1951), which considered the circulation as a series of mixing chambers, provided a derivation of the gamma variate function such that (a

+ 1) is the number of mixing chambers and b the mean time taken to empty each chamber. The product b(a + 1) is thus the mean transit time. Despite the artificial constraints in this derivation, it confirms that mean transit times are additive. Thus, to find the mean transit time through the brain, it is necessary only to measure that of an intravenous bolus as it passes through the head and subtract from this the MTT of the bolus entering the head, for example at the aortic arch (Merrick *et al.* 1991).

Methods for fitting gamma functions to experimental curves are well established (Starmer and Clark 1970). In order to obtain a valid fit to the experimental curves, enough of the first pass must be sufficiently discrete to be distinguished from recirculation. In the normal brain, pertechnetate remains almost entirely intravascular and is acceptable as a blood-pool marker (Bartolini *et al.* 1983, Keyeux and Ochrymowicz-Bemelmans 1983), although this does not remain true in pathological states, when albumin or some other non-diffusible tracer must be used. The MTT calculated at any point in the circulation is of course a summation of the effects of all parts of the circulation between the site of injection and the point of measurement. Thus even a perfect instantaneous bolus into a peripheral vein will have a finite transit time by the time it passes through the aorta, as a result of progressive dilution on passage through the heart and lungs.

The values of a and b can be calculated quite accurately, provided that any random errors (in particular those due to the stoichastic nature of radioactive decay) are uniformly distributed throughout the curve. One of the virtues of this technique, not shared by curve stripping or convolution, is that it produces a single unambiguous solution. MTT can alternatively be calculated from the first pass by a convolution method (Carpentier *et al.* 1982, Britton *et al.* 1985). This, although based on sound mathematical principles, suffers from the disadvantage that convolution is very susceptible to noise (Gamel *et al.* 1973); the data obtained under physiological conditions are very noisy. Convolution effectively involves multiplying two small numbers, *i.e.* the count-rate in the input artery and the count-rate over the brain. The noise in the resultant curve is substantial, and consequently the smallest region which can be examined is comparatively large. In contrast the methods used to fit a gamma variate to the experimental data have the effect of minimising noise present in the data. It is therefore possible to obtain an image by fitting a time-activity curve at each point over the head, and displaying the resultant matrix of transit times as a colour-coded image analogous to a map, each range of values being represented by a discrete colour (Fig. 4.15).

Calculation of bloodflow requires an estimate of the blood volume, in addition to MTT. Some authors (Klingensmith 1983) imply that the area under the first-pass curve is a function of blood volume. Others conclude that this area is a function of the fraction of the cardiac output reaching the volume under investigation (Sapirstein 1956, Mullani and Gould 1983), whilst a third school use the count-rate at equilibrium to estimate the blood volume with ^{11}co, ^{99m}Tc erythrocytes or ^{99m}Tc human serum albumen (Grubb *et al.* 1978), Britton *et al.* 1979, Knapp *et al.* 1986). The formula to calculate perfusion by xenon wash-out (equation 6) can in principle also be employed to measure perfusion from the first pass of a non-diffusible tracer (Lidner *et al.* 1980) by taking as the partition coefficient the fraction of the volume under investigation occupied by blood. Although the mean is 0.04ml/g, the actual value varies widely from region to region and in the same subject from time to time as the result of autoregulation (p. 107). This is thus an inaccurate technique for estimating perfusion (Lassen and Ingvar 1972).

A fall in perfusion pressure normally leads to cerebral vasodilatation, which maintains flow by reducing vascular resistance, but at the price of increasing the volume of blood in the affected region. This is known as autoregulation (Strandgaard and Paulson 1984). It has been shown that the ratio of flow to the volume of blood in the tissue is the most useful parameter in the presence of cerebral vascular disease, to determine the extent to which flow is being maintained at the expense of vasodilatation (Gibbs *et al*. 1984). This has been measured by separate consecutive assay of bloodflow and volume (Gibbs *et al*. 1984, Powers *et al*. 1984, Derlon *et al*. 1986, Knapp *et al*. 1986). However, when using an intravascular tracer:

$$\frac{F}{V} = \frac{(v/\tau)}{v} = \frac{1}{\tau} \tag{22}$$

The reciprocal of the transit time of a wholly intravascular tracer is thus the fraction of the blood in the volume of interest which is replaced per second, which may be termed fractional flow or fractional turnover (Fig. 4.16).

All first-pass techniques suffer from certain limitations. If the patient is suffering from any condition which tends to prolong the central circulation—a right-to-left or a left-to-right shunt, aortic or mitral stenosis or incompetence or low output failure, the first transit may be spread over such a long period that it cannot be clearly separated from recirculation. Under these circumstances this method is not applicable, although these reservations apply to only a very small minority of patients.

To perform this examination, the patient's head is positioned in front of a gamma camera fitted with a very high sensitivity collimator. A large-bore needle or cannula (18G for an adult, smaller for a child) is inserted into a large antecubital vein. The objective is to get the bolus into the superior vena cava as rapidly as possible; it is not possible to influence its behaviour beyond this point by the injection technique. However if the examination is performed with the patient supine, venous return is maximised and the transfer of activity from the superior vena cava to the right atrium accelerated. The radioactivity, in a volume of not more than 1ml, is injected into a short length of wide-bore tubing attached to the cannula and flushed by the rapid injection of an adequate volume, usually 10ml, of normal saline up the arm and into the superior vena cava. At the same time a scintillation detector fitted with a simple cylindrical collimator is positioned just inferior to the angle of Louis; thus directed along the aortic arch it records the count-rate at the entrance to the cerebral circulation. Two clearly separated peaks are usually distinguisable (Fig. 4.14), one due to activity passing through the superior vena cava and the other activity in the aorta. If the injection technique is adequate these should be clearly separated in time. Because of statistical limitations data from the small field gamma camera are acquired as a 32 × 32

104

matrix, at a rate of three frames per second for 60 seconds from the start of the injection.

The vertex projection gives the best over-all view of the cortex. However it is important to position the patient so that the rest of the body is not in the field of view of the camera, placing a lead collar around the neck, which must be as extended as possible, and over the shoulders to minimise scattered radiation from the trunk. If extension is not possible, the posterior or anterior projection can be employed, but under these circumstances the principal vascular territories of the brain are partially superimposed. The lateral view provides a good distinction between the various arterial territories but unfortunately does not permit the simultaneous evaluation of both sides. Moreover, there will always be a certain amount of 'breakthrough' of activity visualised from the contralateral side.

The arterial curve from the aortic arch is identified, a gamma variate fitted (Fig. 4.14) and the values of a and b derived, to calculate the MTT of the bolus as it reaches the arterial supply to the head (the input function). In theory it would be preferable to measure the transit time of the arterial input at the base of the brain. Hedlund *et al.* (1966) were sometimes able to distinguish carotid input from jugular venous output curves obtained from separate collimated detectors directed at the carotid and jugular foraminae.

However, they were only concerned to identify an incisura and did not attempt to fit the curves obtained. In our experience the curves are rarely sufficiently distinct distal to the arch even in children for a gamma variate to be fitted reliably to the input curve, because of the physical proximity of the carotid and jugular vessels and the overlap in time of the arterial and venous curves following intravenous injection. The error introduced by the use of the aortic arch is small because the distance between the two points is comparatively short and the vessels are of large diameter. It is essential, however, to correct for the difference between arrival time at the arch and at the head (equation 21).

The arrival time and first transit through the head are identified by plotting the activity in the whole head region against time. Frames are then summed in sets to give a total of 20, covering the whole of the first transit. Depending on the age and condition of the patient, actual frame duration varies between 0.3 and 3 seconds. The summation is necessary to obtain curves of adequate statistical quality; even so the maximum value in any single curve derived from the summed frames is usually less than 150 counts. The aortic probe, which needs only a simple cylindrical collimator, usually achieves higher count rates. Dead-time correction is important for both aortic and head curves, because losses as low as 10 per cent, by selectively reducing peak values, substantially increase calculated MTTs and thus systematically underestimate fractional flow in the areas of brain with higher rates of turnover.

This series of manipulations produces a 3D matrix of activity against time. The frames are summed to produce a single picture on which the outline of the head can be drawn, so that only pixels within the head are selected for analysis, thus saving time by eliminating pixels which contain only background. For each of the pixels of interest a time/activity curve is produced. The peak value is identified and a gamma variate fitted, starting from the first time point to reach 1 per cent of the peak value.

TABLE 4.III

Nett cerebral mean transit time in 102 normal subjects

| | Left | | Right | |
	Median	Range	Median	Range
Frontal	3.9	1.5–7.2	3.9	1.4–6.9
Antero-central	3.8	1.7–6.5	3.7	1.5–6.2
Postero-central	4.4	2.3–7.7	4.4	2.1–7.7
Occipital	5.6	3.0–12.7	5.8	2.9–12.1

TABLE 4.IV

Central neurotransmitter labels

Dopamine (D1)	^{11}C	Diazepam	Raynaud et al. 1975
		Imipramine	Raynaud et al. 1975
		Flunitrazepam	Comar et al. 1979
		Methyl imipramine	Denutte et al. 1983
		Ro15-1788	Mazière et al. 1983
		Ro15-3890	Halldin et al. 1988b
		Methoxydiazepam	Watkins et al. 1988
	^{18}F	Flurodopa	Garnett et al. 1983
	^{123}I	Ro16-0154	Hoell et al. 1988
		IBZP	Kung et al. 1988
		SCH 23982	Thonoor et al. 1988
(D2)	^{11}C	Spiperidol	Fowler et al. 1982
		Methyl spiperone	Wagner et al. 1983
		Eticlopride	Halldin et al. 1987
		YM-09151-2	Hatano et al. 1989
		Raclopride	Eriksson et al. 1988
	^{18}F	Haloperidol	Tewson et al. 1980
		Spiperidol	Zanzonico et al. 1983
		Pimizole	Baron et al. 1983
		Methyl piperidol	Arnett et al. 1986
		Ethyl fluroraclopride	Halldin et al. 1988a
	^{76}Br	Bromospiperone	Mazière et al. 1984
	^{77}Br	Bromospiperone	Crawley et al. 1986
	^{123}I	Spiperone	Mertens et al. 1987
		IBZM	Chiueh et al. 1988
Re-uptake blockers	^{18}F	GBR13119	Kilbourn et al. 1988
Serotonin (S2)	^{11}C	Ketanserin	Baron et al. 1985
		Methylketanserin	Frost et al. 1987
	^{125}I	Azido-IPAPP	Kung et al. 1987
Opiate	^{11}C	Carfentanil	Frost et al. 1985
		Diprenorphine	Lever et al. 1987
	^{18}F	Cyclofoxy	Carson et al. 1987
		Diprenorphine	Chesis and Welch 1988
Acetylcholine	^{11}C	Scopolamine	Frey et al. 1988
(Muscarinic)		TRB	Mulholland et al. 1988
	^{123}I	4-IQNB	Eckelman et al. 1982
Noradrenaline (α^{-1})	^{123}I	HEAT	Thomas et al. 1987
	^{125}I	DHTP	Efange et al. 1988
	^{11}C	Prazocin	Diksic and Jolly 1988
Histamine (H1)	^{11}C	Pyrilamine	Yanai et al. 1987
N-methyl-D-aspartate	^{18}F	MK801	Mukherjee et al. 1988
(glutamate)			Yang et al. 1988

The last point is determined by identifying the onset of recirculation. The values of a and b are calculated for each pixel, the calculated value of the input function subtracted and both the resultant value and its reciprocal are stored as new matrices. For the purposes of display the original 32×32 matrices are interpolated to 128×128 and displayed using a 20-level colour scale, each colour change calculated to represent a 5 per cent difference in fractional flow or a difference of 0.5 seconds in mean transit time (Figs. 4.15, 4.16).

The median values of MTT and fractional flow for various regions in normal adults are given in Table 4.III. The correlation with age is negligible compared with the normal variation at each age. There is a very strong linear relationship between PCO_2 and fractional flow. The median value of the mean transit time through the aortic arch is 5.8 seconds in normocapnic adults (range 3.5–8.0 seconds). This is much more strongly correlated with age, and in infants values of less than 2 seconds are normal.

Choice of method
Although similar normal global and regional values of perfusion are obtained by all recognised techniques (Table 4.IV), there is no ideal clinical method. The more invasive techniques are impractical in routine practice. Ultrasonic measurement of velocity is simple and painless, but does not always give the information relevant in paediatric patients (or for that matter in adult disease). Xenon inhalation has the advantage in paediatrics of eliminating the need for injections, but many younger children dislike wearing a closely fitting face-mask or mouthpiece, and a loose or poorly fitting one is useless, because escape of the tracer around the mask invalidates the examination. All tomographic methods (PET, SPECT, MRI and CT) require sufficient co-operation for complete immobility throughout the examination, a period which may be anything between five and 90 minutes depending on the technology used. The first-pass method is the simplest from this point of view, requiring immobility for only 30 seconds, but it does require access to a reasonably large vein for the injection, which can be a problem in children who have previously had many operations requiring multiple venous accesses. Moreover, this method gives a measure of perfusion reserves; bloodflow can be derived only if regional blood volume is also measured.

Autoregulation and reactivity
Under normal conditions the bloodflow to the brain remains unchanged over a wide range of arterial pressures. As the input pressure falls, the resistance vessels increase in calibre in an attempt to maintain flow by reducing the vascular resistance. This has the incidental effect of increasing the local blood volume, which can rise to double the mean resting value of 4g/100g/brain. However, once the vessels are fully dilated, no further adaptation can occur and there is thereafter a passive relationship between pressure and flow. Increasing the arterial pressure leads to vasoconstriction. This reflex regulation is impaired for a time following head injury, stroke and in brain tumours, the latter having morphologically abnormal blood vessels which are presumably incapable of responding to the usual

stimuli. The adequacy of cerebral autoregulation has hitherto usually been tested by determining whether there was any global or local change in perfusion on inducing hypotension (Tsuda *et al.* 1985, Voldby 1987). The extent to which cerebral perfusion is being maintained by autoregulation can be determined more easily by measurement of regional mean vascular transit time (p. 100).

Increasing the carbon-dioxide content of the inspired air to between 5 and 7 per cent causes a rise in bloodflow averaging 75 per cent, while a fall is associated with a corresponding decrease, the changes also being mediated through alterations in the vascular resistance of the brain (Kety and Schmidt 1948b). Following head injury and stroke, these responses are preserved much better than when there are changes in arterial pressure (Paulson 1971, Enevoldsen and Jensen 1978). The immediate stimulus is probably the pH of the extracellular fluid (Severinghaus 1965), a fall in PCO_2 causing vasodilatation, and a rise vasoconstriction. In hypercapnic states, as in hypotension, once there is maximal vasodilatation the compensation is abolished and a passive pressure/flow relationship ensues (Harper 1965). Correlations exist between arterial PCO_2, vascular resistance, blood pressure, age, sex and perfusion (Reivich 1964, Gündling *et al.* 1988), and there is a linear relationship between end-tidal PCO_2 and the vascular mean transit time, which increases by 1.4 seconds for each 1 per cent rise in end-tidal PCO_2 (Naylor *et al.* 1991). CBF also responds to changes in PO_2: inhaling 100 per cent oxygen reduces global perfusion by 13 per cent in normal adults, and decreasing the inspired oxygen concentration to 10 per cent has the effect of increasing bloodflow by 35 per cent. Acute hypoxia overrides the vasoconstrictive effect of hypocapnia (Kety and Schmidt 1948b). Perfusion increases in chronic hypoxia, partly because of an increase in the number and diameter of small bloodvessels—capillaries and arterioles (Mayer et al. 1985)—while the basal levels are reset in hypertension (Fujishima *et al.* 1983).

These observations provide the physiological basis for the clinical observation that in most conditions isolated measurements of CBF are of limited practical value (Teasdale and Mendelow 1981). They also form the basis of those tests of cerebral vascular reactivity which measure the fractional change in perfusion on voluntary hyperventilation (Tsuda *et al.* 1985) or induced hypercapnia, the results being expressed as the ratio of the percentage change in perfusion to the alteration in end-tidal or arterial PCO_2. Regions whose flow is being maintained by reflex vasodilatation exhibit a reduction in flow in response to hyperventilation sufficient to induce symptoms of ischaemia (Voldby 1987). No change in a region of low perfusion indicates irreversible changes such as infarction. This test does require active co-operation from the patient, who must be able to maintain a fairly constant level of hyperventilation for several minutes whilst the wash-out is performed.

In experimental animals limb weakness is observed when cerebral perfusion falls below 23ml/100g/min; electrical activity, as determined by EEG activity, ceases below 17ml/100g/min, and failure of the Na^+/K^+ pump (leading to cell death) occurs below 10ml/100g/min. These values vary little between species. There is a rather greater variation between different neurons in the same individual (Heiss 1983). Electrically quiescent but nevertheless viable brain can thus exist, especially adjacent to regions of infarction. The margin between cessation of electrical activity and death is quite narrow but clinically important; it can be identified as a region of increased blood volume and oxygen extraction ratio (Gibbs *et al.* 1984, Powers *et al.* 1984), and may account for the dramatic improvement sometimes observed clinically when blood pressure is restored (Astrup 1981).

In practice the circulation compensates until the conditions are so abnormal that there is a sudden catastrophic failure. The most sensitive index of the extent to which the circulation is being maintained by these mechanisms is the ratio of local bloodflow to blood volume (Gibbs *et al.* 1984). These parameters may be measured separately (Powers *et al.* 1984, Knapp *et al.* 1986). However it is evident from equation 22 that this ratio is the reciprocal of the vascular mean transit time measured by the first-pass method, which is thus the simplest available test of the extent to which autoregulation is occurring. Transit times longer than 11 seconds are associated with an increased oxygen extraction ratio, indicating that the limit of autoregulation has been reached (Levine 1986) and decompensation is imminent. Changes detectable on CT are a late event, occurring only after irreversible infarction of relatively large volumes of tissue (Lassen 1982).

Metabolism
Blood volume can be assayed by PET, with ^{11}co- or c^{15}o-labelled red cells (Phelps *et al.* 1982, Lammertsma *et al.* 1983). The shorter half-life of the latter permits sequential measurements of bloodflow, blood volume and oxygen extraction. The count-rate measured by PET is compared with a peripheral venous blood sample, after correcting for differences in the cerebral and peripheral venous haematocrit. ^{99m}Tc red cells have also been used (Britton *et al.* 1979). Because of the difficulty of adequate attenuation correction this is less accurate than PET and, although it is possible to obtain a reasonable estimate of hemispheric blood volume, the uncertainty increases as the volume defined becomes smaller. Estimation of blood volume on a pixel-by-pixel basis, even for planar parametric imaging, is thus impractical when using single-photon emitting tracers.

Oxygen extraction can be measured only by PET. Because there is no storage of oxygen, extraction is equal to utilisation. Techniques have been described using slow instruments (Jones *et al.* 1976) and fast ones (Mintun *et al.* 1984, Takagi *et al.* 1985). A normal distribution pattern has been described (Lenzi *et al.* 1978), upon which the various physiological or pathological changes are superimposed. Activities such as speech, auditory and visual stimuli and mental activities are associated with increased bloodflow and oxygen consumption in appropriate regions. Bloodflow and oxygen consumption are tightly coupled under most circumstances, and the product of bloodflow and oxygen extraction is the regional metabolic rate of oxygen.

Under normal basal conditions, oxidative metabolism of glucose is the only source of metabolic energy for the brain neurons. They do not store glucose, however, and the amount of energy obtained by glycolysis is small compared with that yielded by oxidation (Siesjö 1984). Therefore oxygen consumption normally alters according to extraction of glucose from the blood. With ischaemia and

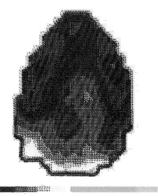

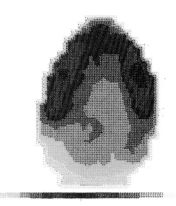

Fig. 4.15. Normal distribution of cortical transit times. The colour scale below the image goes from 0 to 10 seconds. Each shade represents a difference of 0.5 seconds.

Fig. 4.16. The fractional turnover rate or perfusion reserve is the reciprocal of transit time. In this case each shade delineates a difference of 5 per cent.

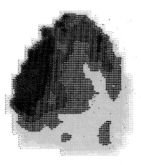

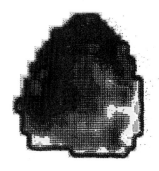

L   FRACTIONAL FLOW   R

L   NETT TRANSIT TIME   R

Fig. 4.17. Distribution of fractional flow (perfusion reserves, see Figure 4.18) following right middle cerebral artery stroke.

Fig. 4.18. Distribution of cortical transit times in nine-year-old girl following right middle cerebral artery stroke. No abnormality was visible on transmission computed tomography until 48 hours after this examination.

tumours this coupling of bloodflow, oxygen consumption and glucose extraction may be lost (Phelps *et al*. 1982). Glial cells are able to metabolise either aerobically or anaerobically, and their activity may be responsible for the 'luxury perfusion' and locally increased oxygen consumption observed after infarction.

Several analogues are used to study glucose metabolism. ^{14}c-2-deoxy-D-glucose (DG) is a competitive substrate of glucose which is transported across the cell membrane and phosphorylated to deoxyglucose-6-phosphate. The next step in metabolism, dephosphorylation, occurs only very slowly. A complex mathematical model has been established to permit the regional metabolic rate for glucose

(CMRGl) to be calculated from the regional concentration of ^{14}c (Sokoloff *et al.* 1977). The equivalent tracer for *in vivo* autoradiography is [^{18}F]-2-fluro-2-deoxy-D-glucose (FDG), the longer half-life of ^{18}F here being an advantage over ^{11}c because of the relatively slow blood-clearance of DG and FDG. The information obtained is similar in most situations to regional oxygen utilisation (Phelps *et al.* 1982) Glucose transport, as distinct from use, can be measured with ^{11}c-methylglucose (Feinende-gen *et al.* 1986). Analogous techniques have been developed using 1-^{11}c-L-leucine or ^{11}c-L-methionine to measure regional protein synthesis.

MRI spectroscopy, by measuring the amount of phosphorus compounds such as ATP, ADP and creatine phosphate, can give some information about the metabolic state of relatively large volumes of brain. Unfortunately the resolution is poor compared with PET, because the signal emitted by phosphorus is very weak compared with the hydrogen signal used for MRI, so that a much larger volume of tissue must be employed. There is no possibility of following the metabolism of any compound present in only trace or even milligram quantities with MRI. In contrast it is possible to measure and follow femtogram quantities of a tracer with PET, if it can be synthesised at a sufficiently high specific activity.

Receptors

At least a dozen neurotransmitters have been identified or postulated in the CNS, and many of them also have peripheral actions. There may be uptake by post-synaptic receptors and re-uptake by presynaptic receptors, which often have an inhibitory function, terminating the release of the transmitter. More than one type of receptor has been identified for many of the transmitters, on the basis of their reaction to a variety of pharmacological stimuli. Radiolabelled agonists or, in a few cases, antagonists of a number of receptor-binding compounds have been synthesised (Table 4.IV). Interpretation of the results is currently hampered by the lack of specificity of many of the available compounds for a single receptor, the absence of any adequate mathematical model of their behaviour, and the difficulty of distinguishing between specific saturable and non-specific non-saturable binding.

Few if any of these compounds are able to use specific transport mechanisms to pass from blood to brain. Initial uptake, especially of those which are lipophilic, is therefore strongly influenced by bloodflow. It may take several hours to distinguish specific from non-specific binding (Crawley *et al.* 1986), which limits the use of very short-lived radio-isotopes such as ^{11}c. The distribution of haloperidol (Tewson *et al.* 1980) is dependent on the specific activity, contrast between specific and non-specific sites decreasing as the total mass of compound administered increases, presumably because of saturation of the finite number of specific receptor sites. Differences have been observed between the distribution of tritiated and fluorinated compounds, which give rise to another problem, which is that the chemical form of the radioactivity cannot be assumed to have stayed the same (Tewson 1983). Tritium is particularly prone to exchange with ubiquitous hydrogen atoms.

There is no established clinical application. Differences in the quantity and distribution of some receptors have been reported at post-mortem examination in

Alzheimer-type dementia, Down's syndrome, schizophrenia and some forms of depressive illness. The role of dopamine in Parkinson's disease is better established. In most cases it is unclear whether the changes found, usually after many years of illness and drug teatment, are the cause or the result of the disease or its treatment.

Changes in disease states
Cerebral vascular disease is rare in childhood, but strokes are occasionally encountered. In 33 children, Gates *et al.* (1982) found dynamic scintigraphy had an accuracy of 94 per cent during the first week after a stroke, compared with a 60 per cent accuracy of CT during this period and 11 per cent for static scintigraphy. MTT and fractional flow images in a nine-year-old girl who had suffered a spontaneous right hemiplegia three days previously (Figs. 4.17, 4.18) showed much more extensively compromised cortex than was evident on the CT scan, in which only a small infarct was evident. However, both investigations are always necessary: CT to distinguish infarctive from haemorrhagic stroke, and transit-time measurement to determine the extent of compromised but potentially recoverable brain, and of regions which—although asymptomatic—are approaching the limits of their vascular reserves.

Diaschisis (change in bloodflow distant from sites of focal brain injury) can present in a number of ways: the cortex ipsilateral to a thalamic region (Metter *et al.* 1981), the thalamus ipsilateral to a cortical infarct (Kuhl *et al.* 1980), the hemisphere contralateral to a supratentorial infarct (Lenzi *et al.* 1982), the visual cortex distal to a lesion anywhere in the visual pathways (Phelps *et al.* 1981), or the contralateral cerebellar hemisphere following supratentorial infarcts in the carotid distribution (Baron *et al.* 1981, Lenzi *et al.* 1982). Crossed cerebellar diaschisis is also observed during the Wada test (internal carotid artery injection of 3mg/kg sodium amytal in order to lateralise speech dominance) (Biersack *et al.* 1987). The phenomenon may be associated with functional interruption of cerebral motor fibres (Graveline *et al.* 1988).

Measurement of perfusion or of metabolism is unnecessary in most patients with epilepsy, but is helpful in a selected minority of those with complex partial seizures either because the diagnosis is difficult to establish by more conventional methods or because the fits have proved refractory to medical management and surgery is contemplated. Interictally, foci of reduced glucose consumption may be identified, which correspond in position to the sites of slowed or abnormal EEG rhythms (Engel *et al.* 1982*a*). The majority of these have no corresponding CT or MRI abnormality (Phelps *et al.* 1988) although pathological examination of the excised specimen, when available, typically reveals lesions which are smaller than the metabolic defect (Engel *et al.* 1982*b*). Not all areas of reduced metabolism are epileptogenic, and there is no correlation between the magnitude of the metabolic and the electrical abnormalities; the significance of any individual lesion must be confirmed electro-encephalographically (Engel *et al.* 1982*c*). Perfusion is also reduced at these sites interictally (Kuhl *et al.* 1980), a finding which can be demonstrated using SPECT as well as PET (Magistretti *et al.* 1983). If the injection of

IMP or HMPAO, or inhalation of ^{133}xe, is made during a period of abnormal electrical activity, uptake or perfusion at the focus is increased rather than decreased (Bonte *et al.* 1982, Royal *et al.* 1985).

Relatively few data are available in other conditions. Following head injury, SPECT with HMPAO demonstrates more abnormalities than CT and shows them earlier (Abdel-Dayem *et al.* 1987). However it cannot demonstrate important abnormalities including fractures, foreign bodies and subdural collections. Its clinical role is not established. Bloodflow is reduced in the affected hemisphere during attacks of classical but not of common migraine (Lauritzen and Olesen 1984) and in the periventricular and centrally in the frontal regions in children with the so-called 'attention deficit disorder' (Henriksen *et al.* 1985). Mean transit times in children with acutely raised ICP correlate with the difference between measured and predicted CPP (Minns and Merrick 1989).

REFERENCES

Aaslid, R., Markwalder, T.-M., Nornes, H. (1982) 'Non-invasive transcranial Doppler ultrasound recordings of flow velocity in basal cerebral arteries.' *Journal of Neurosurgery*, **57**, 769–774.

Abdel-Dayem, H. M., Sadek, S. A., Kouris, K., Bahar, R. H., Higazi, I., Eriksson, S., Englesson, S. H., Berntman, L., Sigurdson, G. H., Fuad, M., Olivecrone, H. (1987) 'Changes in cerebral perfusion after acute head injury: comparison of CT with Tc-99m HM-PAO SPECT.' *Radiology*, **165**, 221–226.

Ahonen, A., Tolonen, U., Koskinen, M., Kallanranta, T., Hokkanen, E. (1981) 'Non-invasive external regional measurements of cerebral circulation time changes in supratentorial infarctions using pertechnetate.' *Stroke*, **12**, 437–444.

Anderson, B. J. (1957) 'Studies on the circulation in organic systems with applications to indicator methods.' *Transactions of the Royal Institute of Technology (Stockholm) Bulletin No. 101, Division of Mechanics*. pp. 1–19.

Arnett, C. D., Wolf, A. P., Shiue, C.-Y., Fowler, J. S., MacGregor, R. R., Christman, D. R., Smith, M. R. (1986) 'Improved delineation of human dopamine receptors using [^{18}F]-*N*-methylspiroperidol and PET.' *Journal of Nuclear Medicine*, **27**, 1878–1882.

Astrup, J., Siesjö, B. K., Symon, L. (1981) 'Thresholds to cerebral ischaemia–the ischaemic penumbra.' *Stroke*, **12**, 723–724.

Aukland, K., Bower, B. F., Berliner, B. W. (1964) 'Measurement of local blood flow with hydrogen gas.' *Circulation Research*, **14**, 164–187.

Axel, L., (1984) 'Blood flow effects in magnetic resonance imaging.' *American Journal of Radiology*, **143**, 1157–1166.

Bailey, D. L., Fulton, R. R., Meikle, S. R., Hutton, B. F. (1987) 'Attenuation correction equations for SPECT. *Journal of Nuclear Medicine*, **28**, 1925–1926.

Baron, J. C., Bousser, M. G., Comar, J., Soussaline, F., Castaigne, P. (1981) 'Non-invasive tomographic study of cerebral bloodflow and oxygen metabolism *in vivo*. Potentials, limitations and clinical applications in cerebral ischaemic disorders.' *European Neurology*, **20**, 273–284.

—— Roeda, D., Zarifian, E., Crouzel, C., Mestelan, G., Loo, H., Agid, Y. (1983) 'An in vivo study of the dopaminergic receptors in the brain of man using ^{11}C-pimozide and positron emission tomography.' *In* Magistretti, P. L. (Ed.) *Functional Radionuclide Imaging of the Brain*. New York: Raven Press. pp. 337–345.

—— Samson, Y., Crouzel, C., Berridge, M., Chretien, L., Deniker, P., Comar, D., Agid, Y. (1985) 'Pharmacologic studies in man with PET: an investigation using ^{11}C-labelled ketanserin, a 5-HT$_2$ receptor antagonist. *In* Hartmann, A., Hoyer, S. (Eds.) *Cerebral Blood Flow and Metabolism Measurement*. New York: Springer. pp. 471–480.

Bartolini, A., Leonardi, A., Albano, A., Primavera, A. (1983) 'Extravasation of pertechnetate in cranial extracerebral tissues during first pass across the cerebral vasculature.' *Bollettino della Società Italiana di Biologia Sperimentale*, **59**, 126–130.

Bassingthwaighte, J. B., Holloway, G. A. (1976) 'Estimation of blood flow with radioactive tracers.' *Seminars in Nuclear Medicine*, **6**, 141–161.

Bellina, C. R., Bottigli, U., Guzzardi, R., Voegelin, M. R., Donato, L. (1980) 'Interactive transit time imaging (ITTI) for improved cardiac and vascular studies in dynamic scintigraphy.' *Journal of Nuclear Medicine*, **24**, 201–207.

Betz, E., Ingvar, D. H., Lassen, N. A., Schmahl, F. W. (1966) 'Regional blood flow in the cerebral cortex measured simultaneously by heat and inert gas clearance.' *Acta Physiologica Scandinavica*, **67**, 1–9.

Biersack, H. J., Linke, D., Brassel, F., Reichmann, K., Kurthen, M., Durwen, H. F., Reuter, B. M., Wappenschmidt, J., Stefan, H. (1987) 'Technetium-99mHM-PAO brain SPECT in epileptic patients before and during unilateral hemispheric anaesthesia (Wada test): report of three cases.' *Journal of Nuclear Medicine*, **28**, 1763–1767.

Bigler, R. E., Kostick, J. A., Gillespie, J. R. (1981) 'Compartmental analysis of the steady-state distribution of $^{15}O_2$ and $H_2^{15}O$ in total body.' *Journal of Nuclear Medicine*, **22**, 959–965.

Blau, M. (1985) 'Radiotracers for functional brain imaging.' *Seminars in Nuclear Medicine*, **15**, 329–334.

Bogren, H. G., Underwood, S. R., Firmin, D. N., Mohiaddin, R. H., Klipstein, R. H., Rees, R. S. O., Longmore, D. B. (1988) 'Magnetic resonance velocity mapping in aortic dissection.' *British Journal of Radiology*, **61**, 456–462.

Bonte, F. J., Stokely, E. M., Devous, M. D. (1982) 'Single-photon tomographic study of regional cerebral blood flow in the seizure disorders.' *In* Raynaud, C. (Ed.) *Proceedings of the Third World Congress of Nuclear Medicine and Biology*. Oxford: Pergamon. pp. 127–130.

Bradley, W. E., Kortman, K. E., Burgoyne, B. (1986) 'Flowing cerebro-spinal fluid in normal and hydrocephalic states: appearance in M-R images.' *Radiology.* **159**, 611–616.

Britton, K. E., Granowska, M., Rutland, M., Lee, T. Y., Nimmon, C. C., Petrosino, I., Lumley, J. S. P. (1979) 'Non-invasive measurement of regional cerebral blood flow before and after microvascular surgery.' *In* Greenhalgh, R. M., Rose, F. C. (Eds.) *Progress in Stroke Research* 1. London: Pitman. pp. 307–318.

—— —— Nimmon, C. C., Horne, T. (1985) 'Cerebral blood flow in hypertensive patients with cerebrovascular disease: technique for measurement and effect of captopril.' *Nuclear Medicine Communications*, **6**, 251–261.

Buell, U., Kazner, E., Rath, M., Steinhoff, H., Kleinhans, E., Lanksch, W. (1979) 'Sensitivity of computed tomography and serial scintigraphy in cerebrovascular disease.' *Neuroradiology*, **131**, 393–398.

Carpentier, P., Lemaire, B., Sulman, C. (1982) 'A non-invasive determination of regional cerebral mean transit time, blood volume and blood flow with single photon emission computed tomography.' *In* Raynaud, C. (Ed.) *Proceedings of the Third World Congress of Nuclear Medicine and Biology*. Oxford: Pergamon. pp. 1727–1730.

Carson, R. E., Channing, M. A., Blasberg, R. G., Milletich, R. S., McManaway, M., Jacobs, G. I., Finn, R. D., Rice, K., Cohen, R. M., Larson, S. M. (1987) 'Effect of naloxone pre-loading on the model parameters of the opiate antagonist [^{18}F]-cyclofoxy.' *Journal of Nuclear Medicine*, **28**, 701P.

Celsis, P., Goldman, T., Henriksen, L., Lassen, N. A. (1981) 'A method for calculating regional cerebral blood flow from emission computed tomography of inert gas concentrations.' *Journal of Computer Assisted Tomography*, **5**, 641–645.

Chesis, P. L., Welch, M. J. (1988) 'Radiosynthesis of [F-18] fluroalkyl diprenorphine analogs for positron emission tomography studies of opiate receptors.' *Journal of Nuclear Medicine*, **29**, 930P.

Chiueh, C. C., Bruecke, T., Singhaniyom, W., McLellan, C., Tsai, Y. F., Cohen, R. M., Kung, H. F. (1988) 'Preclinical trial of a SPECT imaging ligand for denervation induced supersensitive D-2 dopamine receptors: I-123 labeled benzamide (IBZM).' *Journal of Nuclear Medicine*, **29**, 759P.

Choksey, M. S., Costa, D. C., Iannotti, F., Ell, P. J., Crockard, H. A. (1989) '99mTc-HMPAO SPECT and cerebral blood flow: a study of CO_2 reactivity.' *Nuclear Medicine Communications*, **10**, 609–618.

Cohn, J. D., del Guerico, L. R. M. (1967) 'Clinical applications of indicator dilution curves as gamma functions.' *Journal of Laboratory and Clinical Medicine*, **69**, 675–682.

Comar, D., Mazière, M., Godot, J. L., Berger, G., Soussaline, F., Menini, C., Arfel, G., Naquet, R. (1979) 'Visualisation of ^{11}C-flunitrazepam displacement in the brain of the live baboon.' *Nature*, **280**, 239–331.

Crawley, J. C. W., Crow, J. T., Johnstone, E. C., Oldland, S. R. D., Owen, F., Owens, D. G. C., Poulter, M., Smith, T., Veall, N., Zanelli, G. D. (1986) 'Dopamine D_2 receptors in schizophrenia studied *in vivo*.' *Lancet*, **2**, 224–225.

114

Crean, P. A., Pratt, T., Davies, G. J., Myers, M., Lavender, J. P., Maseri, A. (1986) 'The fractional distribution of the cardiac output in man using microspheres labelled with technetium 99^m.' *British Journal of Radiology*, **59**, 209–215.

Creutzig, H., Schober, O., Gielow, P., Friedrich, R., Becker, H., Dietz, H., Hundeshagen, H. (1986) 'Cerebral dynamics of *N*-isopropyl-(^{123}I)*p*-iodoamphetamine.' *Journal of Nuclear Medicine*, **27**, 178–183.

Davenport, R., (1983) 'The derivation of the gamma-variate relationship for tracer dilution curves.' *Journal of Nuclear Medicine*, **24**, 945–948.

Denutte, H., Goethals, P., Cattoir, H., Bogaert, M., Vandewalle, T., Vandercasteele, C., Jonckheere, J., de Leenheer, A. (1983) 'The production in high yield of *N'*-(4-[^{11}C]methyl)-imipramine.' *Journal of Nuclear Medicine*, **24**, 1185–1187.

Derlon, J.-M., Bouvard, G., Lechevalier, B., Dupuy, B., Maiza, D., Hubert, P., Courthéoux, P., Peres, J.-C., Houtteville, J.-P. (1986) 'Haemodynamic study of internal carotid artery stenosis and occlusion: value of combined isotopic measurements of regional cerebral blood flow and blood volume.' *Annals of Vascular Surgery*, **1**, 86–97.

Dischino, D. D., Welch, M. J., Kilbourn, M. R., Raichle, M. E. (1983) 'Relationship between lipophilicity and brain extraction of C-11-labelled radio-pharmaceuticals.' *Journal of Nuclear Medicine*, **24**, 1030–1038.

Diksic, M., Jolly, D. (1988) 'Synthesis of ^{11}C-labelled prazosin, an α-1 adrenoreceptor antagonist.' *Journal of Nuclear Medicine*, **29**, 930P.

van Duyl, W. A., Volkers, A. C. W. (1980) 'Measurement of cerebral blood flow in the pig by the Xe-133 clearance technique.' *European Journal of Nuclear Medicine*, **5**, 89–96.

Eckelman, W. C. (1982) 'Radiolabelled adrenergic and muscarinic blockers for in vivo studies.' *Receptor Binding Radiotracers*, **2**, 25–39.

Efange, S. M. N., Mash, D., Hefti, F., Kung, H., Heal, A. V., Guo, Y.-Z., Billings, J., Pan, S., Dutta, A. (1988) '[I-125]DHTP: a potential radiotracer for mapping central noradrenergic innervation.' *Journal of Nuclear Medicine*, **29**, 777P.

Eiching, J. O., Raichle, M. E., Grubb, R. L., Ter-Pogossian, M. M. (1974) 'Evidence of the limitations of water as a freely diffusible tracer in brain of the rhesus monkey.' *Circulation Research*, **35**, 358–364.

Ell, P. J., Jarritt, P. H., Costa, D. C., Callum, I. D., Lui, D. (1987) 'Functional imaging of the brain.' *Seminars in Nuclear Medicine*, **17**, 214–229.

Enevoldsen, E. M., Jensen, F. T. (1978) 'Autoregulation and CO_2 responses of cerebral blood flow in patients with acute severe head injury.' *Journal of Neurosurgery*, **48**, 689–703.

Engel, J., Kuhl, D. E., Phelps, M. E., Crandall, P. J. (1982*a*) 'Comparative localisation of the epileptic foci in partial complex epilepsy by PCT and EEG.' *Annals of Neurology*, **12**, 529–537.

—— Brown, W. J., Kuhl, D. E., Phelps, M. E., Mazziotta, J. C., Crandall, P. H. (1982*b*) 'Pathological findings underlying focal temporal lobe hypometabolism in partial epilepsy.' *Annals of Neurology*, **12**, 518–528.

—— Engel, J., Kuhl, D. E., Phelps, M. E., Mazziotta, J. C. (1982*c*) 'Interictal cerebral glucose metabolism in partial epilepsy and its relation to EEG changes.' *Annals of Neurology*, **12**, 510–517.

Eriksson, L., Farde, L., Blomquist, G. (1988) 'Kinetic analysis of 11C-raclopride binding to central D2-dopamine receptors.' *Journal of Nuclear Medicine*, **29**, 820P.

Etani, H., Kimura, K., Yoneda, S., Tsuda, Y., Isaka, Y., Asai, T., Nakamura, M., Fukungaga, R., Abe, H. (1983) 'Cerebral perfusion imaging with dual tracer (Tc-99m and In-111) HAM scintigraphy: application for mapping of cerebral function.' *Journal of Cerebral Blood Flow and Metabolism*, **3** (Suppl. 1), 138.

Fazio, F., Fieschi, C., Collice, M., Nardini, M., Banfi, F., Possa, M., Spinelli, F. (1980) 'Tomographic assessment of cerebral perfusion using a single-photon emitter (krypton 81m) and a rotating gamma camera.' *Journal of Nuclear Medicine*, **21**, 1139–1145.

Feinendegen, L. E., Herzog, H., Wieler, H., Patton, D. D., Schmidt, A. (1986) 'Glucose transport and utilisation in the human brain: model using carbon-11 methylglucose and positron emission tomography.' *Journal of Nuclear Medicine*, **27**, 1867–1877.

Fick, A. (1870) 'Über die Messung des Blutquantums in der Herzventrikeln.' *Verhandlungen der Physikalisch-Medizinischen Gesellschaft in Würzburg*, **2**, 16. (*Quoted in translation by* Hoff, H. E., Scott, H. J.) (1948) *New England Journal of Medicine*, **239**, 120–126.

Fowler, J. S., Arnett, C. D., Wolf, A. P., MacGregor, R. R., Norton, E. F., Findley, A. M. (1982) '^{11}C-spiroperidol: synthesis, specific activity determination and biodistribution in mice.' *Journal of Nuclear Medicine*, **23**, 437–445.

Frackowiak, R. S. J., Lenzi, G.-L., Jones, T., Heather, J. D. (1980) 'Quantitative measurement of regional cerebral blood flow and oxygen metabolism in man using ^{15}O and positron emission tomography: theory, procedure, and normal values.' *Journal of Computer Assisted Tomography*, **4**, 727–736.

Frey, K. A., Koeppe, R. A., Mulholland, G. K., Jewett, D. M., Hichwa, R. D. Agranoff, B. W., Kuhl, D. E. (1988) 'Muscarinic receptor imaging in human brain using [C-11]scopolamine and positron emission tomography.' *Journal of Nuclear Medicine*, **29**, 808P.

Frost, J. J., Wagner, H. N., Dannals, R. F. (1985) 'Imaging opiate receptors in the human brain by positron tomography.' *Journal of Computer Assisted Tomography*, **9**, 231–235.

—— Dannals, R. F., Mayberg, H. S., Links, J. M., Ravert, H. T., Kuhar, M. J., Wagner, H. N. (1987) 'Regional localisation of serotonin-2 receptors in man using C-11-*N*-methylketanserin (NMKET) and PET.' *Journal of Nuclear Medicine*, **28**, 600P.

Fujishima, M., Sadoshima, S., Ogata, J., Yoshida, F., Ibayashi, S., Shiokawa, O., Omae, T. (1983) 'Autoregulation of cerebral blood flow during development of spontaneous hypertension.' *Journal of Cerebral Blood Flow and Metabolism*, **3**, Suppl. 1. S668–669.

Gamel, J., Rousseau, W. F., Katholi, C. R., Mesel, E. (1973) 'Pitfalls in digital computation of the impulse response of vascular beds from indicator-dilution curves.' *Circulation Research*, **32**, 516–523.

Garnett, E. S., Firnau, G., Nahmias, C. (1983) 'Dopamine visualised in the basal ganglia of living man.' *Nature*, **305**, 137–138.

Gates, G. F., Fishman, L. S., Segall, H. D. (1982) 'Assessment of cerebral perfusion in childhood strokes.' *Clinical Nuclear Medicine*, **7**, 502–511.

Gibbs, J. M., Wise, R. J. S., Leenders, K. L., Jones, T. (1984) 'Evaluation of cerebral perfusion reserves in patients with carotid artery occlusion.' *Lancet*, **1**, 310–314.

Graveline, R., Soucy, J. P., Lamoureux, J., Lamoureux, F., Danais, S. (1988) 'Study of the anatomical distribution of primary lesions in crossed cerebellar diaschisis (CCD) following acute cerebral infarction: use of Tc-99m hexamethyl propylene amine oxime (HMPAO) scintitomography.' *Journal of Nuclear Medicine*, **29**, 843P.

Grubb, R. L., Raichle, M. E., Higgins, C. S., Eichling, J. O. (1978) 'Measurement of regional cerebral blood volume by emission tomography.' *Annals of Neurology*, **4**, 322–328.

Guldberg, C., Karle, A., Jørgensen P. B. (1977) 'Anger camera imaging of perfused and non-perfused brain tissue with intra-arterial ^{133}Xenon technique.' *European Journal of Nuclear Medicine*, **2**, 205–215.

Gündling, P., Haneder, J., Gaab, M. R. (1985) 'Correlation between CBF, PCO_2, pH, haemoglobin, blood pressure, age and sex.' *In* Hartmann, A., Hoyer, S. (Eds.) *Cerebral Blood Flow and Metabolism Measurement*. New York: Springer. pp. 51–55.

Gur, D., Yonas, H., Wolfson, S. K., Herbert, D., Kennedy, W. H., Drayer, B. P., Shabston, L. (1981) 'Xenon and iodine enhanced cerebral CT: a closer look.' *Stroke*, **12**, 573–578.

Häggendal, E., Nilsson, N. J., Norback, B. (1965) 'On the components of the Kr^{85} clearance curves from the brain of the dog.' *Acta Physiologica Scandinavica*, **66**, Suppl. 258.

Halldin, C., Stone-Elander, S., Farde, L., Sedvall, G. (1987) 'Synthesis of ^{11}C-labelled eticlopride, a new selective D_2-receptor ligand.' *Journal of Nuclear Medicine*, **28**, 625P.

—— Högberg, T., Stone-Elander, S., Farde, L., Hall, H., Printz, G., Solin, O., Sedvall, G. (1988*a*) 'Preparation of (ethyl-^{18}F) fluroraclopride for the *in vivo* study of dopamine D2 receptors using PET.' *Journal of Nuclear Medicine*, **29**, 767P.

—— Stone-Elander, S., Thorell, J-O., Persson, A., Sedvall, G. (1988*b*) '^{11}C-labelling of RO 15-1788 in two different positions and its main metabolite RO 15-3890 for PET studies of benzodiazepine receptors.' *Journal of Nuclear Medicine*, **29**, 931P.

Hamilton, W. F., Moore, J. W., Kinsman, J. M., Spurling, R. G. (1931) 'Studies on the circulation: IV. Further analysis of the injection method, and of changes in hemodynamics under physiological and pathological conditions.' *American Journal of Physiology*, **99**, 534–551.

Harper, A. M. (1965) 'The inter-relationship between $PaCO_2$ and blood pressure in the regulation of blood flow through the cerebral cortex.' *Acta Neurologica Scandinavica*, Suppl. 14, 94–103.

Hatano, K., Ishiwata, K., Kawashima, K., Hatazawa, J., Ito, M., Ido, T. (1989) 'D_2-dopamine receptor specific brain uptake of carbon-II labelled YM-09151-2.' *Journal of Nuclear Medicine*, **30**, 515–522.

Hedlund, S., Ljunggren, K., Kohler, V. (1966) 'Mean cerebral blood transit time obtained by external measurement of an intravenously injected tracer.' *Acta Radiologica Scandinavica*, **4**, 581–591.

Heikkilä, J., Kettunen, R., Ahonen, A. (1983) 'Comparison of the xenon-133 washout method with the microsphere method in dog brain perfusion studies.' *In* Raynaud, C. (Ed.) *Proceedings of the Third*

World Congress on Nuclear Medicine and Biology. Oxford: Pergamon Press. pp. 1752–1754.

Heiss, W. D. (1983) 'Flow thresholds of functional and morphological damage of brain tissue.' *Stroke*, **14**, 329–331.

Hellman, R. S., Collier, B. D., Tikofsky, R. S., Kilgore, D. P., Daniels, D. L., Haughton, V. M., Walsh, P. R., Cusick, J. F., Saxena, V. K., Palmer, D. W., Isitman, A. T. (1986) 'Comparison of single-photon tomography with [^{123}I] iodoamphetamine and xenon-enhanced computed tomography for assessing regional cerebral blood flow.' *Journal of Cerebral Blood Flow and Metabolism*, **6**, 747–755.

Henriksen, L., Lou, H., Bruhn, P. (1985) 'Focal frontal hypoperfusion in children with attention deficit disorder.' *In* Hartmann, A., Hoyer, S. (Eds.) *Cerebral Blood Flow and Metabolism Measurement*, New York: Springer. pp. 278–282.

Herholz, K., Heiss, W. D., Pawlik, G., Ilsen, H. W., Weinhard, K. (1983) 'Detection of compartmental slippage in noninvasive rCBF measurements.' *Journal of Nuclear Medicine*, **24**, 1188–1191.

Herscovitch, P., Martin, W. R. R., Raichle, M. E. (1983a) 'The measurement of regional cerebral blood flow with the classic autoradiographic technique and positron emission tomography: validation studies.' *Journal of Cerebral Blood Flow and Metabolism*, **3**, 95–96.

—— Markham, J., Raichle, M. E. (1983b) 'Brain blood flow measured with intravenous H$_2$^{15}O. 1: Theory and error analysis.' *Journal of Nuclear Medicine*, **24**, 782–789.

Heyman, M. A., Payne, B. D., Hoffman, J. E., Rudolph, A. M. (1977) 'Blood flow measurements with radionuclide-labelled particles.' *Progress in Cardiovascular Disease*, **20**, 55–79.

Hoell, K., Deisenhammer, E., Dauth, J., Loeffler, W., Carmann, H., Schubiger, A., Wagner-Jauregg, K. H. (1988) 'SPECT mapping of human brain benzodiazepine receptors.' *Journal of Nuclear Medicine*, **29**, 759P.

Holman, B. L., Hill, T. C., Magistretti, P. L. (1982) 'Brain imaging with emission computed tomography and radiolabeled amines.' *Investigative Radiology*, **17**, 206–215.

Hoyer, S. (1985) 'Metabolism of the human brain: the principle and limitation of global measurements.' *In* Hartmann, A., Hoyer, S. (Eds.) *Cerebral Blood Flow and Metabolism Measurement*. New York: Springer. pp. 382–390.

Huang, S. C., Phelps, M. E., Hoffman, E. J., Kuhl, D. E. (1979) 'A theoretical study of quantitative flow measurements with constant infusion of short-lived isotopes.' *Physics in Medicine and Biology*, **24**, 1151–1161.

—— Carson, R. E., Phelps, M. E. (1982) 'Measurement of local blood flow and distribution volume with short-lived isotopes: a general input method.' *Journal of Cerebral Blood Flow and Metabolism*, **2**, 99–108.

Iida, H., Kanno, I., Miura, S., Murakami, M., Takahashi, K., Uemura, K. (1986) 'Error analysis of a quantitative cerebral blood flow measurement using H$_2$^{15}O autoradiography and positron emission tomography, with respect to the dispersion of the input function.' *Journal of Cerebral Blood Flow and Metabolism*, **6**, 536–545.

Ingvar, D. H., Cronqvist, S., Ekbert, R., Risberg, J., Høedt-Rasmussen, K. (1965) 'Normal values of regional cerebral blood flow in man, including flow and weight estimates of gray and white matter.' *Acta Neurologica Scandinavica*, Suppl. **14**, 72–78.

—— Lassen, N. A. (1962) 'Regional blood flow of the cerebral cortex determined by Krypton-85.' *Acta Physiologica Scandinavica*, **54**, 325–338.

Jacquy, J., Gerebtzoff, A., Colard, M., Dekoninck, W. J. (1979) 'Assessment of cerebral blood flow by the electrical impedance method.' *In* Greenhalgh, R. M., Rose, F. C. (Eds.) *Progress in Stroke Research*. London: Pitman. pp. 301–306.

Jones, T., Chesler, D. A., Ter-Pogossian, M. M. (1976) 'The continuous inhalation of oxygen-15 for assessing regional oxygen extraction in the brain of man.' *British Journal of Radiology*, **49**, 339–343.

Kanno, I., Uemura, K., Miura, S., Miura, Y. (1981) 'Headtome: a hybrid emission tomograph for single photon and positron emission imaging of the brain.' *Journal of Computer Assisted Tomography*, **5**, 216–226.

Kety, S. S. (1960) 'Measurement of local blood flow by the exchange of an inert diffusible substance.' *Methods in Medical Research*, **8**, 222–238.

—— (1965) 'Observations on the validity of a two compartmental model of the cerebral circulation.' *Acta Neurologica Scandinavica*, Suppl. **14**, 85–87.

—— Landau, W. M., Freygang, W. H., Rowland, L. P., Sokolof, L. (1955) 'Estimation of regional circulation in the brain by the uptake of an inert gas.' *Federation Proceedings*, **14**, 85.

—— Schmidt, C. F. (1945) 'The determination of cerebral blood flow in man by the use of nitrous oxide in low concentrations.' *American Journal of Physiology*, **143**, 53–66.

117

—— —— (1948*a*) 'The nitrous oxide method for the quantitative determination of cerebral blood flow in man: theory, procedure and normal values.' *Journal of Clinical Investigation*, **27**, 476–483.

—— —— (1948*b*) 'The effects of altered arterial tensions of carbon dioxide and oxygen on cerebral blood flow and cerebral oxygen consumption of normal young men.' *Journal of Clinical Investigation*, **27**, 484–492.

Keyeux, A., Ochrymowicz-Bemelmans, D. (1983) 'Early behaviour of 99mTc-pertechnetate in the head after intravenous bolus injection: its relevance to the cerebral blood circulation.' *European Journal of Nuclear Medicine*, **8**, 196–200.

—— Laterre, C., Beckers, C. (1988) 'Resting and hypercapnic rCBF in patients with unilateral occlusive disease of the internal carotid artery.' *Journal of Nuclear Medicine*, **29**, 311–319.

Kilbourn, M. R., Haka, M. S., Ciliax, B. J., Kuhl, D. (1988) 'Synthesis and regional brain uptake of [F-18]GBR 13119, a dopamine uptake blocker.' *Journal of Nuclear Medicine*, **29**, 767P.

Kinsman, J. M., Moore, J. W., Hamilton, W. F. (1929) 'Studies on the circulation: 1: injection method: physical and mathematical considerations.' *American Journal of Physiology*, **89**, 322–331.

Kirkos, L. T., Carey, J. E., Keyes, J. W. (1987) 'Quantitative organ visualisation using SPECT.' *Journal of Nuclear Medicine*, **28**, 334–341.

Klingensmith, W. C. (1983) 'Regional blood flow with first circulation time-indicator curves: a simplified, physiologic method of interpretation.' *Radiology*, **149**, 281–286.

Knapp, W. H., von Kummer, R., Kübler, W. (1986) 'Imaging of cerebral blood flow to volume distribution using SPECT.' *Journal of Nuclear Medicine*, **27**, 465–470.

Koeppe, R. A., Holden, J. E., Ip, W. R. (1985) 'Performance comparison of parameter estimation techniques for the quantitation of local cerebral blood flow by dynamic positron computed tomography.' *Journal of Cerebral Blood Flow and Metabolism*, **5**, 224–234.

—— Hutchins, G. D., Rothley, J. M., Hichwa, R. D. (1987) 'Examination of assumptions for local cerebral blood flow studies in PET.' *Journal of Nuclear Medicine*, **28**, 1695–1703.

Kuhl, D. E., Phelps, M. E., Kowell, A. P., Mettler, E. J., Selin, C., Winter, J. (1980) 'Effects of stroke on local cerebral metabolism and perfusion—mapping by emission computed tomography of ^{18}FDG and ^{13}NH$_3$.' *Annals of Neurology*, **8**, 47–60.

Kuikka, J., Lehtovirta, P., Kuikka, E., Rekonen, A. (1974) 'Application of the modified gamma function to the calculation of cardiopulmonary blood pools in radiocardiography.' *Physics in Medicine and Biology*, **19**, 692–700.

—— Ahonen, A., Koivula, A., Kallantranta, T., Laitinen, J. (1977) 'An intravenous isotope method for measuring regional cerebral blood flow (rCBF) and volume (rCBV).' *Physics in Medicine and Biology*, **22**, 958–970.

Kung, H. F., Shih, J., Chumpradit, S., Guo, Y.-Z., Yang, W., Billings, J. (1987) 'Preparation of I-125 Azido IPAPP: an irreversible CNS serotonin receptor agonist.' *Journal of Nuclear Medicine*, **28**, 725P.

—— Alavi, A., Billings, J., Kung, M. P., Pan, S., Reilley, J. (1988) '[^{123}I] IBZP: a potential CNS D-1 dopamine receptor imaging agent: in vivo biodistribution in a monkey.' *Journal of Nuclear Medicine*, **29**, 758P.

Lammertsma, A., Wise, R., Heather, J., Rhodes, C., Gibbs, J., Jones, T. (1983) 'The correction for intravascular Oxygen-15 in the steady state technique for measuring regional oxygen extraction ratio.' *Journal of Cerebral Blood Flow and Metabolism*, **3**, Suppl. 1, S19–20.

Lassen, N. A. (1965) 'Blood flow of the cerebral cortex calculated from 85-krypton beta-clearance recorded over the exposed surface: evidence of inhomogeneity of flow.' *Acta Neurologica Scandinavica*, Suppl. 14, 24–28.

—— (1982) 'Incomplete cerebral infarction—focal incomplete ischaemic tissue necrosis not leading to emollision.' *Stroke*, **13**, 522–523.

—— (1985) 'Cerebral blood flow tomography with Xenon-133.' *Seminars in Nuclear Medicine*, **15**, 347–356.

—— Ingvar, D. H. (1972) 'Radioisotopic assessment of regional cerebral blood flow.' *Progress in Nuclear Medicine*, **1**, 376–409.

Lauritzen, M., Olesen, J. (1984) 'Regional cerebral blood flow during migraine attacks by xenon–133 inhalation and emission tomography.' *Brain*, **107**, 447–461.

Lenzi, G. L., Jones, T., McKenzie, C. G., Buckingham, P. D., Clark, J. C., Moss, S. (1978) 'Study of regional cerebral metabolism and blood flow relationships in man using the method of continuously inhaling oxygen–15 and oxygen-15-labelled carbon dioxide.' *Journal of Neurology, Neurosurgery, and Psychiatry*, **41**, 1–10.

—— Frackowiak, R. S., Jones, T. (1982) 'Cerebral oxygen metabolism and blood flow in human cerebral ischaemic infarction.' *Journal of Cerebral Blood Flow and Metabolism*, **2**, 321–335.

Leonard, J.-P., Nowotnik, D. P., Neirinckx, R. D. (1986) 'Technetium-99m-d,1-HM-PAO: a new radiopharmaceutical for imaging regional brain perfusion using SPECT—a comparison with iodine-123 HIPDM.' *Journal of Nuclear Medicine*, **27**, 1819–1823.

Léveillé, J., Demonceau, G., Rigo, P., De Roo, M., Taillefer, R., Burgess, B. A., Morgan, R. A., Walovitch, R. C. (1988) 'Brain tomographic imaging with Tc-9m-ethyl cysteinate dimer (Tc-ECD): a new stable brain perfusion agent.' *Journal of Nuclear Medicine*, **29**, 758P.

Lever, J. R., Dannals, R. F., Wilson, A. A., Ravert, H. T., Frost, J. J., Wagner, H. N. (1987) 'Radiosynthesis of carbon-11 labelled diprenorphine for positron emission tomography studies of opiate receptors.' *Journal of Nuclear Medicine*, **28**, 635P.

Levine, R. L. (1986) 'The study of cerebral ischaemic reversibility: part 1: A review of positron imaging studies.' *American Journal of Physiology: Imaging*, **1**, 54–58.

Lidner, P., Wolf, F., Schad, N. (1980) 'Assessment of regional blood flow by intravenous injection of 99m-technetium pertechnetate.' *European Journal of Nuclear Medicine*, **5**, 229–235.

Lindegaard, M. W., Skretting, A., Hager, B., Watne, K., Londegaard, K.-F. (1986) 'Cerebral and cerebellar uptake of ^{99m}Tc-(d,1)-hexamethyl-propyleneamine oxime (HM-PAO) in patients with brain tumour studied by single photon emission computerised tomography.' *European Journal of Nuclear Medicine*, **12**, 417–420.

Lucignani, G., Rossetti, C., Ferrario, P., Zecca, L., Guardi, M. C., Zito, F., Perani, D., Lenzi, G. L. (1990) 'In vivo metabolism and kinetics of ^{99m}Tc-HMPAO.' *European Journal of Nuclear Medicine*, **16**, 249–255.

Magistretti, P. L., Uren, R. F., Parker, J. A., Royal, H. D., Front, D., Kolodny, G. M. (1983) 'Monitoring of regional cerebral blood flow by single photon emission tomography of I123-n-isopropyl iodoamphetamine in epileptics.' *Annals of Radiology*, **26**, 68–71

Mallett, B. L., Veall, N. (1965) 'The measurement of regional cerebral clearance rates in man using Xenon-133 inhalation and extracranial recording.' *Clinical Science*, **29**, 179–191.

Mayer, H.-M., Fritschka, E., Cervòs-Navarro, J. (1985) 'Regional cerebral blood flow in experimental chronic hypoxic hypoxia.' *In* Hartmann, A., Hoyer, S. (Eds.) *Cerebral Blood Flow and Metabolism Measurement*. New York: Springer. pp. 498–503.

Mazière, M., Prenant, C., Sastre, J., Crouzel, M., Comar, D., Hantraye, P., Kaïsima, M, Grubert, P., Naquet, R. (1983) '^{11}C-RO 15 1788 et ^{11}C-flunitrazépam, deux coordinats pour l'étude par tomographie par positons des sites de liaisons des benzodiazépines.' *Comptes Rendus de l'Académie des Sciences de Paris*, **286**, 871–876.

—— Loc'h, C., Hantraye, H., Guillon, R., Duquesnoy, N., Soussaline, F., Naquet, R., Comar, D. (1984) '^{76}Br-bromospiperidol: a new tool for quantitative in vivo imaging of neuroleptic receptors.' *Life Sciences*, **35**, 1349–1356.

Mazoyer, B. M., Raynaud, C., Tzourio, N. Verrey, B., Chiron, C., Bussy, E., Dulac, O., Lassen, N., Bourguignon, M., Syrota, A. (1988) 'Error analysis of regional cerebral blood flow (rCBF) measured in children by SPECT with ^{133}Xe.' *Journal of Nuclear Medicine*, **29**, 869P.

Meier, P., Zierler, K. L. (1954) 'On the theory of the indicator-dilution method for measurement of blood flow and volume.' *Journal of Applied Physiology*, **6**, 731–744.

Merrick, M. V., Ferrington, C. M., Cowan, S. J. (1991) 'Parametric imaging of regional cerebral vascular reserves: 1. theory, validation and normal values.' *European Journal of Nuclear Medicine (in press)*.

Mertens, J., Terrière, D., Laysen, J., Ingles, M. (1987) 'NCA 4-1-123 (125)-spiperone, new high yield labelling coupled to *in vitro* and SPECT animal studies.' *Journal of Nuclear Medicine*, **28**, 570–571.

Metter, E. J., Wasterlain, C. G., Kuhl, D. E., Hanson, W. R., Phelps, M. E. (1981) '^{18}FDG-positron emission computed tomography: a study of aphasia.' *Annals of Neurology*, **10**, 173–183.

Meyer, E., Yamamoto, Y. L. (1984) 'The requirement for constant arterial radioactivity in the $C^{15}O_2$ steady-state blood-flow model.' *Journal of Nuclear Medicine*, **25**, 455–460.

Meyer, J. S., Hayman, A., Amano, T., Nakajima, S., Shaw, T., Lauzon, P., Derman, S., Karacan, I., Harati, Y. (1981) 'Mapping local blood flow of human brain by CT scanning during stable xenon inhalation.' *Stroke*, **12**, 426–436.

—— Okayasu, H., Tachibana, H., Takashi, O. (1984) 'Stable xenon CT CBF measurements in prevalent cerebrovascular disorders (stroke).' *Stroke*, **15**, 80–90.

Minns, R. A., Merrick, M. V. (1989) 'Cerebral perfusion pressure and nett cerebral mean transit time in childhood hydrocephalus.' *Journal of Pediatric Neuroscience*, **5**, 69–77.

Mintun, M. A., Raichle, M. E., Martin, W. R. W., Herscovitch, P. (1984) 'Brain oxygen utilisation measured with 0-15 radiotracers and positron emission tomogoraphy.' *Journal of Nuclear Medicine*, **25**, 177–187.

Moss, D. C., James, E., Strauss, H. W. (1972) 'Regional cerebral blood flow estimation in the diagnosis of cerebrovascular disease.' *Journal of Nuclear Medicine*, **13**, 135–141.

Mukherjee, J., Murphy, S. N., Hartwig, W., Miller, R. J., Cooper, M. D. (1988) 'N-(3-F-18 fluropropyl)MK 801: a PET tracer for *in-vivo* studies of N-methyl-D-aspartate receptors.' *Journal of Nuclear Medicine*, **29**, 932P.

Mulholland, G. K., Otto, C. A., Jewett, D. M., Kilbourn, M. R., Sherman, P. S., Koeppe, R. A., Wieland, D. M., Frey, K. A., Kuhl, D. E. (1988) 'Synthesis and preliminary evaluation of [C-11]-(+)-2α-tropanyl benzilate (C–11 TRB) as a ligand for the muscarinic receptor.' *Journal of Nuclear Medicine*, **29**, 932.

Mullani, N. A., Gould, K. (1983) 'First pass measurements of blood flow with external detectors.' *Journal of Nuclear Medicine*, **24**, 577–581.

Naylor, A. R., Merrick, M. V., Slattery, J., Notghi, A., Ferrington, C. M., Miller, J. D. (1991) 'Parametric imaging of regional cerebral vascular reserves: 2. Reproducibility, response to CO_2 and correlation with middle cerebral artery velocities.' *European Journal of Nuclear Medicine (in press)*.

Newman, E. V., Merrell, M., Genecin, A., Monge, C., Milnor, W. R., McKeever, W. P. (1951) 'The dye dilution method for describing the central circulation: an analysis of factors shaping the time-concentration curves.' *Circulation*, **4**, 735–746.

Nowotnik, D. P., Canning, L. R., Cumming, S. A., Harrison, R. C., Higley, B., Nechvatal, G., Pickett, R. D., Piper, I. M., Bayne, V. J., Forster, A. M., Weisner, P. S., Neirinckx, R. D., Volkert, W. A., Troutner, D. E., Holmes, R. A. (1985) 'Development of a $^{99}Tc^m$-labelled radiopharmaceutical for cerebral blood flow imaging.' *Nuclear Medicine Communications*, **6**, 499–506.

O'Brien, M. D., Veall, N. (1974) 'Partition coefficients between various brain tumours and blood for ^{133}Xe.' *Physics in Medicine and Biology*, **19**, 472–475.

Obrist, W. D., Thompson, H. K., King, C. H., Wang, H. S. (1967) 'Determination of regional cerebral blood flow by inhalation of 133-Xenon.' *Circulation Research*, **20**, 124–135.

—— —— Wang, H. S., Wilkinson, W. E. (1975) 'Regional cerebral blood flow estimated by $^{133}Xenon$ inhalation.' *Stroke*, **6**, 245–256.

—— Wilkinson, W. E. (1985) 'Stability and sensitivity of CBF indices in the non-invasive ^{133}Xe method.' *In* Hartmann, A., Hoyer, S. (Eds.) *Cerebral Blood Flow and Metabolism.* New York: Springer. pp. 30–36.

Oldendorf, W. H. (1962) 'Measurement of the mean transit time of cerebral circulation by external detection of an intravenously injected radioisotope.' *Journal of Nuclear Medicine*, **3**, 382–398.

Paulson, O. B. (1971) 'Cerebral apoplexy (stroke): pathogenesis, pathophysiology and therapy as illustrated by regional blood flow measurements in the brain.' *Stroke*, **2**, 327–360.

Phelps, M. E., Kuhl, D. E., Mazziotta, J. C. (1981) 'Metabolic mapping of the brain's response to visual stimulation: studies in humans.' *Science*, **211**, 1445–1448.

—— Mazziotta, J. C., Huang, S.-C. (1982) 'Study of cerebral function with positron computed tomography.' *Journal of Cerebral Blood Flow and Metabolism*, **2**, 113–162.

—— Chungani, H. T., Mazziotta, J. C., Shewman, D. A. (1987) 'Refractory neonatal seizures: use of PET in surgical selection.' *Journal of Nuclear Medicine*, **28**, 646P.

—— —— —— —— Peacock, W. J., Shields, W. D. (1988) 'The role of PET in pediatric epilepsy surgery.' *Journal of Nuclear Medicine*, **29**, 831P.

Podreka, I., Goldenberg, G., Binder, H., Roszuczky, A. (1983) 'Clinical reliability of noninvasive CBF measurements with the scintillation camera.' *Journal of Cerebral Blood Flow and Metabolism*, **3**, Suppl. 1, 45–46.

—— Suess, E., Goldenberg, M., Steiner, T., Brüke, T., Müller, Ch., Lang, W., Neirinckx, R. D., Deecke, L. (1987) 'Initial experience with technetium-99m HM-PAO brain SPECT.' *Journal of Nuclear Medicine*, **28**, 1657–1666.

Powers, W. J., Grubb, R. L., Raichle, M. E. (1984) 'Physiologic responses to focal cerebral ischaemia in humans.' *Annals of Neurology*, **16**, 546–552.

Raichle, M. E., Martin, W. R. W., Herscovitch, P., Mintun, M. A., Markham, J. (1983) 'Brain blood flow measured with intravenous $H_2^{15}O$. II. Implementation and validation.' *Journal of Nuclear Medicine*, **24**, 790–798.

Raynaud, C., Todd-Pokropek, A. E., Comar, D., Pizer, S. M., Kacperek, A., Mazière, M., Marazano, C., Kellershohn, C. (1975) 'A method for investigating regional variations of the cerebral uptake rate of ^{11}C-labelled psychotropic drugs in man.' *Dynamic Studies with Radioisotopes*. Vienna: International Atomic Energy Authority. pp. 45–59.

Reid, R. H., Gulenchyn, K. Y., Ballinger, J. R., Ventureyra, E. C. G. (1988) 'Clinical use of cerebral perfusion imaging with Tc-99m HMPAO in paediatric patients.' *Journal of Nuclear Medicine*, **29**, 919P.

Reivich, M. (1964) 'Arterial PCO_2 and cerebral haemodynamics.' *American Journal of Physiology*, **206**, 25–35.

Rezai, K., Kirchner, P. T., Armstrong, C., Ehrhardt, J. C., Heistad, D. (1988) 'Validation studies for brain blood flow assessment by radioxenon tomography.' *Journal of Nuclear Medicine*, **29**, 348–355.

Ridgway, J. P., Turnbull, L. W., Smith, M. A. (1987) 'Demonstration of pulsatile cerebrospinal fluid flow using magnetic resonance phase imaging.' *British Journal of Radiology*, **60**, 423–428.

Rosenthall, L., Martin, R. H. (1970) 'Cerebral transit of pertechnetate given intravenously.' *Radiology*, **94**, 521–527.

Rowan, J. O., Cross, J. N., Tedechi, G. M., Jennett, W. B. (1970) 'Limitations of circulation time in the diagnosis of intracranial disease.' *Journal of Neurology, Neurosurgery and Psychiatry*, **33**, 739–744.

Royal, H. D., Hill, T. C., Holman, B. L. (1985) 'Clinical brain imaging with isopropyl-iodoamphetamine and SPECT.' *Seminars in Nuclear Medicine*, **15**, 357–376.

Sapirstein, L. A. (1956) 'Fractionation of the cardiac output of rats with isotopic potassium.' *Circulation Research*, **4**, 680–692.

Schmidt, C. F., Kety, S. S., Pennes, H. H. (1945) 'The gaseous metabolism of the brain of the monkey.' *American Journal of Physiology*, **143**, 33–52.

Schroeder, T., Vorstrup, S., Lassen, N. A., Engell, H. C. (1986) 'Noninvasive Xenon-133 measurements of cerebral blood flow using stationary detectors compared with dynamic emission tomography.' *Journal of Cerebral Blood Flow and Metabolism*, **6**, 739–746.

von Schulthess, G. K., Higgins, C. B. (1985) 'Blood flow imaging with MR: spin-phase phenomena.' *Radiology*, **157**, 687–695.

Severinghaus, J. W. (1965) 'Role of cerebrospinal fluid pH in normalization of cerebral blood flow in chronic hypocapnia.' *Acta Neurologica Scandinavica,* Suppl. 14, 116–120.

Siesjö, B. K. (1984) 'Cerebral circulation and metabolism.' *Journal of Neurosurgery*, **60**, 883–908.

Sokoloff, L. (1976) 'Circulation and energy metabolism of the brain.' *In* Siegel, G. J., Albers, R. W., Katzman, R., Agranoff, B. W. (Eds.) *Basic Neurochemistry*. Boston: Little Brown. pp. 388–413.

Spencer, M. (Ed.) (1987) *Ultrasonic Diagnosis of Cerebrovascular Disease*. The Hague: Martinus Niehoff.

Starmer, C. F., Clark, D. O. (1970) 'Computer computations of cardiac output using the gamma function.' *Journal of Applied Physiology*, **28**, 219–220.

Steinling, M., Baron, J. C., Mazière, B., Lasjaunias, P., Loc'h, C., Cabanis, E. A., Guillon, B. (1985) 'Tomographic measurement of cerebral blood flow by the ^{68}Ga-labelled-microsphere and continuous-$C^{15}O_2$-inhalation methods.' *European Journal of Nuclear Medicine*, **11**, 29–32.

Stewart, G. N. (1894) 'Researches on the circulation time in organs and on the influences which affect it.' *Journal of Physiology*, **15**, 1–30.

Stokely, E. M., Sveinsdottir, E., Lassen, N. A., Rommer, P. (1980) 'A single photon dynamic computer assisted tomograph (DCAT) for imaging brain function in multiple cross sections.' *Journal of Computer Assisted Tomography*, **4**, 230–240.

Strandgaard, S., Paulson, O. B. (1984) 'Cerebral autoregulation.' *Stroke*, **15**, 413–416.

Swartz, B. E., Halgren, E., Ropchan, J., Mandelkern, M., Blahd, W. H. (1988) 'F-18 FDG PET scanning in frontal lobe epilepsy.' *Journal of Nuclear Medicine*, **29**, 831P.

Szabo, Z., Ritzl, F. (1983) 'Mean transit time image—a new method of analysing brain perfusion studies.' *European Journal of Nuclear Medicine*, **8**, 201–205.

Takagi, S., Ehara, K., Kenny, P. J., Gilson, A. J. (1985) 'Theory for non-invasive measurement of oxygen extraction fraction by intravenous bolus injection or bolus inhalation of 15-oxygen.' *In* Hartmann, A., Hoyer, S. (Eds.) *Cerebral Blood Flow and Metabolism Measurement*. New York: Springer. pp. 442–445.

Taylor, G. (1953) 'Dispersion of soluble matter in solvent flowing slowly through a tube.' *Proceedings of the Royal Society, A.*, **219**, 186–203.

Teasdale, G., Mendelow, D. (1981) 'Cerebral blood flow measurements in neurosurgery.' *Journal of Cerebral Blood Flow and Metabolism*, **1**, 357–359.

Ter-Pogossian, M. M., Herscovitch, P. (1985) 'Radioactive oxygen-15 in the study of cerebral blood flow, blood volume and oxygen metabolism.' *Seminars in Nuclear Medicine*, **15**, 377–392.

Tewson, T. J. (1983) 'Radiopharmaceuticals for receptor imaging.' *Journal of Nuclear Medicine*, **24**, 442–443.

—— Welch, M. J., Raichle, M. E. (1980) 'Preliminary studies with [^{18}F]-haloperidol: a radioligand for in vivo studies of the dopamine receptor.' *Brain Research*, **192**, 291–298.

Thomas, K. D., Greer, D. M., Couch, M. W., Williams, C. M. (1987) 'Radiation dosimetry of iodine-123 HEAT, an alpha-1 receptor imaging agent.' *Journal of Nuclear Medicine*, **28**, 1745–1750.

Thompson, H. K., Starmer, C. F., Whalen, R. E., McIntosh, H. D. (1964) 'Indicator transit time considered as a gamma variate.' *Circulation Research*, **14**, 502–515.

Thonoor, C. M., Couch, M. W., Greer, D. M., Thomas, K. D., Williams, C. M. (1988) 'Biological distribution and radiation dosimetry of radio-iodinated SCH 23982.' *Journal of Nuclear Medicine*, **29**, 803–804P.

Tsuda, Y., Kimura, K., Iwata, Y., Hayakawa, T., Etani, H., Asai, T., Nakamura, M., Yoneda, S., Abe, H. (1985) 'Effect of STA-MCA bypass on hemispheric CBF and CO_2 reactivity in patients with haemodynamic TIA's and watershed-zone infarctions.' *In* Hartmann, A., Hoyer, S. (Eds.) *Cerebral Blood Flow and Metabolism Measurement*. New York: Springer. pp. 23–29.

Veall, N., Mallett, B. L. (1965*a*) 'The partition of trace amounts of xenon between human blood and brain tissues at 37°C.' *Physics in Medicine and Biology*, **10**, 375–380.

—— —— (1965*b*) 'Regional cerebral blood flow determination by ^{133}Xe inhalation and external recording: the effect of arterial recirculation.' *Clinical Science*, **30**, 353–369.

Voldby, B. (1987) 'Alterations in vasomotor reactivity in subarachnoid haemorrhage.' *In* Wood, J. H. (Ed.) *Cerebral Blood Flow*. New York: McGraw Hill. pp. 402–412.

Wagner, H. N., Burns, H. D., Dannals, R. F., Wong, B. F., Langstrom, B., Duelfer, T., Frost, J. J., Ravert, H. T., Links, J. M., Rosenbloom, S. B., Lukas, S. E., Kramer, A. V., Kuhar, M. J. (1983) 'Imaging dopamine receptors in the human brain by positron tomography.' *Science*, **221**, 1264–1266.

Watkins, G. L., Jewett, D. M., Kilbourn, M. R. (1988) '3-[C-11]methoxybenzodiazepines: new radioligands for PET studies of benzodiazepine receptors.' *Journal of Nuclear Medicine*, **29**, 755P.

Winchell, H. S., Horst, W. D., Braun, L., Oldendorf, W. H., Hattner, R., Parker, H. (1980) 'N-isopropyl-[^{123}I]p-iodoamphetamine. Single pass brain uptake and washout: binding to brain synaptosomes and localisation in dog and monkey brain.' *Journal of Nuclear Medicine*, **21**, 947–952.

Yamamoto, Y. L., Meyer, E., Thompson, C., Feindel, W. (1980) '[77]Kr clearance technique for measurement of regional cerebral blood flow (rCBF) by positron emission tomography (PET).' *In* Kuhl, D. H. (Ed.) *Positron and Single Photon Emission Tomography*. New York: G. & T. Management.

Yang, D. J., Ciliax, B. J., Pirat, J.-L., Gildersleeve, D. L., van Dort, M. E., Young, A. B., Wieland, D. M. (1988) 'Mapping glutamate receptor channels: synthesis and auto-radiography of MK-801 analogs.' *Journal of Nuclear Medicine*, **29**, 930P.

Yipintsoi, T., Dobb, W. A., Scanlon, P. D. (1973) 'Regional distribution of diffusible tracers and carbonised microspheres in the left ventricle of isolated dog hearts.' *Circulation Research*, **33**, 573–587.

Yanai, K., Dannals, R. F., Wilson, A. A., Ravert, H. T., Scheffel, U., Tanada, S., Wagner, H. N. (1987) 'Synthesis and in vivo biodistribution of carbon-11 labelled pyrilamine, a potential histamine H-1 receptor tracer.' *Journal of Nuclear Medicine*, **28**, 624–625P.

Yonekura, Y., Nishizawa, S., Mukai, T., Fujita, T., Saji, H., Fukuyama, H., Ishikawa, M., Kikuchi, H., Konishi, K., Torizuka, K. (1988) 'Evaluation of Tc-99m HMPAO as a cerebral perfusion tracer with SPECT: comparison with cerebral blood flow measured with PET.' *Journal of Nuclear Medicine*, **29**, 843–844.

Young, W. (1980) 'H$_2$ clearance measurement of blood flow: a review of technique and polarographic principles.' *Stroke*, **11**, 552–564.

Zanzonico, P. B., Bigler, R. E., Schmall, B. (1983) 'Neuroleptic binding sites: specific labelling in mice with [^{18}F]-haloperidol, a potential tracer for positron emission tomography.' *Journal of Nuclear Medicine*, **24**, 408–416.

Zierler, K. L. (1962) 'Theoretical basis of indicator-dilution methods for measuring flow and volume.' *Circulation Research*, **10**, 393–407.

—— (1965) 'Equations for measuring blood flow by external monitoring of radioisotopes.' *Circulation Research*, **16**, 309–321.

5
INTRACRANIAL PRESSURE MONITORING–CURRENT METHODS

J. R. S. Leggate and R. A. Minns

Although intermittent measurements of ICP have been performed in patients for many years (Blackfan *et al.* 1929, Carmichael *et al.* 1937, Antoni 1946, Ryder *et al.* 1951), continuous ICP monitoring was not carried out as part of routine management of the neurological patient till more recently (Guillaume and Janny 1951, Lundberg 1960, Keegan and Evans 1962). The main indications for ICP monitoring remained the investigations of altered conscious level in those patients suffering from head injury, brain tumours, intracranial haemorrhage, acute encephalopathies or hydrocephalus. The place of ICP monitoring in anoxic-ischaemic injury to the brain is still the subject of debate. The principal sites of ICP monitoring remain the anterior fontanelle before its closure in the infant, the ventricular cavity, the subarachnoid space and the extradural space (Table 5.I). When continuous ICP monitoring is carried out, systemic blood pressure (SBP) must also be measured continuously so that CPP (mean SBP minus mean ICP) can be recorded.

Ventricular catheter
Continuous ICP monitoring became clinically useful in the early 1960s. The use of the ventricular catheter placed through a burrhole into the frontal horn of the right lateral ventricle linked by a fluid-filled coupling system to an external transducer became the gold standard against which all other ICP monitoring devices are assessed (Lundberg 1960). The main advantages of such a system are that it can be calibrated and zeroed to an external reference point whilst *in situ*. It allows CSF drainage to be carried out on a limited basis when the ICP remains high despite therapy. Dynamic studies, such as pressure-volume index (PVI) and dynamic and static outflow resistance (Ro) (Miller *et al.* 1973, 1977; Miller and Pickard 1974; Marmarou and Shulman 1976) can also be carried out through such a device, and in certain situations drug installation may be carried out through this catheter. The main disadvantages of such a system are that it requires puncture of the brain cortex. In addition there is a real risk of infection. In one large series, definite infections caused by ventricular fluid pressure (VFP) recording were found in 4.3 per cent of 540 patients. These were almost exclusively in patients on prolonged drainage of haemorrhagic fluid, and definite infections in other cases were found in 1.3 per cent (Sundbärg *et al.* 1988). In a further study of 255 patients from four institutions in one area, the presence of an ICP monitor with craniotomy was associated with an 11 per cent infection rate whereas craniotomy alone was associated with a 6 per cent infection rate. Infection in this series was twice as likely

TABLE 5.I

Sites for ICP monitoring

Ventricle	Catheter (percutaneous AF)
	Catheter (via burrhole)
	Reservoir
	Transducer (camino)
	Telemetry (± inline with shunt)
Subarachnoid (and	Bolt (Leeds, Richmond, Newell, Philadelphia)
subdural)	Catheter (cordis via burrhole)
	Catheter (teflon via AF)
	Transducer (catheter tipped-Gaeltec ICTb)
	Transducer (miniaturised, fitment to burrhole)
	Lumbar space (at LP or cannula)
Extradural	Catheter tip transducers
	Transducer (similar to subdural)
	Sensors (Ladd)
Brain parenchyma	Fibreoptic transducer (brain tissue pressure)
Fontanelle	Fontanometers (aplanation especially pneumatic)
Tympanic membrane	Impedance test of TM tension

in those patients with open trauma or haemorrhage (Aucoin *et al.* 1986). For cases of ICP monitoring only, the incidence of intracranial infection in experienced hands is 1 or 2 per cent (Langfitt 1973). Throughout the literature, the over-all incidence of infection from VFP monitoring is reported from less than 1 per cent to greater than 5 per cent. Obviously the infection rate is influenced by the number of times the system is opened, the duration of monitoring, and the possible use of prolonged steroids. The incidence of infection can be minimised by care with insertion of the ventricular catheter, and also by stabilising it by passing it through about 7cm of subgaleal tunnel before it emerges through the scalp wound.

A further disadvantage of VFP monitoring occurs in situations in which ICP monitoring is desired but may be difficult or impossible on account of the cerebral oedema and compression of the lateral ventricles. The risk of intracranial haemorrhage from ventricular puncture or from opening the dura is less than 1 per cent. Finally the method suffers from the major drawback of all fluid-coupled devices, namely that of dampening of the ICP waveform. This can be overcome to a certain extent by inserting devices such as the accudynamic tap* to optimise the dampening, but these devices have to be adjusted to suit the characteristics of each individual monitoring system.

Contra-indications to VFP monitoring include patients with bleeding diatheses or on anticoagulants or if there is a significant scalp infection. If trained medical and nursing personnel are not available to supervise the monitoring around the clock, it should not be undertaken.

Poor quality or false recordings may result from a defective or malfunctioning transducer or amplifier, or from the catheter coming out of the ventricle, or from excessive CSF drainage with consequent ventricular collapse and occlusion of the

---

*An adjustable damping device used to correct underdamping in fluid-filled catheter transducer systems to ensure an optimally damped flat frequency response. Manufactured by Abbott Critical Care Systems, Chicago, Illinois.

124

catheter. To prevent ventricular collapse it is important to lose as little CSF as possible during puncture, and the drainage manoeuvre should be performed against a positive pressure head of approximately 15mmHg in the older child or adult. False mean pressure readings may also be recorded when there is complete occlusion of the catheter, *e.g.* from being clogged with blood clot, brain tissue or fibrinous debris, or a kink or airbubble in the catheter. False pulse pressures may result from changes in the internal diameter (tolerance) of the catheter from partial blockage, kinking, or the use of distensible catheter material. False pressure recordings may be caused by priming the catheter to ensure that there are no airlocks, or by the infusion and extraction of fluid necessary for hydrodynamic calculations.

While most clinicians will use individually made-up sterile packs of the necessary equipment for VFP monitoring, a complete 'closed' system (Becker ICP system) is a commercially available sterile non-pyrogenic system for monitoring CSF pressure from either the lateral ventricle or the cerebral subarachnoid space. This system is compatible with electronic pressure-monitoring equipment or disposable transducers. The system comprises a ventricular catheter, a manifold with stopcocks and ports, and a CSF drainage bag with volumetric graduations.

The ideal pressure transducer

The *frequency response* is defined in terms of the frequency band over which the transducer system's gain does not vary by more than 3dB. For waveforms with a cardiac component (such as ICP), the frequency response should be flat up to about 30Hz.

If the pressure output from a transducer is plotted against the actual pressure, the deviation should be less than 1 per cent. This is the *linearity* and should therefore be within 1 per cent over the full scale working range.

If one measures the pressure with a transducer by coming up from zero, it may be a slightly different reading than that coming down from a higher pressure to the same pressure. This is the *hysteresis* and should be within 1 per cent.

The *thermal sensitivity* is the difference in recorded pressures for change in temperature. For arterial BP transducers, the temperature coefficient of sensitivity is 0.1 per cent per degree centigrade.

The *general sensitivity* is measured in μv/v/mmHg. If 10mmHg pressure is put in to the transducer representing so many microvolts, then the general sensitivity is the voltage output.

Methodology
Via burrhole
The burrhole is made through a 2.5cm incision just anterior to the coronal suture, in line with the pupil (or inner edge of the iris). After opening the dura and coagulating and incising the underlying pia, a Jefferson brain cannula is inserted into ventricle. The first pass is directed to the inner canthus of the ipsilateral eye. The second pass is directed to the bridge of the nose. The third pass is directed to the inner canthus of the contralateral eye. These landmarks can be palpated

through the drape. At no stage should the cannula be inserted to a depth of more than 6cm. No more than three passes should be attempted.

Via fontanelle
In children with a patent fontanelle, the ventricle may be cannulated percutaneously using the same landmarks.

A further modification which has been applied is to attach a *subcutaneous reservoir* to the end of the ventricular catheter and leave it as a permanent installation under the skin. This allows the ventricles to be accessed for monitoring and/or therapy on a long-term basis, and when repeated series of measurements are needed, *e.g.* in cases of hydrocephalus treated by shunting procedures (Leggate *et al.* 1988).

Rapid bedside technique for vfp monitoring
Where neurosurgical assistance is not available for the management of non-traumatic encephalopathies, then a bedside percutaneous technique for intraventricular catheter placement in children with fused cranial bones has been described (McWilliam and Stephenson 1984). This technique is performed when the child is paralysed, sedated and ventilated. The puncture site is a quarter of the distance from the nasion to the external occipital protuberance, 5cm from the midline. The skull and dura are perforated at right angles to the surface with a small bore (1.5mm diameter) disposable marrow-aspiration needle with a guard set at 5mm. A catheter (Leder-Cath, 8cm × 0.9mm diameter, Vygon) is then introduced and directed to a point 1cm ipsilateral to the midline and to the depth (equal to half the distance from the puncture site to a line between the ears) of the frontal horns. The catheter contains a guide wire which is bent at the proximal end (to prevent its advancement beyond the catheter tip) and marked along its length by a silk thread to indicate the maximum depth to be inserted. If difficulty is encountered in entering the ventricle, the catheter is fluid-coupled to a pressure transducer and an oscilloscope, to detect the maximum csf pulse signal, indicating that the catheter tip is in the ventricle.

Ventricular transducer
One solution to the disadvantage of using fluid-coupled systems is to place a pressure-sensitive transducer inside the ventricle. Such devices rely on a catheter tip transducer reflecting pressure alterations along either a fibre-optic coupling or along an electrical coupling to an external recording device. Whilst this has the advantages of a fast-frequency response combined with faithful reproduction of the true ventricular pressure waveform, it suffers from two main disadvantages. Such a system still requires brain puncture, with the associated risks of haemorrhage and/or infection, and currently zero checks and calibration cannot be carried out with such transducers in place. Furthermore, as mentioned above, cannulation of the ventricles may be difficult in certain circumstances. However these systems also appear to work when placed intra-parenchymally, and some may be deliberately placed there, to measure brain-tissue pressure, through the lumen of an 18 gauge

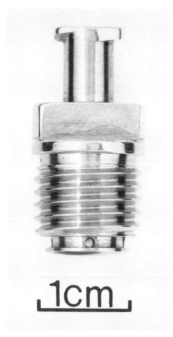

Fig. 5.1. Newell subarachnoid screw with side holes for communication with CSF. A finely tapered thread enables the screw to fit snugly into a burrhole. Luer connection for transducer or three-way tap.

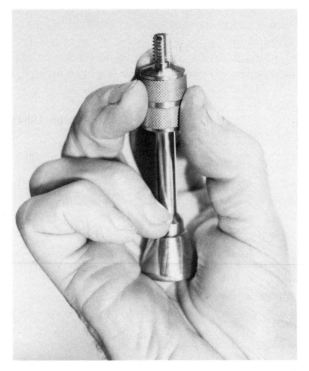

Fig. 5.2. Tapping device for trephining a burrhole of appropriate dimensions to accept the screw.

Teflon intravenous cannula (Ostrup *et al*. 1987). In certain circumstances placement of the Teflon IV Cannula through the patent anterior fontanelle into the brain parenchyma may be used to monitor ICP after removal of the stilette, by using a fluid-filled coupling to an external transducer.

Subarachnoid bolt

This popular device for monitoring ICP has frequently been employed as an alternative to the use of a ventricular catheter. There are many types available (Richmond, Leeds, Newell and Philadelphia) but the principle is the same in all of them (Fig. 5.1). A metal or plastic bolt is inserted through a burrhole which has already been threaded, using a tapping device (Fig. 5.2) to receive it. The dura mater is opened to enter the subarachnoid space. All bleeding is stopped. The bolt, which has a series of side holes or a terminal hole, enables the fluid-coupled system to link the subarachnoid space to an externally placed transducer. Its main advantage over the ventricular catheter is that it avoids the necessity for brain puncture. However, it has certain mechanical disadvantages. It may be difficult to seat the device in the thin skull of an infant and the Philadelphia bolt is contraindicated in children less than one year old. It is imperative to have no CSF leakage.

127

Successful recordings (reliable and low risk) were obtained using the subarachnoid screw in 92 per cent of 650 patients who were monitored for an average of five days (Winn *et al.* 1977). There is increasing evidence that at higher pressures the device tends to underread even when there is no leak of CSF: this fall-off in accuracy also appears to be related to the duration of the ICP recording. Because the subarachnoid space has been opened, there is as much risk of infection as with ventricular catheter methods and this has been assessed specifically for screws as 0.7 per cent (Winn *et al.* 1977).

Lumbar CSF space
In certain circumstances, *e.g.* after CT scanning or where the patient is fully conscious without neurological deficit, it may be safe to monitor ICP from the lumbar subarachnoid space. The safety and validity of this approach depends upon knowledge that there is communication throughout the craniospinal CSF axis and no mass present. In practice this means a full CT examination. The traditional method of using a manometer attached to the lumbar puncture needle provides a measurement of CSF pressure over too short a time and allows fluid displacements to occur and is, therefore, not desirable. By using an external pressure transducer coupled to the lumbar puncture needle, a non-displacement pressure recording can be achieved (Minns 1984, Minns and Engleman 1988, Minns *et al.* 1989). This can be carried out over a prolonged period by inserting a flexible catheter through the lumbar puncture needle into the subarachnoid space. The main advantage of this method is that it is easily performed; it suffers from the traditional disadvantages of a fluid-coupled system, however, and the lumbar CSF pressure does not always reflect the true ICP.

Methodology
With the patient in a lateral supine position, with the lumbar spine flexed, the iliac crest is palpated and the anterior superior iliac spine located. The line vertically joining the two spines lies over the L3/4 interspace. After preparing and draping the skin, a 23 gauge spinal needle is inserted into the subarachnoid space (local anaesthetic may be used but in our experience this is not always necessary). Either a prefilled manometer and, three-way tap is attached to the needle or a non-displacement transducer (Gaeltec) is attached directly onto the needle via a three-way tap for pressure monitoring.

Subdural catheter
The earliest ICP measurements from the subdural space involved the insertion of balloons or tambours in the subdural space, *e.g.* Hoppenstein's balloon (Rothballer 1963, Hoppenstein 1965). These were followed by more refined implantable switches (Numoto *et al.* 1966, 1969) and a pressure-indicating bag with a metal frame, which could correct for baseline shift (Numoto *et al.* 1973).

The subdural catheter method involves the placement of a silicon catheter through a burrhole into the subarachnoid space overlying the cortical surface. The main advantage over the subarachnoid bolt is its easy insertion, and in comparison it appears less likely than the subarachnoid bolt to underread ICPS above 30mmHg and less likely to obstruct. Once again, however, there are the disadvantages of infection and fluid coupling, and CSF may leak along the catheter tract when the ICP is very high. This can be minimised by tunnelling the catheter for some distance away from the incision site, before bringing it out through the skin.

Percutaneous placement of subdural or subarachnoid teflon catheters in neonates and small infants
Because of the frequency with which RICP occurs in the newborn, modalities for the ready measurement of ICP have been described which make use of the open fontanelle by percutaneous placement of teflon catheters in either the subdural or subarachnoid space. For subdural monitoring, the catheter (Quick-Cath) placement follows conventional subdural-tap procedures through the lateral angle of the anterior fontanelle and is connected to a monitoring system. This method is accurate, safe and easy to perform, and can be performed even when the fontanelle admits only one fingertip (Goitein and Amit 1982). The method for subarachnoid monitoring is similar. A 16 gauge Medicut (Sherwood Medical Industries) is inserted through the lateral margin of the anterior fontanelle on the right-hand side, in an anterior direction and aiming at a point 1cm above the right eye. After CSF is obtained, the needle is removed and a saline-primed round-ended polyethylene 16 gauge Portex epidural catheter is threaded through the cannula, to lie over the right frontal lobe. The cannula is then removed. The catheter is inserted to a maximum of 3cm from the scalp puncture and secured with a suture or tape (Levene and Evans 1983).

Subdural transducer
To overcome the disadvantages of the fluid coupling, it is possible to place the pressure monitor in the subdural space directly. Such devices are easy to insert through a burrhole after opening the dura and they avoid puncture of the brain. They have a fast-frequency response and reflect the true waveform of the ICP. Various types have been developed: Hulme and Cooper (1966) used a 3mm diameter pressure transducer in a stainless steel housing which fitted into a burrhole. For long-term continuous ICP monitoring, Richardson *et al.* (1970) employed a miniature pressure transducer with its casing vented to the exterior by nylon tubing. An inflatable compartment was added in front of the pressure-sensitive diaphragm.

The *Gaeltec ICTb transducer* incorporates a double-lumen tube with a silastic membrane covering the pressure sensor. It can be zeroed *in situ* using a null displacement reference, and can also be calibrated *in situ* by the application of back pressures of known magnitude. However, these devices tend to be fragile and require delicate handling. A failure rate of 25 per cent has been recorded. Some devices do not allow *in situ* calibration or zero checks to be carried out, and as a group they are expensive. Their use outside specialist centres is therefore limited. They give an accurate ICP value when correlated with ventricular catheter recordings, and they may be left *in situ* for long periods of recording (up to three weeks).

TABLE 5.II

Non-invasive ICP monitoring

Type	Reference	Method/principle
Oscillographic (tambours)	Purin (1964)	Tambours were originally applied directly to dura (Riechert and Heines 1950). Applied to AF, pressures measured via tambours were similiar to ventricular or lumbar CSF pressure
	Barashnev and Leontiev (1967)	Used similiar fontanometers in preterm and full-term babies with and without birth injury
	Picton-Warlow and Robinson (1970)	Investigated and discounted tambours as lacking scientific accuracy
	Wealthall and Smallwood (1974)	Investigated latex-covered tambours held by velcro over the AF and suggested they were only applicable to patients with large AFs
Tonometers	Davidoff and Chamlin (1959)	Adapted a schiotz tonometer to the AF
	Edwards (1974)	Specially adapted ICP tonometers with a spring-loaded outer ring which enabled readings by minimising head-movement artefact
	Wealthall and Smallwood (1974)	Investigated tonometers and considered them theoretically and practically inaccurate
Stethoscope	Blaauw *et al.* (1974)	Used stethoscope diaphragm with pulse pick-up to give qualitative information about fontanelle pulsations over one to three hours
Aplanation transducers	Wealthall and Smallwood (1974)	A pressure-sensitive plunger detects the pressure required to prevent a membrane from bulging into the centre of a guard ring surrounding the plunger. Hewlett Packard APT 16 transducer (expensive)
	Salmon *et al.* (1977)	Applied the above to clinical situation
	Robinson *et al.* (1977)	Refined the above instrument
	Whitelaw and Wright (1982)	Pneumatic aplanation, fixed to AF
	Kaiser and Whitelaw (1987)	Found a good correlation between values from pneumatic aplanation with CSF pressures
	Rochefort *et al.* (1987)	Variant of pneumatic aplanation in which a semiflexible thermoplastic was securely fixed to AF. Useful for continuous monitoring. Good correlation with CSF pressure ($p<0.001$) over one week. Separates pressure measurement from continuous gas flow
	Mehta *et al.* (1988)	A similiar pneumatic system consists of air supply, pressure gauge, and fontanometer
Pressure-activated fibreoptic sensor	Vidyasagar and Raju (1977) Donn and Philip (1978)	Ladd ICP monitoring device is based on optical principals: when the pressure acting on the contact surface of the sensor tilts a mirror, uneven reflection of light is fed back to the monitor. The monitor then balances the air pressure in the pneumatic tube to equalise the pressure on the transducer surface
Impedance method	Kast (1985)	This relies on tympanic membrane tension. CSF and perilymph communicate through cochlear aqueduct. RICP causes pressure on stapes foot plate, transmitted to TM by ossicles and detected by impedance testing
	Marchbanks *et al.* (1987)	Clinical application of the above

TABLE 5.III
Preferred method of monitoring ICP

	Ventricular dilatation	*Ventricles small/shifted*
AF open	1. Percutaneous AF puncture of ventricles *2. If repeated, use reservoir 3. Ventricular transducer	1. Percutaneous AF puncture with S/D or S/A catheter 2. Ventricular transducer (or brain-tissue pressure)
AF closed	*1. Insert reservoir	*1. Surface 'cordis' catheter 2. Ventricular catheter via marrow gauge needle puncture of skull and dura

*Requires neurological assistance.

Extradural monitors

To avoid the need of opening the dura, and thereby decreasing significantly both the rate and the severity of infection, transducers (some miniaturised) were developed in the late 1970s specifically for placement in the extradural space through a burrhole (Gobiet *et al.* 1974, Beks *et al.* 1977, Dietrich *et al.* 1977, Gaab *et al.* 1978). These devices are either transducers such as the Gaeltec system (Gaab *et al.* 1978) or sensors such as the Ladd and cardio-search pressure devices. The intracranial extradural transducers are identical to the subdural transducers. The main difficulty with recording from the extradural space is that the pressure recording can be significantly altered by the compliance of the dura (Dorsch and Symon 1975). Furthermore, sensors which rely in principle on a pleinum chamber* linked to an external air pump suffer from inherent problems of zero drift, temperature instability, slow-frequency response and difficulty with *in situ* calibration. In general, pressures observed by the extradural route appear to be 1 or 2mmHg higher than VFP at normal ICP, but at high ICP the extradural value is considerably higher (Coroneos *et al.* 1972, Gobiet *et al.* 1972, Jorgensen and Riishede 1972, Sundbarg and Nornes 1972).

Fontanometry

In neonates and infants, the presence of a patent anterior fontanelle acts as a window onto the intracranial contents and hence ICP. However, in practice accurate measurement of ICP has proved very difficult with fontanometry (Riechert and Heines 1950, Davidoff and Chamlin 1959). The principals used for measuring ICP by the anterior fontanelle consist of placement of a detector system mounted over the anterior fontanelle, the pulsations of which are picked up by the detector and either calibrated via a known pressure/deflection calibration curve, or by the application of a known back pressure through the detector to stop the pulsations leaving the anterior fontanelle in a plainer configuration to the detector system (Table 5.II).

*A trapped air or fluid volume chamber to enable movement of the sensor diaphragm to be reflected.

There is a need for reliable, continuous and routine non-invasive monitoring in the newborn and young infant who is at risk of developing RICP rather than one with known or established raised pressure, which we would consider an indication for direct monitoring (Table 5.III). The more recent types of *pneumatic aplanation* (Whitelaw and Wright 1982, Rochefort *et al.* 1987, Mehta *et al.* 1988) are more accurate and inexpensive and have overcome many of the coplanimetry problems by fixing a small plastic device to the anterior fontanelle (by collodion). They are useful for continuous surveillance of the infant at risk (which is their main indication), but still the recordings lack the accuracy of direct tracings. More importantly, we consider the pulse-pressure measurements from fontanometers to be inaccurate.

Using fontanometers, the normal full-term neonatal ICP via fontanometry has been demonstrated to be approximately 7.4mmHg (Peabody *et al.* 1977, Robinson *et al.* 1977, Salmon *et al.* 1977, Vidyasagar and Raju 1977). This ICP is substantially different from the normal range of neonatal lumbar CSF pressures, and this difference is almost certainly related to the mechanical difficulties of measurement.

Telemetric devices

A number of experimental telemetric devices have been developed in recent years, none of which has found its way into routine practice. There are advantages in a pressure-balanced radio-telemetry system for the measurement of ICP, which is incorporated in a ventricular shunt system. This system (Zervas *et al.* 1977, Cosman *et al.* 1979) is fully implantable, non-invasive, and can be placed in line with a shunt, or separately from it. It contains an electronically passive implant and can detect proximal shunt malfunction if placed in line. It is a rapid method of estimating ICP by a pressure-balanced telemetric method, and involves a radio antenna and cuff held over the implanted pressure sensor in the shunt system. It would be a useful outpatient check on the ICP of children with CSF shunts *in situ*. It is possible with this system to have an *in vivo* zero point calibration. When compared to simultaneous direct ICP measurements via a contralateral reservoir, there was a significant correlation between the two measurements (Minns and Shaw 1986). Theoretically it should allow exclusion of RICP in shunted patients with obscure symptoms. The disadvantages are that the measurement is a single instantaneous value and ICP recordings in shunted children should be prolonged and ideally overnight. Cosmetically the system is more obtrusive than a single shunt system, and an expensive removal of everything is necessary if infection (ventriculitis) occurs. Despite the over-all good correlation, the telesensor is less accurate at high ICP values. The length of the implant compared to the size of an infant's head means there is a lot of tunnelling necessary. In summary, the telesensor is less accurate when there is RICP than when ICP is in the normal range. Developments in this area are continuing.

ICP data collection and analysis

Continuous ICP monitoring by its nature generates large amounts of raw data, which must be interpreted with care by the clinician. Continuous chart recordings were at

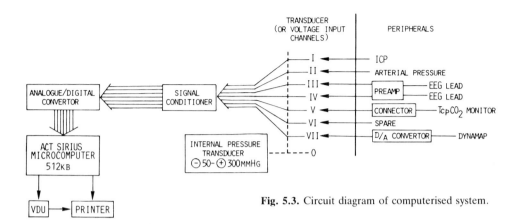

Fig. 5.3. Circuit diagram of computerised system.

first the most common form of data collection and enabled the display of pressure recordings to be quickly and easily visualised. While they are of tremendous help in the management of the individual child, it can be difficult to make objective measurements of over-all mean values, mean maximum pressures and opening pressures for accurate analysis, and frequently one had to resort to scrutinising the ICP trace to describe the different waveforms, or select several epochs of the record to manually measure the mean pressures. These laborious measurements are fraught with inaccuracies, particularly when correlations are attempted between two or more monitored parameters. For this reason, pressure waveform displays and pressure trend recordings have been used for the recognition of temporal trends in the ICP following pharmacologic interventions. More useful still, for later analysis of the recording, are pressure-frequency distributions on a histogram or frequency polygon (Kullberg 1972). A few attempts have been reported of computerised ICP monitoring (Schedl *et al.* 1983). A computerised neuromonitoring unit suitable for bedside use has been described (Gaab *et al.* 1985).

The following description is of a computerised monitoring system developed by Gaeltec specifically for our use in the paediatric neurology unit in Edinburgh, which is mobile but ordinarily housed in a neuro-intensive monitoring room.

Description of patient monitoring system

This unit comprises the circuitry to drive up to seven transducers and one internal transducer against which the working transducers are calibrated. Voltage inputs may be received from other equipment and monitored in place of the pressure channels.

Figure 5.3 shows a block diagram illustrating a ribbon cable which provides the 11 Bit digital conversion of each channel output voltage to an interface on a microcomputer. There is a signal conditioner which contains trim potentionemeters controlling the gain and zero of each channel, and these do not require adjustment by the user since all calibration is normally carried out automatically by the computer software. The calibration of the transducers is by reference to the internal reference transducer. There is a transducer port at the side of the cabinet which is connected to an airline and to all the pressure transducers being used, and to a syringe which is used to pressurise them over the working pressure-range in a routine which takes only a few seconds.

Peripherals and lagging

1. EEG

Adapted standard EEG preamplifiers are used with a high-frequency cut of 3dB down at 30Hz and a time constant of 0.3 seconds, sensitivity of 5μv per mm. Silver/Silver chloride electrodes are applied. The real-time EEG is processed to show a peak to peak value sampled at 50/sec. and maximum, minimum and mean values are calculated on this basis and put to disc every 10 seconds. This provides an envelope-type write-out of EEG over a long period. While the frequency is indiscernible on this compressed record, the amplitude gives a wide envelope record which is recognisable as either 'slow-wave' sleep or the low amplitudes of awake or REM sleep. In 'real time', the EEG record is comparable with conventional EEG speeds of 15mm/sec (*i.e.* half the normal EEG paper speed).

2. ICP

The ICP transducer is connected to a channel input. In the ordinary mode this channel is inputed from a Gaeltec miniature strain-gauge transducer which can measure from ventricular puncture or reservoir, or may be directly computed from the Gaeltec ICTb epidural non-fluid displacing catheter tip transducer for brain surface measurement. It is also possible to connect this to a fibre-optic catheter system. The 'real-time' ICP is initially produced on the screen again by sampling the signal 50 times per second. All subsequent computations are done on the basis of this record, *i.e.* the average values over 10 seconds of the maximum, minimum and true mean pressures are put to disc. Calculation of the average values of ICP excludes transient artefacts associated with coughing and movement.

3. BP/CPP

The system may accept intravascular blood pressure, pulmonary wedge pressure and JVP when the clinical situation dictates. For most overnight monitoring on hydrocephalic patients, the BP is recorded as the mean arterial pressure via a Dynamap. The Dynamap is equipped with a rear chassis accessory connector for a printer, and these printer lines are a convenient source of serially formated pressure-measurement signals for interfacing with the computer monitoring system. Using a digital/analogue convertor the mean arterial pressure is extracted and converted to a voltage signal which is the put into the ICP system. This signal is is recorded as a mean value and updated every minute. The software has written into it the computations for the automatic display of the CPP. Previously one calculated the CPP by taking one third of the distances between the diastolic and systolic value, and subtracting from that the ICP. Such approximations are not necessary with this system, since it is a true mean BP and a true mean ICP that are being recorded and therefore an accurate CPP.

4. T_cCO_2

The CO_2 tension is measured continuously and non-invasively by transcutaneous CO_2

monitor with a D/A convertor and enters as a voltage input. The reason for choosing transcutaneous rather than an end-tidal measurement is that it is more readily applicable to infants, and more importantly, pressure often causes respiratory irregularities and apnoea, making end-tidal measurements unreliable just when one wants to know the CO_2. The signal, sampled continuously 50 times per second, is seen in real time on the screen, and the average value is stored on disc.

Analysis and display

1. REAL-TIME RECORDING (VDU)

During recording, the ICP and other parameters are displayed continuously on the screen together with the derived curve of the CPP. The sampling rate may be changed during the recording in much the same way that the paper speed may be changed in a chart recording system. In this way a transient event observed during monitoring may be retained in full detail without unduly shortening the total recording space available. The recording can be halted at any time and there is an event marker. A 'comments file' is for nursing staff to record observations during the recording. The recording is in two parts, a full record of the last minute's input, and an extracted record of maximum, minimum and mean pressures written onto disc at 10-second intervals. This latter recording can extend over several days, if necessary, although the period is reduced if disc space is taken up by the optional dumping of short periods of full record. This means that there is a facility for saving interesting pieces of real-time recording one wants to keep in full, and this is written on the disc for later printout.

2. PLAYBACK OF THE LAST MINUTE OF RECORD

The recorded data are displayed initially on the same time-scale as originally recorded, to show one minute across the screen (Fig. 5.4). A cursor may be moved to concentrate on interesting parts of the recording. The record may be expanded or contracted by as much as four times the real-time picture. A printout of the screen display may be made at any time.

3. PLAYBACK OF LONG-TERM RECORD

As previously mentioned, the data extracted from the incoming signal are written to disc every 10 seconds and playback of these data, using the long-term record mode, shows the last five hours of the recording (Fig. 5.5). This also can be expanded or contracted. When the recording is complete, details may be selected using the cursor and displayed in an expanded or contracted form, together with digital information of the pressures, gradients and areas as required. With this long-term playback mode, the record shows the first five hours of recorded data on the screen, and by moving the cursor forwards the whole of the night's ICP recording can be viewed screen by screen. At the completion of the recording, it is possible to print out the whole uninterrupted tracing.

4. ADDITIONAL ANALYTICAL FACILITY

(a) *Histograms or frequency polygons.* Using the long-term record, it is possible to

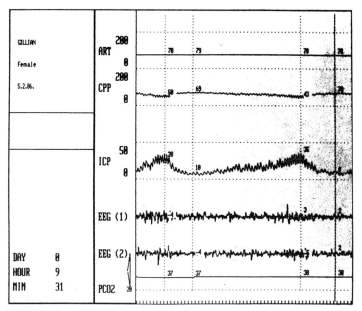

Fig. 5.4. Short-term playback mode (as seen in real time) of ICP fluctuations in early sleep in hydrocephalus.

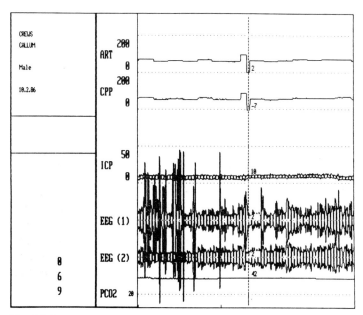

Fig. 5.5. Long-term playback mode of last few hours of recording showing persistently normal levels of ICP in arrested hydrocephalus.

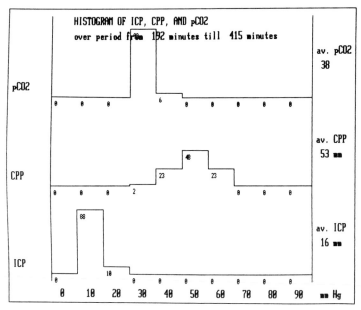

Fig. 5.6. Histogram of mean values of ICP, CPP and carbon dioxide tension for a 220-minute section of recording. 88 per cent of this epoch was accompanied by an ICP between 10 and 20mmHg.

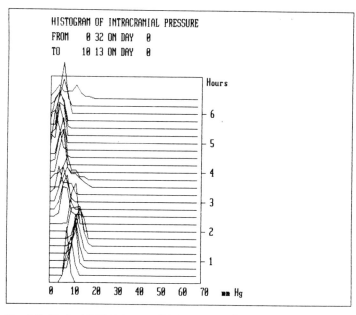

Fig. 5.7. Stacked ICP histogram (histogram array).

137

set cursor points which cause a histogram to be produced with maximum, minimum and mean ICP values over a stipulated time period, for example REM sleep. These histograms are plots of percentage time on the y-axis and pressure bands (0 to 10, 10 to 20 and so on) on the x-axis. These data, together with an over-all mean computed for that period, are shown on the histogram analysis (Fig. 5.6). Histograms may also be produced of CO_2 levels, EEG amplitude, BP and CPP, together with a graphic display of a stacked ICP histogram (histogram array) which may be useful when visualising trends over lengthy recording periods (Fig. 5.7).

(b) *Other facilities.* There are possibilities for correlating any two recorded parameters. With a sampling rate of 50 per second for ICP and BP, it is possible to carry out Fast Fourier analysis with sufficient harmonies to analyse the ICP waveform, although ideally non-fluid filled transducer systems should be used to provide pressure recording for Fourier analysis.

It is possible to write pattern recognition of the different ICP waveforms into the software programme, for example plateau waves, ramp and sinus B waves, C waves and tonic D waves, which would automatically be recognised by the computer. It is also possible to use the mathematical ability of the computer to measure pulse pressures. In summary, this computerised logging system has been developed for continuous monitoring of ICP, BP, CPP, CO_2 and EEG. It is especially useful in children with acute encephalopathies and for evaluation of hydrocephalus. The system provides continuous visual display together with storage facility for later retrieval and analysis of data. The value of the automated system is in the accuracy of ICP and CPP measurement over short or long recording periods with automatically calculated mean values. The apparatus is mobile, relatively inexpensive and provides good quality hard copy.

REFERENCES

Antoni, N. (1946) 'Pressure curves from the cerebrospinal fluid.' *Acta Medica Scandinavica* (Suppl.), **170**, 439–462.

Aucoin, P. J., Kotilainen, H. R., Gantz, N. M., Davidson, R., Kellogg, P., Stone, B. (1986) 'Intracranial pressure monitors. Epidemiologic study of risk factors and infections.' *American Journal of Medicine*, **80**, 369–376.

Barashnev, Y. I., Leontiev, A. F. (1967) 'Cerebrospinal fluid pressure in premature infants with and without intracranial birth injury.' (*Abstract.*) *Developmental Medicine and Child Neurology*, **8**, 117.

Beks, J. W. F., Albarda, S., Gieles, A. C. M., Kuypers, M. H., Flanderijn, H. (1977) 'Extradural transducer for monitoring intracranial pressure.' *Acta Neurochirurgica*, **38**, 245–250.

Blaauw, G., van der Bos, J. L., Mus, A. (1974) 'On pulsations of the fontanelle.' *Developmental Medicine and Child Neurology*, **16**, Suppl. 32, 23–32.

Blackfan, K. D., Crothers, B., Ganz, R. N. (1929) 'Transmission of intracranial pressure in hydrocephalus in infancy.' *American Journal of Diseases of Children*, **37**, 893–899.

Carmichael, E. A., Doupe, J., Williams, D. J. (1937) 'The cerebrospinal fluid pressure of man in the erect posture.' *Journal of Physiology*, **91**, 186–201.

Coroneos, N. J., Turner, J. M., Gibson, R. M., McDowall, D. G., Pickerodt, V. W. A., Keaney, N. P. (1972) 'Comparison of extradural with intraventricular pressure in patients after head injury.' *In* Brock, M., Dietz, H. (Eds.) *Intracranial Pressure, Vol. I.* Berlin: Springer. pp. 51–58.

Cosman, E. R., Zervas, N. T., Chapman, P. H., Cosman, B. J., Arnold, M. A. (1979) 'A telemetric pressure sensor for ventricular shunt system.' *Surgical Neurology*, **11**, 287–294.

Davidoff, L. M., Chamlin, M. (1959) 'The "Fontanometer" adaption of the Schiotz Tonometer for the determination of intracranial pressure in the neonatal and early periods of infancy.' *Pediatrics*, **24**, 1065–1068.

Dietrich, K., Gaab, M., Knoblich, O. E., Schupp, J., Ott, B. (1977) 'A new miniaturized system for monitoring the epidural pressure in children and adults.' *Neuropädiatrie*, **8**, 21–28.

Donn, S. M., Philip, A. G. S. (1978) 'Early increase in intracranial pressure in preterm infants.' *Pediatrics*, **61**, 904–907.

Dorsch, N. W. C., Symon, L. (1975) 'The validity of extradural measurement of the intracranial pressure.' *In* Lundberg, N., Ponten, U., Brock, M. (Eds.) *Intracranial Pressure, Vol. II.* Berlin: Springer. pp. 403–408.

Edwards, J. (1974) 'An intracranial pressure tonometer for use on neonates: preliminary report.' *Developmental Medicine and Child Neurology*, **16**, Suppl. 32, 38–39.

Gaab, M., Knoblich, O. E., Dietrich, K., Gruss, P. (1978) 'Miniaturized methods of monitoring intracranial pressure in craniocerebral trauma before and after operation.' *Advances in Neurosurgery*, **5**, 5–11.

—— Ottens, M., Busche, F., Moller, G., Trost, H. A. (1985) 'Routine computerised neuromonitoring.' *In* Miller, J. D., Teasdale, G. M., Rowan, J. O., Galbraith, S. L., Mendelow, A. D. (Eds.) *Intracranial Pressure, Vol. VI.* Berlin: Springer. pp. 240–247.

Gobiet, W., Bock, W. J., Liesegang, J., Grote, W. (1972) 'Long term monitoring of epidural pressure in man.' *In* Brock, M., Dietz, H. (Eds.) *Intracranial Pressure, Vol. I.* Berlin: Springer. p. 14.

—— —— —— —— (1974) 'Experience with an intracranial pressure transducer readjustable in vivo.' *Journal of Neurosurgery*, **39**, 272–276.

Goitein, K., Amit, Y. (1982) 'Percutaneous placement of subdural catheter for measurement of intracranial pressure in small children.' *Critical Care Medicine*, **10**, 46–48.

Guillaume, J., Janny, P. (1951) 'Manometrie intracranienne continue.' *Revue Neurologique*, **84**, 131–142.

Hoppenstein, R., (1965) 'A device for measuring intracranial pressure.' *Lancet*, **1**, 90.

Hulme, A., Cooper, R. (1966) 'A technique for the investigation of intracranial pressure in man.' *Journal of Neurology, Neurosurgery and Psychiatry*, **29**, 154–156.

Jorgensen, P. B., Riishede, J. (1972) 'Comparative clinical studies of epidural and ventricular pressure.' *In* Brock, M. Dietz, H. *Intracranial Pressure, Vol. I.* Berlin: Springer. p. 41.

Kaiser, A., Whitelaw, A. G. L. (1987) 'Non-invasive monitoring of intracranial pressure—fact or fancy?' *Developmental Medicine and Child Neurology*, **29**, 320–326.

Kast, R. (1985) 'A new method for non-invasive measurement of short-term cerebrospinal fluid pressure changes in humans.' *Journal of Neurology*, **232**, 260–261.

Keegan, H. R., Evans, J. P. (1962) 'Studies of cerebral swelling. III: Long term recordings of cerebrospinal fluid pressure before and following parenteral urea.' *Acta Neurochirurgica*, **10**, 466–472.

Kullberg, G. (1972) 'A method for statistical analysis of intracranial pressure recordings.' *In* Brock, M., Dietz, H. (Eds.) *Intracranial Pressure, Experimental and Clinical Aspects.* New York: Springer. pp. 65–69.

Langfitt, T. W. (1973) 'Summary of First International Symposium on Intracranial Pressure, Hannover, Germany, July 27–29, 1972.' *Journal of Neurosurgery*, **38**, 541–544.

Leggate, J. R. S., Baxter, P., Minns, R. A., Steers, A. J. W., Brown, J. K., Shaw, J. F., Elton, R. A. (1988) 'Role of a separate subcutaneous cerebro-spinal fluid reservoir in the management of hydrocephalus.' *British Journal of Neurosurgery*, **2**, 327–337.

Levene, M. I., Evans, D. H. (1983) 'Continuous measurement of subarachnoid pressure in the severely asphyxiated newborn.' *Archives of Disease in Childhood*, **58**, 1013–1025.

Lundberg, N. (1960) 'Continuous recording and control of ventricular fluid pressure in neurosurgical practice.' *Acta Psychiatrica et Neurologica Scandinavica*, **36**, Suppl. 149, 1–193.

Marchbanks, R. J., Reid, A., Martin, A. M., Brightwell, A. P., Baheman, D. (1987) 'The effect of raised intracranial pressure on intracochlear fluid pressure: three case studies.' *British Journal of Audiology*, **21**, 127–130.

Marmarou, A., Shulman, K. (1976) 'Pressure–volume relationships—basic aspects.' *In* McLaurin, R. L. (Ed.) *Head Injuries: Chicago Symposium on Neurological Trauma 2nd Edn.* New York: Grune & Stratton. pp. 233–236.

McWilliam, R. C., Stephenson, J. B. P. (1984) 'Rapid bedside technique for intracranial pressure monitoring.' *Lancet*, **2**, 73–75.

Mehta, A., Wright, B. M., Shore, C. (1988) 'Clinical fontanometry in the newborn.' *Lancet*, **1**, 754–758.

Miller, J. D., Garibi, J., Pickard, J. D. (1973) 'Induced changes in cerebrospinal fluid volume. Effects during continuous monitoring of ventricular fluid pressure.' *Archives of Neurology*, **28**, 265–269.

—— Pickard, J. D. (1974) 'Intracranial volume pressure studies in patients with head injury.' *Injury*, **5**, 265–268.

—— Becker, D. P., Ward, J. D., Sullivan, H. G., Adams, W. E., Rosner, M. D. (1977) 'Significance of intracranial hypertension in severe head injury.' *Journal of Neurosurgery*, **47**, 503–516.

Minns, R. A. (1984) 'Intracranial pressure monitoring.' *Archives of Disease in Childhood*, **59**, 486–488.

—— Shaw, J. F. (1985) 'Clinical evaluation of the Cosman telesensor in children.' *In* Miller, J. D., Teasdale, G. M., Rowan, J. O., Galbraith, S. L., Mendelow, A. D. (Eds.) *Intracranial Pressure, Vol. VI*. Berlin: Springer. pp. 125–127.

—— Engleman, H. M. (1988) 'The use of CSF pressure recordings in acute purulent meningitis.' *Zeitschrift für Kinderchirurgie*, **43**, Suppl. II, 28–29.

—— —— Stirling, H. (1989) 'Cerebrospinal fluid pressure in pyogenic meningitis.' *Archives of Disease in Childhood*, **64**, 814–820.

Numoto, M., Slater, J. P., Donaghy, R. M. P. (1966) 'An implantable switch for monitoring intracranial pressure.' *Lancet*, **1**, 528.

—— —— (1969) 'An automatic method of measuring and recording intracranial pressure.' *Medical Research and Engineering*, **8**, 38–39.

—— Wallman, J. K., Donaghy, R. M. P. (1973) 'Pressure indicating bag for monitoring intracranial pressure.' *Journal of Neurosurgery*, **39**, 784–787.

Ostrup, R. C., Luerssen, T. G., Marshall, L. F., Zornow, M. H. (1987) 'Continuous monitoring of intracranial pressure with a miniaturized fibreoptic device.' *Journal of Neurosurgery*, **67**, 206–209.

Peabody, J. L., Philip, A. G. S., Lucey, J. F. (1977) '"Disorganized breathing". An important form of apnoea and cause of hypoxia.' *Pediatric Research*, **11**, 540. (Abstract.)

Philip, A. G. S. (1979) 'Noninvasive monitoring of intracranial pressure. A new approach for neonatal clinical pharmacology.' *Clinics in Perinatology*, **6**, 123–137.

Picton-Warlow, C. G., Robinson, R. J. (1970) 'Evaluation of a method of indirect measurement of intracranial pressure in infants.' *Developmental Medicine and Child Neurology*, **12**, 507–511.

Purin, V. R. (1964) 'Measurement of the cerebrospinal fluid pressure in the infant without puncture. A new method.' *(Russian) Pediatriya*, **43**, (5), 82–85.

Richardson, A. Hide, T. A. H., Everden, I. D. (1970) 'Long-term continuous intracranial-pressure monitoring by means of a modified subdural pressure transducer.' *Lancet*, **2**, 687–690.

Riechert, T., Heines, K. D. (1950) 'Über zwei Untersuchungsmethoden zur Beurteilung der Hirndurchblutung.' *Nervenarzt*, **21**, 9.

Robinson, R. O., Rolfe, P., Sutton, P. (1977) 'Non-invasive method for measuring intracranial pressure in normal newborn infants.' *Developmental Medicine and Child Neurology*, **19**, 305–308.

Rochefort, M. J., Rolfe, P., Wilkinson, A. R. (1987) 'New fontanometer for continuous estimation of intracranial pressure in the newborn.' *Archives of Disease in Childhood*, **62**, 152–155.

Rothballer, A. B. (1963) *Communications to the Harvey Cushing Society, Philadelphia, April 18*.

Ryder, H. W., Espey, F. F., Kristoff, F. V., Evans, J. P. (1951) 'Observations on the inter-relationships of intracranial pressure and cerebral blood flow.' *Journal of Neurosurgery*, **8**, 46–58.

Salmon, J. H., Hajjar, W., Bada, H. S. (1977) 'The fontogram: a non-invasive intracranial pressure monitor.' *Pediatrics*, **60**, 721–725.

Schedl, R., Benzer, H., Fasol, P., Mutz, N., Sebek, W., Spangler, H., Strickner, M. (1983) 'Computerised monitoring of ICP.' *In* Ishii, S., Nagai, H., Brock, M. (Eds.) *Intracranial Pressure, Vol. 5*. Berlin, Heidelberg: Springer. pp. 145–149.

Sundbärg, G., Nornes, H. (1972) 'Simultaneous recording of the epidural and ventricular fluid pressure.' *In* Bock, M., Dietz, H. (Eds.) *Intracranial Pressure, Vol. I*. Berlin: Springer. p. 46.

—— Nordstrom, C., Soderstrom, S. (1988) 'Complications due to prolonged ventricular fluid pressure recording.' *British Journal of Neurosurgery*, **2**, 485–495.

Vidyasagar, D., Raju, T. N. K. (1977) 'A simple non-invasive technique of measuring intracranial pressure in the newborn.' *Pediatrics*, **59**, 957–961.

Wealthall, S. R., Smallwood, R. (1974) 'Methods of measuring intracranial pressure via the fontanelle without puncture.' *Journal of Neurology, Neurosurgery and Psychiatry*, **37**, 88–96.

Whitelaw, A. G. L., Wright, B. M. (1982) 'A pneumatic applanimeter for intracranial pressure measurement.' *Journal of Physiology*, **336**, 3–4.

Winn, H. R., Dacey, R. G., Jane, J. A. (1977) 'Intracranial subarachnoid pressure recording: experience with 650 patients.' *Surgical Neurology*, **8**, 41–47.

Zervas, N. T., Cosman, E. R., Cosman, B. J. (1977) 'A pressure-balanced radio-telemetry system for the measurement of intracranial pressure. A preliminary design report.' *Journal of Neurosurgery*, **47**, 899–911.

6
PHYSIOLOGICAL ASSESSMENT OF THE ASPHYXIATED NEWBORN INFANT

Malcolm I. Levene

Asphyxia during the birth process is the single most important cause of permanent functional injury of the immature brain. Unfortunately, the term 'asphyxia' itself is imprecise and there is little consensus as to what it means. The Oxford English Dictionary defines it as 'a stoppage of the pulse or suffocation', and in a sense this provides the essence for the meaning of perinatal asphyxia. The fetus relies for gas exchange on the placenta rather than the lungs, and any process which significantly impairs placental gas exchange will cause the fetus to suffocate.

Although the clinical meaning of asphyxia may be obscure, the clinician usually uses the term to describe its effect on the newborn rather than to imply a precise aetiology. Clinical observation or investigative procedures provide evidence for asphyxia, but this information may differ quite considerably depending on the severity of the asphyxial insult and the maturity of the fetus. Asphyxia is an unhelpful diagnosis unless placed in the context of gestational age.

Birth asphyxia is a common clinical problem. General management includes maintenance of the infant in optimal condition: but more recent neurospecific methods offer exciting possibilities for protecting the neuron following the asphyxial injury. These methods are discussed in some detail below.

At a cellular level, asphyxia represents a combination of hypoxia together with reduction in the delivery of metabolic substrates. This pathophysiological process results in anaerobic metabolism with local production of metabolic acids. The metabolic acidosis is the fundamental result of asphyxia. The term 'hypoxic-ischaemic encephalopathy' has been widely used in the United States to refer to this process and encapsulates the fundamental pathophysiological and clinical features of the condition.

Mechanisms exist in the fetus to protect the immature organism from the early effects of asphyxia. Initially the response of the fetus to hypoxia and reduced perfusion is a fall in heart-rate and an increase in blood pressure. There is an increase in myocardial contractility and cardiac output with redistribution of flow in favour of the brain, coronary arteries and adrenals primarily at the expense of the gut, kidneys, muscles and skin (Cohn *et al.* 1974, Edelstone *et al.* 1977, Peeters *et al.* 1979, Fisher *et al.* 1980).

These control mechanisms exist to provide adequate metabolic subtrates to the cells of vital organs for as long as possible. When these circulatory mechanisms fail, the brain (like other organs) switches to anaerobic metabolism in order to continue production of energy-rich ATP molecules. Anaerobic metabolism is a very wasteful process, providing only two molecules of ATP for every mole of glucose burnt, compared with the 38 molecules of ATP when aerobic metabolism occurs. Lactic acid is produced by anaerobic metabolism, and this may be directly toxic to the brain.

Complete ischaemic anoxia for a period of less than five minutes is sufficient to deplete the cell of ATP totally (Ljunggren *et al.* 1974). The concentration of minerals (including sodium, potassium and calcium) is maintained at vastly different concentrations inside and outside the cell by 'pumps' dependent on high-energy ATP molecules for their function. The direct result of severe asphyxia is failure of these membrane pumps, with consequent imbalance of intracellular electrolytes.

It has been known for over 300 years that the brain of immature animals is considerably more resistant to the effects of asphyxia than that of the more mature animal (Boyle 1670). There is a variety of reasons for this, but the most important is probably the lower metabolic rate of the fetal brain, which is therefore more resistant to the effects of hypoxic ischaemic insult.

Although the effects of asphyxia at a cellular level are reasonably well understood, the effects on the infant vary considerably and depend on the anatomical and functional development of the brain. The brain of the preterm infant is particularly susceptible to damage as the result of vascular insufficiency, and two forms of pathology may be seen: germinal matrix haemorrhage and periventricular leukomalacia (see below). These forms of pathology are very uncommon in the brains of term infants, but there are other forms of vascular injury, such as subcortical leukomalacia which are more characteristic of vascular compromise to the mature brain.

Diagnosis
Fetal asphyxia
Meconium staining of the liquor amnii is a particularly well-recognised feature associated with fetal asphyxia, but is poorly specific and relatively insensitive. Monitoring of the fetal heart-rate in response to uterine activity is widely used as a method of assessing fetal well-being in labour. Decelerations of the fetal heart-rate at the time of contractions (Type I dips) are due to vagal stimulation (Beard *et al.* 1971) and are considered a benign feature. Late fetal heart-rate decelerations (Type II dips) following the contraction are more ominous and may be associated with fetal distress, but if they are present as an isolated observation, they are poorly sensitive to fetal distress (Bissonette 1975). The fetal heart-rate usually shows beat-to-beat variability, and loss of this feature may occur in association with hypoxia. Like the other features it is unreliable if used alone. In general, cardiotocographic abnormalities are not particularly sensitive to fetal asphyxia with acidosis (Beard *et al.* 1971, Bissonette 1975). In a controlled study of continuous fetal heart-rate monitoring compared with intermittent auscultation, cardiotocography appears neither to save fetal lives, nor to protect the fetal brain from severe injury (MacDonald *et al.* 1985, Grant *et al.* 1989).

Because of the imprecision of fetal heart-rate monitoring, an estimate of fetal acidosis has been adopted as a clinical method for assessing fetal asphyxia with acidosis (Saling and Schneider 1967). In this test a specimen of blood from the fetal scalp is collected in a capillary tube, and its pH measured. (This is only possible following cervical dilatation and membrane rupture.) A pH value below 7.20 is suggestive of fetal acidosis, and delivery should be expedited.

Delay in establishing spontaneous respiration
Donald (1959) was the first to define 'asphyxia neonatorum' as failure to establish spontaneous ventilation at birth. Unfortunately the time to establish spontaneous respiration is dependent on factors other than intrapartum asphyxia, including maternal sedation, anaesthesia, preterm birth and neuromuscular disease. Many preterm infants are born apnoeic and require resuscitation, but this may not be due to intrapartum asphyxia. This significantly limits the value of this criterion in immature infants.

Depression of the Apgar score
The Apgar score is widely used as a method for determining the condition of the infant at the time of birth or shortly afterwards. Unfortunately it has become used as a method for diagnosing asphyxia, which Virginia Apgar—who described the method—never intended (Apgar 1953). A score of 3 or less at five minutes has been used by some as a diagnostic indicator of severe asphyxia (Nelson and Ellenberg 1981, Ergander *et al.* 1983), but like depression of respiration, a low Apgar score may also reflect a variety of non-asphyxial causes. In particular the very preterm infant is likely to be born with a depressed Apgar score for no other reason than his immaturity. Many of these infants are intubated early for apnoea, thus rendering the Apgar score extremely unreliable for the diagnosis of asphyxia.

As metabolic acidosis is a fundamental marker of asphyxia, Sykes *et al.* (1982) have suggested that cord blood pH estimates may be a particularly sensitive measure of intrapartum asphyxia. Unfortunately this is not a practicable method for universal use in obstetric units.

Post-asphyxial encephalopathy (PAE)
As discussed above, the fetus has a number of compensatory mechanisms to preserve cerebral function despite quite marked placental dysfunction. If the brain is compromised, however, some abnormality may be seen on clinical examination if the insult is severe enough to affect cerebral function. Encephalopathy is the term used to describe the abnormal neurological behaviour, and a number of schemes have been described to document these abnormalities in term infants (Table 6.I) (Sarnat and Sarnat 1976, Fenichel 1983, Levene *et al.* 1985a).

In mild encephalopathy, the infant has usually recovered fully within 48 hours of birth, and in moderate encephalopathy the infant shows signs of improvement by the end of the first week of life. But in the most severe form, the infant may not recover and abnormal clinical signs may persist for many weeks. Unfortunately this method is of limited value in preterm infants, because the immature and the mature brain is susceptible to different forms of pathology. The immature brain may show separate, subtle or even no abnormal clinical or physical signs. We have recently reported classical PAE in an infant of 29 weeks' gestation who had severe

TABLE 6.I
Clinical severity of post-asphyxial encephalopathy

Mild (Grade I)	Moderate (Grade II)	Severe (Grade III)
Irritability 'Hyperalert'	Lethargy	Comatose
Some hypertonia	Hypertonia with differential limb tone	Severe hypotonia
Poor sucking	Requires tube-feeding	Failure to maintain spontaneous respiration
No seizures	Seizures	Prolonged seizures

(After Levene *et al.* 1985*a*.)

intrapartum asphyxia and marked metabolic acidosis (Niijima and Levene 1988), but this is very uncommon. Nevertheless PAE is a valuable clinical method when applied to mature infants.

We have compared PAE with depression of the Apgar score in defining intrapartum asphyxia (Levene *et al.* 1986), and found a poor correlation. Unfortunately severity of PAE can only be determined retrospectively, which limits the method when an early assessment of asphyxia is necessary.

Incidence

The incidence of asphyxia depends on the criteria by which it is diagnosed. For the purpose of comparing incidence of perinatal asphyxia between populations or time periods, it is only possible to make proper comparisons between term infants. Two studies have reported the incidence of PAE in term deliveries. In Edinburgh, 5.9 per 1000 babies showed clinical signs associated with intrapartum asphyxia (Brown *et al.* 1974), and in Leicester an incidence of 6 per 1000 has been reported (Levene *et al.* 1985*a*). In the latter study, moderate and severe encephalopathy was found in 1.1 and 1.0 per 1000 liveborn infants respectively.

There appears to have been a reduction in the reported incidence of birth asphyxia recently. Infant mortality due to intra-uterine hypoxia has fallen from 253 per 1000 births in 1970 to 39 per 1000 in 1981 (Wegman 1984). These figures from the United States refer to all birthweights, but their definition of intra-uterine hypoxia is not clear.

There is evidence, based on a clinical definition of asphyxia, that its incidence has fallen in recent years. In infants weighing more than 2500g at birth, the incidence of convulsions considered to be due to birth asphyxia has fallen from 1.8 per 1000 in 1960 to 0.7 per 1000 in 1978 to 1980 (Cyr *et al.* 1984). In Paris the incidence of mild and moderate encephalopathy occurring in term infants has fallen from 18.9 per 1000 in 1974 to 3.9 per 1000 between 1976 and 1978 (Amiel-Tison *et al.* 1980). There was, however, no change in the numbers of mature infants born with severe encephalopathy.

There is also evidence that the outcome following intrapartum asphyxia has improved with time (Finer *et al.* 1983). Svenningsen *et al.* (1982) reported that 50

144

per cent of term infants surviving asphyxia between 1973 and 1976 had significant neurodevelopmental sequelae, in contrast to only 17 per cent with similar findings in equivalently mature infants born between 1976 and 1979. This has been attributed to the introduction of 'neuro-intensive care', but other studies show an over-all decline in the incidence of birth asphyxia over the past 20 years, and this is probably related to improved obstetric techniques and supportive care of the newborn, rather than to the specific effects of small doses of phenobarbitone.

Pathology
The pathological effects of intrapartum asphyxia on the preterm infant's brain are much less well documented than in the brain of the term fetus. Periventricular haemorrhage and periventricular leukomalacia are the two most important pathological lesions that occur in the immature brain and both usually develop as postnatal events. Studies of risk-factors for these conditions have not convincingly shown that either can be related to intrapartum events. Complications of mechanical ventilation are the best recognised associated factors. As both these conditions are common in preterm infants and occur within the first few days of life, they will be considered here as 'asphyxial' events, using this term in a somewhat wider sense.

Periventricular haemorrhage (PVH)
This condition occurs in 50 per cent of very low-birthweight infants, and is even commoner in those infants born below 28 weeks of gestation. PVH arises in the region of the germinal matrix, an area of rapid glial cell proliferation situated in the floor of the lateral ventricle and closely related to the caudate nucleus. In 80 per cent of cases there is rupture through the ependyma into the lateral ventricle, hence the term 'intraventricular haemorrhage'. Unfortunately this is an unhelpful description, as the original lesion does not develop *de novo* in the ventricle, and ventricular haemorrhage may arise from sites other than the germinal matrix, including the choroid plexus. The term 'periventricular haemorrhage' is a much better one to describe the germinal matrix-IVH lesion, and will be used throughout this chapter.

PVH is most likely to occur in infants with respiratory complications who require mechanical ventilation. Two factors are necessary for PVH to occur. Initially the germinal matrix capillary wall is injured followed by fluctuations in CBF which cause the damaged vessel wall to rupture and produce germinal matrix haemorrhage. A third factor involves impairment of the clotting mechanisms, so that bleeding from capillary vessel rupture is more likely to extend and involve the ventricles. Insults which may damage the capillary include asphyxia, hypoxia, acidosis and cerebral ischaemia. It is thought that sudden increases in CBF are likely to cause the vessel to rupture, and babies who actively breathe against a mechanical ventilator have been shown to be very much at risk of PVH (Perlman *et al.* 1983). Haemorrhage may also be caused by complications of mechanical ventilation, including pneumothorax or rapid infusions of plasma. These complications produce an acute rise in CBF, capillary rupture and germinal matrix haemorrhage.

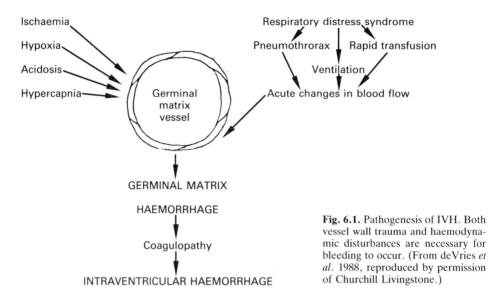

Vessel factors
Haemodynamic factors

Ischaemia

Hypoxia

Acidosis

Hypercapnia

Germinal
matrix
vessel

Respiratory distress syndrome

Pneumothrorax   Rapid transfusion

Ventilation

Acute changes in blood flow

GERMINAL MATRIX

HAEMORRHAGE

Coagulopathy

INTRAVENTRICULAR HAEMORRHAGE

Fig. 6.1. Pathogenesis of IVH. Both vessel wall trauma and haemodynamic disturbances are necessary for bleeding to occur. (From deVries *et al.* 1988, reproduced by permission of Churchill Livingstone.)

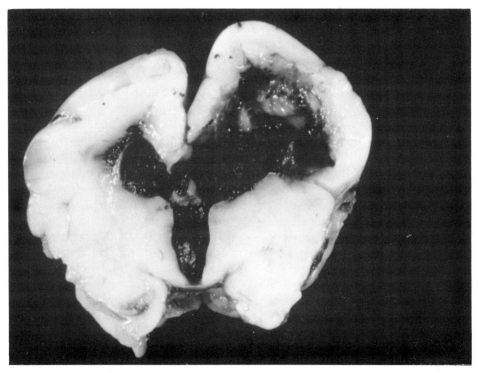

Fig. 6.2. Coronal cut through the brain of an extremely preterm infant showing clot distending the left lateral ventricle and extensive parenchymal haemorrhage in the right hemisphere.

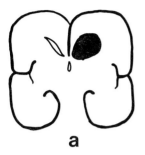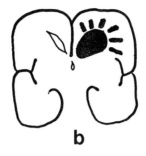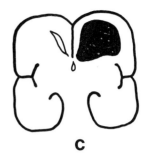

a **b** **c**

Fig. 6.3. Diagram to illustrate the development of venous cerebral infarction. Clot distends the lateral ventricle (*a*) followed by engorgement of veins draining the periventricular white matter (*b*). Finally the engorged area becomes infarcted due to impaired perfusion (*c*).

Hypercapnia, hypoxia and acidosis cause cerebral vasodilatation, with a rise in CBF and an increased risk of germinal matrix haemorrhage. Coagulopathy is more likely to be present in infants at risk of PVH than in those who do not develop the condition (McDonald et al. 1984). Figure 6.1 summarises the pathogenetic factors involved in the development of PVH.

In approximately 20 to 30 per cent of infants with PVH, haemorrhage also occurs into the cerebral parenchyma (Fig. 6.2). It was once thought that this was the direct result of the initial germinal matrix lesion extending through the ventricles into the periventricular white matter. This seems unlikely, as it is difficult to explain how the initial lesion (capillary oozing) can generate sufficient pressure then to rupture into normal periventricular white matter. The most likely explanation for this process is venous infarction (Gould *et al.* 1987, deVries *et al.* 1988), which is usually a unilateral condition. The initial event involves distension of a lateral ventricle by a clot, which in some cases causes impairment of venous return from the periventricular white matter with venous stasis and subsequent venous infarction due to reduced perfusion pressure (Fig. 6.3). In a number of cases of parenchymal haemorrhage, bleeding into an area of ischaemic infarction may be the cause of the parenchymal lesion (see below).

Periventricular leukomalacia
This term was introduced by Banker and Larroche (1962) to describe a pathological process involving white matter just lateral to the angle of the lateral ventricles. The lesions vary in macroscopic appearance, from discrete 'white spots' to extensive cavities which may be multiple throughout the periventricular white matter. There are three areas of predilection: the white matter in front of the anterior pole of the lateral ventricle, the centrum semiovale, and the area around the occipital pole of the lateral ventricle.

These lesions occur in a vascular watershed distribution. This may be in the region between the vascular territories of the three major cerebral arteries, or in the region between the ventriculopetal and ventriculofugal arteries of the periventricular white matter. PVL occurs predominantly in preterm infants, and the mature term baby appears to be much more resistant to this form of pathology. The

TABLE 6.II

Factors implicated in the pathogenesis of periventricular leukomalacia

Complications of mechanical ventilation
Antepartum haemorrhage
Intrapartum asphyxia
Cardiac arrhythmia
Anaesthesia and surgery
Severe necrotising enterocolitis
? Hypotension
Monozygotic twin

cerebral hemispheres go through a period of rapid growth in the second half of pregnancy. Between 24 and 34 weeks' gestation the periventricular white matter is vulnerable to ischaemia due to the vascular watersheds in this region. Anastomoses become more secure with increasing maturity, and ischaemic infarction of the periventricular white matter becomes progressively less likely by the time the infant reaches term.

A variety of factors have been implicated in the pathogenesis of PVL (Table 6.II). PVL lesions are well recognised in the immature fetus, and prenatal asphyxia or maternal collapse may be recognised in some cases. Monozygotic twins are particularly vulnerable to PVL (Szymonowicz *et al.* 1985), particularly if one twin dies. Intrapartum asphyxia and particularly antepartum haemorrhage may also be important factors in the development of PVL (Sinha *et al.* 1985, Weindling *et al.* 1985, Calvert *et al.* 1987). Although hypotension is considered to be the final common pathway for the development of PVL, there is very little evidence to support this. A number of studies assessing the risk factors for PVL have failed to find an association with hypotension (Weindling *et al.* 1985, Trounce *et al.* 1987, Watkins *et al.* 1987). Sudden episodes of transient but severe cerebral hypoperfusion, such as cardiac arrythmia, may cause PVL in some cases (Shortland *et al.* 1987). Late-onset PVL has been well documented in some infants, particularly those with severe gastro-intestinal complications and those requiring surgery (deVries *et al.* 1986).

Cerebral pathology of the term infant
Brain pathology detected in term infants, and directly related to birth asphyxia, is better documented than pathological lesions affecting the immature brain. The pathological appearances depend on the duration of time between the asphyxial event and death. Initially the brain may appear normal, but within 24 to 48 hours swelling occurs with flattening of the gyri and obliteration of the sulci. On section, the lateral ventricles appear slit-like with little CSF present within them. Rarely, other mechanical effects of cerebral swelling may be seen: *e.g.* herniation of the uncus, infundibulum into the interpeduncular cistern, or cerebellar vermis through the foramen magnum (Larroche 1977).

Injury to the mature brain following asphyxia is usually global, but some areas of the brain may be more vulnerable than others. The cortex may be specifically damaged, and ulegyria (gyral sclerosis with widening of the sulci) has been recognised for many years. The hippocampus is also particularly vulnerable to asphyxial injury, probably related to its relatively higher metabolic rate compared with other areas of the brain. Subcortical structures may also be prone to perinatal asphyxia. This is related to another vascular watershed within the subcortical region. In immature infants this area was well vascularised by primitive leptomeningeal vessels, but by term these vessels have regressed to leave a triangular watershed area in the subcortical region at the depths of the sulci (Takashima *et al.* 1978). Status marmoratus is the classical neuropathological lesion affecting the basal ganglia; it has been recognised for many years, but appears to be very rare. Protective mechanisms exist to preserve bloodflow to the brainstem and basal ganglia when CBF is compromised. It is therefore very uncommon to see lesions affecting the basal ganglia alone without involvement of other parts of the brain.

Clinical signs

The term infant shows a consistent pattern of clinical signs following birth asphyxia (Table 6.I). The preterm infant has far less impressive clinical signs of encephalopathy, but consistent clinical abnormalities have been recognised in infants with PVH and PVL. On clinical examination, four items have been found to correlate with blood in the lateral ventricles: impairment of visual tracking, abnormal popliteal angle, decrease in tone with poor motility, and roving eye movements (Dubowitz *et al.* 1981). This latter feature was usually not seen for some weeks after the haemorrhage. The same group have also reported consistent clinical abnormalities which correspond to the development of PVL. These include extreme irritability, with either persistent fisting or a consistent pattern of abnormal finger posturing. These infants also showed poor trunk- and limb-tone and generally felt stiff. These abnormal signs were often not present until the infant reached 40 weeks of post-menstrual age (deVries *et al.* 1988).

Imaging

Two methods are readily available for investigating brain structure of the asphyxiated infant: ultrasound and computerised x-ray tomography (CT). In term infants, CT is the more valuable technique. The characteristic abnormality is an appearance of extensive low attenuation, through the periventricular white matter or involving most of the brain (Fig. 6.4). Moderate or severe involvement affecting white matter or cortex occurs in approximately 40 per cent of asphyxiated term infants examined by CT (Flodmark *et al.* 1980, Magliner and Wertheimer 1980, Schumpf *et al.* 1980, Fitzhardinge *et al.* 1981, Gerard *et al.* 1981, Finer *et al.* 1983, Adsett *et al.* 1985, Lipp-Zwahlen *et al.* 1985*a*). Lesions of the thalamus have also been reported on CT examination and MRI (Shewman *et al.* 1981, Morimoto *et al.* 1985, Voit *et al.* 1985). It is possible that the 'bright' thalamus seen on CT may be mistaken for the site of cerebral injury whereas it appears bright only in comparison with the surrounding brain which shows markedly low attenuation (Fig. 6.4). Asphyxiated mature infants also show a high incidence of intracranial haemorrhage

149

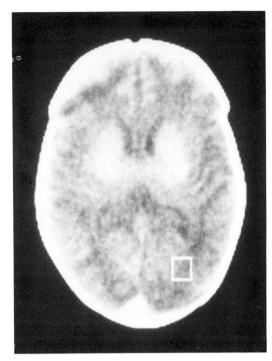

Fig. 6.4. CT scan of a severely asphyxiated term infant showing extensive areas of low attenuation involving the cerebral hemispheres. It is the basal ganglia that retain their normal CT density.

on CT examination. Analysis of cumulative data gives an over-all risk of haemorrhage in around 30 per cent of infants with clinical evidence of significant birth asphyxia (Levene 1988).

Real-time ultrasound is an extremely effective method for diagnosing intracranial pathology in preterm infants (Levene *et al.* 1985*b*). Regular scanning will allow the PVH lesion to be reliably diagnosed and its onset accurately timed. Criteria for the diagnosis of PVL (Fig. 6.5) are now well described (Trounce *et al.* 1986*a*), and with autopsy findings the diagnostic accuracy has been reported to be 90 per cent (Trounce *et al.* 1986*b*).

Pathophysiological assessment
Clinical examination and assessment will give useful information for diagnosis and prognosis, but more precise information may be obtained only by resorting to technological methods for assessment of brain function following asphyxia. The methods depend on the questions asked about cerebral function. The most important information concerns the presence of RICP, CPP level, the presence of subclinical seizures and an index of CBF. These methods are reviewed below.

ICP
Cerebral oedema is thought to be an important complication of perinatal asphyxic cerebral injury, and information about intracranial hypertension may be useful in managing the infant. The open fontanelle offers the possibility of measuring ICP

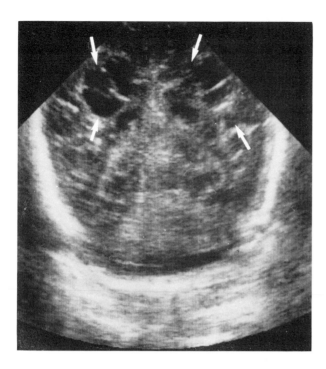

Fig. 6.5. Posterior coronal ultrasound scan of a preterm infant showing extensive but discrete echolucent cavities in the periventricular white matter (*arrows*).

indirectly and non-invasively through the anterior fontanelle, and various such methods have been devised (Levene 1987), but doubt has been thrown on the validity of these techniques. A number of studies have shown that the application pressure of the device influences the perceived pressure (Horbar *et al.* 1980, Walsh and Logan 1983), thus making accurate measurement of ICP unreliable. Kaiser and Whitelaw (1987) carefully assessed a number of transfontanelle devices, and found accurate recording of ICP to be unreliable.

The alternative method is a direct and invasive approach, whereby a mechanical device or catheter is inserted through the skull. Many such devices are used in the older child and are reviewed elsewhere in this book. Few have been undertaken in the newborn infant, and the best evaluated are the subarachnoid catheter (Levene and Evans 1983) and the subdural cannula (Goitein and Amit 1982).

The subarachnoid catheter is inserted through the lateral angle of the anterior fontanelle, usually over the right hemisphere. First the hair is shaved, and careful skin preparation is applied using a solution of 10 per cent povidone iodine. The skin of the fontanelle through which the cannula is to be inserted is infiltrated with 1 per cent lignocaine, and the scalp and galeal membranes nicked with a scalpel blade. An 18G Oxford Tuohy needle is inserted through the path of the scalpel blade with its bevel uppermost and directed towards a point 1cm above the infant's right eye. When the tip of the needle is just under the frontal bone it is then lifted up and advanced so that the bevel is lying in the subarachnoid space just below the bone.

151

TABLE 6.III

'Normal' data for intracranial pressure measurement in preterm and term infants. These studies were all performed using indirect transfontanelle aplanation devices

Authors	Gestational age	Intracranial pressure (mmHg)
Robinson *et al.* 1977	Term	8.2 ± 2.4
Salmon *et al.* 1977	Term	7.4 ± 1.5
Philip *et al.* 1981	Term	9.7 ± 2.2
Menke *et al.* 1982	Term	7.0 ± 1.9
Philip *et. al.* 1981	Preterm	7.9
Raju and Vidyasagar 1982	Preterm	7.4 ± 1.5

The stylet is then removed and CSF may be seen to drip from the needle, though this does not always happen, particularly if the brain is swollen. A fine Portex epidural catheter primed with saline is advanced 5cm through the Tuohy needle so that its tip lies over the frontal lobe of the brain. The needle is then withdrawn and the catheter attached to a fluid-filled pressure transducer. If the catheter is situated in the subarachnoid space, pressure waves corresponding to both cardiac and respiratory impulses are seen on the trace.

I have performed this technique on over 50 infants, and the risk of trauma has been carefully evaluated. Most infants who died had autopsy examination, and only one infant was found to have evidence of subdural haemorrhage. It is believed that the bleeding occurred prior to insertion of the catheter. No infant showed evidence of cerebral trauma related to the catheter placement. All the surviving infants had either ultrasound or CT examinations, and none showed evidence of trauma related to the technique. No infants developed local infection or meningitis.

All infants with moderate or severe PAE have routine measurements of arterial blood pressure from the aorta (via an umbilical artery catheter) or radial artery. These measurements are recorded simultaneously with ICP, and the cerebral perfusion pressure (CPP) is calculated from the formula:

$$CPP = MAP - ICP$$

A low CPP may be due to raised ICP with no compensatory rise in mean arterial blood pressure, or a fall in MAP. The CPP is assumed to measure the driving force of blood through the brain, although this is clearly an oversimplification. Management of a falling CPP depends on evaluation of both MAP and ICP.

There are few data on normal values of ICP in the newborn infant and these are summarised in Table 6.III. Most of these values are probably an overestimate and in my view the figure of 2mmHg for normal ICP given by Minns (1984) is more realistic. Measurement of CSF pressure at lumbar puncture has been reported to vary between 0.5 to 5mmHg (Kaiser and Whitelaw 1986). The normal CPP is also open to question due to the unreliability of indirect methods to measure ICP. The only 'normal' data are from Raju *et al.* (1982), who suggest that the mean CPP for infants during the first week of life is roughly equal to gestational age in weeks.

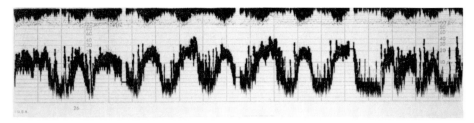

Fig. 6.6. Cerebral function monitor (CFM) trace showing regular seizures (*arrowed*) lasting for approximately two minutes and occurring every four minutes.

Electrodiagnostic tests

There are two types of investigation: analysis of spontaneously generated EEG signals, and recording of evoked electrical potentials. The former has been traditionally derived from 12 lead EEG recordings, but these have obvious limitations in intensive care. For that reason, techniques have been derived to record the EEG signal, or a function of it, in real-time.

Eyre *et al.* (1983) described the use of a two-channel continuous EEG system for the recording of cortical activity. This system records the raw signals onto audio tape for later interpretation on playback through an analysis system. Unfortunately this system in its commercial form is of little clinical value, as on-line analysis is not possible. Nevertheless, use of this system has shown that approximately 50 per cent of infants with electroconvulsive seizures show few or no signs of clinically recognised seizures (Eyre *et al.* 1983). A simpler technique is the cerebral function monitor, which records electrical activity from a single pair of biparietal electrodes and then electronically converts these signals to a read-out showing voltage and frequency. Some machines are more sophisticated and break frequency down into component parts, and may also display raw EEG data. These machines produce a continuous rolling average trace showing voltage in real-time, and seizure activity can be readily recognised providing the seizure lasts at least 20 seconds (Fig. 6.6).

Evoked potentials have been used in a limited way in the assessment of asphyxiated infants. Auditory evoked potentials (Hecox and Cone 1981), visual and somatosensory evoked responses (Hrbek *et al.* 1977) have been reported to become progressively abnormal with more severe degrees of asphyxia.

Assessment of CBF

Accurate measurement of CBF is of fundamental importance to understanding both the cause and effects of perinatal asphyxia. Unfortunately there is no reliable and safe method, and several indirect techniques have been employed (Greisen 1988). Doppler ultrasound gives some information on the cerebral circulation, and it is a safe and easily used technique which has been applied to the asphyxiated newborn infant (Evans and Archer 1988).

The velocity of blood cells in major cerebral arteries can be measured by detecting the difference between the transmitted frequency and the reflected frequency. If the angle of insonation is known, and the speed of the ultrasound impulse through the tissue assumed, then velocity is calculated from a relatively

153

TABLE 6.IV
Systemic complications of asphyxia

Cardiovascular	Cardiac failure
	Myocardial ischaemia
	Hypotension
Renal	Acute tubular necrosis
	Oliguria
Pulmonary	Meconium aspiration
Metabolic	Hypoglycaemia
	Inappropriate ADH secretion
Haematological	Disseminated intravascular coagulation
Gastro-intestinal	Stress ulceration
	Necrotising enterocolitis

simple formula. Archer *et al.* (1986) showed that some infants with moderate and severe asphyxia have abnormally low pulsatility on the Doppler frequency spectrum, and that this abnormal pattern is 100 per cent sensitive and also relatively specific (81 per cent) for adverse outcome. The advantage of this technique is that the waveform becomes abnormal at a median time of 28 hours and at a considerably earlier age than other techniques. There is a rise in cerebral bloodflow velocity (CBV) at about the time that the waveform becomes abnormally pulsatile. If a CBV measurement above 3SD from the mean is taken as abnormal, then this has a 94 per cent positive predictive value for adverse outcome (death or severe handicap) following birth asphyxia (Levene *et al.* 1989).

The reason for the change in pulsatility and increased velocity is not known, but it must reflect some change in the cerebral vascular bed, probably due to vasoparalysis. This relates to the degree of injury sustained by the brain in term infants, and may provide further clues to the basic pathophysiology of birth asphyxia. Unfortunately Doppler methods are currently of no value in the prediction of outcome in very immature infants.

Management
The management of asphyxiated infants can be divided into general supportive methods and neurospecific techniques. Although we are most concerned about the effects of asphyxia on the brain, the initial insult involves the whole organism, and complications may occur in many different systems (Table 6.IV). Careful attention must be paid to anticipation of these complications and their appropriate management. Many preterm infants require respiratory support and must be managed in neonatal units experienced in the treatment of these infants. Equally, those infants with severe asphyxia should be managed in units experienced in neuro-intensive care. At present there are no specific methods with which to intervene in the management of preterm infants who have sustained acute PVH or PVL lesions, unless ventricular dilatation with RICP develops (see below).

Fluids and glucose
Most mature infants with birth asphyxia are managed with fluid restriction. The

reason for this appears to be an effort to prevent circulatory overload and minimise cerebral oedema. Although there is no evidence to support this practice, we manage the infant with 20 per cent less fluid than his normal requirements based on postnatal age. Serum and urinary electrolytes should also be carefully monitored in order to detect inappropriate ADH secretion, and fluid restriction should be instituted if this occurs.

There is considerable evidence that infusion of glucose prior to experimental asphyxia in newborn animals exacerbates cerebral injury due to accumulation of intracellular lactate (Myers *et al.* 1983). These authors suggest that infusion of glucose following asphyxia may also be potentially dangerous, but the evidence for this is much less good. Glucose is an essential metabolic substrate of the neuron, and hypoglycaemia may have a devastating effect on the brain. For this reason asphyxiated infants should have regular blood glucose stick-test estimations, and if the blood glucose falls below 2mmol/l an infusion of 10 per cent dextrose should be given to correct the hypoglycaemia. Rapid bolus injections of concentrated glucose must be avoided.

Barbiturates
Barbiturates have multiple effects on the brain and have been extensively evaluated in adult human and animal studies. Beneficial effects have been shown in these studies only if the drug was given prior to the period of asphyxia (Campbell *et al.* 1968, Cockburn *et al.* 1969, Goodlin and Lloyd 1970). The only study assessing a barbiturate (thiopentone) following a period of cardiac arrest in adults showed no differences in outcome between the treated and non-treated groups (Abramson *et al.* 1983). Svenningsen *et al.* (1982) recommended routine use of phenobarbitone (10mg/kg) within an hour of delivery in all severely asphyxiated infants and claimed to have reduced the mortality and incidence of neurodevelopmental handicap in a group of infants compared with a group treated earlier. It seems unlikely that the relatively low dose of phenobarbitone used in this study had any significant beneficial effect in protecting the brain. It is more likely that the careful attention paid to the infant generally was the factor that was most likely to have improved the outcome.

Recently two studies have been published, reporting the outcome in term asphyxiated infants of early treatment with thiopentone. Eyre and Wilkinson (1986) used a continuous infusion of thiopentone sufficient to suppress the EEG in six severely asphyxiated infants, but did not feel that this form of therapy benefited the infants. The three survivors were moderately or severely disabled. In an American study, thiopentone was continuously infused in 32 severely asphyxiated term infants and the results were no better than a control non-treated group (Goldberg *et al.* 1986). Both studies reported hypotension to be a common complication of thiopentone infusion.

Monitoring of ICP
There are good theoretical reasons to monitor ICP and treat intracranial hypertension. However, there are fundamental differences between RICP that

TABLE 6.V

Regime to treat severe birth asphyxia with raised intracranial pressure

Respiratory system	If spontaneous respiration then ensure $PaCO_2$ does not exceed 6.5kPa. If mechanically ventilated maintain $PaCO_2$ between 3.5 and 4.0kPa. Maintain PaO_2 10 to 12kPa.
Fluids	Maintain infants on 20 per cent less fluids than their normal daily requirement. If inappropriate ADH secretion further reduce fluids.
Seizures	Phenobarbitone 20mg/kg loading dose and maintenance 3mg/kg 12 hourly. Paraldehyde 0.1mg/kg as required. Clonazepam 0.25mg loading dose and 0.05mg 12 hourly. In severe cases 5-10µg/kg/hr can be infused continuously.
Raised intracranial pressure	Mannitol 20 per cent solution 0.5–1g/kg infused 20 minutes four-hourly as required.

occurs with birth asphyxia, and that which develops in association with post-haemorrhagic hydrocephalus. In the former case there is global brain-swelling with compression of the ventricular system. The oedema is both cytotoxic and vasogenic (Klatzo 1967) and is secondary to the underlying asphyxial process. Intracranial hypertension occurring after intracranial haemorrhage is due to obstruction to the passage of CSF through the ventricular system. In this case the surrounding brain is often normal and injury may occur only as the result of compression, quite unlike the situation following asphyxial injury.

Birth asphyxia

There is little information concerning the management of RICP in the term infant who has suffered birth asphyxia. Only about 50 per cent of babies born at term with birth asphyxia develop intracranial hypertension (Levene *et al.* 1987), but there appears to be no way of predicting which infants will do so. Table 6.V summarises a recommended regime to manage intracranial hypertension in the term infant. Infants should be maintained in a stable condition and blood gases carefully monitored. Elective mechanical ventilation should be undertaken if the $PaCO_2$ exceeds 6.5kPa (45mmHg), and when the infant is mechanically ventilated, we maintain the $PaCO_2$ between 3.5 and 4.0kPa. There is a close relationship between arterial carbon dioxide tension ($PaCO_2$) and CBF. In adults, for every 0.13kPa (1mmHg) change in $PaCO_2$ there is approximately a 3 per cent change in CBF over the physiological range for $PaCO_2$ (Bruce 1984), but this diminishes for $PaCO_2$ levels below 2.7kPa (23mmHg). This effect is mediated by changes in tone of the cerebral arterioles, and it has been shown that term infants can alter their arteriolar resistance in response to changing levels of carbon dioxide tension (Archer *et al.* 1985).

We have abandoned the use of corticosteroids in birth asphyxia. There is no evidence in perinatal animal studies that the administration of steroids *after* the asphyxial insult reduces subsequent brain swelling (DeSouza and Dobbing 1973). We could not show that dexamethasone had any effect on improving CPP in a six-hour period immediately following dexamethasone injection (Levene and Evans 1985). In addition, there is a body of evidence reporting the adverse effects of steroids on the developing brain (Weichsel 1977); and measurable differences in the cerebral function of children who had received hydrocortisone early in life have been reported (Fitzhardinge *et al.* 1974).

There is little evidence to support the concept that monitoring ICP makes any difference to the outcome of infants who have suffered severe birth asphyxia. Although there are no controlled studies available, an analysis of our own data suggests that in only 9 per cent of infants in whom direct measurement of ICP was made from the subarachnoid space could this information have altered management to the benefit of the infant (Levene *et al.* 1987). I do not recommend the routine measurement of ICP in birth asphyxia.

Cerebral perfusion pressure

As well as RICP impairing CPP it is important to be aware of the role of systemic hypotension in reducing the CPP. Hypotension—a mean arterial blood-pressure below 40mmHg—is a common event in severely asphyxiated term infants. The severity and duration of hypotension may not be recognised unless continuous monitoring of arterial blood pressure is performed. Hypotension is treated with plasma (10ml/kg) or an inotropic agent such as dopamine (5 to 10µg/kg/hr) or dobutamine (2.5µg/kg/hr).

Post-haemorrhagic ventricular dilatation (PHVD)

This is a common condition in preterm infants following PVH, but may occur in children of any age following intracranial haemorrhage. Hydrocephalus with RICP also occurs commonly following neonatal meningitis.

The prevalence of PHVD depends on its diagnostic criteria. We define this condition when measurement of the distance from the midline to the lateral-most extent of the lateral ventricle (referred to as the ventricular index or VI) exceeds the 97th centile (Levene *et al.* 1985b). We have reported an incidence of PHVD diagnosed by regular examinations with real-time ultrasound to be 34 per cent (Levene and Starte 1981). In this study, only three of the 15 infants with PHVD actually required a ventricular shunt. Others have reported incidences of PHVD between 10 per cent (Ment *et al.* 1984) and 54 per cent (Allan *et al.* 1982). The incidence of PHVD varies with the severity of the haemorrhage and is three times as frequent in infants with parenchymal haemorrhage compared to haemorrhage confined to the region of the germinal matrix (Levene 1987).

The site of blockage to CSF flow is most commonly at the arachnoid granulations over the surface of the brain, and in our experience non-communicating obstruction due to blockage at the outlet of the fourth ventricle is the cause of PHVD in only 18 per cent of cases (Levene 1987). Distinction between PHVD and cerebral atrophy may be extremely difficult. On scanning the ventricles of a child with pressure-driven PHVD the ventricles are ballooned in shape, with loss of the normal

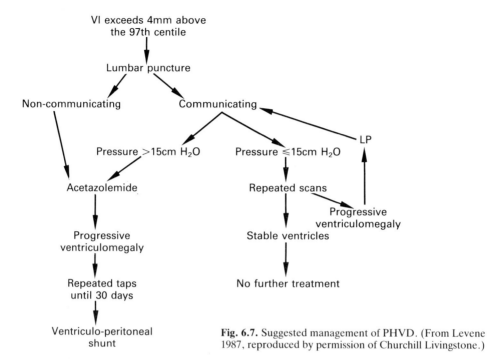

Fig. 6.7. Suggested management of PHVD. (From Levene 1987, reproduced by permission of Churchill Livingstone.)

angles of the lateral ventricles. In cerebral atrophy the ventricles are enlarged but retain their usual configuration. A diagnostic criterion for pressure-driven PHVD, as opposed to atrophy, is to show an increase in ICP. We perform this by measuring the CSF-opening pressure at lumbar puncture. A pressure of more than 15cm of water is taken to confirm significant intracranial hypertension.

There are three methods of treatment: regular lumbar punctures, drugs such as acetazolamide, and ventriculoperitoneal shunting. We avoid placing a shunt in an infant following intracranial haemorrhage until at least 30 days after the bleed to reduce the risk of the valve blocking. At diagnosis of PHVD and in the presence of intracranial hypertension we start acetazolamide (25mg/kg/day rising to a maximum of 100mg/kg/day) orally (Shinnar *et al.* 1985). This drug is a carbonic anhydrase inhibitor and induces metabolic acidosis. The infant's acid-base status must be carefully monitored and base replacement given as a matter of routine. It is claimed that regular lumbar punctures prevent the need for shunting (Goldstein *et al.* 1976, Papile *et al.* 1980), but this has not been confirmed by others (Anwar *et al.* 1985). It may, however, temporarily ameliorate progressive ventricular dilatation (Kreusser *et al.* 1985). In babies treated by this method we remove CSF equivalent in volume to 1 per cent of the infant's birthweight. Figure 6.7 summarises our approach to the management of PHVD.

Doppler assessment of cerebral haemodynamics
We initially used Doppler ultrasound to try to determine non-invasively whether the infant was likely to develop RICP. Unfortunately there appears to be no

correlation between Doppler signals and ICP, but we did find that changes in the Doppler signals correlated with adverse outcome (Archer *et al*. 1986). This method may be used to determine which infants should have invasive monitoring of ICP (see below).

A practical approach to the management of birth asphyxia
There are few clear-cut rules related to how long resuscitative attempts should continue after birth in a child born with no signs of life. My recommendation is that resuscitation should be abandoned if an infant has no cardiac output for 10 minutes after birth, or if he fails to breathe 30 minutes after establishing cardiac output. If there is any doubt, then treatment should be continued and the child admitted to the neonatal intensive care unit. Careful systematic clinical examination should be performed at regular intervals. Doppler assessment of the cerebral circulation appears to be a useful method for predicting outcome, and consistently low Pourcelot resistance index (PRI) values or very high CBV are very poor signs. In my view, direct measurement of ICP does not have a role in the clinical management of severe birth asphyxia. If the infant survives into the second week of life, CT scanning may be of further use in guiding prognosis. Care should be withdrawn in severely asphyxiated infants only after careful and repeated explanation to the parents. They may need quite some time to come to terms with the information and its consequences. It is the duty of medical and nursing staff to continue to give the parents maximum support, although there is nothing positive to be done for their infant.

Prognosis
Depression of the Apgar score has traditionally been used for predicting outcome. Nelson and Ellenberg (1981) found that in term infants the risk of death or cerebral palsy becomes high only if the Apgar score is 3 or less at 20 minutes. A score of 3 or less at 15 minutes is associated with a lower than 10 per cent risk of cerebral palsy in surviving infants. Thomson *et al*. (1977) reported that 93 per cent of infants with an Apgar score of 0 at one minute or less than 3 at five minutes were normal at follow-up examination. A score of 5 or less at 10 minutes is the most sensitive predictor of adverse outcome, but is still much less reliable than the degree of PAE (Levene *et al*. 1986).

PAE is the best clinical method of predicting neurodevelopmental outcome. Although mild PAE is defined slightly differently by different groups, the published studies show remarkable consensus when it is used to predict outcome. In a recent review of these studies (Levene 1988), no infant with mild PAE developed significant neurodevelopmental handicap as the result of asphyxia. In the Leicester study, 25 per cent of infants with moderate encephalopathy died or were severely disabled compared to 75 per cent of infants with severe PAE (Levene *et al*. 1986). Sarnat and Sarnat (1976) showed that a good outcome was seen in infants with moderate PAE (lethargy, hypotonia and seizures) if the abnormal clinical signs had disappeared within five days of birth. Scott (1976) found that cerebral palsy developed only in infants who had persistent neurological abnormality for more

159

than six weeks. Two particular patterns of neurological abnormality were found to correspond with adverse outcome. These were persistent hypotonia and the pattern of early hypotonia evolving to hypertonus (Brown *et al.* 1974).

CT appears to be a useful prognostic test in term infants. Hypodensity is thought to correlate with cerebral oedema, and the majority (76.5 per cent) of infants with extensive areas of hypodensity had major neurodevelopmental sequelae (Fitzhardinge *et al.* 1981). Adsett *et al.* (1985) also found low attenuation on CT to be both sensitive (90 per cent) and specific (80 per cent) for major handicap or death. CT appears to be reliable for prognostic purposes only if performed in the second week after birth (Lipp-Zwahlen *et al.* 1985*b*).

A sustained rise in ICP of 15mmHg or more, lasting for an hour or more, is associated with a very poor prognosis (Levene *et al.* 1987). No infant with intracranial hypertension of this degree survived without very severe neuro-developmental sequelae. Low CPP, however, did not predict adverse outcome with the same sensitivity as RICP, and we had some normal survivors with a sustained fall in CPP to 25mmHg for an hour or more.

Doppler ultrasound is a reliable prognostic tool in asphyxiated term infants. A low PRI reading of less than 0.55 predicted adverse outcome with a sensitivity of 100 per cent and specificity of 81 per cent (Archer *et al.* 1986). The over-all accuracy of this technique in predicting adverse outcome was 86 per cent. The PRI became abnormal within 62 hours of birth and at a median time of 28 hours.

Real-time ultrasound is a particularly good method of predicting outcome in preterm infants. Most recent studies using high-quality ultrasound equipment agree that it is the PVL lesions that are most likely to be correlated with adverse outcome (Bozynski *et al.* 1985, deVries *et al.* 1985, Fawer *et al.* 1985, Weindling *et al.* 1985, Graziani *et al.* 1986, Graham *et al.* 1987). In a follow-up study of 157 very low-birthweight infants who all had careful and repeated ultrasonic examinations in the newborn period, cavitating PVL was found to be 94 per cent accurate in predicting cerebral palsy (Graham *et al.* 1987). If the ultrasonic cavities were multiple or in the region of occipital periventricular white matter, then the children were at very high risk of severe cerebral palsy. It is now accepted that uncomplicated PVH (providing there is no parenchymal extension) does not put the infant at significantly greater risk of disability than if the infant had normal scans (Graham *et al.* 1987, Stewart *et al.* 1987).

Cerebral protection
There has been considerable interest in recent years in the pharmacological management of the brain both before and after insult. In the newborn infant, these methods can be divided into the prevention of PVH and drug use after a period of global asphyxia. To date there has been little work specifically related to the asphyxiated perinatal animal, and none at all in the human neonate, but as these methods hold great promise they will be briefly reviewed here.

Calcium channel blockers
Imbalance between intracellular and extracellular calcium occurs after severe

cerebral compromise, and elevated levels of intracellular calcium are extremely toxic to the neuron and may also cause intense cerebral arteriolar vasospasm. Entry of calcium into the cell may be blocked by certain drugs and some have been shown to be particularly successful if used prior to the asphyxial event (Bircher and Safar 1983, Steen *et al.* 1983, White *et al.* 1983). Recently two studies have reported on the effect of calcium channel blockers in newborn animals after a severe asphyxial event. Thiringer *et al.* (1987) described an improvement in outcome in a group of lambs treated with lidoflazine (together with an oxygen-free radical scavenger) compared with a control group. In a study of newborn beagle puppies the calcium antagonist, nimodipine, did not improve CBF in asphyxiated animals (Ment *et al.* 1987). These two studies varied considerably in their methodology, and it is difficult to draw conclusions with any clinical implications in mind.

We have recently studied the effects of nicardipine, a water-soluble calcium channel blocker, in four severely asphyxiated term newborn infants. The infants all had abnormal Doppler studies indicating a poor prognosis, but in two infants severe hypotension developed with marked tachycardia within hours of the start of the infusion (Levene *et al.* 1990). We suggest that calcium channel blockers may cause hypotension in newborn infants by means of a systemic vasodilatory action, and these drugs should be very carefully evaluated prior to their routine use for birth asphyxia.

Oxygen-free radical scavengers
Oxygen-free radical (OFR) scavengers are produced on reperfusion following a period of asphyxia. They are extremely reactive and damage intracellular membranes, causing secondary compromise to cellular metabolism. Thiringer *et al.* (1987) used OFR scavengers (mannitol, l-methionine and magnesium sulphate) together with a calcium channel blocker after experimental asphyxia in lambs, to beneficial effect. It is not clear whether the OFR scavengers alone were the protective agent. Vitamin E is also a potent OFR scavenger, and this agent has been used in the prevention of PVH (p. 163).

Excitatory amino acid neurotransmitters
Certain excitatory synaptic neurotransmitters, such as aspartate and glutamate, may accumulate following asphyxia and cause neuronal damage (Meldrum 1985). Agents which act as inhibitors of neurotransmitters may prevent neuronal death in tissue culture during asphyxia (Rothman 1984). To date there are few experimental data on the use of these agents in the perinatal period.

Prostaglandin inhibitors
During periods of asphyxia and ischaemia there is production of intracellular arachidonic acid, a precursor of prostaglandins. During reperfusion, oxidation occurs with the production of vaso-active compounds including thromboxane (a vasoconstrictor) and prostacyclin (a vasodilator). Indomethacin is a prostaglandin synthetase inhibitor and causes a fall in CBF in preterm infants (Evans *et al.* 1987). Indomethacin and prostacyclin, when infused into dogs following experimental

TABLE 6.VI

Agents that have been reported to reduce the incidence of periventricular haemorrhage in infants or immature animals

Phenobarbitone
Ethamsylate
Pancuronium
Vitamin E
Indomethacin
Prolactin
Plasma infusion

ischaemic cerebral injury, prevents the impairment in CBF normally seen following this procedure (Hallenbeck and Furlow 1979). Neither indomethacin nor prostacyclin when given alone had a similar beneficial effect.

Indomethacin has been used in preterm infants to prevent PVH but has not been used following perinatal asphyxia.

Naloxone
The specific opiate antagonist naloxone, when given after asphyxia, has been shown to improve bloodflow to the brainstem in lambs (Lou *et al.* 1985). Chernick and Craig (1982) have shown that naloxone improves the short-term outcome of rabbits if given before the asphyxial event, but others have found that naloxone exacerbates cerebral injury in the neonatal rat (Young *et al.* 1984) and the newborn rabbit (Goodlin 1981). The routine use of naloxone following birth asphyxia cannot be recommended.

Prevention of periventricular haemorrhage
A relatively large number of drugs have been shown to reduce the incidence of PVH in newborn human infants or animals (Table 6.VI) and these studies are discussed in detail elsewhere (deVries *et al.* 1988). A few agents will be mentioned here.

Phenobarbitone
Donn *et al.* (1981) first suggested that phenobarbitone given in the first few hours after birth may prevent PVH, and others have shown that prenatal use of this drug may also reduce the incidence of PVH (Shankaran *et al.* 1986, Morales and Koerten 1986). In contrast, four other studies have failed to reproduce these results (Morgan *et al.* 1982, Whitelaw *et al.* 1983, Bedard *et al.* 1984, Kuban *et al.* 1986). The Boston group (Kuban *et al.* 1986) designed the study to have a 90 per cent power of showing a 50 per cent reduction in the occurrence of PVH and actually found the pretreated infants to have a statistically higher incidence of haemorrhage! The balance of evidence does not support the routine use of phenobarbitone in preterm infants.

Ethamsylate
This drug reduces capillary bleeding and also has an effect on reducing

prostaglandin synthesis. Morgan *et al.* (1981) showed that its early use in preterm infants reduces the incidence of PVH, and this has been subsequently confirmed in a multicentre controlled double-blind study (Benson *et al.* 1986).

Vitamin E

There are conflicting data on the use of vitamin E in preventing PVH. A number of studies have suggested that it reduces the incidence of haemorrhage (Chiswick *et al.* 1983, Speer *et al.* 1984, Sinha *et al.* 1987), but another study showed that in a group of extremely low-birthweight infants weighing less than 1000g there was an increased incidence of PVH (Phelps 1984). It is suggested that its effect is mediated through stabilisation of endothelial membranes but that it also has an effect as an OFR scavenger.

Indomethacin

This agent is discussed above, and it has been shown that if administered shortly after birth to immature animals (Ment *et al.* 1983) and human infants (Ment *et al.* 1985) it reduces the incidence of haemorrhage. It inhibits the vasodilatory prostaglandins and limits acute changes in blood pressure. It also causes a fall in CBF in preterm infants (Evans *et al.* 1987) and causes dissociation between cerebral metabolism and flow (Pickard and Mackenzie 1973), and both of these factors may not be of benefit to the immature infant.

At present, I do not believe that there is any indication for the routine use of any of these agents in the prevention of PVH in preterm infants. The important question is not 'Can we prevent PVH?' but 'Can we prevent subsequent disability and handicap?' To date, there is no evidence to suggest that we can.

REFERENCES

Abramson, N.S., Safer, P., Detre, K., Kelsey, S., Monroe, J., Reinmuth, U., Snyder, J., Mullie, J., Hedstrand, U., Tammisto, T., Lund, J., Breivik, H., Lind, B., Jastremski, M. (1983) 'Thiopental loading in cardiopulmonary resuscitation (CPR) survivors: a randomized collaborative study.' *Anesthesiology*, **59**, A101.
Adsett, D.B., Fitz, C.R., Hill, A. (1985) 'Hypoxic-ischaemic cerebral injury in the term newborn: correlation of CT findings with neurological outcome.' *Developmental Medicine and Child Neurology*, **27**, 155–160.
Allan, W.C., Holt, P.J., Sawyer, L.R., Tito, A.M., Meade, S.K. (1982) 'Ventricular dilation after neonatal periventricular-intraventricular hemorrhage.' *American Journal of Diseases of Children*, **136**, 589–593.
Amiel-Tison, C., Dalisson, C., Henrion, R. (1980) 'L'évolution de la pathologie cérébrale du nouveau-né à terme.' *Archives Françaises de Pédiatrie*, **37**, 87–92.
Anwar, M., Kadam, S., Hiatt, I.M., Hegyi, T. (1985) 'Serial lumbar punctures in prevention of post-hemorrhagic hydrocephalus in preterm infants.' *Journal of Pediatrics*, **107**, 446–450.
Apgar, V. (1953) 'A proposal for a new method of evaluation of the newborn infant.' *Current Research in Anesthesia and Analgesia*, **32**, 260–267.
Archer, L.N.J., Evans, D.H. (1988) 'Doppler assessment of the neonatal cerebral circulation.' *In* Levene, M.I., Bennett, M.J., Punt, J. (Eds.) *Fetal and Neonatal Neurology and Neurosurgery.* Edinburgh: Churchill Livingstone.
—— —— Paton, J.Y., Levene, M.I. (1985) 'Controlled hypercapnia and neonatal cerebral artery Doppler ultrasound waveforms.' *Pediatric Research*, **20**, 218–221.

—— Levene, M.I., Evans, D.H. (1986) 'Cerebral artery Doppler ultrasonography for prediction of outcome after perinatal asphyxia.' *Lancet*, **2**, 1116–1118.

Banker, B.Q., Larroche, C.-L. (1962) 'Periventricular leukomalacia of infancy.' *Archives of Neurology*, **7**, 386–410.

Beard, R.W., Filshie, G.M., Knight, C.A., Roberto, G.M. (1971) 'The significance of the changes in the continuous fetal heart rate in the first stage of labour.' *Journal of Obstetrics and Gynaecology of the British Commonwealth*, **78**, 865–881.

Bedard, M.P., Shankaran, S., Slovis, T.L., Pantoja, A., Dayal, B., Poland, R.L. (1984) 'Effect of prophylactic phenobarbital on intraventricular hemorrhage in high-risk infants.' *Pediatrics*, **73**, 435–439.

Benson, J.W.T., Drayton, M.R., Hayward, C., Murphy, J.E., Osborne, J.P., Rennie, J.M., Schulte, J.E., Speadel, B.D., Cooke, R.W.I. (1986) 'Multicentre trial of ethamsylate for prevention of periventricular haemorrhage in very low birthweight infants.' *Lancet*, **2**, 1297–1300.

Bircher, N.G., Safar, P. (1983) 'Cerebral preservation during cardiopulmonary resuscitation (CPR) in dogs.' *Anesthesiology*, **59**, A93.

Bissonette, J.M. (1975) 'Relationship between continuous fetal heart rate patterns and Apgar score in the newborn.' *British Journal of Obstetrics and Gynaecology*, **82**, 24–28.

Boyle, R. (1670) 'On the phenomena afforded by a newly kittened kitling in the exhausted receiver.' *Philosophical Transactions of the Royal Society*, **5**, 2017–2019.

Bozynski, M.E., Nelson, M.N., Matalon, T.A.S., Genaze, D.R., Rosati-Skertich, C., Naughton, P.M., Meier, W.A. (1985) 'Cavitary periventricular leukomalacia: incidence and short term outcome in infants weighing <1200 grams at birth.' *Developmental Medicine and Child Neurology*, **27**, 572–577.

Brown, J.K., Purvis, R.J., Forfar, J.O., Cockburn, F. (1974) 'Neurological aspects of perinatal asphyxia.' *Developmental Medicine and Child Neurology*, **16**, 567–580.

Bruce, D.A. (1984) 'Effects of hyperventilation on cerebral blood flow and metabolism.' *Clinics in Perinatology*, **11**, 673–680.

Calvert, S.A., Hoskins, E.M., Fong, K.W., Forsyth, S.C. (1987) 'Etiological factors associated with the development of periventricular leukomalacia.' *Acta Paediatrica Scandinavica*, **76**, 254–259.

Campbell, A.M., Milligin, J.E., Talner, N.S. (1968) 'The effect of pretreatment with pentobarbital, meperidine or hyperbaric oxygen on the response to anoxia and resuscitation in newborn rabbits.' *Journal of Pediatrics*, **72**, 518–527.

Chernick, V., Craig, R.J. (1982) 'Nalaxone reverses neonatal depression caused by fetal asphyxia.' *Science*, **216**, 1252–1253.

Chiswick, M.L., Johnson, M., Woodhall, C., Gowland, M., Davies, J., Tomer, W., Sims, D.G. (1983) 'Protective effect of vitamin E (*dl*-alpha-tocopherol) against intraventricular haemorrhage in premature babies.' *British Medical Journal*, **287**, 81–84.

Cockburn, F., Daniel, S.S., Dawes, G.S., James, L.S., Myers, R.E., Niemann, W. (1969) 'The effect of pentobarbital anesthesia on resuscitation and brain damage in fetal rhesus monkeys asphyxiated on delivery.' *Journal of Pediatrics*, **75**, 281–291.

Cohn, H.E., Sacks, E.J., Heymann, M.A., Rudolph, A.M. (1974) 'Cardiovascular responses to hypoxemia and acidemia in fetal lambs.' *American Journal of Obstetrics and Gynecology*, **120**, 817–824.

Cyr, R.M., Usher, R.H., McLean, F.H. (1984) 'Changing patterns of birth asphyxia and trauma over 20 years.' *American Journal of Obstetrics and Gynecology*, **148**, 490–498.

DeSouza, S.W., Dobbing, J. (1973) 'Cerebral oedema in developing brain. III. Brain water and electrolytes in immature asphyxiated rats treated with dexamethasone.' *Biology of the Neonate*, **22**, 388–397.

deVries, L.S., Dubowitz, V., Kaiser, M., Lary, S., Silverman, M., Whitelaw, A., Wigglesworth, J.S. (1985) 'Predictive value of cranial ultrasound: a reappraisal.' *Lancet*, **2**, 137–140.

—— Regev, R., Dubowitz, L.M.S. (1986) 'Late onset cystic leukomalacia.' *Archives of Disease in Childhood*, **61**, 298–299.

—— Larroche, J.-C., Levene, M.I. (1988) 'Cerebral ischaemic lesions.' *In* Levene, M.I., Bennett, M.J., Punt, J. (Eds.) *Fetal and Neonatal Neurology and Neurosurgery*. Edinburgh: Churchill Livingstone.

Donald, I. (1959) 'Birth. Adaptation from intrauterine to extrauterine life.' *In* Holland, E., Bourne, A. (Eds.) *British Obstetric Practice*. London: Heinemann.

Donn, S.M., Roloff, D.W., Goldstein, G.W. (1981) 'Prevention of intraventricular hemorrhage in preterm infants by phenobarbitone. A controlled trial.' *Lancet*, **2**, 215–217.

Dubowitz, L.M.S., Levene, M.I., Morante, A., Palmer, P., Dubowitz, P. (1981) 'Neurologic signs in neonatal intraventricular hemorrhage: a correlation with real-time ultrasound.' *Journal of Pediatrics*, **99**, 127–133.

Edelstone, D.I., Rudolph, A.M., Heymann, M.A. (1977) 'Liver and ductus venosus blood flow in fetal lambs in utero.' *Circulation Research*, **42**, 426.

Ergander, U., Ericksson, M., Zetterstrom, R. (1983) 'Severe neonatal asphyxia. Incidence and prediction of outcome in the Stockholm area.' *Acta Paediatrica Scandinavica*, **72**, 321–325.

Evans, D.H., Levene, M.I., Archer, L.N.J. (1987) 'The effect of indomethacin on cerebral blood-flow velocity in premature infants.' *Developmental Medicine and Child Neurology*, **29**, 776–782.

Eyre, J.A., Wilkinson, A.R. (1986) 'Thiopentone induced coma after severe birth asphyxia.' *Archives of Disease in Childhood*, **61**, 1084–1089.

—— Oozeer, R.C., Wilkinson, A.R. (1983) 'Diagnosis of neonatal seizure by continuous recording rapid analysis of the electroencephalogram.' *Archives of Disease in Childhood*, **58**, 785–790.

Fawer, C-L., Calame, A., Furrer, M-T., (1985) 'Neurodevelopmental outcome at 12 months of age, related to cerebral ultrasound appearances of high risk preterm infants.' *Early Human Development*, **11**, 123–132.

Fenichel, G.M. (1983) 'Hypoxic-ischaemic encephalopathy in the newborn.' *Archives of Neurology*, **40**, 261–266.

Finer, N.N., Robertson, O.M., Peters, K.L., Coward, J.H. (1983) 'Factors affecting outcome in hypoxic-ischaemic encephalopathy in term infants.' *American Journal of Diseases of Children*, **137**, 21–25.

Fisher, D.J., Heymann, M.A., Rudolph, A.M. (1980) 'Myocardial oxygen and carbohydrate consumption in fetal lambs in utero and adult sheep.' *American Journal of Physiology*, **238**, H399–H405.

Fitzhardinge, P., Eisen, E., Lejtonyi, C., Metrakos, K., Ramsay, M. (1974) 'Sequelae of early steroid administration to the newborn infant.' *Pediatrics*, **53**, 877–883.

—— Flodmark, O., Fitz, C.R., Ashby, S. (1981) 'The prognostic value of computed tomography as an adjunct to assessment of the term infant with postasphyxial encephalography.' *Journal of Pediatrics*, **99**, 777–781.

Flodmark, O., Becker, L.E., Harwood-Nash, D.C., Fitzhardinge, P.M., Fitz, C.R., Chuang, S.H. (1980) 'Correlation between computed tomography and autopsy in premature and full-term neonates that have suffered perinatal asphyxia.' *Radiology*, **137**, 93–103.

Gérard, P., Verheggen, P., Bachy, A., Langhandries, J-P. (1981) 'Intérêt de la tomodensitometrie cérébrale chez les infants nés asphyxiés.' *Archives Françaises de Pédiatrie*, **38**, 591–596.

Goitein, K.J., Amit, Y. (1982) 'Percutaneous placement of subdural catheter for measurement of intracranial pressure in small children.' *Critical Care Medicine*, **10**, 46–48.

Goldberg, R.N., Moscoso, P., Bauer, C.R., Bloom, P.L., Curless, R.G., Burke, R., Bancalari, E. (1986) 'Use of barbiturate therapy in severe perinatal asphyxia: a randomized controlled trial.' *Journal of Pediatrics*, **109**, 851–856.

Goldstein, G.W., Chaplin, E.R., Maitland, J., Norman, D. (1976) 'Transient hydrocephalus in premature infants: treatment by lumbar punctures.' *Lancet*, **1**, 512–514.

Goodlin, R.C. (1981) 'Nalaxone administration and newborn rabbit response to asphyxia.' *American Journal of Obstetrics and Gynecology*, **140**, 340–341.

—— Lloyd, D. (1970) 'Use of drugs to protect against fetal asphyxia.' *American Journal of Obstetrics and Gynecology*, **107**, 227–231.

Gould, S.J., Howard, S., Hope, P.L., Reynolds, E.O.R. (1987) 'Periventricular intraparenchymal cerebral haemorrhage in preterm infants: the role of venous infarction.' *Journal of Pathology*, **151**, 197–202.

Graham, M., Levene, M.I., Trounce, J.Q., Rutter, N. (1987) 'Prediction of cerebral palsy in very low birthweight infants: prospective ultrasound study.' *Lancet*, **2**, 593–596.

Grant, A., O'Brien, N., Joy, M-T., Hennessy, E., MacDonald, D. (1989) 'Cerebral palsy among children born during the Dublin randomised trial of intrapartum monitoring.' *Lancet*, **2**, 1233–1236.

Graziani, L.J., Pasto, M., Stanley, C., Pidcock, F., Desai, H., Desai, S., Branca, P., Goldberg, B. (1986) 'Neonatal neurosonographic correlates of cerebral palsy in preterm infants.' *Pediatrics*, **78**, 88–95.

Greisen, G. (1988) 'Methods of assessing cerebral blood flow.' *In* Levene, M.I., Bennett, M.J., Punt, J. (Eds.) *Fetal and Neonatal Neurology and Neurosurgery*. Edinburgh: Churchill Livingstone.

Hallenbeck, J.M., Furlow, T.W. (1979) 'Prostaglandin 12 and indomethacin prevent impairment of post-ischaemic brain reperfusion in the dog.' *Stroke*, **10**, 629–637.

Hecox, K.F., Cone, B. (1981) 'Prognostic importance of brainstem auditory evoked responses after asphyxia.' *Neurology*, **31**, 1429–1433.

Horbar, J.D., Yeager, S., Philip, A.G.S., Lucey, J.F. (1980) 'Effect of application force on noninvasive measurements of intracranial pressure.' *Pediatrics*, **66**, 455–457.

165

Hrbek, A., Karlberg, P., Kjellmer, I., Olsson, T., Riha, M. (1977) 'Clinical application of evoked electroencephalographic responses in newborn infants. I. Perinatal asphyxia.' *Developmental Medicine and Child Neurology*, **19**, 34–44.

Kaiser, A.M., Whitelaw, A.G. (1986) 'Cerebrospinal fluid pressure during post haemorrhagic ventricular dilatation in newborn infants.' *Archives of Disease in Childhood*, **60**, 920–924.

—— —— (1987) 'Noninvasive monitoring of intracranial pressure—fact or fancy?' *Developmental Medicine and Child Neurology*, **29**, 320–326.

Klatzo, I. (1967) 'Neuropathological aspects of brain damage.' *Journal of Neuropathology and Experimental Neurology*, **26**, 1–14.

Kreusser, K.L., Tarby, T.L., Kovnar, E., Taylor, D.A., Hill, A., Volpe, J.J. (1985) 'Serial lumbar punctures for at least temporary amelioration of neonatal posthemorrhagic hydrocephalus.' *Pediatrics*, **75**, 719–724.

Kuban, C.K., Leviton, A., Krishnamoorthy, K.S., Brown, E.R., Teele, R.L., Baglivo, J.A., Sullivan, K.P., Huff, K.R., White, S., Cleveland, R.H., Allred, E.N., Spritzer, K.L., Skouteli, H.N., Cayea, P., Epstein, M.C. (1986) 'Neonatal intracranial hemorrhage and phenobarbital.' *Pediatrics*, **77**, 443–450.

Larroche, J-C. (1977) *Developmental Pathology of the Neonate*. Amsterdam: Excerpta Medica.

Levene, M.I. (1987) *Current Reviews in Paediatrics. 3. Neonatal Neurology*. Edinburgh: Churchill Livingstone.

—— (1988) 'Birth asphyxia—management and outcome.' *In* Levene, M.I., Bennett, M.J., Punt, P. (Eds.) *Fetal and Neonatal Neurology and Neurosurgery*. Edinburgh: Churchill Livingstone.

—— Evans, D.H. (1983) 'Continuous measurement of subarachnoid pressure in the severely asphyxiated newborn.' *Archives of Disease in Childhood*, **58**, 1013–1015.

—— —— (1985) 'The medical management of raised intracranial pressure following severe birth asphyxia.' *Archives of Disease in Childhood*, **60**, 12–16.

—— Starte, D.R. (1981) 'A longitudinal study of post-haemorrhagic ventricular dilatation in the newborn.' *Archives of Disease in Childhood*, **56**, 905–910.

—— Kornberg, J., Williams, T.H.C. (1985a) 'The incidence and severity of post-asphyxial encephalopathy in full-term infants.' *Early Human Development*, **11**, 21–26.

—— Williams, J.L., Fawer, C-L. (1985b) *Ultrasound of the Infant Brain. Clinics in Developmental Medicine No. 92.* London: S.I.M.P. with Blackwell Scientific; Philadelphia: Lippincott.

—— Sands, C., Grindulis, H., Moore, J.R. (1986) 'Comparison of two methods of predicting outcome in perinatal asphyxia.' *Lancet*, **1**, 67–69.

—— Evans, D.H., Forde, A., Archer, L.N.J. (1987) 'Value of intracranial pressure monitoring of asphyxiated newborn infants.' *Developmental Medicine and Child Neurology*, **29**, 311–319.

—— Fenton, A.C., Evans, D.H., Shortland, D.B., Gibson, M.A. (1989) 'Severe asphyxia and abnormal cerebral blood-flow velocity.' *Developmental Medicine and Child Neurology*, **31**, 427–434.

—— Gibson, N.A., Fenton, A.C., Papathoma, E., Barnett, D. (1990) 'The use of a calcium-channel blocker, nicardipine, for severely asphyxiated newborn infants.' *Developmental Medicine and Child Neurology*, **32**, 567–574.

Lipp-Zwahlen, A.E., Deonna, T., Micheli, J.L., Calame, A., Chrzanowski, R., Cêtre, E. (1985a) 'Prognostic value of neonatal CT scans in asphyxiated term babies: low density score compared with neonatal neurological signs.' *Neuropediatrics*, **16**, 209–217.

—— Chrzanowski, R., Micheli, J.L., Calame, A. (1985b) 'Temporal evolution of hypoxic-ischaemic brain lesions in asphyxiated full-term newborns as assessed by computerized tomography.' *Neuroradiology*, **27**, 138–144.

Ljunggren, B., Schultz, H., Siesjo, B.K. (1974) 'Changes in energy state and acid-base parameters of the rat brain during complete compression ischaemia.' *Brain Research*, **73**, 277–289.

Lou, H.C., Tweed, W.A., Davies, J.M. (1985) 'Preferential blood flow increase to the brain stem in moderate neonatal hypoxia: reversal by naloxone.' *European Journal of Pediatrics*, **144**, 225–227.

MacDonald, D., Grant, A., Sheridan-Pereira, M., Boylan, P., Chalmers, I. (1985) 'The Dublin randomized controlled trial of intrapartum fetal heart rate monitoring.' *American Journal of Obstetrics and Gynecology*, **152**, 524–539.

Magliner, A.D., Wertheimer, I.S. (1980) 'Preliminary results of a computed tomography study of neonatal brain hypoxia-ischemia.' *Journal of Computer Assisted Tomography*, **4**, 457–463.

McDonald, M.M., Johnson, M.L., Rumack, C.M., Koops, B.L., Guggenheim, M.A., Babb, C., Hathaway, W.E. (1984) 'Role of coagulopathy in newborn intracranial hemorrhage.' *Pediatrics*, **74**, 26–31.

Meldrum, B. (1985) 'Possible therapeutic applications of antagonists of excitatory amino acid neurotransmitters.' *Clinical Sciences*, **68**, 113–122.

Menke, J.A., Miles, R., McIlhany, M., Bashiru, M., Chua, C., Schweid, E., Menten, T.G., Khanna, N.N. (1982) 'The fontanelle tonometer: a noninvasive method for measurement of intracranial pressure.' *Journal of Pediatrics*, **100**, 960–963.

Ment, L.R., Stewart, W.B., Scott, D.T., Duncan, C.C. (1983) 'Beagle puppy model of intraventricular hemorrhage: randomized indomethacin prevention trial.' *Neurology*, **33**, 179–184.

—— Duncan, C.C., Scott, D.T., Ehrenkranz, R.A. (1984) 'Posthemorrhagic hydrocephalus. Low incidence in very low birth weight neonates with intraventricular hemorrhage.' *Journal of Neurosurgery*, **60**, 343–347.

——— Ehrenkranz, R.A., Kleinman, C.S., Pitt, B.R., Taylor, K.J.W., Scott, D.T., Stewart, W.B., Gettner, B. (1985) 'Randomized indomethacin trial for prevention of intraventricular hemorrhage in very low birth weight infants.' *Journal of Pediatrics*, **107**, 937–943.

—— Stewart, W.B., Duncan, C.C., Pitt, B.R. (1987) 'Beagle pup model of perinatal asphyxia: nimodipine studies.' *Stroke*, **18**, 599–605.

Minns, R.A. (1984) 'Intracranial pressure monitoring.' *Archives of Disease in Childhood*, **59**, 486–488.

Morales, W.J., Koerten, J. (1986) 'Prevention of intraventricular hemorrhage in very low birth weight infants by maternally administered phenobarbital.' *Obstetrics and Gynecology*, **68**, 295–299.

Morgan, M.E.I., Benson, J.W.T., Cooke, R.W.I. (1981) 'Ethamsylate reduces the incidence of periventricular haemorrhage in very low birth weight infants.' *Lancet*, **2**, 830–831.

—— Massey, R.F., Cooke, R.W.I. (1982) 'Does phenobarbitone prevent periventricular hemorrhage in very low birth weight babies? A controlled trial.' *Pediatrics*, **70**, 186–189.

Morimoto, K., Sumita, Y., Kitajima, H., Mogami, H. (1985) 'Bilateral, asymmetrical hemorrhagic infarction of the basal ganglia and thalamus following neonatal asphyxia.' *No To Shinkei*, **37**, 133–137.

Myers, R.E., Wagner, K.R., Courten-Myers, G.M. (1983) 'Brain metabolic and pathologic consequences of asphyxia.' *In* Milunsky, A., Friedman, E.A., Gluck, L. (Eds.) *Advances in Perinatal Medicine, Vol. 3.* New York: Plenum.

Nelson, K.E., Ellenberg, J. (1981) 'Apgar scores as predictors of chronic neurological disability.' *Pediatrics*, **68**, 36–44.

Niijima, S., Levene, M.I. (1989) 'Post-asphyxial encephalopathy in a preterm infant.' *Developmental Medicine and Child Neurology*, **31**, 395–397.

Papile, L., Burstein, J., Burstein, R., Koffler, H., Koops, B.L., Johnson, J.D. (1980) 'Post-hemorrhagic hydrocephalus in low birth weight infants: treatment by serial lumbar punctures.' *Journal of Pediatrics*, **97**, 273–277.

Peeters, L.L., Sheldon, R.E., Jones, M.D., Makowski, E.L., Meschia, G. (1979) 'Blood flow to fetal organs as a function of arterial oxygen content.' *American Journal of Obstetrics and Gynecology*, **135**, 637–646.

Perlman, J.M., Hill, A., Volpe, J.J. (1983) 'Fluctuating cerebral blood flow velocity in respiratory distress syndrome. Relation to the development of intraventricular haemorrhage.' *New England Journal of Medicine*, **309**, 204–209.

Phelps, D.L. (1984) 'Vitamin E and CNS hemorrhage.' *Pediatrics*, **74**, 1113–1114.

Philip, A.G.S., Long, J., Donn, S.M. (1981) 'Intracranial pressure. Sequential measurements in full-term and preterm infants.' *American Journal of Diseases of Children*, **135**, 521–524.

Pickard, J.D., Mackenzie, E.T. (1973) 'Inhibition of prostaglandin synthesis and the response of baboon cerebral circulation to carbon dioxide.' *Nature*, **245**, 187–188.

Raju, T.N., Vidyasagar, D. (1982) 'Intracranial and cerebral perfusion pressure: methodology and clinical considerations.' *Medical Instruments*, **16**, 154–156.

—— Doshi, U.V., Vidyasagar, D. (1982) 'Cerebral perfusion pressure studies in healthy preterm and term newborn infants.' *Journal of Pediatrics*, **100**, 139–142.

Robinson, R.O., Rolfe, P., Sutton, P. (1977) 'Non-invasive method for measuring intracranial pressure in normal newborn infants.' *Developmental Medicine and Child Neurology*, **19**, 305–308.

Rothman, S. (1984) 'Synaptic release of excitatory amino acid neurotransmitter mediates anoxic neuronal death.' *Journal of Neuroscience*, **4**, 1884–1891.

Saling, E., Schneider, D. (1967) 'Biochemical supervision of the fetus during labour.' *Journal of Obstetrics and Gynaecology*, **74**, 799–811.

Salmon, J.H., Hajjar, W., Bada, H.S. (1977) 'The fontogram: a noninvasive intracranial pressure monitor.' *Pediatrics*, **60**, 721–725.

Sarnat, H.B., Sarnat, M.S. (1976) 'Neonatal encephalopathy following fetal distress.' *Archives of Neurology*, **33**, 696–705.

Schumpf, J.D., Sehring, S., Killpack, S., Brady, J.P., Hirata, T., Mednick, J.P. (1980) 'Correlation of early neurologic outcome and CT findings in neonatal brain hypoxia and injury.' *Journal of Computer Assisted Tomography*, **4**, 445–450.

Scott, H. (1976) 'Outcome of very severe birth asphyxia.' *Archives of Disease in Childhood*, **51**, 712–716.

Shankaran, S., Cepeda, E.E., Ilagan, N., Mariona, F., Hassan, M., Bhata, R., Ostrea, E., Bedard, M.P., Poland, R.L. (1986) 'Antenatal phenobarbital for the prevention of neonatal intracerebral hemorrhage.' *American Journal of Obstetrics and Gynecology*, **154**, 53–57.

Shewmon, D.A., Fine, M., Masdeu, J.C., Palacios, E. (1981) 'Postischemic hypervascularity of infancy: a stage in the evolution of ischemic brain damage with characteristic CT scan.' *Annals of Neurology*, **9**, 358–365.

Shinnar, S., Gammon, K., Bergman, E.W., Epstein, M., Freeman, J.M. (1985) 'Management of hydrocephalus in infancy: use of acetazolemide and furosemide to avoid cerebrospinal fluid shunts.' *Journal of Pediatrics*, **107**, 31–37.

Shortland, D., Trounce, J.Q., Levene, M.I. (1987) 'Hyperkalaemia, cardiac arrhythmias, and cerebral lesions in high risk neonates.' *Archives of Disease in Childhood*, **62**, 1139–1143.

Sinha, S.K., Davies, J.M., Sims, D.G., Chiswick, M.L. (1985) 'Relation between periventricular haemorrhage and ischaemic brain lesions diagnosed by ultrasound in very preterm infants.' *Lancet*, **2**, 1154–1155.

——— Toner, N., Bogle, S., Chiswick, M. (1987) 'Vitamin E supplementation reduces the frequency of periventricular haemorrhage in very preterm babies.' *Lancet*, **1**, 466–471.

Speer, M.E., Blifeld, C., Rudolph, A.J., Chadda, P., Holbein, B.M., Hittner, H.M. (1984) 'Intraventricular hemorrhage and vitamin E in very low birth weight infants: evidence for efficacy of early intramuscular vitamin E administration.' *Pediatrics*, **74**, 1107–1112.

Steen, P.A., Newberg, L.A., Milde, J.H., Michenfelder, J.D. (1983) 'Nimodipine improves cerebral blood flow and neurologic recovery after complete cerebral ischemia in the dog.' *Journal of Cerebral Blood Flow and Metabolism*, **3**, 38–42.

Stewart, A.L., Reynolds, E.O.R., Hope, P.L., Hamilton, P.A., Baudin, J., Costello, A.M., Bradford, B.C., Wyatt, J.S. (1987) 'Probability of neurodevelopmental disorders estimated from ultrasound appearance of brains of very preterm infants.' *Developmental Medicine and Child Neurology*, **29**, 3–11.

Svenningsen, N.W., Blennow, G., Lindroth, M., Gäddlin, P.O., Ahlström, H. (1982) 'Brain-orientated intensive care treatment in severe neonatal asphyxia. Effects of phenobarbitone protection.' *Archives of Disease in Childhood*, **57**, 176–183.

Sykes, G.S., Molloy, P.M., Johnson, P., Gu, W., Ashworth, F., Stirrat, G.M., Turnbull, A.C. (1982) 'Do Apgar scores indicate asphyxia?' *Lancet*, **1**, 494–496.

Szymonowicz, W., Preston, H., Yu, V.Y.H. (1985) 'The surviving monozygotic twin.' *Archives of Disease in Childhood*, **61**, 454–458.

Takashima, S., Armstrong, D., Becker, L.E. (1978) 'Subcortical leukomalacia. Relationship to development of the cerebral sulcus and its vascular supply.' *Archives of Neurology*, **35**, 470–472.

Thiringer, K., Hrbek, A., Karlsson, K., Rosen, K.G., Kjellmer, I. (1987) 'Postasphyxial cerebral survival in newborn sheep after treatment with oxygen free radical scavengers and a calcium antagonist.' *Pediatric Research*, **22**, 62–66.

Thomson, A.J., Searle, M., Russell, G. (1977) 'Quality of survival after severe birth asphyxia.' *Archives of Disease in Childhood*, **52**, 620–626.

Trounce, J.Q., Rutter, N., Levene, M.I. (1986a) 'Periventricular leucomalacia and intraventricular haemorrhage in the preterm neonate.' *Archives of Disease in Childhood*, **61**, 1196–1202.

—— Fagan, D., Levene, M.I. (1986b) 'Intraventricular haemorrhage and periventricular leucomalacia: ultrasound and autopsy correlation.' *Archives of Disease in Childhood*, **61**, 1203–1207.

——Shaw. D.E., Levene, M.I., Rutter, N. (1988) 'Clinical risk factors and periventricular leukomalacia.' *Archives of Disease in Childhood*, **63**, 17–22.

Voit, T., Lemburg, P., Stork, W. (1985) 'NMR studies in thalamo-striatal necrosis.' *Lancet*, **2**, 445.

Walsh, P., Logan, W.J. (1983) 'Continuous and intermittent measurement of intracranial pressure by Ladd monitor.' *Journal of Pediatrics*, **102**, 439–442.

Watkins, A., West, C., Cooke, R.W.I. (1987) 'Blood pressure and cerebral injury in sick very low birthweight infants.' *Archives of Disease in Childhood*, **62**, 648–649.

Wegman, M.E. (1984) 'Annual summary of vital statistics—1983.' *Pediatrics*, **74**, 981–990.

Weichsel, M.E. (1977) 'The therapeutic use of glucocorticoid hormones in the perinatal period. Potential neurological hazard.' *Annals of Neurology*, **2**, 364–366.

Weindling, A.M., Wilkinson, A.R., Cook, J., Calvert, S.A., Fok, T-F., Rochefort, M.J. (1985) 'Perinatal events which precede periventricular haemorrhage and leukomalacia in the newborn.'

British Journal of Obstetrics and Gynaecology, **92**, 1218–1223.

White, B.C., Winegar, C.D., Wilson, R.P., Krause, G. (1983) 'Calcium blockers in cerebral resuscitation.' *Journal of Trauma*, **23**, 788–793.

Whitelaw, A., Placzek, M., Dubowitz, L.M.S., Lary, S., Levene, M.I. (1983) 'Phenobarbitone for prevention of periventricular haemorrhage in very low birth weight infants.' *Lancet*, **2**, 1168–1170.

Young, R.S.K., Hessert, T.R., Pritchard, G.A., Yagel, S.K. (1984) 'Naloxone exacerbates hypoxic-ischemic brain injury in the neonatal rat.' *American Journal of Obstetrics and Gynecology*, **150**, 52–56.

7

INFECTIOUS AND PARAINFECTIOUS ENCEPHALOPATHIES

R. A. Minns

Acute encephalopathy is a clinical label denoting a nonspecific brain insult in a patient admitted with a combination of seizures, decerebration and coma, and less commonly with ataxia, hemiplegia or cardio/respiratory arrest. Encephalopathies may be due to infection, anoxic-ischaemia, intracranial haemorrhage, toxic/metabolic illness, or epilepsy. Those cases due to infection are the infectious or parainfectious encephalopathies, while those mediated by a circulating 'toxic' substance (exogenous or endogenous) are labelled toxic encephalopathy. Those due to accidental or non-accidental head injury are labelled traumatic encephalopathy.

While the remainder of this chapter will specifically deal with the infectious and parainfectious encephalopathies, *i.e.* tuberculous meningitis, pyogenic meningitis and Reye's syndrome, the presentation is inevitably with coma and it is important to see how these individual disease entities fit into the over-all clinical presentation of coma.

Coma

The MRC definition (1941) was 'the absence of any psychologically understandable response to external stimuli or "inner need"'. This is no more useful in clinical practice than attempting to define 'thought' as the content of consciousness. In practical terms, coma is defined as an impairment of arousal or absence of sleep-wake cycles.

The almost universally accepted method of recognising and grading degrees of coma in adults is that of the Glasgow coma scale (Teasdale and Jennett 1974). The original scale was based on observations of eye-opening and the best verbal and motor response, with a total score of 14 points (Table 7.I). This has been subsequently modified to include an extra grading in the motor response section, by adding flexor withdrawal to abnormal flexion posture (Jennett and Teasdale 1977).

While these are applicable to older children, for those less than five years of age Simpson and Reilly (1982) modified the original Glasgow coma scale so that normal developmental milestones would be taken into account. Therefore, for a normal infant of less than six months the total score would be 9 points; 11 points for an older infant up to 12 months, and so on to a total of 14 points for the child of five or above.

Several other coma scales have been devised for children—the Children's coma score (CCS) (Raimondi and Hirschauer 1984), the Children's Orthopaedic Hospital and Medical Center scale (Morray *et al.* 1984), the 0–IV scale

170

TABLE 7.I

Coma scales

GCS (original) adult (Teasdale and Jennett 1974)	Modified GCS (adults) (Jennett and Teasdale 1977)	Children < 5 years (Simpson and Reilly 1982)
Eye opening — 4 spontaneous — 3 to speech — 2 to pain — 1 nil	Eye opening — 4 (same) — 3 — 2 — 1	Eye opening — 4 (same) — 3 — 2 — 1
Verbal response — 5 oriented/conversant — 4 confused/disoriented — 3 inappropriate words — 2 non-specific sounds — 1 nil	Verbal response — 5 (same) — 4 — 3 — 2 — 1	Verbal response — 5 oriented — 4 words — 3 vocal sounds — 2 cries — 1 nil
Motor response — 5 obeys commands — 4 localises pain — 3 flexion — 2 extension — 1 nil	Motor response — 6 obeys commands — 5 localises pain — 4 flexor withdrawal — 3 flexion — 2 extension — 1 nil	Motor response — 5 (same) — 4 — 3 — 2 — 1
Total 14 points	Total 15 points	(Normal developmental milestones taken into account) 0–6mths 9 points >6mths–12mths 11 points >12mths–2yrs 12 points >2yrs–5yrs 13 points >5yrs 14 points

CSS (Children's coma score) (Raimondi and Hirschauer 1984)	COHMC (Children's Orthopaedic Hospital and Medical Center scale) (Morray et al. 1984)
Ocular response — 4 pursuit — 3 EOM intact pupils reactive — 2 EOM impaired or pupils fixed — 1 EOM paralysed and pupils fixed (EOM = external ocular movements)	Cortical function — 6 purposeful, spontaneous movements — 5 purposeful, voice-evoked movements — 4 painful stimuli localised — 3 non-purposeful movements/global withdrawal — 2 decorticate posturing — 1 decerebrate posturing — 0 flaccidity
Verbal response — 3 cries spontaneous — 2 respirations — 1 apnoeic	Brainstem function — 3 intact — 2 depressed — 1 absent but breathing spontaneously — 0 absent and apnoeic
Motor response — 4 flexes and extends — 3 withdraws from painful stimuli — 2 hypertonic — 1 flaccid	Total 9 points
Total 11 points	*(Table continues over page.)*

171

0–IV scale *(Seshia et al. 1977)* *(Huttenlocher 1972)*	Jacobi scale *(Gordon et al. 1983)*

0 — Arouses spontaneously and to stimuli	Best verbal response
	  — 5 fixes, follows, recognises, laughs
	  — fixes and follows inconstantly, recognition uncertain

I — Stuperose. Spontaneous arousal rare
    Roused readily but briefly by stimuli
    Cough/gag present
	— 3 arouses at times
	  — 2 motor restlessness—unarousable
	  — 1 complete unresponsiveness

II — Spontaneous arousal absent
    Semipurposive/avoidance motor
    response to stimuli
    Cough/gag depressed
	Best motor response
	  — 5 obeys
	  — 4 localises

III — Arousal in form of motor response
    only to intense, sustained, painful
    stimuli
    Cough/gag absent.
	— 3 flexion
	  — 2 extension
	  — 1 none

IV — Not aroused even by intense/sustained
    painful stimuli
    Cough/gag absent
	Eyes open
	  — 4 spontaneous
	  — 3 to speech
	  — 2 to pain
	  — 1 none

	Oculo-vestibular response
	  — 5 normal
	  — 4 tonic-conjugate
	  — 3 minimal dysconjugate
	  — 2 no eye movements
	  — 1 pupils non-reactive

	Total 19 points

(Huttenlocher 1972, Seshia *et al.* 1977) and the 'Jacobi' scale (Gordon *et al.* 1983) (Table 7.I). It has become common to sum the items in the Glasgow coma scale (Starmark *et al.* 1988). Levy *et al.* 1981 did not find it useful to generate a coma score in their study of non-traumatic coma in adults because many of their patients were intubated. Teasdale *et al.* (1979, 1983) considered that a summated score conveyed less information than was available in the individual responses and that the responses were not equally weighted. They felt that information was lost when the scores were summed. Teasdale *et al.* (1979) considered that the individual responses should be supplemented by other neurological data. In point of fact, the Glasgow coma scale is a mini neurological examination and is not a pure assessment of unconsciousness. The only one of the above scales which is not summated is the 0–IV scale. The inter-observer variability for the six coma scales was assessed prospectively on a sample of 15 comatose children (Yager *et al.* 1990). The disagreement rate was least for the 0–IV scale, and for all items in the Simpson and Reilly scale and the 'Jacobi' scale. The disagreement rate was relatively high for the verbal responses in the Glasgow coma and Children's coma scales, reflecting difficulty in assessing verbal responses in comatose children.

The differential diagnosis of coma includes aphasia, acute autism or psychosis, sudden deafness or headache in the 'withdrawn' child, persistent vegetative state (sleep-wake cycles without awareness) and akinetic mutism (locked-in, sleep-wake cycles, awareness but no motor response).

Apart from grading coma for the purposes of audit and comparison between centres, outcomes also need to be standardised. Jennett and Bone (1975) graded outcome as follows: (i) death, (ii) persistent vegetative state, (iii) severe disability (totally dependent), (iv) moderate severity (neurologically or intellectually impaired, but independent), and (v) good recovery (full independent life).

The outcome from childhood coma has also been graded on a five-point scale: (i) normal (fits if present are controllable), (ii) minimal (minimal motor problems, isolated cranial nerve palsies, ataxia and fits partially controlled), (iii) moderate (moderate weakness or ataxia, behaviour problems, multiple cranial abnormalities and seizures moderately controlled), (iv) severe (severe weakness or ataxia, tetraplegia and uncontrolled fits), and (v) death (Seshia et al. 1983). All outcome scales documented the best achievement attainable.

Clinical aspects of coma

Coma scale

The neurological examination of a comatose patient will determine the severity of coma, and whether there is a brainstem lesion, bilateral hemispheric lesion or transtentorial herniation. It has to be carried out on a patient who is often ventilated, paralysed and unco-operative. After the first examination, it is important to repeat the examination frequently: not only to detect changes in the level of consciousness, but also to detect any progression of signs, such as finding a rapidly decreasing level of consciousness with progressive dilatation of one pupil, which would indicate imminent uncal herniation due to RICP.

Diminished consciousness may be due to depression of the reticular activating system (in the deep and medial structures of the brainstem). This may be due to RICP with midbrain compression from herniations, or it may be unrelated to pressure and due to involvement of the reticular formation by anoxic/toxic/metabolic or parenchymatous involvement of this area by infection, trauma, demyelination or vascular lesions.

If the reticular activating system is intact, but there are very large areas of the hemisphere which have been damaged and therefore cannot be alerted by the reticular system, then consciousness will be depressed. Localised areas of hemispheric damage (e.g. from infarcts) will not necessarily give rise to diminished consciousness whereas more global hemispheric insults, such as anoxia, ischaemia and poisoning, will result in coma.

Conditions which commonly cause a brief loss of consciousness must be differentiated from those with a more serious prolonged coma. The patient found in coma is commonly suffering from one of the following: Addison's disease, epilepsy, intracranial haemorrhage and head injury, uraemia, diabetes and hypoglycaemia, drug effects (alcohol, barbiturates, tricyclic antidepressants), meningitis or myxoedema. For the patient with a *brief loss of consciousness* the cause is most likely due to seizures, hypoglycaemia, short-term concussive head injury, syncopal attacks from infundibular spasm in Fallot's tetralogy, atrial myxoma, or a short-term drug effect. Many of these will be brief interferences with consciousness and will be obvious on admission or diagnostically resolve themselves within a short time. Prolonged coma, however, will require an urgent CT scan, which in most instances will be possible within an hour of arrival at hospital, so that ICP monitoring and full invasive monitoring should be possible within two hours of admission.

Brainstem reflexes
1. OCULAR
Pupillary constriction is a function of the intact third nerve, the nucleus for which is near the top of the brainstem. Afferent stimulation of the pupil, with light, results in a direct connection with the lateral geniculate body which stimulates the third nerve to constrict.

If the pupils are regular, in mid-position and unreactive to light, this is due to a midbrain lesion involving the pretectal region. Fixed, dilated pupils also occur in midbrain damage from tentorial herniation or destructive lesions. A unilateral dilated pupil results from a third-nerve palsy and may indicate uncal herniation. Pinpoint constriction of the pupils is seen in pontine lesions and in narcotic overdose. A Horner's syndrome may be seen in a lateral medullary infarct.

Apart from this function, the third nerve is also responsible for medial, upward and inferior movements of the eye, and the third-nerve nucleus is connected by means of the medial longitudinal bundle to the sixth-nerve nucleus, 1½ inches below. Therefore the *position of the eyes* at rest, whether there is conjugate or dysconjugate *deviation*, and *roving eye movements*, will be reflecting extra-ocular motor palsies.

The *oculocephalic reflex*, or 'doll's eyes', is tested by passive head movement. The examiner stands at the top of the patient, holds the head and raises the eyelids. The head is rotated briskly to one side for three or four seconds, and then through 180° to the other side. Movements of the head will cause conjugate deviation of the eyes to the opposite side. Apart from its use as a test of third- or sixth-nerve palsies, paralysis of gaze and internuclear ophthalmoplegia, the doll's eye reflex is really stimulating the labyrinths. If there is conjugate deviation of the eyes to the opposite side, this is spoken of as an intact doll's eye response. It means that the area from the midbrain to the pons is intact and you are looking at damaged hemispheres as the cause for the coma. In newborn infants less than two weeks of age, it is intact and is normally present, whereas in the dead brainstem it is negative or absent.

Ocular bobbing is due to pontine infarction or haemorrhage, in which there is intermittent brisk dipping of the eyeballs for a few minutes, before they return to the original position. *Blinking* may be normal, increased or decreased in response to a light stimulus, menace, draught, corneal reflex elicitation, noise or pain. An exaggerated response in a tonic repetitive fashion suggests bilateral supratentorial damage.

The *corneal reflex* is well represented throughout the stem in young children and is quite sensitive. Its early absence indicates poisoning or other toxic cause. It may be absent because of hemispheric or pontine lesions, or it may relate to the severity of coma.

If a patient is in deep coma with impaired pupillary, oculocephalic and vestibulo-ocular responses, it is impossible to be sure whether this is due to RICP with herniation or if it is a manifestation of diffuse cerebral injury.

2. BULBAR REFLEXES

A cough reflex, a gag reflex and spontaneous respiratory status are the best ways of assessing the status of the lower pons and medulla.

A patient with skewed deviation of the eyes, depressed corneal reflexes, pupillary abnormalities and an abnormal vestibulo-ocular response or decerebration is really showing isolated injury to the brainstem. However, drugs can also interfere with brainstem responses, and in metabolic coma (hepatic or renal) the half-life of drugs such as sedatives and anticonvulsants may be prolonged.

3. MOTOR

In a flexor position (decorticate), there is loss of inhibition on the red nucleus and therefore unimpeded action of the rubrospinal tract with an increase in muscle tone. On the other hand, in an extensor posturing (decerebrate) there is loss of inhibition on the vestibular nuclei in the pons, with uninhibited vestibulospinal tract function and extensor tone and movement pattern. These posturing patterns specify where the lesion is absent, and may occur following large extensive or small discrete lesions.

If the pupillary light reflex and extra-ocular movements are normal, and the patient is posturing, one can be sure that the problem is *metabolic* or *toxic* and not related to a mass lesion. Because the areas of the third-nerve nucleus and the red and vestibular nuclei are close together, if the pupils are intact this cannot be due to a mass lesion. This does not mean that in coma following poisoning the eye movements are always normal. In severe poisoning there may be absence of eye movements and pupillary responses, but this may still be compatible with the patient's full recovery if intensive care support is provided.

One of the greatest sources of confusion is that of *post-hypoxic rigidity*. These patients are in an extensor posture (usually decorticate), but significantly there are no other brainstem signs. This only follows hypoxia, the best example of which is carbon monoxide poisoning, with rigidity and opisthotonos, followed later by dyskinesia, and much later still by a return to normal. It is important therefore to distinguish the mid-collicular level compression of tentorial herniation with opisthotonus and decerebration, from the transient post-hypoxic rigidity following an hypoxic insult. Clearly this has implications for treatment because in post-hypoxic rigidity, the patient will need ventilating, but not necessarily ICP monitoring, unless cerebral oedema from severe hypoxia supervenes.

The decerebrate patterns may be preceded in young infants by bicycling movements of the upper and lower limbs (doggy paddling), and by a return of primitive reflexes (ATNR). The cycling and posturing may be spontaneous, or occur

175

TABLE 7.II

Strategy for coma management

Diagnostic investigations		Supportive investigations (independent of cause of coma)	Monitoring neurology and coma state
Obvious cause	Non-obvious cause		
— HI	— CT — ultrasound	*— Gases (4-hourly)	1. GCS
— D. Ketoacidosis	— LP (including immunofluorescence)	*— Pulse oximeter (O_2 saturation)	2. Ocular (pupils, external ocular movements)
— Poisoning	— EEG	— CVP ± wedge	3. Bulbar reflexes
— Infections	— Toxicology (barbiturates, toluene, benzodiazepines, salicylates, iron, lead, anticonvulsants, antidepressants)	*— Dextrostix (4-hourly)	4. Temperature, pulse rate, respiratory rate, blood pressure
— Drowning	— Metabolic (ammonia, liver function tests, porphyrins, amino acids, organic acids, dicarboxylic acids, urine sugars, lactate/pyruvate/acidosis, urea/creatinine, calcium, T_4/TSH)	*— Osmolality (8-hourly)	
— Burns/scalds	— Tuberculin test	*— Calcium/phosphate (b.d.)	
— CRA	— Virology	— EEG (continuous)	
	— Technetium scan	— ICP/CPP (continuous)	
	— X-rays (skull, skeletal)	— (mean pressure, pulse pressure, periodic waves)	
	— Brain biopsy	— BP arterial (continuous)	
		— Coagulation (once then prn)	
		*— Temperature	
		*— Fluid balance (u. output, weight, labstix)	
		*— Hb and white blood cell count count	
		*— Chest radiograph (portable)	
		— Anticonvulsant levels	
		*— ECG (continuous)	
		*— Urea and electrolytes (b.d.)	
		*— Infection screen	
		— VEP	
		— BSEP	
		— Liver function tests (once/day)	
		— $AVDO_2$ or JVO sat. (continuous)	
		— CBF (initial + change) (autoregulation, CO_2 resp. and perfusion)	
		— CBFv. (continuous, intermittent, daily)	

*All coma regardless of cause.

only after stimulation of an uninhibited brainstem (e.g. to the trigeminal area, or snout stimulation). Supraorbital compression or pinching of the skin may cause decorticate posturing in internal capsular lesions, with decerebrate posturing when there is insipient tentorial herniation. With foramen magnum herniation, the decerebrate posture is replaced by profound hypotonia or return of spinal flexion, exaggerated 'withdrawal reflexes' and apnoea.

Apart from these postures there may be *focal weakness* with eversion of one foot, unilateral hypotonia and hyporeflexia. It is important to contrast the tone on both sides of the body; the limbs on the hemiplegic side fall heavily when dropped, and do not respond to painful stimuli. Asymmetry of the reflexes is also noted.

4. VEGETATIVE FUNCTION

These are irregularities of brainstem function causing disturbances of pulse, blood pressure, temperature and respiration. Cheyne-Stokes respiration is seen in metabolic disorders, and in bilaterally situated lesions deep in the cerebral hemisphere and basal ganglia. Central neurogenic hyperventilation is seen in lesions around the lower midbrain and pontine reticular formation. Ataxic respiration (*i.e.* irregular breathing) indicates a medullary lesion. Apneustic respiration (sustained inspiratory effort) is a terminal gasping pattern.

General examination will also include evidence of external or internal injuries, skin petechiae suggesting infection with Neisseria meningitidis, Haemophilus influenzae, Rickettsia and Streptococcus pneumoniae or a bleeding disorder or NAI. The patient should be examined for neck stiffness, the presence or absence of intracranial bruits, and irregularities of the eyes, eardrums and mastoids (for Battle's sign*), mouth and nose, cranium, heart, lungs, abdomen, major vessels and for epileptic phenomena, which may be generalised or focal, or may represent brainstem fits with vegetative and respiratory features.

Ongoing neurological surveillance in the comatose patient should assess (i) the Glasgow coma scale, (ii) the ocular findings (pupils and eye movements), (iii) bulbar reflexes, and (iv) abnormalities of temperature, pulse, blood pressure and respiration.

Strategy for approach to coma management

When initially managing a comatose patient, the physician must institute supportive care and investigations, as well as search for the possible cause (Gordon *et al.* 1983). Table 7.II suggests an outline for routine coma management.

Reasons for ICP monitoring

General reasons

(1) Many acute diseases of the nervous system will result in secondary brain-swelling, which is then responsible for mortality and morbidity.

(2) RICP is treatable independent of the cause of the coma, and therefore monitoring is necessary for effective management.

*Mastoid haematoma indicative of basal skull fracture.

TABLE 7.III

Pathophysiological basis for coma in 72 children

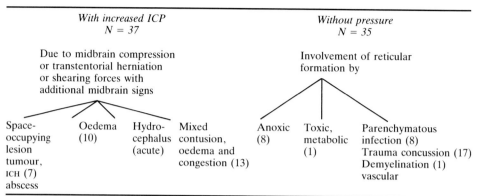

| With increased ICP N = 37 | Without pressure N = 35 |

*Excluding patients with chronic hydrocephalus, tumours and other space occupation with diminished conscious state.

There was mixed pathology in 14 cases (extra 2 with oedema and pressure, 3 with anoxia and no pressure, 2 with toxic/metabolic. and no pressure, 6 parenchymatous-infective and no pressure, 1 demyelination-parenchymatous and no pressure).

TABLE 7.IV

Methods of ICP recording in non-traumatic coma

	Method of ICP measurement in non-traumatic coma (N = 36)	
Ventricle	(Direct ventricular cannulation or ventriculostomy reservoir)	19
Surface	(Subarachnoid [Leeds] screw, cordis or subdural epidural catheter)	9
Lumbar (after CT)	Lumbar puncture	8
	Total	36

Specific reasons

(1) To give warning of impending brain shifts.

(2) To allow continuous assessment of cerebral perfusion.

(3) To prognosticate on outcome.

(4) Because in the comatose, paralysed and ventilated patient, the neurological function is not easily monitored, and physiological monitoring of brain function is necessary.

(5) Because the clinical signs of RICP are unreliable, and when present indicate that RICP has already occurred.

(6) To test shunt malfunction.

(7) To evaluate 'arrested' or 'progressive' hydrocephalus.

(8) To facilitate in the titration of therapy for RICP.

Edinburgh Coma Series (original data)

A total of 72 comatose children with ICP monitoring were included in this study of coma. Fourteen were due to encephalitis, nine to meningitis, and 13 had anoxic-ischaemic injury. Thirty-six patients, reported with traumatic coma (courtesy of Dr John Ward, Head Injury Unit, Medical College of Virginia), are discussed

TABLE 7.V

Coma and anoxic ischaemia

Patient	Age (years, months)	Primary pathology	Secondary pathology	Presumed pathogenesis of coma	ICP units	Outcome
1	0.3	Apparently life threatening event	Brain-swelling	Anoxia	<20	Cerebral atrophy, CP, MR
2	5.9	Disseminated tuberculosis	CRA pleural effusion, immune deficiency	Anoxia	<20	Dead
3	0.14	Fallot's tetralogy	CRA	Anoxia	<20	Dead
4	0.4	Choroid plexus papilloma	CRA, renal failure, hyperosmolality	Anoxia, parenchymatous, metabolic	<20	Deficit (visual, motor)
5		Lead encephalopathy	Status epilepsy	Anoxia, parenchymatous, toxic	<20	No deficit
6	0.3	Status epilepsy	(L) hemisphere oedema	Mid-brain compression, anoxia	20 to 40	Dead
7	2.9	Acute lymphoblastic leukaemia	Radiotherapy-induced seizures	Anoxia	<20	No deficit
8	9.7	Acute lymphoblastic leukaemia	Necrotising leuco-encephalopathy, seizures, cerebral oedema	Anoxia	20 to 40	No deficit
9	6.9	Acute lymphoblastic leukaemia	Asparaginase encephalopathy with deposits in corpus callosum	Parenchymatous-demyelination vascular	<20	No deficit
10	1.0	Smoke inhalation	Tentorial herniation seizures	Anoxia	<20	No deficit
11	7.0	Para-infectious encephalopathy	Cerebral infarction	Ischaemic	20 to 40	Spastic, quadriplegia, seizures, blind
12	6.7	Status epilepsy (ataxic diplegia with mental retardation)	Cerebral oedema	Anoxia, mid-brain compression	<20	Dead
13	0.16	Reye-like syndrome, medium chain acyl-co A dehydrogenase deficiency	Cerebral oedema	Mid-brain oedema	<20	Normal

179

TABLE 7.VI

Coma and meningitis

Patient	Age (years, months)	Primary pathology	Secondary pathology	Presumed pathogenesis of coma	ICP	Outcome
1	2.3	Tuberculous meningitis	Acute ventricular dilatation basal adhesions	Mid-brain compression	20 to 40	No deficit
2	1.8	Tuberculous meningitis	Acute ventricular dilatation	Mid-brain compression	>40	No deficit
3	9.6	Tuberculous meningitis	IV ventricle dilatation	Mid-brain compression	20 to 40	No deficit
4	0.1	Escherichia coli meningitis	Acute (mod.) ventricular dilatation	Mid-brain compression	<20 (18mm/Hg = raised for age)	Deficit (double hemiplegia, epilepsy, micro-cephaly)
5	12.0	Meningococcal meningitis		Mid-brain compression	20 to 40	No deficit
6	3.5	Haemophilus influenza meningitis	Respiratory arrest, intermittent seizures	Parenchymatous-infective	<20	No deficit
7	4.5	Chronic neoplastic meningitis	Adhesive arachnoiditis (Froin's syndrome), acute ventricular dilatation, stem adhesions	Mid-brain compression	>40	Died
8	4.6	Meningococcal meningitis	Enlarged ventricles, periventricular leukomalacia	Parenchymatous-infective	<20	No deficit
9	0.1	Haemophilus influenza meningitis		Parenchymatous-infective	<20	Evolving severe cerebral palsy

separately. There were an additional five patients with space occupation and 30 patients with hydrocephalus and diminished conscious state not included in the statistical analysis. Table 7.III shows the presumed pathogenesis of all patients.

The method of ICP measurement in the 36 patients with non-traumatic coma is seen in Table 7.IV. The aetiology in these patients was categorised as head injury, anoxic ischaemia, meningitis, encephalitis, space occupation and hydrocephalus, as previously mentioned. Tables 7.V to 7.IX show the clinical details, together with the pathology, ICP levels (less than 20mmHg, 20 to 40mmHg and greater than 40mmHg) and outcome. The percentage of children with RICP in the various aetiological groups is seen in Tables 7.X and 7.XI.

The children with severe head injury included in this study were aged from two to 15 years. There was a total of 36 patients, eight of whom required surgical decompression for a mass lesion. 28 were in the non-surgical group (Table 7.XII). The majority of patients with an intracranial mass lesion had RICP; five of them died, and two made a good recovery. By contrast, fewer than half the patients not operated for a mass lesion had raised pressure, and 24 out of the 28 made a good or moderate recovery. The relationship between ICP level and outcome is significant (Table 7.XIII).

In the non-traumatic group, 36 patients had encephalitis, meningitis, or anoxic-ischaemic damage. The mean ICP level was used for statistical analysis, together with the calculated CPP levels (Seshia *et al.* 1983). ICP was accurately known in 30 patients, and CPP was known in 26 patients. The exact outcome was known in 33 patients.

Statistics were run separately, firstly on the whole group and secondly the infected group. For both groups correlation of the ICP or CPP and outcome was performed. Both groups had t-tests to test the effective ICP and CPP thresholds on outcome, and the effects of outcome threshold on ICP and CPP.

These significant results are shown in Table 7.XIV. There was no correlation between ICP and outcome. The threshold for outcome used was > 1, < 2 and > 2. The threshold for CPP was above and below 50mmHg and the threshold for ICP was above and below 15mmHg. In summary therefore, for these 36 patients with non-traumatic coma, the CPP correlated with outcome at the 5 per cent level, and 50mmHg was the significant critical point. For the subgroup (infections) there was a significant correlation of CPP with outcome, and again 50mmHg CPP was critical for outcome. Testing the effects of outcome thresholds on the CPP showed non-significance for the total group, but significance at the 5 per cent level for the infected group.

ICP/CPP in non-traumatic coma in childhood

In an earlier series from this Unit—64 infants and children with acute encephalopathies presenting with decerebrate rigidity—clinical features of RICP were found in 87 per cent of cases (Brown *et al.* 1973). In a series of 16 cases of prolonged non-traumatic coma (greater than five days), reviewed retrospectively, RICP was found in nine, although it was objectively measured in only six cases (Margolis and Shaywitz 1980).

TABLE 7.VII

Coma and encephalitis

Patient	Age (years, months)	Primary pathology	Secondary pathology	Presumed pathogenesis of coma	ICP	Outcome
1	8.10	Viral encephalitis	Minimal dilatation (L), temporal horn and low density in (L) posterior temporal region (scarring from previous-L-temporal abscess complicating meningitis)	Parenchymatous-infective	<20	No deficit
2	11.3	Viral encephalitis	Cerebral oedema with multi-focal infarction	Parenchymatous-infective, mid-brain compression	20 to 40	Deficit (epilepsy, MR, dyskinetic CP)
3	2.11	Acute disseminated encephalomyelitis	Diffuse demyelination, cerebral oedema (died without RICP and no evidence of oedema or hydrocephalus)	Mid-brain compression, parenchymatous-demyelination	>40	Died
4	6.1	Meningo-encephalitis	No evidence of brain-swelling or shift	Parenchymatous-infective	<20	No deficit
5	6.0	Mumps encephalitis	Nil	Parenchymatous-infective	<20	No deficit
6	1.5	Measles encephalitis		Parenchymatous-infective	<20	No deficit
7	6.1	Herpes simplex virus encephalitis	Status epilepsy (90 mins) (L) hemisphere oedema	Mid-brain compression, anoxia	>40	Died
8	9.6	SSPE	Ventricular dilatation following IT. drugs	Mid-brain compression	20 to 40	Died
9	6.0	Acute lymphoblastic leukaemia	Inclusion body encephalitis	Parenchymatous-infective	<20	Died
10	6.0	Acute lymphoblastic leukaemia	Immune-suppressed measles, encephalitis (mild ventricular dilatation and brain-swelling at post-mortem examination)	Mid-brain compression, parenchymatous-infective	20 to 40	Died
11	5.7	Viral encephalitis	Brain-swelling	Mid-brain compression, parenchymatous-infective	<20	Died

TABLE 7.VII, *contd.*

Patient	Age (years, months)	Primary pathology	Secondary pathology	Presumed pathogenesis of coma	ICP	Outcome
12	6.6	Viral meningo-encephalitis	Hydrocephalus	Mid-brain compression parenchymatous-infective	>40	Minimal hand-function problems
13	8.0	Meningo-encephalitis	Brain-swelling, seizures	Mid-brain compression, parenchymatous-infective	20 to 40	No deficit
14	1.3	Herpes simplex virus encephalitis	Oedema and vasculitis	Parenchymatous-infective, mid-brain compression	20 to 40	Dyskinetic spastic quadriparesis

TABLE 7.VIII

Coma and space occupation

Patient	Age (years, months)	Primary pathology	Secondary pathology	Presumed pathogenesis of coma	ICP	Outcome
1	4.0	Cerebral staphylococcal abscess following tonsillectomy	Cerebral oedema and shift	Mid-brain compression	>40	Deficit (tetraplegia and PVS)
2	6.3	Arterio-venous malformation	Intracerebral haemorrhage with surrounding oedema and and brain shift	Mid-brain compression	20 to 40	Deficit (ataxic, hemiplegia, speech)
3		Grade III astrocytoma	Secondary hydrocephalus with space occupation	Mid-brain compression	>40	No deficit
4	10.10	Cerebellar cystic astrocytoma	Space occupation with large IVth ventricle	Mid-brain compression	20 to 40	No deficit
5	11.7	Abscess, chronic pneumococcal meningitis	IVth ventricle adhesions and obstruction	Parenchymatous-infective mid-brain compression	20 to 40	Deficit hemiplegia

TABLE 7.IX

Coma and hydrocephalus

Pathology	No. of patients	ICP			Outcome			Comment
		<20	20 to 40	>40	No deficit	Deficit	Dead	
Shunted post-meningitic hydrocephalus	4	1	1	2	3	3	0	One patient with congenital toxoplasmosis had periventricular calcification and low intracranial compliance
Shunted post-haemorrhagic hydrocephalus	3	1	0	2	3	0	0	
Shunted hydrocephalus assoc. tumour (astrocytoma)	1	0	0	1	1	0	0	Blocked T/P and cystoperitoneal shunts
Shunted hydrocephalus assoc. myelomeningocele	13	3	5	5	11	2	0	
Shunted hydrocephalus assoc. occipital meningocele	2	0	1	1	2	0	0	
Shunted congenital hydrocephalus	6	1	1	4	2	4	0	Diffuse aetiological group with shunt malfunction
Acute idiopathic hydrocephalus	1	0	1	0	1	0	0	Pre-operative
	30	6	9	15	23	9	0	

T-test CPP $\leq 50/>50$

TABLE 7.X

Percentage of comatose children with RICP

No.	Aetiology	% RICP
36	Head injury	53
13	Anoxic-ischaemia	23
9	Meningitis	66
14	Encephalitis	57
5	Space occupation	100
30	Hydrocephalus	80
107		

TABLE 7.XI

Frequency of RICP in traumatic and non-traumatic coma

	N	% RICP
Medical coma (infective, anoxic-ischamia)	36	47
Traumatic coma (± mass lesion)	36	53

TABLE 7.XII

Outcome in severe childhood head injury in 36 patients aged between two and 15

Surgical decompression of mass lesion			Non-surgical group	
Died	Severe	Good	Severe	Good/moderate
5	1	2	4	24
(88% RICP)			(43% RICP)	

TABLE 7.XIII

Relationship of ICP to outcome in severe childhood head injury

ICP	Good/moderate	Severe/vegetative	Dead	Total
0–20mmHg	17	0	0	17
20–40mmHg	8	4	1	13
>40mmHg	1	1	4	6

N = 36
p < 0.001 (K.R. correl.)
(Courtesy of Dr J. Ward, Medical College Virginia, Richmond, USA)

TABLE 7.XIV

Relationship of CPP to outcome in non-traumatic coma

	Whole group	Infected group
Correlation of CPP and outcome	r = −0.393, n = 26 p < 0.05	r = −0.498, n = 18 p < 0.05
T-test CPP ≤50/>50 on outcome	t = −2.92, n = 26 p < 0.01	t = −2.21, n = 18 p < 0.05
T-test outcome ≤2/>2 on CPP	NS	t = −2.42, n = 18 p < 0.05

185

Tasker *et al.* (1988) monitored the ICP of 49 children in non-traumatic coma, for a median duration of three days. The ICP was charted half-hourly, or at the time of acute rises of ICP (or decreased CPP), although no account was taken of the duration of low perfusion. The maximum ICP did not correlate with outcome, although all children with an ICP above 55mmHg had a poor outcome. On the other hand, the lower minimum CPP was related to poor outcome, 40mmHg being considered the critical value. All patients with a CPP less than 40mmHg had a poor outcome, while some with CPPs above 40mmHg still had a poor outcome. Some of these cases were due to multi-system failure. Twenty-one of the 49 children had a good outcome, five had a moderate and 23 a poor result, based on their neurological state.

In summary, therefore, from both studies the mean or maximum ICP does not correlate with outcome. CPP, however, does correlate with outcome, and the lowest CPP ($\leqslant$40mmHg) correlates with poor outcome.

ICP/CPP in traumatic coma in childhood

There are two separate sets of events that produce brain damage from trauma in childhood: firstly a biomechanical effect with the *primary head injury* (acceleration/deceleration injury to neurons or glia is likely to cause a diffuse injury, whereas direct blows to the head are likely to cause haematomas, *e.g.* epidural haematomas), and secondly the *secondary head injury* due to hypotension, hypoxia, hypocarbia, RICP and infection. A 'lucid interval' suggests that a secondary injury is occurring. All of the latter are preventable, and therefore the aim of treatment is to prevent the secondary head injury.

The primary head injury is thought in children to be different from that in adults and to be due to diffuse brain-swelling from diffuse hyperaemia with a raised CBV (Bruce *et al.* 1979, 1981). The secondary damage was then considered to be ischaemic, which could occur within hours of the injury and was caused by RICP. This meant that hyperventilation with a diminished PaCO$_2$ would lead to cerebro-vasoconstriction with a lowering of the RICP and appeared to be the treatment of choice rather than mannitol with its known effect of increasing CBF (Muizelaar *et al.* 1983). CO$_2$ responsiveness in head injury is usually well preserved, and hyperventilation results in the cerebro-vasoconstriction with lowering of intravascular blood volume. Some investigators have suggested that CO$_2$ reactivity is affected by trauma, and others that there may be a regional response in CO$_2$ reactivity.

Hyperaemia, however, cannot be defined by absolute CBF criteria alone; the AVDO$_2$ and CMRO$_2$ in relationship to the depth of the coma must also be taken into account (Obrist *et al.* 1984). In a most thorough study, Muizelaar *et al.* (1989*a*) made 72 measurements of CBF on 32 severely head-injured children. They also measured AVDO$_2$, CMRO$_2$, PVI, GCS, ICP and outcome. The AVDO$_2$ is the ratio of metabolism to flow, and high values indicate an insufficient flow for the metabolism present (*i.e.* ischaemia), while subnormal values indicate a relative excess of flow for the metabolic needs (*i.e.* hyperaemia or luxury perfusion). The CMRO$_2$ is calculated by the following equation:

$$CMRO_2 = CBF \times AVDO_2$$

(normal range $= 3$ to $3.5\text{ml}/100\text{g}^{-1}$ min^{-1}). Early after the injury (less than 12 hours) the CBF was low in patients with a low Glasgow coma score and there was a mild uncoupling of CBF above the metabolic demands (low AVDO$_2$). Twenty-four hours post-injury, there was significant hyperaemia with low Glasgow coma score and now the flow and metabolism were completely uncoupled (very low AVDO$_2$). In contrast, the mean CMRO$_2$ at all times correlated positively with the Glasgow coma score and outcome. 88 per cent of patients showed a hyperaemia at some point in their management. Although three of their patients with the most hyperaemia had the stiffest brains (PVI), there was no correlation between the degree of hyperaemia and the ICP or PVI. Nor was there any correlation between the level of ICP and the level of CBF (Muizelaar et al. 1989a).

Autoregulation is impaired in severe head injury (Lewelt et al. 1980) and this may be a global or a regional impairment. When not present it means that CBF is pressure-passive and any drop in systemic arterial pressure is likely to result in ischaemic brain damage. Autoregulation has been found to be present in 59 per cent of severely head-injured children although its presence or absence did not correlate with coma score, early or late assessment, or outcome (Muizelaar et al. 1989b).

The CSF is a compensatory compartment in head injury and therefore anything which diminishes this compartment will have the potential for increasing ICP. CSF formation, outflow resistance and absorption may all be affected by severe head injury. The formation is decreased when there is shock or cerebral ischaemia (Weiss and Werlman 1978), although measurements which show an apparent increase are probably reflecting a clearing of brain oedema via the ventricular CSF. Outflow resistance is increased on account of blood in the ventricles or a shift of the brain or infections (Dacey et al. 1983). Absorption may be decreased on account of subarachnoid haemorrhage or blood in the cisterns. Head injury results in a subsequent hydrocephalus in 15 per cent of cases (Kishore et al. 1978).

At the initial resuscitation it is best to assume that RICP is present and avoid factors which might cause a rise in pressure. Intubation therefore is done after the patient is anaesthetised and is first hyperventilated with a mask. It is generally accepted that pressures less than 15mmHg are normal in adults and older children but pressures above 20mmHg need treatment, and this level obviously needs adjusting depending on the age of the child. Certainly if there is any neurological deterioration at any level of ICP, then treatment should be commenced immediately to lower the ICP. Usually in older children and adults, neurological change will not occur until the pressure is approximately 40 to 50mmHg, but by then it may be irreversible. It is best therefore to begin treatment at about 20mmHg.

Available evidence suggests that while hyperventilation has been the mainstay of treatment in the past, it should have a more restricted use. Hyperventilation results in a significant increase in the AVDO$_2$ and a change in the Pcr/Pi ratio, indicative of ischaemia. There is undoubtedly a 10 per cent decrease in cerebral vessel diameter with hyperventilation and this vasoconstriction, alteration of pH, bicarbonate and improved CO$_2$ reactivity are not maintained for longer than 24 hours. Hyperventilation should therefore not be used as a preventative measure in head injury but used only to treat intermittent rises in ICP for short periods. The effect of hyperventilation on systemic blood pressure is not known. By contrast, however, mannitol has four main actions: (i) to increase cerebro-vasoconstriction (the CBF remains normal, and the CBV is decreased), (ii) to decrease blood viscosity, (iii) to withdraw brain water due to the hyperosmolar dehydration, and (iv) to scavenge free radicals. Mannitol may be used whether or not autoregulation is intact and is therefore effective in the acute head injury of childhood. The normal CBV is 4 to 4.5ml per 100g. This is approximately 50ml in an adult, 20ml of which is on the arterial side of the circuit. It should be remembered that with an intact cerebrovascular autoregulation a drop in the systemic blood pressure results in a normal CBF (*i.e.* preserved flow) but an increase in CBV.

ICP in traumatic coma in childhood is significantly related to outcome (*vide supra*). In a further series of 29 comatose children with head injury, 59 per cent had an ICP greater than 20mmHg in the first three days and ICP was significantly related to outcome (Bruce *et al.* 1981). ICP is after all the end result of the interaction of the CSF circulation, the cerebral metabolism, the bloodflow to the brain, and the compliance of the brain, and therefore is not as discriminating as correlations of CBF with outcome; however, the ICP and CPP are the parameters most commonly and easily measured. The normal cerebral perfusion is considered to be 80 to 100mmHg (Rosner and Becker 1984). It is adversely affected by changes in blood pressure or ICP. If the patient has an intracranial mass lesion and is shocked then he has both RICP and a low blood pressure with a resultant precipitate drop in CPP. CBF is dependent on CPP and falls off rapidly with CPP levels below 50 to 60mmHg in the older child.

Prognosis of coma
Since unconsciousness may occur transiently, or may be a sign of impending death, it is imperative to define the length of time after which prognostic signs may be applied. Six hours appears to be the most universally agreed time for prognostication. There is a poor prognosis for adult patients still in medical coma at six hours; only 10 per cent make a full recovery, and only 5 per cent achieve a level of independence with disability (Levy *et al.* 1981).

As mentioned above, the CPP in non-traumatic coma may give a guide to the poor outcome at the time the patient is in intensive care, particularly when levels are below 40 or 50mmHg. In a further series of 16 patients with prolonged non-traumatic coma (Margolis and Shaywitz 1980), six were normal, six had minor handicaps and four had major sequelae. It has been suggested (although not statistically proven) that RICP lasting more than two days is an indication of abnormal outcome.

Multiple rather than isolated variables are the best way of assessing the prognosis of medical coma patients. If two of the following are abnormal on admission—corneal reflexes, pupillary and vestibulo-ocular responses—then the patient will not achieve active independent function (Levy *et al.* 1981). Seshia *et al.* (1983) assessed multiple clinical variables in children (omitting investigative and diagnostic labels as well as the duration of the coma) and considered that non-

188

traumatic coma patients examined within the first two to three minutes of admission (before paralysis and ventilation) could have their outcome predicted with a 75 to 79 per cent rate of accuracy, based on severity of coma, extra-ocular movements, pupil responses, motor function, blood pressure, temperature and seizures. If the patient was still in coma 24 hours later, then the depth of coma, motor findings, blood pressure and seizures produced a 67 per cent predictability. With both examinations taken in conjunction, outcome could be predicted with more than 90 per cent accuracy.

Pyogenic meningitis

Infectious encephalopathies account for about one third of all acute encephalopathies. With regard to pyogenic meningitis, the particular organism will define the clinico-pathological features; it is not the intention to proceed through each pathogenic organism, but rather to define (i) the evidence for raised pressure in meningitis, (ii) the pathophysiology of raised pressure in meningitis, (iii) the methods of measurement that have been employed, and (iv) how pressure and other neurological complications fit into the over-all scheme of investigation of the child with therapeutic failure in pyogenic meningitis.

Evidence for RICP in pyogenic meningitis

1. PRESSURE CONES

In one series, necropsy evidence of a 'pressure cone' was found in four of 13 children who died from meningitis (Benjamin *et al.* 1988). The relative risk of coning was greater when the child presented with fits and impaired consciousness. Horwitz *et al.* (1980) investigated 302 children with bacterial meningitis. Coning was suspected in 27 of them; 10 died, three of whom had signs of coning at postmortem examination. The authors could not identify any features on presentation that would have predicted the likelihood of coning. Slack (1980) found evidence of coning in six of 90 deaths from meningococcal infection in all age groups in England and Wales in 1978. In Glasgow at least five of 11 deaths in 248 children with bacterial meningitis were thought to be associated with brain-swelling and coning (Stephenson 1985). Addy (1987) assessed from the available literature that coning contributed to the outcome in 30 per cent or more deaths from bacterial meningitis.

The inevitable question is whether the raised pressure itself produced the coning, or whether the lumbar puncture predisposed to the coning. Either way, it seems that raised pressure is present in at least a percentage of cases.

There are a number of *potential complications from lumbar punctures* themselves. The more common complications are transient low back pain; post-lumbar puncture headache (postural); transient sixth-nerve palsy; and a traumatic tap from puncture of an epidural vein or epidural venous plexus. Uncommon complications include vertebral osteomyelitis; intervertebral disc puncture; and the possible installation of pathogenic organisms in a bacteraemic patient (from infected or burned skin), with the subsequent development of meningitis (Fischer *et al.* 1975). There is experimental work to reinforce this belief (Petersdorf *et al.* 1962); epithelial rests resulting in neoplasms from introducing skin through a nonstiletted needle may occur years later (Findlay and Kemp 1943, Choremis *et al.* 1956); there may be cardiac arrest in patients with cardiorespiratory disease (Margolis and Cook 1973); but tonsillar or tentorial coning induced by lumbar puncture is the most dramatic and serious complication.

Most difficulties arise when considering the child who presents with meningococcaemia with CNS, CVS and skin or mucous membranes being affected simultaneously. A positive culture from blood, or a gram stain of an imprint smear taken after scraping a typical skin infarct, will show the intracellular gram-negative diplococci. Death in this condition may be due to cardiac arrhythmias with cardiovascular collapse secondary to myocardial dysfunction (from endogenous endotoxaemia or massive endotoxaemia from the use of bactericidal antibiotics —Rao *et al.* 1978), or to adrenal failure or brainstem haemorrhages. There is always the possibility, however, of acute or delayed coning induced by lumbar puncturing in the presence of cerebral oedema: so lumbar puncture should not be performed in patients presenting with a typical petechial rash, especially if new haemorrhages are appearing or there is peripheral vascular collapse. An infant or child presenting with any suspected meningitis, with decreased conscious state or in epileptic status, should not have a lumbar puncture because there may be cerebral oedema and lumbar puncture may precipitate coning. There are existing reports of *Haemophilus influenzae* meningitis with brain-swelling and coning following lumbar puncture (Lorber and Sunderland 1980, MacVicar and Symon 1985). The absence of papilloedema does not exclude cerebral oedema, and early death may be from cerebral oedema and not from the meningitis.

A CT scan is required with the unconscious patient, and a lumbar puncture may be done only after the cisterns have been shown to be open and there is no evidence of space occupation or acute hydrocephalus. If raised pressure is found, mannitol and frusemide may be given intravenously to reduce the pressure. It does not appear to matter how much CSF is removed at the initial lumbar puncture in the presence of raised pressure, because a continuing leak of CSF through a dural hole may still result in a slow leak and subsequent compartmental differences with coning.

In summary, therefore, an immediate lumbar puncture is *contraindicated*: (i) where there is evidence that this is meningococcal septicaemia and meningitis, (ii) in any comatose child (Glasgow coma score of 8 or less), (iii) where there is evidence of poor peripheral perfusion and cardiac output together with respiratory abnormalities, all of which necessitate cardio-respiratory support, (iv) where there is known or suspected intracranial space occupation, or known non-communicating hydrocephalus, (v) where there are clinical signs of incipient herniation (posturing, return of primitive reflexes, unequal pupils, systemic hypertension with bradycardia), (vi) with retinal haemorrhages with or without papilloedema, and (vii) where there is acute sutural separation.

Having defined these contraindications, one should be aware of the instances where a *repeat lumbar puncture* is required: (i) where the clinical situation deteriorates, despite having had a previously normal CSF from lumbar puncture (normal results from a single LP should not satisfy the paediatrician when the

TABLE 7.XV

Frequency of symptoms and signs in 35
cases of pyogenic meningitis

	No.
Symptoms:	
Fever	31
Headache/irritability	29
Vomiting	22
Anorexia	17
Seizure	14
Lethargy	10
Diarrhoea	9
Photophobia	5
Stridor	4
Signs:	
Neck stiffness	22
Drowsiness	21
Respiratory dysfunction	19
Abnormal tone	18
Pallor	18
Tense anterior fontanelle	13
Rash	12
Opisthotonos	11
Squint	8
Positive Kernig's sign	8
Papilloedema	8

patient is bacteraemic, or if there is a change in the clinical condition of the patient), (ii) where any unusual organism is involved in CNS infection, (iii) where there is failure to respond adequately to an otherwise normal antibiotic regime, and (iv) where the first CSF, done in the course of presentation of meningitis, has produced organisms in the CSF but no cells (inflammatory response).

2. CLINICAL

There are some signs of the child presenting with pyogenic meningitis which are unequivocally due to RICP: *e.g.* a tense distended fontanelle (which occurs in about one third of newborns and infants), intracranial bruit, squint, retinal venous congestion or papilloedema. Seizures themselves are not an unequivocal sign of RICP, although they may both produce RICP and be a sign of it (Minns and Brown 1978). About 40 per cent of newborns and infants will have seizures with pyogenic meningitis (Klein *et al.* 1986). The frequency of symptoms and signs in 35 cases of pyogenic meningitis is seen in Table 7.XV (Minns *et al.* 1989). Meningitis can occur without neck stiffness, and neck stiffness can occur without meningitis when it is a sign of RICP with herniation of the cerebellum. Neck stiffness may not be elicitable in the comatose patient.

Cranial bruits over the anterior fontanelle and posterior temporal areas have been found in 82 per cent of patients with purulent meningitis between the ages of three months and five years (Mace *et al.* 1968). They also occur in febrile convulsions and in afebrile children. With meningitis they are usually transitory and

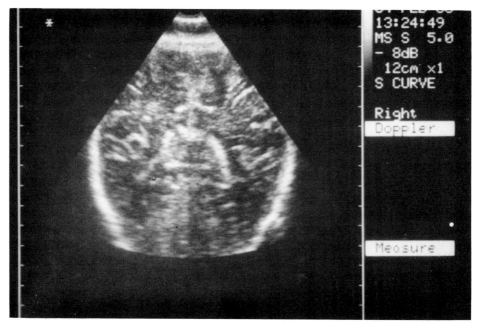

Fig. 7.1. Ultrasound scan of infant with pyogenic meningitis showing widespread increase in parenchymal echogenicity.

last no more than one to four days after starting treatment, although their reappearance may herald the devvelopment of a subdural effusion. They may be due to inflamed meninges, with increased CBF, or they may be similar to a Korotkoff sound in the head due to a wide pulse from RICP. The bruit often disappears after lumbar puncture.

Spontaneous retinal venous pulsations disappear at 14mmHg. There is no correlation between the pulsations and blood pressure. While the presence of spontaneous venous pulsations is a reliable indicator that ICP is below 14mmHg, the absence of pulsations may be found with normal or increased ICP (Levin 1978).

3. IMAGING

Ventriculomegaly is the most common abnormality on CT scan occurring in pyogenic meningitis. It has been recognised for some time (Adams *et al.* 1948), Smith and Landing 1960, Dodge and Swartz 1965, Poser and Kuiken 1968, Stovring and Snyder 1980, Bodino *et al.* 1982, Fisher *et al.* 1984, Snyder 1984). No particular infecting organism is found more than another in these patients with ventriculomegaly. The over-all incidence of seizures in bacterial meningitis is 51 per cent, while in patients with meningitis and ventriculomegaly, 92 per cent have seizures. The ventriculomegaly is progressive during the acute illness. While this may be due to an active or intermittently active hydrocephalus, it may be that some of the later ventricular dilatation represents loss of brain parenchyma with atrophy due to vasculitis, infarction or necrosis, hypoxic ischaemic damage, ventriculitis, encephalitis, bacterial neurotoxins or an immunologic response.

192

Transfontanellar sonography in children with pyogenic meningitis shows *early patterns* of increased echogenicity of the interhemispheric circonvolutions due to inflammatory cell infiltration of the arachnoid, plus exudate deposition at the cerebral base and vault.

There is also a widespread increase in parenchymal echogenicity due to cerebral oedema or cerebritis (Fig. 7.1). There are circumscribed areas of increased parenchymal echogenicity due to vasculitis, increased intraventricular echogenicity, increased ependymal echogenicity and ventricular dilatation.

The *late* ultrasound patterns are of an increased echogenicity of the interhemispheric circonvolutions, circumscribed areas of decreased parenchymal echogenicity, ventricular dilatation or hydrocephalus, subdural effusions, and intraventricular septa (Angonese and Zorzi 1986).

Cerebral abscess initially features on ultrasound as focal hyperechoic areas, but later evolves into a hypo-echoic image with a thin, well-defined hypo-echogenic rim.

With ependymitis, the oedema infiltration of the subependymal region and the presence of exudate and blood in the ventricles correspond to the sonographic images of increased ependymal echogenicity, with a characteristic 'double border' image at the roof of the ventricle. Within the ventricle there is low echogenicity or hyperechoic intraventricular haemorrhage. Later, fibrin membranes in the ventricle appear as hyperechogenic bands.

In a study of 74 infants with bacterial and eight infants with viral meningitis, 55 (two thirds) had abnormal sonographic appearances (Fisher *et al.* 1984). These abnormal appearances were in the subdural space, parenchyma, and ventricles. Subdural effusions were present in 15 cases, ventriculomegaly in 47 cases, ventriculitis in four cases, and debris, septa and strands within the ventricles in nine cases. Parenchymal changes included oedema in 18 cases, infarction in seven cases, parenchymal cysts in 11 cases, abscesses in two cases, and calcification in one case.

4. EVIDENCE FROM DIRECT ICP MEASUREMENTS

The ICP has been measured in 14 children with severe CNS infections who presented deeply comatose (Goitein *et al.* 1983). The mean opening pressure was 33mmHg and significantly different from the mean maximum ICP, which was 57mmHg. A minimum CPP above 30mmHg was a significant pointer to survival. The mean opening and maximal pressures were significantly different in those who survived and those who did not. The opening pressure is therefore an unreliable indicator of the subsequent maximal ICP, suggesting the need for continuous monitoring. The difference between the opening pressure and the later pressure in CNS infection is due to the fact that the pressure increases occur early. The mean ICP value is often not used for prognostication, since rapid and effective treatment means that over-all means are not accurate.

The normal CPP in newborns has been reported as 30mmHg, but the minimum adequate value has not been established (Raju *et al.* 1982). In older children and adults, 40mmHg is thought to be the lower limit of normal (Miller *et al.* 1972). Pyogenic meningitis patients with a CPP of 30 to 40 mmHg survived intact with easily

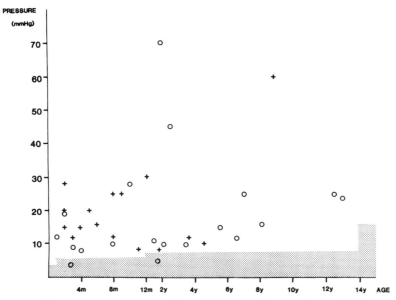

Fig. 7.2. CSF pressure measurements from 35 children with pyogenic meningitis compared with normal upper limits as previously defined (open circles [O] = pressure level without mannitol; closed circles [●] = pressure level after mannitol plus frusemide).

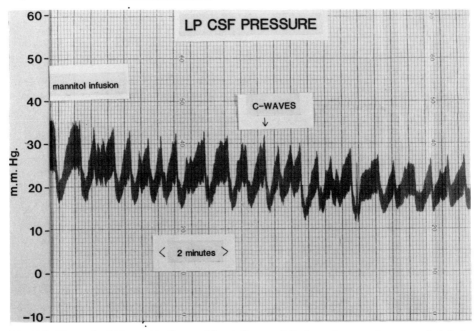

Fig. 7.3. 12-month-old boy with *Haemophilus influenzae* infection who was given mannitol during recording CSF pressure at lumbar puncture, with slow return of pressure from 30mmHg to normal, and who required intravenous frusemide. The recording shows typical C waves with ramped appearance.

194

reducible ICP. Four of the five who died, however, had intractable RICP that could not be reduced (Goitein *et al.* 1983).

The Ladd ICP monitor was applied to the anterior fontanelle in four newborns and four older infants with meningitis (McMenamin and Volpe 1984). In the older infants (mean age 5.75 months) the ICP was markedly elevated (mean peak pressure 17mmHg) with a low CBF velocity in the first two days of the illness, but in the newborns there was no marked elevation of ICP or depression of CBF velocity.

The CSF pressure has also been measured at lumbar puncture by objective strain-gauge recording in 35 infants and children with pyogenic meningitis (Minns *et al.* 1989). The pressure was raised in 33 cases. The median pressure was 15mmHg in all age-groups, but ranged from 4 to 70mmHg. Higher pressures were found on the day of admission (19mmHg). Figure 7.2 shows the results of the CSF pressure measurements from 35 children with pyogenic meningitis, compared to the normal upper limits as defined from the literature.

Despite the high CSF pressures, the CPP values were below 30mmHg in only two children. The high CPPs reflect a compensatory Cushing response of increased systemic pressure and hence cerebral perfusion. In severe infections of the CNS, cerebrovascular autoregulation is defective.

'c' waves (4 to 8/min. 0 to 20mmHg) are often seen on plateau waves, and probably reflect vasomotor waves from systemic blood pressure transmitted to the intracranial pulse. Their frequent presence in patients with pyogenic meningitis is consistent with an intact Cushing response and preservation of the CPP (Fig. 7.3). It was concluded from this study that raised pressure accompanied childhood pyogenic meningitis much more frequently than is suggested by the number of children dying from coning. Raised pressure requires treatment in its own right, independent of the infection.

5. THERAPEUTIC EVIDENCE OF RICP IN PYOGENIC MENINGITIS

It has been observed occasionally that acute purulent meningitis may produce brain-swelling, brainstem herniation and death before antibiotic therapy can interrupt the process. Intravenous urea was used immediately in the treatment of six patients with acute purulent meningitis whose ages ranged from nine weeks to four years. All had *Haemophilus influenzae* meningitis and received adequate antibiotic therapy (Williams *et al.* 1964). In a typical case cited, a child of seven months was conscious on admission, but later developed generalised clonic convulsions, and gradually became semi-comatose. 2½ hours after further fits there was eye deviation, sluggish pupillary reactions, unresponsiveness to painful stimuli and an absent gag reflex. Respirations were irregular, with intermittent 15-second apnoeic episodes. Following intravenous urea (0.55g/kg as a 20 per cent solution over a 40-minute period), the child became more active, breathing well and spontaneously, crying, and responding to painful stimuli with appropriate withdrawal. The fontanelle was now depressed and convulsions ceased, and 10 hours after admission the child was alert, moving about, whimpering and sucking her thumb. In this case the level of consciousness had deteriorated from stupor to semi-coma to coma, the respirations had progressed from hyperventilation to ataxic

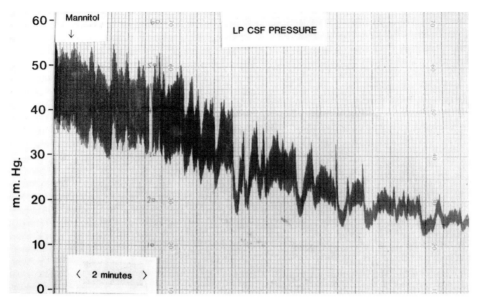

Fig. 7.4. 2½-year-old boy with meningococcal meningitis and septicaemia whose CSF pressure at lumbar puncture decreased from 43mmHg to normal values in approximately 12 minutes with mannitol infusion.

and then became apnoeic. The pupils became dilated and fixed and finally mid-sized and fixed, and 'doll's eye' movements became sluggish and then disappeared.

Two children who were moribund, with bulging fontanelle, coma, poor reactive pupils, deteriorating respiration and convulsions, had a dramatic response to infusion of urea, with improvement of consciousness, respiration, pupillary signs and cessation of convulsions. Two further children had a less dramatic response to urea, but were definitely improved. Two were thought to have had possible benefit, and no child showed deleterious effects from treatment with urea (Williams *et al.* 1964). Our own observations on the effect of mannitol and frusemide in the acutely ill child are similar (Fig. 7.4). After mannitol, in a child presenting with irritability, resentment of handling, vital sign abnormalities and pupillary abnormalities, one sees an improvement in the patient's general responsiveness, confirming that it is often the raised pressure which is responsible for the clinical picture.

Pathophysiology of RICP in pyogenic meningitis
A. *Hydrocephalus*
1. Choroid plexitis (increased production)
2. Ventriculitis
3. Ependymitis
4. Obstruction at the foramina of Luschka and Magendie
5. Arachnoiditis (occlusion of arachnoid granulations)
6. Subdural effusion/hygroma
7. Subdural empyema

B. *Space occupation*
Abscess (from suppurative encephalitis)

C. *Brain swelling*
1. Oedema
   (i) Cerebritis
   (ii) Encephalitis
   (iii) Generalised inflammatory brain oedema
   (iv) White-matter oedema
   (v) Inappropriate ADH secretion
   (vi) Necrotic oedema (due to perfusion failure, vasculitis, or major vessel infarct).

2. Congestion
   (i) Vasculitis
   (ii) Thrombophlebitis
   (iii) Seizures (status)
   (iv) Constriction and strangulation of cerebral veins.

A. *Hydrocephalus*
1. CHOROID PLEXITIS (INCREASED CSF PRODUCTION)
Isolated choroid plexus studies have suggested the choroid plexus produces between 60 and 80 per cent of the CSF (Rougement *et al.* 1960, Welch and Friedman 1960, Davson 1976), but all agree that 20 to 40 per cent arises from extra-choroidal sites, such as brain parenchmya. The ependymal cells produce an insignificant contribution to over-all bulk CSF formation (Pollay and Curl 1967). The normal CSF production is 0.3 to 0.5cc per minute, or 20cc per hour, or 500cc per day (Cutler *et al.* 1968, Lorenzo *et al.* 1970). The CSF from the choroid plexus is produced by two mechanisms: firstly, dependent on choroidal capillary flow, an ultrafiltrate is formed through lax choroidal capillary endothelium and then an active process secretes sodium into and out of the apical villi. The raised osmotic pressure is followed passively by water (Welch 1975). The second production method is a direct neurogenic stimulation of choroidal epithelium, independent of choroidal capillary perfusion. Stimulation of adrenergic fibres or cholinergic fibres will reduce or increase the CSF production accordingly. Beta 2 adrenergic receptors have been identified in human choroid plexus (Juncos *et al.* 1982).

Although the CSF production rate is very constant, ventricular outflow rate is pulsed and there is most likely a mirror-image pulsed absorption (Minns *et al.* 1987). The production I_f is the same in infants and newborns as in adults (possibly due to different maturation rates of the enzyme systems despite a different-sized choroidal area), however a number of factors influence it, including increased production from a choroid plexus papilloma (Milhorat 1975, McComb 1983); acetazolamide and frusemide will reduce production (Rubin *et al.* 1966, Cutler *et al.* 1968, McCarthy and Reed 1974). Hypothermia will reduce the production (Snodgrass and Lorenzo 1972). Under normal physiological conditions CSF production is independent of ICP, but when sufficiently high ICP occurs there is a fall-off in choroidal perfusion pressure and the formation-rate drops (Welch 1975, Sklar *et al.* 1980).

Experimentally, other factors may change CSF secretion: for example, corticosteroid in the dog will reduce the rate of CSF production by 50 per cent; vasopressin decreases the CSF production rate; hypoglycaemia and hypoxia reduce production. Prolonged VP shunting probably reduces the rate of CSF production.

Hypersecretion of CSF occurs with choroid plexus papillomas, and in isolated hydrocephalic children without papillomata. Few other situations result in an increase. It is my impression, however, that patients with ventriculitis, on external drainage, produce increased volumes of CSF; and this, together with the imaging evidence from ultrasound of plexus 'brightup' with ventriculitis and meningitis, suggests that an inflammatory choroid plexitis occurs with an increased CSF production and possible increase in ICP. There is experimental evidence that rabbits given increasing doses of gentamicin show a progressive development from initially no abnormality, to clinical ventriculitis, followed by ependymitis and choroid plexitis and eventually ventricular dilatation.

2. VENTRICULITIS

Ventriculitis is most likely to complicate gram-negative neonatal meningitis (Berman and Banker 1966) or CSF shunt infections. Shunt infection is usually with coagulase negative staphylococci (especially *Staphylococcus epidermidis* or *Staphylococcus aureus* (usually beta lactamase positive). Occasionally other skin flora gain entry through the surgical incision. Ventriculitis in the newborn may be associated with a depressed anterior fontanelle if the infant is dehydrated and it may be full and/or boggy rather than tense and may not become bulging until the very late stages of the disease. The head circumference can increase rapidly (normally 1mm per day 'except on Sunday'). There is no neck stiffness or positive Kernig's sign, and no papilloedema or focal neurological signs until late. Intrathecal treatment is always required. While the ventricular CSF in spinal meningitis may be crystal clear, because there is little reflux of CSF back into the ventricles, it is possible to have ventriculitis complicating spinal meningitis or ventriculitis without spinal meningitis. Ventriculitis must be considered as a possible cause for late relapse after apparent sterilisation of the CSF. The possibility of ventriculitis should be raised in newborn infants if organisms are still cultured from the lumbar CSF 48 to 72 hours after treatment has commenced for spinal meningitis.

Apart from organisms entering the ventricular CSF from the lumbar CSF, studies of fluorescent labelled specific anti-sera in experimental animals suggest that after intranasal inoculation, bacteria enter the nasal mucosa and the circulation and spread to the meninges from the dural sinuses (Moxon *et al.* 1974). Bacteraemia accompanies neonatal meningitis in a high proportion of cases (Davies 1977).

Ventriculitis secondary to CSF shunt infection occurs mostly in the immediate postoperative period and 70 per cent of all cases occur within the first month and 80 per cent by four months postoperatively. Cases of later ventriculitis are usually associated with ventriculo-atrial shunts. In ventriculo-atrial shunt infection, the

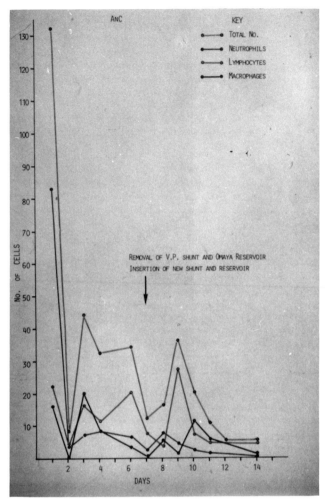

Fig. 7.5. A 15-year-old girl with neurofibromatosis and shunt for hydrocephalus: ventriculitis for 14 days before shunt revision.

bacterial endocarditis may also be associated with recurrent pneumonia and pulmonary hypertension, but more commonly results in nephrotic syndrome and shunt nephritis. The diagnosis of ventriculitis requires identification of bacteria in the ventricular CSF and the diagnosis of colonisation requires bacterial isolation from the shunt CSF or the shunt. In situations where mixed infection is detected in CSF shunts (especially gram-negative and anaerobic bacteria), one should be alerted to the possibility of bowel perforation by the shunt.

CSF shunts are colonised frequently by *Staphylococcus epidermidis*, which produces a 'slime' (Bayston and Penny 1972, Gray *et al.* 1984). This is a mucoid substance which acts as a nutrient for the bacteria and promotes colony formation of the staphylococcus. It is also antiphagocytic, which is a barrier to opsonisation and antibiotic activity.

The cell types vary in ventriculitis, but with removal of the shunt and effective

199

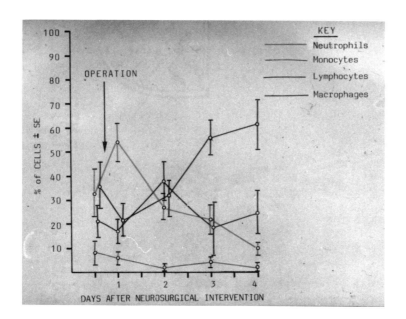

Fig. 7.6. Course of 12 cases of ventriculitis.

therapy, the cells (in particular the lymphocytes and macrophages) show a mirror-image pattern (Figs. 7.5, 7.6) (Kontopolous *et al.* 1986). Intrathecal antibiotics via the lumbar route may only sterilise the lumbar CSF and the antibiotics may not rise to the basal cisterns.

Treatment with intraventricular antibiotics by repeated puncture tracts through developing brain, particularly if the intraventricular pressure is raised, produces a real risk of porencephalic cyst formation and secondary infection. There appears to be no significant risk associated with insertion of a ventriculostomy reservoir for the control of pressure and installation of drugs (flucloxacillin and gentamicin or vancomycin and gentamicin). Although systemic and intraventricular antibiotics alone are said to produce a cure for ventriculitis in some 30 per cent of cases (McLaurin 1973), this is not our experience and complete removal of the shunt system and reservoir is usually required, as well as the use of intravenous and intraventricular antibiotics. The timing of shunt removal is crucial. While a degree of CSF sterilisation can occur with the neurosurgical hardware *in situ*, total sterilisation is unlikely to occur until the shunt (and reservoir) is removed. If the CSF is sterilised before removal of the old infected shunt, then it is possible to do a removal and re-insertion at the same operation. Usually, however, the second stage of re-insertion of a new shunt system will require to be delayed until the cell count has fallen and the percentage of macrophages is dominant in any persisting CSF pleocytosis. During this interval a second reservoir may be required for the duration of treatment, which would also require to be removed before re-insertion of a definitive shunt and reservoir.

The use of intraventricular antibiotics is imperative for sterilisation of ventricular CSF. Peak and trough levels are performed and if the trough level is too

200

low the frequency of the medication is increased; if the peak levels are too low then the dose is increased. As a measure of the antibiosis in the CSF, 'back titration' is used with CSF rather than serum. In the laboratory the organism is challenged with serial dilutions of CSF. The CSF antibiotic activity is sufficient for sterilisation if the CSF remains bactericidal at a dilution of 1 : 4.

3. EPENDYMITIS
Apart from the usual pyogenic organisms, cerebral cysticercosis is one form of granulomatous meningitis which may result in ependymitis as well as focal granulomata, cysts and hydrocephalus.

4. OBSTRUCTION AT THE FORAMINA OF LUSCHKA AND MAGENDIE
Partial or total obstruction to CSF flow by purulent or organised exudate occluding the aqueduct, the foramina or even the spinal canal is relatively common.

5. ARACHNOIDITIS (OCCLUSION OF ARACHNOID GRANULATIONS)
Failure of adequate absorption of CSF from the subarachnoid space may result in communicating hydrocephalus, and measurement of the head circumference at diagnosis, three times a week, with repeated ultrasounds, is a necessary monitor in the neonate. A rapid increase in head size, separation of the sutures or a rising CSF protein suggests obstruction or malabsorption of CSF.

6. SUBDURAL EFFUSION/HYGROMA
Fifteen per cent of patients with *Haemophilus influenzae* Type b meningitis develop subdural effusions in the fronto-parietal region, which are frequently bilateral (Bell and McCormick 1981), and 18 per cent of all types of pyogenic meningitis have a subdural effusion (Fisher *et al.* 1984). They are recognised when a raised temperature reappears or fails to drop in three to five days after treatment. There is a reappearance of vomiting, irritability, a fit or focal signs, and the effusion may be responsible for an increase in head circumference. It is better detected with ultrasound and a 'stand-off'*. A thin rim of subdural fluid requires no treatment. Tapping of subdurals should be continued until the symptoms subside. Neurosurgery is seldom necessary, but if there is a large, persistent effusion despite tapping, a subdural-peritoneal shunt is needed. The subdural collection may be responsible for RICP, and if asymmetrical may result in brain shifts. In some cases, persistent effusions will be associated with membrane formation similar to recurrent subdural haemorrhages.

7. SUBDURAL EMPYEMA
True empyema (pus) is very rare, compared with effusion, and occurs in conjunction with a sinusitis and otitis. It produces the same clinical signs as a subdural effusion, but with a more severe fever. Surgical treatment is necessary.

---

*A fluid-containing sac or attachment to set back the transducer, so that the object to be viewed is in the focal plane of the ultrasound beam.

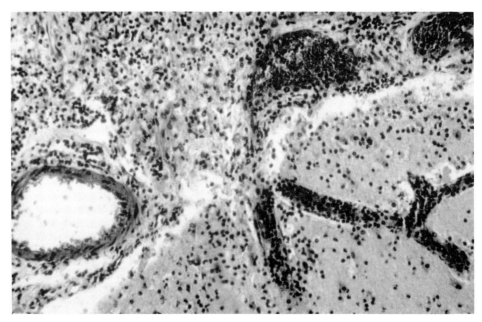

Fig. 7.7. Subarachnoid cells and inflammatory cells surrounding blood vessels in the subarachnoid space and being carried into the cerebrum resulting in cerebritis in case of *Haemophilus influenzae* meningitis.

B. *Space occupation*
ABSCESS (FROM SUPPURATIVE ENCEPHALITIS)

Cerebral abscesses are rare. They may complicate pyogenic meningitis, and in a study of 82 infants with infectious meningitis (74 pyogenic, eight viral) one third had normal ultrasound appearances and the remaining two thirds had abnormalities in the subdural space, parenchyma and ventricles. Ventricular dilatation was the commonest abnormality and was present in 57 per cent of the infants with pyogenic meningitis (Fisher *et al.* 1984). Cerebral abscesses (due to *Escherichia coli* and *Proteus mirabilis*) were present in two cases (2.5 per cent).

Abscesses usually occur in the cerebral hemispheres, the frontal lobe being most commonly affected, and less commonly the cerebellum. Small early abscess formation, multiple abscesses, or abscesses at unusual sites, for example the subdural or interhemispheric space, may not be recognised with imaging. In the newborn infant, cerebral abscesses may be silent and require ultrasound or other imaging for detection. Abscess formation may be another cause for a slow or poor response to treatment. In infants abscesses are distinguished by their relatively large size and by the relative poor capsule formation in unmyelinated white matter.

Two major clinical syndromes are associated with neonatal brain abscesses. The first is seen as a subacute evolution with signs of RICP, which may be mistakenly diagnosed as hydrocephalus because of the rapid head expansion, and the second is that associated with an acute onset of a fulminating bacterial meningitis (*e.g. Citrobacter* and *Proteus*), which by their nature have a capacity to invade nervous tissue and cause necrosis.

202

Abscesses may follow a bacteraemia which causes a localised thrombophlebitis, followed by a suppurative encephalitis, and then abscess formation. Or it may be secondary to an empyema with a parameningeal focus, such as otitis, mastoiditis, sinusitis and osteomyelitis. Enzmann *et al.* (1979) have described four stages in the evolution of experimental brain abscesses. The *early cerebritis stage* is characterised by necrotic tissue infiltrated by inflammatory cells with oedema in the surrounding brain. The *late cerebritis stage* is characterised by the necrotic area becoming better defined, and encapsulation begins as blood vessels proliferate on the periphery and deposit more inflammatory cells, reticulin, and some collagen. The third stage of *early capsule formation* is associated with increasing amounts of collagen and reticulin forming a wall surrounding the necrotic centre. The *late capsule formation* stage is characterised by a thick collagen capsule, more substantial on the cortical side than on the ventricular side. For all cerebral abscesses surgical drainage is necessary.

A case of multiple small ring-enhancing hypodensities consistent with cerebral abscesses, with symptoms of RICP, proved to be due to *Haemophilus paraphrophirus*, and autopsy disclosed disseminated micro-abscesses with an associated endocarditis (Habib *et al.* 1984). In the newborn, extensive suppuration may occur with relatively minor changes in the CSF (Raimondi and DiRocco 1979).

C. *Brain swelling*

1. OEDEMA

Cerebritis. Haemophilus influenzae meningitis is particularly associated with cerebritis and therefore encephalitis. The inflammatory cells and organisms in the subarachnoid space become carried on to the surface of the brain around penetrating vessels, and an inflammatory response and oedema occurs in the grey matter (Fig. 7.7). *Haemophilus influenzae* Type B is the common offending organism in children. *Listeria monocytogenes* meningitis requires a minimum of two weeks' treatment (with ampicillin and an aminoglycoside), which is in part related to the organism's potential to produce a superficial cerebritis for which more prolonged treatment is indicated.

Encephalitis. Fits, decerebration and coma may be the presenting features of encephalitis accompanying *Haemophilus influenzae* meningitis; meningism need not be present and there may be scanty CSF pleocytosis, despite positive cultures there and in the blood. 30 per cent of newborn infants with group B streptococcal and 4 per cent of newborns with *Escherichia coli* meningitis will have normal lumbar CSF white-cell counts (Klein *et al.* 1986). Bacteria causing gastro-enteritis may directly invade the CNS, causing encephalitis or meningitis (*e.g. Salmonella* sp.), or may release a neurotoxin (*e.g. Shigella* sp. or *Helicobacter*), causing fits and coma without direct invasion of the brain. From the dehydration, hyperviscosity may occur with venous sludging and thrombosis and complicate the picture. Cerebral oedema may occur also from osmotic imbalance during treatment and low calcium and magnesium may cause additional fits.

Generalised inflammatory brain oedema. There is evidence that even in the absence of meningitis, cerebral swelling is a concomitant of meningococcal septicaemia (Conner and Minielly 1980, Brandtzeac and Skulberg 1987, Sinclair *et al.* 1987); and this raised pressure from oedema, which may be severe enough to cause herniation of the brain through the anterior fontanelle (Gibson *et al.* 1975), together with the severe hypotension, may be responsible for critically low CPPs. Aggressive attempts therefore have to be made to maintain the CPP. This is a different sort of primary vasogenic oedema which causes cerebral damage, from the posthypoxic and post-traumatic oedema and rises in ICP which follow cerebral damage. *Haemophilus influenzae, Neisseria meningitidis* and *Escherichia coli* are also known to be associated with endotoxin release. The presence of endotoxin directly correlates with the recovery of gram-negative bacteria from the CSF, and may also be detected in the brain, meninges, subdural and ventricular fluid (McCracken and Sarff 1976). The endotoxin (measured by the *Limulus* amoebocyte lysate assay) may be instrumental in producing this oedema.

White-matter oedema. Some infections produce a clearly delineated white-matter oedema. One such condition is neurocysticercosis, which produces intracranial hypertension almost invariably related to white-matter oedema. Focal cystic lesions or hydrocephalus may dominate some cases. A strong inflammatory response with oedema due to the dying larvae, may result in the increased ICP during treatment (Danziger and Bloch 1975, Mervis and Lotz 1980, Kalra *et al.* 1987).

Inappropriate ADH secretion. Neonatal meningitis may occasionally be associated with a syndrome of inappropriate ADH secretion (Reynolds *et al.* 1972, Mendoza 1976) and the hyponatraemia, increased urine osmolality, increased renal excretion of sodium, all subside with the acute stage of the disease. The most effective and safest treatment of the hyponatraemia is fluid restriction to 60ml/kg/day for the first two or three days.

Necrotic oedema (due to perfusion failure, vasculitis, or major vessel infarct). Intense *vasculitis* with infarction and necrosis of brain tissue may occur in pyogenic meningitis and has been particularly associated with the *Enterobacteriaceae* (Shortland-Webb 1968). The development of arthritis and cutaneous vasculitis in meningococcaemia, thought to be due to immune complex deposition in synovium and skin and gut, is probably accompanied by a similar cerebral vasculitis.

Type B is responsible for most meningococcal infections in Britain. Bacteraemia is probably the primary event in all forms of this infection, although it has been suggested that the meninges might be infected by direct spread through the cribriform plate (Christie 1980). Penicillin should be given to patients with suspected meningococcal infection before transfer to hospital. Certainly at hospital presentation, patients with suspected meningococcaemia should have a blood culture taken, with intravenous penicillin (500,000 units) injected before removing the needle. The antibiotic cover should then be intravenous benzylpenicillin (30,000 units/kg/day) and chloramphenicol (100mg/kg/day) given four-hourly. The chloramphenicol is to cover *Haemophilus influenzae* meningitis which may present in a similar fashion. Mild petechial rashes may also occur in pneumococcal, Rickettsial and enteroviral infections. Initial cardiovascular resuscitation is aimed at maximum tissue oxygen delivery, including volume loading with 20ml/kg of fresh

204

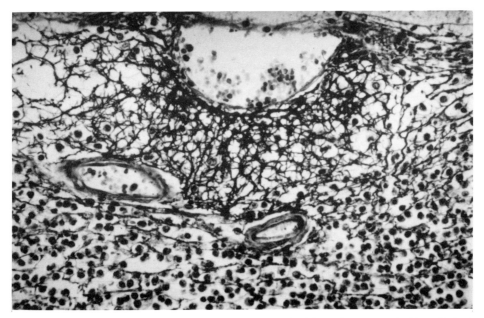

Fig. 7.8. Case of pyogenic meningitis in which fibrin and protein-rich exudate surrounds thin-walled vein adjacent to the pia (*top*) seen on high-power PTAH stain.

frozen plasma, or blood and albumin, supplementary oxygen and non-invasive monitoring. The fresh frozen plasma, in addition to coagulation factors, contains protease inhibitors, (alpha-1 antitryspin and antithrombin 111), which may limit neutrophil damage to the capillary endothelium. A significant difference between the survivors and non-survivors in this overwhelming infection is the pulmonary function and oxygen utilisation variables (Sinclair 1988). Malaria may result in coma from convulsions associated with fever or from cerebral malaria with severe petechial haemorrhages and cerebral oedema (especially that due to *Plasmodium falciparum*).

Perfusion defects may result from an overwhelming meningococcal infection (especially Type c), with gram-negative shock, DIC and coma. The rapid progression of purpura usually heralds the DIC and shock from endotoxaemia, sometimes with bacterial embolisation of the lungs. Perfusion defects may also result from an accompanying myocarditis, particularly with Type b and c infections when severe hypotension results in a loss of cerebrovascular autoregulation.

2. CONGESTION

Vasculitis. Arteritis occurs in all bacteriological varieties of meningitis and affects arteries of varying sizes; it is particularly related to basilar inflammation. It was previously demonstrated well on angiography and results in hemiparesis, hemianopsia and focal seizures. Encephalopathy with proliferative vasculitis, perivascular inflammation and thrombotic occlusions may accompany Rickettsial infections such as tick typhus and Rocky Mountain spotted fever.

205

Thrombophlebitis. Venous occlusion as a complication is now infrequently seen because of careful fluid management and prevention of dehydration. The signs are of intractable focal seizures and a hemiparesis, often involving the arm more than the leg. Red cells in the CSF may herald the thrombosis, because of the associated haemorrhagic infarction.

Seizures (status). In 253 attacks of pyogenic meningitis, seizures occurred in 33 per cent of cases and were a presenting feature in 22 per cent of those between six months and six years (Stephenson 1985). The incidence is greater in pneumococcal meningitis. If seizures continue, they may be reflecting RICP and also contributing to it. On the other hand, persistent focal seizures suggest a focal inflammatory collection. Treatment is by intravenous phenytoin (15 to 20mg/kg) over a 30-minute period with ECG control. Particular care is needed that the 'dead space' and the 'chasing fluid' are free of dextrose since phenytoin is incompatible with dextrose.

Constriction and strangulation of cerebral veins. Histological sections of pia and cortex show dense fibrous and inflammatory network of cells surrounding the surface veins (Fig. 7.8).

D. *Iatrogenic from treatment*
This includes fluid overload resulting in cerebral oedema, fits and coning, and the controversial concept of glucose use and cerebral damage.

E. *Hypertensive encephalopathy*
Although acute transient hypertension occurs with RICP, the association with acute meningitis is not common. A 21-month-old child who presented with a hypertensive encephalopathy due to *Haemophilus influenzae* Type B meningitis was reported (Waters and Gillis 1987). Blood pressure was 200/100mmHg, and treatment with frusemide and diazoxide resulted in a fall in blood pressure to 150/80mmHg over the next 30 minutes, with an associated improvement in her conscious state.

In this case the CSF was under normal pressure and there were no symptoms of RICP, although the diuretic may have relieved RICP that was not clinically evident.

The pathophysiology of hypertensive encephalopathy may involve blood-pressure regulation centres in the hypothalamus and medulla affected by changes in bloodflow or mechanical compression. It would be unlikely that ADH secretions from increased blood volume or sympathetic overactivity would be responsible. RICP may be responsible, and as with RICP occurring in the course of meningitis, systemic hypertension will need treatment of itself. Clearly significant hypertension could open the blood-brain barrier and cause secondary brain infection, rather than the reverse (Robinson 1986).

Systemic hypertension is associated with cerebral vasoconstriction until the breakpoint for the blood-brain barrier is reached outside the limits of autoregulation, when local vasospasms and dilatations result in leakage through the vessel walls (van Vught 1976) with cerebral oedema and hypertensive encephalopathy and

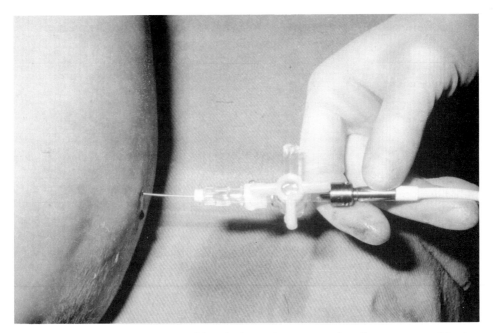

Fig. 7.9. A small Luer fitting sensor with a sloping surface connected to three-way tap and lumbar puncture needle.

the clinical picture of fits, coma, headache, vomiting, aphasia, blindness and hemiplegia. It is difficult in patients with hypertension and neurological symptoms to differentiate between hypertensive encephalopathy, cerebral complications due to hypertension, and hypertension secondary to RICP. According to Taylor *et al.* (1954), intracranial hypertension occurs in 39 per cent of cases of hypertensive encephalopathy.

Measurement of ICP in meningitis
Two series of ICP measurements in pyogenic meningitis have been reported. One method used in comatose infants involves a percutaneously placed subdural catheter (Goitein and Amit 1982). The same technique is used as for subdural taps, *i.e.* a 22 gauge Quickcath is introduced into the subdural space, then connected via non-compliant tubes to a pressure transducer whose signal is displayed on a bedside monitor. Simultaneous arterial blood pressure is displayed on the same monitor. The above series recorded ICP and blood pressure hourly, or when acute changes took place.

Treatment was commenced if the pressure exceeded 20mmHg, or if the CPP fell below 40mmHg, but acute short-term changes were not treated. Prior to any procedures that might increase ICP, prophylactic thiopentone sodium (5mg/kg, single dose) was given.

A treatment protocol was devised for managing the RICP initially with frusemide and hyperventilation; if this failed to bring the ICP below 20mmHg within

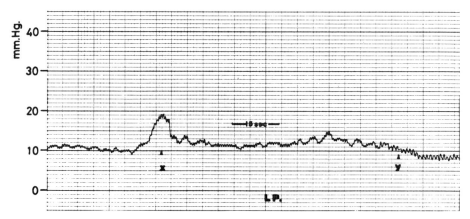

Fig. 7.10. A lumbar CSF pressure recording showing effects of Queckenstedt's test (X) and hyperventilation (Y).

20 minutes, or if the CPP was below 40mmHg then mannitol was added and finally barbiturates. Treatment was continued until the ICP had been normal for 24 hours and the subdural catheter remained in place for an additional 24 hours to ensure continued normal ICP.

The more routine measurement of CSF pressure in pyogenic meningitis has been reported (Minns 1984, Minns and Engleman 1988, Minns *et al.* 1989). The technique involved measurement of pressure at the time of lumbar puncture. A non-displacement method of measurement was used by connecting a strain-gauge pressure transducer with a Luer fitting, attached to a three-way tap, to the end of the spinal needle after the stilette had been cautiously removed and CSF had reached the mouth of the spinal needle. A specially designed pressure transducer with a sloping diaphragm means that air-bubbles are not introduced between the sensor and the liquid column (Fig. 7.9). Should air-bubbles be introduced then there would be attenuation of the signal from liquid to gas before the signal was received at the sensor and this would invalidate the reading. The presence of a respiratory and cardiac pulse-wave verifies that the needle is in the spinal subarachnoid space and therefore measuring the CSF pressure (Fig. 7.10).

The transducer, amplifier and recorder are located permanently in the ward treatment room and calibrated before the procedure, using an anaeroid sphygmo-manometer over the range 0 to 50mmHg. Staff become familiar with this technique after a very short time. The transducer is sterilised beforehand in a 2 per cent solution of glutaraldehyde. A minute or more of recording is obtained while the patient is encouraged to relax after the initial insertion of the needle, and to slightly deflex the head and neck and back into a more neutral position, without undue compression of the neck or abdomen. Following the initial apprehension and struggle, the pressure drops to its true mean level. With free communication in the CSF spaces, the pressure recorded then reflects the ICP. The mean CSF pressure is taken as one third of the pulse pressure above diastolic. It must be mentioned that these lumbar recordings are only obtained when a lumbar puncture is indicated,

TABLE 7.XVI

Mean upper limit of normal ICP derived from studies where ICP was objectively measured

	Normal pressure (mmHg)	Method	Mean upper normal limit (mmHg)
Neonates:			
Welch 1980	0.29–4.41	Fontanometry	
Welch 1978	<2.94	Fontanometry	
Kaiser and Whitelaw 1986	2.8 (1.4) (SD)	Lumbar puncture	
Gerlach *et al.* 1967	0.74–1.03	Lumbar puncture	<3.5
Infants:			
Welch 1980	1.84–12.15	Fontanometry	
Gaab *et al.* 1980	5 (2) (SD)	Fontanometry	
von Wild and Porksen 1980	−2–5	Fontanometry	
Sidbury 1920	2.21–5.15	Lumbar puncture	
Levinson 1928	1.47–5.15	Lumbar puncture	<5.8
Munro 1928	2.12–5.88	Lumbar puncture	
Children:			
Quincke 1891	2.94–4.41	Lumbar puncture	
Levinson 1923	3.31–6.99	Lumbar puncture	
Levinson 1928	2.94–5.88	Lumbar puncture	
Lups and Haan 1954	2.94–7.35	Lumbar puncture	<6.4
Gerlach *et al.* 1967	2.94–7.35	Lumbar puncture	
Adults:			
Merritt and Fremont-Smith 1937	<13.24	Lumbar puncture	
Masserman 1934	10.9 (2.5) (SD)	Lumbar puncture	
Masserman 1935	11.1 (2.1) (SD)	Lumbar puncture	
Spina-Franca 1963	3–14.5	Cisternal puncture	
Tourtellotte *et al.* 1964	11 (2.4) (SD)	Lumbar puncture	<15.3
Gilland *et al.* 1974	11.5 (2.6) (SD)	Lumbar puncture	
Ekstedt 1978	10.3 (1.5) (SD)	Lumbar puncture	
Ferris 1941	<17.6	Lumbar puncture	

and should the patient be in coma, have decerebration, papilloedema, or retinal haemorrhages, then a CT scan is performed first and, if necessary, intracranial methods are used. This method is potentially safer and more accurate than using an open-ended manometric tube. It is more accurate, in that CSF is not displaced from a closed cavity into a capillary column to record the pressure. It is potentially safer in that if raised pressure is found, then without removing CSF, mannitol (7ml/kg of a 20 per cent solution) and frusemide (1mg/kg) can be given immediately to reduce the pressure.

Such direct measurement is unequivocal and is done at the time of diagnostic lumbar puncture or whenever subsequent lumbar punctures are indicated, or if intrathecal antibiotics are being used. At the same time, a blood-pressure measurement allows calculation of the cerebral perfusion pressure, *i.e.* CPP = SAP − ICP.

The normal CSF pressure reported by various investigators from objective measurements at different ages has been outlined in the following table together with the calculated mean upper normal limit for the various age-groups from neonates to adults (Table 7.XVI).

Neurosurgery in pyogenic meningitis

Occasionally in the course of pyogenic meningitis, severe exudate in the cisterns and over the surface of the brain or in the sulci produces severe adhesive arachnoiditis and an obstruction to bulk flow of CSF which may be virtually impermeable to otherwise adequate concentrations of intrathecal and systemic antibiotics, and resistant to intrathecal steroids. The following three cases illustrate the use of neurosurgical procedures for these complications of pyogenic meningitis.

CASE 1 This was a 3½-month-old male admitted with a two-day history of pyrexia, who was generally lethargic, unwell and off his feeds. There was no significant past or family history of note. At the time of admission his anterior fontanelle was slightly full, he was irritable and disliked neck flexion. An opening pressure at lumbar puncture was 12mmHg, which is elevated for a 3½-month-old child. Fluid was turbid and antibiotic treatment commenced with penicillin and chloramphenicol. Pneumococci sensitive to penicillin were isolated from this first CSF. CSF protein at this time was 3.62g/l.

Anticonvulsants were prophylactically added to his regime but he subsequently developed clonic fits and opisthotonos. He became apnoeic during this fit and required mannitol and elective ventilation. He continued to have seizures for the first two days and a subdural tap was performed. This revealed 530 WBC/mm^3, 95 per cent of which were neutrophils. No organisms were cultured. He continued to require daily subdural taps for the next seven days. IPPV was continued for three days, followed by CPAP and extubation. Ten days after admission he still had a persistent low-grade pyrexia, was slightly hypertonic with fisting, and had a squint. By this time there had been a definite increase in the size of the lateral and the third ventricles on ultrasound, along with the subdural midline collection.

A reservoir was inserted 13 days after admission; at this time the ventricular fluid contained 650WBC/mm^3, 50 per cent of which were neutrophils. At the same time, his lumbar CSF persisted with 1200WBC/mm^3, predominantly neutrophils, but without organisms seen. He was commenced on intrathecal benzylpenicillin given in split doses between the lumbar route and Rickham reservoir. His temperature decreased following the start of the intrathecal penicillin, although there remained a low-grade pyrexia with persistent WBCs in the CSF. A second change of antibiotics was started, which again produced an initial response in the CSF, but the child remained persistently irritable.

Twenty-six days after admission he became lethargic, pyrexial and pale again, with a resurgence of cells in the lumbar and ventricular CSF (980 WBC/mm^3 with 90 per cent neutrophils from lumbar CSF and 68 WBC/mm^3 from the reservoir). An air encephalogram was performed with 5cc of air introduced into the lumbar space. This settled in the basal cisterns and did not enter the ventricular system, confirming a block in the CSF circulation around the basal cisterns. Treatment was commenced with intrathecal

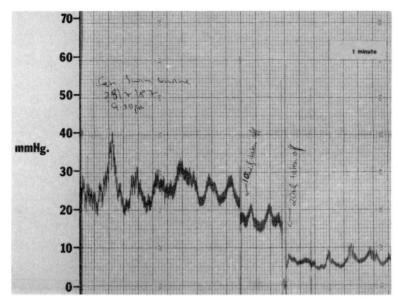

Fig. 7.11. Control of RICP by CSF removal.

hydrocortisone into both lumbar and ventricular CSF. Initially this seemed to have effect, and was continued for seven days. Unfortunately the cell count again rebounded with further pyrexia and irritability. By one month after admission there had been a further marked increase in the size of the third and lateral ventricles on ultrasound and a parasagittal subdural collection was present. A further change of antibiotics to intravenous and intrathecal chloramphenicol produced a similar transient response in the white cell count and general condition. RICP developed at this time, necessitating continuous overnight pressure monitoring with withdrawal of CSF to control the pressure (Fig. 7.11). An MRI scan 41 days after admission showed the presence of pus in the cisterna magna, and it was decided that should a further relapse occur after the chloramphenicol, he would require *posterior fossa exploration and débridement.*

Forty-three days after admission he became pale again, with vomiting and septicaemia. The following day, at posterior fossa exploration, infected tissue was removed from the cisterna magna. Following surgery he breathed spontaneously but remained on continual drainage from his Rickham reservoir, and 54 days after admission the frontal reservoir was changed and a ventriculo-peritoneal shunt inserted. There was a gradual improvement in his condition, as he became apyrexial and began feeding spontaneously. Two years later he uses a phonic ear on account of cochlea damage with profound deafness. Although on anticonvulsants, he has had no further seizures, but he is globally developmentally delayed and is developing an ataxic cerebral palsy. He has normal vision and his hydrocephalus is well controlled with a CSF shunt.

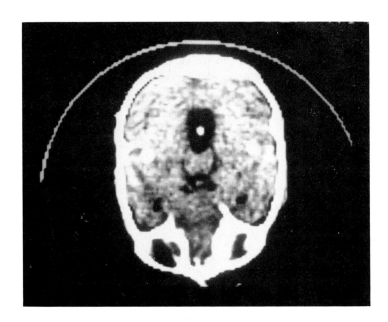

Fig. 7.12. CT scan with encysted fourth ventricle.

CASE 2 This child was born preterm at 34 weeks' gestation; he suffered birth asphyxia and necrotising enterocolitis with a perforated gut. He also sustained an IVH and developed a post-haemorrhagic hydrocephalus, for which a ventriculo-peritoneal CSF shunt was inserted. He was admitted at the age of 6½ years with symptoms of shunt malfunction.

On arrival he was alert and afebrile, with long-standing dysarthria, optic atrophy, bilateral sixth-nerve palsy, left-sided seventh-nerve palsy, and dystonic tetraplegia. He was microcephalic, with a right-sided VP shunt.

A CT scan revealed markedly dilated and encysted fourth ventricle and posterior fossa (Fig. 7.12). He underwent a cysto-peritoneal shunt. Post-operatively he developed a ventriculitis with a more extensive posterior fossa hydrocephalus. Over the next few months he had recurrent episodes of ventriculitis and clinical deterioration associated with RICP, requiring repeated revisions of the ventriculo-peritoneal and cysto-peritoneal shunt. He then developed a peritonitis-like illness which responded to conservative management with antibiotics. He again deteriorated after a few weeks with RICP and brainstem signs. He underwent a *posterior fossa exploration* which revealed thickened fibrinous tissue running tightly across the brainstem. This was removed together with fragments of cerebellar tissue. A drain was left in the posterior fossa for external drainage. He continued to have a fluctuating clinical state with irregular respiration and bradycardia.

He required further shunt revisions for persistent ventriculitis, and on one occasion he required external drainage from his posterior fossa shunt system. The cyst slowly disappeared in the posterior fossa. His neurological state, and in particular bulbar function and speech, slowly improved. Nine months later he still had severe bulbar weakness, but was beginning to take food by mouth and was nutritionally coping. By this time he had good protective bulbar reflexes, and the nasogastric tube had been removed.

This was an 11-year-old boy who had been well until one month prior to **CASE** admission, when he complained of early morning headaches, particularly **3** in the right temporal region. He was given several courses of antibiotics for this, but then became dysphasic and was admitted to a local hospital as an emergency for scanning and lumbar puncture. CSF revealed over 2000 wbc/mm^3, predominantly neutrophils, which had risen to 17,000 three days later. No organisms were seen at any time. Seven days into treatment he developed a facial weakness and an urgent CT scan was arranged, which showed a small focal, non-enhancing, low-density area in the right thalamic region, and evidence of basal meningitis.

On admission he was apyrexial and oriented, but obviously in pain, with a left hemiparesis, left hemianopia and left supranuclear seventh-nerve palsy. Over the following 24 hours his paresis became denser, with intermittent drowsiness and bradycardia. A subarachnoid bolt was inserted and the ICP recorded between 20 and 25mmHg. He showed some improvement with antibiotics, pressure control and dexamethasone, but five days after admission he deteriorated again. A CT scan on this occasion showed a swollen right hemisphere, suggesting a cortical thrombophlebitis. Mannitol and fluid restriction were continued, and the pressure problems resolved. The screw was removed eight days after admission. Three weeks after admission he had further intermittent headaches and a repeat lumbar puncture revealed a fluid pressure of 18 to 20mmHg, with 67 wbc/mm^3, glucose of 0.4mmol/l and protein of 153g/l. Further CT scan showed a small low-density abnormality in the right internal capsular region and evidence of an inflammatory process affecting the right temporo-parietal cortex and basal cisterns. An isotope scan confirmed the vascularity. Apart from antibiotics and metronidazole, he required mannitol for his increased ICP. He developed a third-nerve palsy, and an emergency reservoir was inserted. External ventricular drainage was then set up from his reservoir, with intermittent pressure monitoring, which showed a consistent level of 15 to 20mmHg. Comparison of the CSF pressure from the lumbar puncture and the reservoir revealed different pressures, different cell counts and different protein levels. Despite the commencement of intrathecal vanco-mycin, he developed nystagmus, severe vomiting and hyporeflexia, and had an emergency posterior fossa craniotomy five weeks after initial admission.

An operation revealed stringy, spaghetti-like pus, which showed inflammatory slough under the microscope. Immunofluorescence was

213

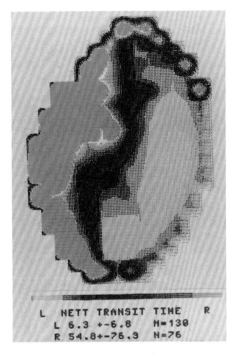

L METT TRANSIT TIME   R
L 6.3 +-6.8   M=130
R 54.8+-76.3 N=76

Fig. 7.13. Mean transit time study showing excessively prolonged transit times for the right hemisphere and virtually no cerebral perfusion.

strongly positive for pneumococcal antigens. Intrathecal cefuroxime was added but, despite this, he developed further infarcts in the right internal capsular region, considerable shrinkage in the right fronto-temporal region and selective dilatation of the right lateral ventricle. A suprasellar abscess also developed. He improved after being started on intrathecal hydrocortisone and intravenous sulphadiazine in high doses, although an allergic rash interrupted this therapy. The CT scan showed gradual improvement. There was dilatation of the lateral ventricles, but disappearance of the abscess. His neurological state remained fairly stable thereafter, with a dense left hemiparesis, facial palsy and hemianopia.

He subsequently developed early-morning vomiting and fasciculation of the tongue, so that a fourth ventricular syndrome was thought possible, and an NMR scan showed pus organising around the fourth ventricle. There was also shadowing in the sphenoidal and paranasal sinuses; they were washed out, and inspissated pus was revealed. Gradually, with the help of the reservoir and lumbar puncture, CSF pressure and cell count, protein and glucose returned to normal. CBF studies, using a mean transit-time isotope investigation, revealed virtually absent cerebral perfusion in the right hemisphere (Fig. 7.13). Three years later his facial movements are more symmetrical and cranial nerves relatively intact. His main residual difficulty is dystonia in the right arm. He walks with a heel/toe gait, a good stance and swing, and has normal speech.

Neurosurgical involvement in these three cases of pyogenic meningitis

214

was very useful in *removal of exudate and adhesions in the posterior fossa cisterns, freeing adhesive strangulation of the brainstem*, and extracting long strands of organised pus and inflammatory slough, which would never be penetrated by antibiotics given intrathecally or intravenously. All three cases were associated with pneumococcal infection: meningitis, abscess and ventriculitis. There are no existing reports in the literature of such surgical involvement in pyogenic meningitis, which in these cases was vital.

Therapeutic failure
The outcome from pyogenic meningitis in childhood has not changed appreciably over the last 14 years (McCracken 1984) and there is still a significant mortality and morbidity in the form of neurological sequelae, for two main reasons.

1. *Delay in initial diagnosis*
Young infants and newborns have fairly non-specific symptoms and there may be delay in making the original diagnosis. Similarly, older children with vague non-specific symptomatology are likely to present late with fits and coma (*i.e.* an encephalopathic presentation). When the interval from onset of symptoms to the commencement of treatment is greater than 24 hours the mortality and morbidity increase dramatically.

2. *Delay in diagnosing a cause for failure to respond to an otherwise adequate therapeutic regime*
This failure of optimal response may be due to *problems with the organism or antibiotic*: for instance if the organism has been wrongly identified; if there has been mixed infection; if it is a particularly virulent strain (*e.g. Haemophilus influenzae* may be resistant to ampicillin and chloramphenicol); if the wrong antibiotic has been used, or in an insufficient dose, or it is not being administered via the right route to reach the appropriate locus in sufficient concentration. Alternatively, the antibiotic kinetics may not have been taken into account: for example, the normal chloramphenicol preparation is the palmitate or succinate form, which if given orally is broken down by esterases in the gut to 'free chloramphenicol', which gets into the CSF very well. Intravenous chloramphenicol may get into the CSF less well on account of too little esterase in the blood. Intrathecal (free) chloramphenicol is difficult to procure, but is very effective in small doses (1mg) compared to the 40mm/kg intravenous dose. Alternatively, the serum chloramphenicol levels may be unreliable if phenobarbitone or phenytoin are being concurrently used or if there is systemic hypotension with renal and hepatic inflammation. Failure to recognise this optimal response (ensuring that viable organisms are no longer present, that the cell count is responding, and that the antibiotic levels in the CSF are adequate) means that lumbar punctures should be redone in any case in which steady improvement is not occurring.

The failure of optimal response may also be due to a *neurological complication*. It might be that there is loculation of the organisms, as we have demonstrated with a subdural effusion or adhesive arachnoiditis, adhesive pus in pneumococcal infection, a hydrocephalus, abscess, cerebritis, suppurative enceph-alitis, seizures, oedema, ventriculitis or raised pressure. Meningitis is an infection of and around the brain, and the most important sequelae of meningitis are always neurological. It is therefore important to pay attention to the possible neurological complications which might be responsible for therapeutic failure, and to measure the lumbar CSF or intraventricular pressure, to involve a neurosurgeon, to use intrathecal penicillin for all newly diagnosed pneumococcal meningitis, to use intrathecal steroids where indicated and generally to be aware of the possible accompaniment of RICP with pyogenic meningitis, which will need treatment in its own right. In our series no one type of organism (*Haemophilus influenzae, Neisseria meningitidis* or *Streptococcus pneumoniae*) was more responsible for raised pressure than another. Apart from pressure due to the various neurological complications, it may also be iatrogenic, *e.g.* from fluid overload or the inappropriate use of glucose, which may contribute to the raised pressure and hence morbidity and mortality.

Tuberculous meningitis
Tuberculosis may affect the central and peripheral nervous system in a number of ways, one of which is a presentation with an acute encephalopathy, either with a sudden hemiparesis due to vasculitis or with acute hydrocephalus and RICP. Tuberculous meningitis is now rare in the United Kingdom (Naughten *et al.* 1981). In other parts of the world, particularly the Indian subcontinent and parts of Africa, the incidence is very much higher. The highest incidence in children is between six and 24 months of age. While the BCG vaccine has prevented tuberculous meningitis or miliary tuberculosis in the United Kingdom, in other parts of the world tuberculous meningitis has been described in children who have had BCG vaccination in the neonatal period (Paul 1961, Myint 1980).

The classical presentation of tuberculous meningitis is with a three-week history. Younger children may have a shorter presenting history. In the first week there is a gradual onset with temperature, irritability, listlessness, headache, vomiting and abdominal pains. In the second week the symptoms become more pronounced, with neck stiffness and positive Kernig's sign. The conscious state begins to decline and there may be cranial nerve signs, such as facial palsy, ptosis, extra-ocular muscle palsies and papilloedema. In the third week there is frank coma, decerebrate rigidity, convulsions, papilloedema and multiple cranial nerve palsies (particularly third-, fourth-, sixth- and eighth-nerve palsies). Choroid tubercles (in up to 50 per cent of cases) are seen only in association with miliary tuberculosis (66 per cent of cases). Untreated, this condition has a natural history to death within three to five weeks. Many of the symptoms and signs at presentation may be features of RICP, for example, pressure-induced convulsions, hemiparesis, photophobia and diplopia, opisthotonos and expanding head circum-ference, tense fontanelle, high-pitched cry and false localising cranial-nerve palsies.

Diagnosis
For a definitive diagnosis, a Mantoux Test 1:1000 should be used. Tuberculin

sensitivity is usually present even in very ill children. A chest x-ray may aid in the diagnosis, but tuberculous meningitis is not excluded by a normal chest x-ray. Sometimes there is difficulty in demonstrating acid fast bacilli (AFBS) in the CSF (Lincoln *et al*. 1960), although Smith and Vollum (1954) identified AFBS in 90 per cent of their patients with tuberculous meningitis. An increased CSF protein is a consistent finding.

The CSF characteristics, apart from the raised protein, are of a lympho-cytosis, up to 400 cells/mm^3, but occasionally a predominance of polymorphs may be found in the first few days (Smith 1975). The glucose is normal in the early stages, but then becomes low and frequently undetectable. Rarely the cell count and glucose are normal; however, the CSF protein is invariably raised. As mentioned, the search for tubercle bacillus in the CSF can be quite time-consuming and the institution of therapy before the CSF is obtained does not preclude subsequent identification of bacilli. Cultures, however, provide the diagnosis, either from the CSF or gastric washings, usually only after several weeks in 40 to 75 per cent of patients.

The bromide partition test is used to study the integrity of the blood-brain barrier. There is a relative concentration of bromide in the blood and CSF 24 hours after a loading-dose of sodium bromide. In normal individuals the ratio is 3 : 1. This ratio approaches 1 : 1 when the blood-brain barrier is damaged. The test is safe, and bromide estimations are easily performed by most laboratories. This test is supportive of the diagnosis but is not conclusive. The bromide partition test is more reliable than adenosine deaminase activity or the enzyme-linked immunosorbent assay in detecting tubercle and differentiating tuberculous from viral and pyogenic meningitis. The test remains abnormal for up to five months (Coovadia *et al*. 1986). Tuberculostearic acid estimation of the CSF is another rapid and specific test for tuberculous meningitis, and it can be used for retrospective diagnosis in patients who have been started on therapy (French *et al*. 1987).

The differential diagnosis includes viral encephalitis, in particular herpes simplex virus (HSV) encephalitis and mumps meningitis, cryptococcal meningitis, pyogenic brain abscess, partially treated pyogenic meningitis, sarcoidosis, and lead encephalopathy.

Pathogenesis
The temporal relationship of tuberculous meningitis with miliary tuberculosis has suggested haematogenous dissemination. They were found to coexist among 297 cases of tuberculous meningitis in 68 per cent of cases (Blacklock and Griffin 1935). Direct spread is suggested by small (3 to 5mm) caseous tuberculous foci which have been found in the meninges or in the brain adjacent to the subarachnoid space in 77 of 82 cases examined (Rich and McCordock 1933).

1. TUBERCULOUS EXUDATE AND ACUTE HYDROCEPHALUS
Early studies with air encephalography found a 62 per cent incidence of hydrocephalus in tuberculous meningitis (Lorber 1951). Later studies showed it to be more common in children than in adults (Dastur *et al*. 1970; Tandon *et al*. 1973, 1975). A significant study of 60 cases of tuberculous meningitis in children and

217

adults found that only three patients had a normal CT scan (Bhargava *et al.* 1982), *i.e.* severe hydrocephalus was present in 87 per cent of children. For all children less than 10 years of age, the incidence of hydrocephalus was 71 per cent compared to 12 per cent for adults. The incidence of hydrocephalus increased in a linear relationship with the duration of the illness, and decreased with age. In another series hydrocephalus was present in 59 per cent of 26 childhood cases of tuberculous meningitis, and was linked to the development of neurological deficit and a fall in consciousness (Gelabert and Castro-Gago 1988).

The hydrocephalus is mostly the 'communicating' type and due to blockage of the basal cisterns by exudate in the acute stage, and possibly impaired CSF absorption due to high CSF protein levels, and adhesive leptomeningitis in the chronic stage. There are some cases of 'obstructive' hydrocephalus because of obstruction of the outlet foramina of the fourth ventricle or obstruction of the aqueduct. The aqueduct occlusion may be caused both by internal narrowing and circumferential compression of the brainstem by exudate. Only rarely does an intraluminal tuberculoma result in obstruction of the aqueduct.

Patients with non-enhancing exudates tend to have a good prognosis, while those with enhancing exudates, despite medical and surgical treatment, even if the ventricles return to normal, have a poor prognosis (Bhargava *et al.* 1982). Visual loss due to organised exudate in the basal cisterns, involving the optic nerve or chiasm, tends not to recover. The commonest cisterns involved are the suprasellar, cisterna ambiens, and sylvian fissures.

Early exudate is gelatinous and later is a grey, thick, firm mass of connective tissue consisting of lymphocytes, plasma cells, giant cells within areas of caseation necrosis, obliterating the subarachnoid space and adherent to the brain (Levison *et al.* 1950, Horne 1951). Later the granulation tissue is replaced by hyalinised tissue in some areas, whereas in other areas frank granulomatous meningitis may continue (Auerbach 1951, Tandon and Tandon 1975).

The *relationship between the CSF pressure and the degree of hydrocephalus* in different stages of experimental hydrocephalus has been studied. Drapkin and Sahar (1978) found that the ICP rises acutely and immediately after the CSF obstruction. The second stage was of periventricular oedema with expanded ventricles. The third stage is the increase in the CSF absorption (absorption is pressure-dependent), and the fourth stage is the decrease in CSF pressure. They concluded that the speed of ventricular dilatation and the eventual size was dependent on the external support of the brain. In experimentally induced congenital hydrocephalus there is widening of the extracellular space in the periventricular white matter, which occurs before the ventricular dilatation becomes progressive (Sato 1986). The white matter which supports the ventricular walls is also under the process of myelination and contributes to the lack of structural support. The intraventricular pressure in 'obstructive' hydrocephalus is higher than in 'communicating' hydrocephalus (McCullough 1980).

According to Laplace's Theorem*, one expects the pressure to be high to

$$*P = \frac{2t}{R}$$

initiate ventricular dilatation, and the pressure to become relatively less as the radius increases. Ordinarily physiological buffers come into play, such as (i) shutting down of cerebral veins, (ii) increasing the CSF absorption at the sagittal sinus and also increasing absorption around spinal nerve roots and paranasal sinuses, (iii) shunting of CSF from the ventricular into the spinal compartment, and (iv) in infants, expansion of the skull. Loss of central substance due to tuberculous infection, aiding the ventricular dilatation, may contribute to the ventriculomegaly in tuberculous meningitis (Schoeman *et al.* 1985).

The ICP has been thought by some to be at a normal level in young infants with hydrocephalus (5 to 12mmHg) and therefore to be of little use (McCullough 1980). This seems to be confirmed in the early stages of hydrocephalus in rats and mice (Jones 1987); however, higher values were obtained in 24 pre-shunted hydrocephalic infants in which a true mean value was obtained by computerised analysing systems and values of 12.1 ± 4.1mmHg found (Sato *et al.* 1988). In a further study of 25 hydrocephalic children who had direct ICP measurements, Hayden *et al.* (1970) found a range of mean intraventricular pressures of 3.67 to 5.5mmHg in the infants and near 7.35mmHg in all the children.

Measured pressure levels, however, must be considered in the light of what is a normal ICP level in term infants. The upper limit of normal ICP at term is no more than 3.5mmHg (Minns *et al.* 1989), so the reported pressure levels are still important in the pathogenesis of ventricular dilatation, together with the known increased outflow resistance in young animals with hydrocephalus (Jones 1987) and a very much higher PVI than predicted (on the volume of the cranial and spinal axis) (Shapiro *et al.* 1985). In term and preterm infants, we often see pressure levels of 5 to 12mmHg (above normal for age), which are sufficient to interfere with the CBF velocity (increased Resistance Index), and if not relieved will result in ischaemia, infarcts, brain shifts and extensive astrocytosis of white matter.

2. CEREBRAL INFARCTS

These were seen in 28 per cent of cases of tuberculous meningitis (Bhargava *et al.* 1982). The infarcts involve the middle cerebral territory alone in most cases, and both middle and anterior cerebral in 12 per cent. The middle cerebral artery is involved, because exudate surrounds it and the origins of the thalamoperforating and lenticulo-striate arteries in the suprasellar and parasellar cisterns. The basal ganglia on the left tend to be frequently involved. There develops a gradual dilatation of the ipsilateral anterior horn and displacement of the septum pellucidum due to shrinkage of the gliosed brain.

Ischaemic infarcts may occur as a direct result of the hydrocephalus, and raised endoventricular tension will distort the cerebral vasculature with stretching of the supraclinoid portion of the internal carotid artery, anterior displacement and bowing of the vertical segment of the anterior cerebral artery, stretching and bowing of the pericallosal artery, a vertical positioning of the main trunk of the middle cerebral artery, and flattening and unfolding of the Sylvian complex (Belloni and Di Rocco 1975). Vascular abnormalities also occur in the brainstem as a result of a progressive increase in ICP. Usually microscopic stasis is seen first, and with an increase in pressure this is followed by microhaemorrhages (especially about the tectum). Finally, with prolonged untreated pressure macrocirculation, haemorrhages occur—especially in the tegmentum (Goodman and Becker 1973).

3. TUBERCULOMATA
These are now rarer than tuberculous meningitis itself. They are solid, granulomatous and relatively avascular lesions, which may be round, oval or lobulated, single or multiple, and usually bounded by a thin capsule. They contain giant cells, epithelioid cells and caseation necrosis, and may have microscopic calcification. They may be supra- or infra-tentorial and, if less than 1cm in size, may not be visible on CT scan. The density on pre-contrast scans may be high or low, but they show enhanced density with contrast medium. Before anti-tuberculous treatment was introduced they were found in the majority of post-mortem studies. Now, with anti-tuberculous treatment, both large and small tuberculomata show a marked reduction in size, and even complete clearing with medical treatment. Cranial tuberculomata may develop during treatment of tuberculous meningitis with coexisting miliary tuberculosis (Lees *et al.* 1980). Clinical features of tuberculomata are similar to other space-occupying lesions.

4. VASCULITIS (ARTERITIS)
Vasculitis occurs in various infections including tuberculous meningitis, and it may be the pathological forerunner of tuberculomata. Vasculitis is responsible for a presentation with hemiparesis, or additional cranial-nerve deficits that occur in the course of the meningitis. The vascular changes progress from a necrotising panarteritis in the acute stage through to a fibrous obliterative endarteritis in the latter stages. The vessels are therefore subjected on the outside to the circumferential compression from exudate at the same time as fibrous thickening of the intima with vascular impairment from the inside.

5. ALLERGIC TUBERCULOUS ENCEPHALOPATHY
The frequency of white-matter oedema varies from only 3.3 per cent of cases in one series (Bhargava *et al.* 1982), to 27 per cent in others (Dastur and Udami 1966). Tuberculous encephalopathy is a possible allergic phenomenon, due to a hypersensitivity or allergic response of the brain and meninges during the initial phase of tuberculous meningitis. The morphological changes seen in the brain, the white-matter oedema with myelin depletion and astrocytic proliferation, are consistent with a hypersensitivity response to tuberculous protein.

Low attenuation on CT scan is evidence of white-matter oedema, whereas high-attenuation lesions outlining the gyrus are compatible with encephalitis. This is different from the periventricular lucencies accompanying distended ventricles. Two-thirds of hydrocephalic cases have periventricular lucency (especially about anterior horn) indicating transependymal migration of fluid from the ventricle into the white matter from high intraventricular pressure.

6. TUBERCULOUS BRAIN ABSCESS
Tuberculous brain abscess is rarer than tuberculoma.

7. CALVARIAL INVOLVEMENT

Calvarial involvement is more common in children and young adults, but remains very rare. This bone infection produces an osteolytic picture, particularly in the fronto-temporal regions, similar to that seen with histiocytosis (Danziger *et al.* 1976).

8. ENCEPHALITIS

This may occur in the same sort of way that pyogenic infections (*e.g. Haemophilus influenzae*) get carried into the substance of the brain by penetrating bloodvessels from the infected subarachnoid space. A distinct brain infection with brain-swelling will result.

9. INAPPROPRIATE ADH SECRETION

This has been documented in a single case report of a two-year-old boy with tuberculous meningitis (Scheidemantel and Weis 1983), and obviously contributes to the pathological picture of brain-swelling and the clinical features of seizures and coma.

Management

There is no universally agreed combination of antituberculous drugs for management. 'First-line' drugs include a combination of rifampicin (10 to 20mg/kg/day orally, up to a maximum of 600mg per day), streptomycin (10 to 20mg/kg/day) intramuscularly, up to a maximum of 1g per day for the first two months), and isoniazid (10mg/kg/day orally, up to a maximum of 300mg per day). 'Second-line' drugs include pyrazinamide (40mg/kg/day), ethionamide (15mg/kg/day) and ethambutol (15 to 20mg/kg/day). Some of these antituberculous drugs have serious side effects; for example, high-dose rifampicin and isoniazid may be associated with hepatotoxicity. It is important therefore to monitor the transaminases regularly. Isoniazid may also result in a myelinoclastic brain oedema. Streptomycin is ototoxic and pyrazinamide therapy should be monitored with regular liver-function tests and uric acid estimations. Ethambutol may result in optic neuritis. Ethambutol and ethionamide penetrate inflamed meninges, and ethionamide will also penetrate normal meninges. The other antituberculous drugs all penetrate the CSF well. Treatment should be maintained for two years.

The value of steroids in tuberculous meningitis has long been debated. Most clinicians keep them for severe systemic disease, such as miliary tuberculosis, and do not generally include them as part of routine treatment of tuberculous meningitis. However, in the case of rapid deterioration in conscious state and an encephalopathic presentation, their use could be justified in inhibiting the allergic brain-swelling response to tuberculo-protein. Some authors have used them empirically in the belief that they prevent or suppress the development of arteritis (Escobar *et al.* 1975).

CT scan

Children presenting with suspected tuberculous meningitis should have an immediate CT scan. Of the various pathologies responsible for brain damage from tuberculous meningitis, the hydrocephalus and associated RICP is eminently treatable; and early detection and treatment (to avoid the deleterious effects of cerebral ischaemia and herniations) is one way of significantly improving outcome, which has not improved despite newer antituberculous medication.

There are various indices for assessing the severity of ventricular dilatation: Huckman index (maximum plus minimum diameter of the frontal horns); ventricular index (diameter of the posterior horns divided by the maximum diameter of the frontal horns—Skjodt *et al.* 1987); cella media index (maximum diameter of lateral ventricles divided by the maximum biparietal diameter); ventricular size index (maximum diameter of the frontal horns divided by the bifrontal diameter at the same level—Heinz *et al.* 1980); maximum diameter of posterior horns divided by the biparietal diameter; the frontal horn radius; the maximum diameter of the temporal horns; the total brain area divided by ventricular area in a single CT cut using image analysis or graticule; or the summated ventricular area multiplied by the slick thickness using CT image analysis. The actual cranial CSF volume can be measured by MRI scan, which shows variable volumes between male and female. The normal total CSF volume is 146cc in males and 114cc in females, and the ventricular volume varies between 7 and 30cc. The posterior fossa CSF volume is between 5 and 27cc (Grant *et al.* 1984).

The index most commonly in use is a V/P ratio, *i.e.* the ventricular diameter at the mid-portion of the lateral ventricles divided by the biparietal diameter from inner table to inner table. Hydrocephalus is then defined as a ratio greater than 0.26 (Liechty *et al.* 1983). Schoeman *et al.* (1985) found that all of their patients with a mean baseline pressure above 15mmHg had periventricular lucencies on CT scan, and the degree of oedema measured was between 4 and 16mm. There was no correlation between the level of pressure and the extent of the oedema. There was, however, a significant correlation between the degree of periventricular low density and the outcome, and a measurement of more than 5mm was associated with a significantly higher mortality and morbidity. Indirectly, this relates to the level of pressure which is not being treated. In summary, therefore, apart from the ventricular dilatation, the presence and extent of periventricular low densities should be assessed, the presence of cerebral oedema without hydrocephalus, enhancing or non-enhancing exudates, and the presence or absence of tuberculomata.

ICP

Following the CT scan and demonstration of an acute hydrocephalus, it is our practice to have a frontal ventriculostomy reservoir inserted (see Chapter XX), and to control the intraventricular pressure by means of continuous intraventricular pressure measurement and CSF removal, intermittently or by means of continuous closed ventricular drainage. It has been recognised that shunting the comatose child with tuberculous meningitis may restore consciousness within a couple of days (Bhagwati and George 1986). Others have suggested the need for continuous ICP monitoring in tuberculous meningitis (Kocen 1977, Bullock and Van Dellen 1982),

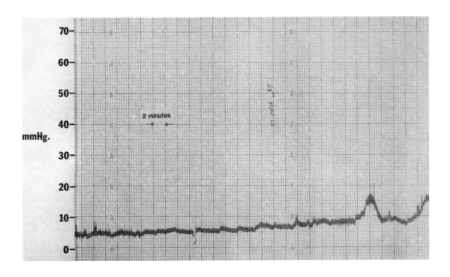

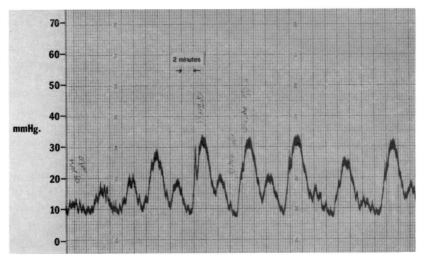

Fig. 7.14 (*top*) and **Fig. 7.15** (*bottom*). ICP tracings of paralysis with atracurium berylate and following its withdrawal.

but Schoeman *et al.* (1985) published the results of such ICP monitoring. In a relatively large study of 24 children with tuberculous meningitis, at a mean age of two years, the mean duration of their initial pressure recording was 50 minutes. A cut-off point of 15mmHg indicated elevated ICP, and a pulse-wave amplitude more than 3mm. The mean baseline pressure for those with elevated pressure was 32.6mmHg with a mean pulse-pressure of 7.3mmHg. Three subgroups were identified on the basis of the ICP recordings. The first had B-waves dominating the ICP tracing; the second had plateau waves, and the third had elevated baseline pressure together with a wide pulse-pressure, but no abnormal waveforms.

223

V. P. M.

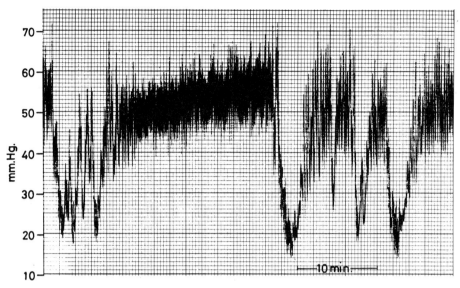

Fig. 7.16. Plateau or A wave.

B waves (½ to 2/min, 0 to 50mmHg) may be due to oscillations of cerebral vessels when the pressure is raised (Auer and Sayama 1983), or may be due to variations in systemic blood pressure within the cardiovascular bed and may occur during periodic breathing. Figure 7.14 shows a paralysed and ventilated patient with no abnormal waveforms, and Figure 7.15 shows the appearance of beta-waves after the muscle relaxant atracurium besylate is withdrawn.

Plateau waves (5 to 20/min, 50 to 100mmHg), on the other hand, are due to intrinsic vasomotor-control problems, and indicate a serious compliance problem, with acute non-compliance and imminent herniation (Fig. 7.16). Plateau waves may occur alone and on a normal baseline, so a single opening pressure is not totally helpful, and continuous ICP monitoring is required. Plateau waves appear to result from an intact autoregulation response to changes in CPP in a patient with poor compliance (Rosner and Becker 1984). Four distinct phases of plateau waves were described. The first phase is the premonitory drift phase where the ICP gradually increases; it is caused by a slow decline in the systemic arterial blood pressure, and results in an autoregulatory vasodilatation and a reduction in CPP. The second phase is the plateau phase, initiated at a CPP of 70mmHg, and as the ICP shows a rapid rise the CPP falls to 40 to 50mmHg. The third phase is the ischaemic response characterised by the CPP returning towards normal by increases in the systemic blood pressure in response to very low CPP. The fourth resolution phase is characterised by a rapid decline in ICP with stabilisation of the systemic blood pressure and the CPP from autoregulatory vasoconstriction. Mori *et al.* (1986) studied the epidural ICP recordings of 10 patients with hydrocephalus associated with myelomeningocoele, five of whom were thought to be compensated (shunt-

224

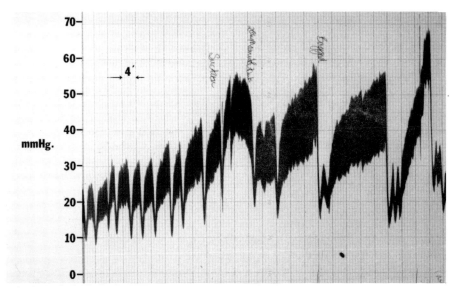

Fig. 7.17. Ramped B waves building up to plateau wave.

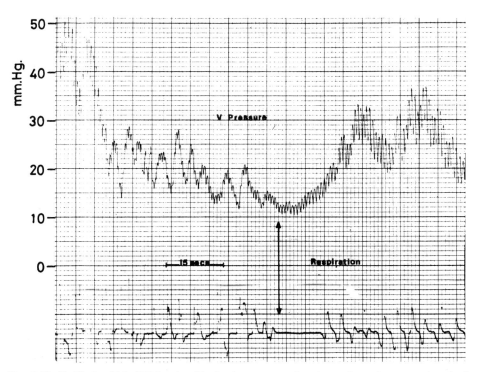

Fig. 7.18. Oscillating high ICP levels with simultaneous nasal catheter show short apnoeic episode preceding further build-up in pressure level.

225

dependent) and five who had arrested (shunt-independent) hydrocephalus. The ICP recordings were classified as Type I (normal baseline, no pressure waves)—no shunt required; Type II (normal baseline pressure with intermittent high-pressure waves during sleep)—shunt if symptomatic; and Type III (high baseline pressure plus or minus pressure waves)—shunt or revise. There must be continuous monitoring of the ICP, noting the baseline pressure, any abnormal waveforms and the pulse pressure, as any one of these features may predominate, and even a wide pulse pressure in the presence of a normal mean level of ICP may result in hydrocephalus, at least experimentally (Di Rocco *et al.* 1978).

The usual sequence of events in hydrocephalus is that high enough RICP level results in B waves (or B like, Ramp B or slow tonic D waves) occur. If these persist for more than about 10 minutes, then plateau waves (A-like or typical plateaux) occur (Fig. 7.17). These waveforms are accompanied by the respiratory changes of bradypnoea, ataxia (see Chapter 3) and then apnoea (Fig. 7.18). These typical waves are modulated by the open structure of the cranium and immature brain, with wide extracellular spaces and myelinating periventricular white matter in the newborn and young infants, so that the waves are smaller and less frequent.

There is no significant relationship between the level of raised pressure and the outcome. This is not surprising because when raised pressure occurs, it is treated immediately. This does not mean that raised pressure is not important in terms of mortality or morbidity. Raised pressure will occur in those patients who die, and will also occur in those patients who survive with no deficit, although uncontrolled pressure would be likely to correlate strongly with outcome.

The advantage of inserting a reservoir, and using this to measure and control the ICP, is that one is not committing the patient to long-term shunting or, indeed, to short-term shunting with the possibility of shunt infection. It is, however, an option for controlling the pressure in acute tuberculous meningitis when there are no facilities for continuous direct monitoring. With control of the raised intraventricular pressure and anti-tuberculous therapy, many of the exudates will clear from the cisterns and result in an arrested communicating hydrocephalus. Severe adhesive arachnoiditis and spinal CSF blocks were particularly common with tuberculous meningitis, and resulted in a strangulated brainstem and spinal cord. The use of intrathecal steroids for this now uncommon situation was particularly effective in 'dissolving' the adhesions within two or three days (Lorber 1961, 1980). Alternatively one could use intraventricular hyaluronidase, 1500u (Bhagwati and George 1986), intrathecal streptokinase (Cathie and McFarlane 1950) or Purified Protein Derivative (American Trudeau Society 1954) for these adhesions.

While tuberculous meningitis must always be suspected in children who present with encephalopathy, communicating hydrocephalus and RICP, it is not always the cause. The following case is sited as an example of a presentation with chronic meningo-encephalitis, hydrocephalus with RICP, chronic arachnoiditis and Froin's syndrome, and ultimately with progressive brainstem and spinal compression, which although treated for tuberculous meningitis, proved at autopsy to be a primary subarachnoid microglioma confined to the CNS, in the absence of congenital or acquired immune deficiency syndrome.

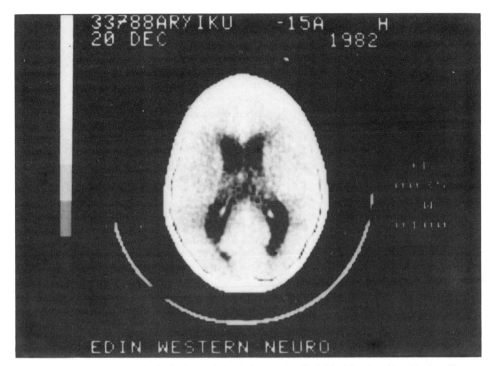

Fig. 7.19. An acute panventricular hydrocephalus in four-year-old child with subarachnoid microglioma.

This four-year-old African boy had had two recent admissions in the CASE previous fortnight with headache, vomiting, increasing tiredness and 4 occasional irrational speech. On admission he was febrile and had minimal neck stiffness, with 56 wbc/mm³ in the csf (which included 10 macrophages, 30 lymphocytes and 13 neutrophils), with a slight increased uptake on technetium scan in the temporal lobes and with negative results for investigations for tuberculosis and hsv. He settled on each of these occasions.

On this admission he was confused and increasingly drowsy, with headache, vomiting, abdominal pain, right-sided ptosis, squint, a dilated unresponsive right pupil, dilated fundal veins on the right and a right hemiparesis.

An urgent ct scan showed a four-ventricle hydrocephalus (Fig. 7.19). Under the same general anaesthetic, a reservoir was inserted which showed clear ventricular csf under high pressure, necessitating external ventricular drainage. After normalisation of the ventricular pressure, a lumbar puncture was performed and csf showed 600 wbc/mm³ and 7700mg/l of protein. Treatment was commenced with antibiotics and anti-tuberculous therapy. The icp trace showed pressure plateaux developing (Fig. 7.20), and a vp shunt was inserted eight days into the admission. There followed an intercurrent distal shunt block which required revision.

227

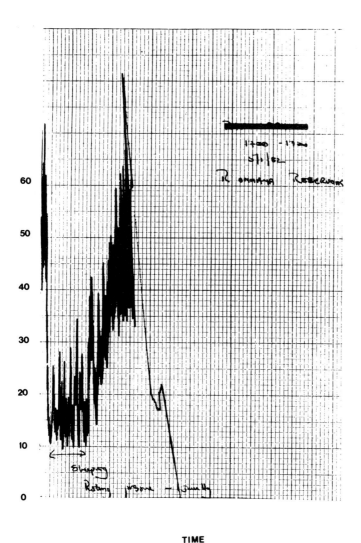

TIME

Fig. 7.20. From arresting pressure of 15mmHg a sudden development of plateau wave aborted by CSF drainage.

Three-and-a-half weeks after the anti-tuberculous drugs were commenced, he developed a spinal paraparesis. Myelography showed chronic arachnoiditis and a total spinal block. Treatment was begun with intrathecal streptomycin and hydrocortisone via lumbar puncture. One week later, after hallucinations, increasing deterioration of consciousness, right-sided epileptic discharges, and a right third- and sixth cranial-nerve palsy, he was given intrathecal hydrocortisone hemisuccinate (10mg daily) for 10 days via a c_{1-2} tap in an attempt to 'dissolve' the adhesions (Fig. 7.21). Raised pressure necessitated further external drainage.

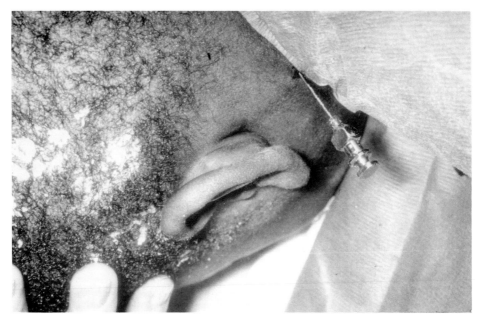

Fig. 7.21. Needle *in situ* for C 1/2 puncture and administration of intrathecal steroids.

There followed progressive brainstem dysfunction, with intermittent apnoea and bradycardia requiring ventilation. He developed an ophthalmoplegia, then fixed dilated pupils with absent corneal reflexes and loss of all maintenance of thermoregulation and blood pressure control, until he died seven weeks after admission. At autopsy, the subarachnoid space was totally occluded with pink tissue up to 1cm thick, extending from the subarachnoid space into the brain and into the spinal cord, which was necrotic and swollen. Microscopy showed two predominant cell types: the first was a lymphocyte and the second a larger, paler cell with fine granular nucleus of microglial origin (Fig. 7.22). There were additional anoxic ischaemic changes at the surface of the brain due to occlusion of penetrating vessels.

General indications for shunting
Hydrocephalus results from an imbalance between the formation and absorption of CSF. Various forms of investigation of the production, outflow resistance, ventricular effluent rates, absorption and ICP have been undertaken by several investigators in an attempt to define closely the precise indications for shunting devices.

1. *CSF absorption* can be studied in a number of ways, the most popular being the lumbar subarachnoid constant infusion test (Katzman and Hussey 1970), and the results of this form an indication for surgery (Bird *et al.* 1973, Di Rocco *et al.* 1977). This test involves an infusion of normal saline at a rate of 0.76ml/min into the lumbar subarachnoid space with CSF pressures measured at one-minute

229

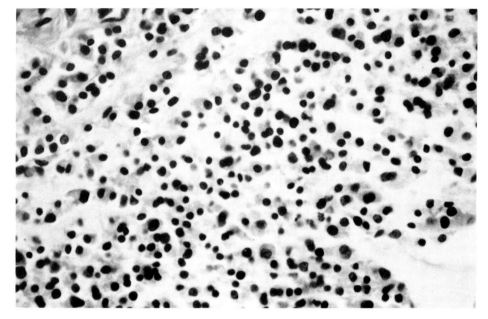

Fig. 7.22. Light microscopy of subarachnoid material showing predominantly two cell types, lymphocytes and microglial cells.

intervals. A negative (normal) response occurs when the CSF pressure remains below 300mm of water (20mmHg). Various types of bisegmental response curve (P/V) are seen, consistent with the two proposed types of absorption defects: CSF absorption may be defective in the low pressure range and normal at high pressures, or it may be normal in the low pressure range and defective at high pressures. When the CSF pressure attains a steady equilibrium above 300mm of water, this appears to indicate impairment of absorption with a slowly progressive hydrocephalus. Normal absorption is found in cerebral atrophy, well shunted patients, and microcephaly. A bolus injection technique, to study CSF absorption in a number of pre-shunted hydrocephalic patients whose mean steady state pressure was 11.7 ± 5.7mmHg, found that absorption did not occur at the steady state but readily ocurred above 16mmHg (Shapiro *et al*. 1985).

2. *The Pressure Volume Index (PVI)* is the compliance parameter, and a high PVI indicates a propensity for progressive ventricular dilatation, *i.e.* the volume buffering is increased enabling volume to be stored without significant elevation of intraventricular pressure. The PVI has been found to be more than double the normal predicted values (8.2 to 30.1ml) (Shapiro *et al*. 1979) in progressive infantile hydrocephalus, and this—together with an absorptive defect—is responsible for the progression (Shapiro and Fried 1986). Another measure of intracranial compliance is obtained by spectral analysis of the CSF pulse waveform by Fast Fourier Transformation (FFT). An increase in the amplitude of the first harmonic occurs before any rise in ICP. This increased amplitude of the first harmonic is probably brought about by impairment of cerebral circulation (Maira *et al*. 1987).

230

3. *Outflow resistance (Ro)*. The biomechanical properties of the brain are different in the unshunted and the shunted patient. Before shunting, the outflow resistance (CSF absorptive resistance) is 7.2mmHg, about double what it should be (Shapiro *et al.* 1985). After shunting, some children with shunt malfunction develop an acute deterioration, while others appear stable with mild ventricular dilatation. Again, the outflow resistance is different in these two groups of patients.

4. *Amplitude of the ICP trace*. The amplitude of the ICP trace is considered by some to be a reliable method of indicating active hydrocephalus, and more so than the mean ICP level (Foltz and Aine 1981).

5. *Ventricular size*. When the decision to operate is based totally on ventricular size, the results are unpredictable (Bullock and Van Dellen 1982) because there is no direct correlation between the level of ICP and the ventricular size (Minns 1977, 1979). While an active process is indicated by an increasing ventricular dimension on sequential imaging—calling for shunting—it could be argued that the parenchymal damage has already occurred at this time, and is less than optimal.

6. As mentioned earlier, Mori *et al.* (1986) shunted patients on the basis of ICP *recordings*. They were shunted if there was elevated baseline ± intermittent pressure waves, or normal baseline pressure with intermittent pressure waves if patients were symptomatic.

Indications for shunting in tuberculous meningitis

Some authors have considered that a progressive communicating hydrocephalus may be treated by *periodic lumbar punctures* and acetazolamide (Visudhiphan and Chiemchanya 1979), while a progressive obstructive hydrocephalus should be treated with a diversionary CSF shunting procedure. I still maintain that communicating or non-communicating hydrocephalus, with or without spinal block, is an indication for a *reservoir and tapping*, because the CSF pathways may clear in time, and also because the presence of some ventricular pressure will enhance absorption and further help to clear CSF bulk-flow passages. In summary, the options are (i) to insert a permanent ventriculo-peritoneal shunt; (ii) to insert a temporary ventriculo-peritoneal shunt, as a *transient hydrocephalus* may occur with tuberculous meningitis as with subarachnoid haemorrhage, head injury, or following other bacterial meningitides; and (iii) to insert a reservoir with continuous ICP monitoring and intermittent tapping or continuous ventricular drainage, followed by a shunt if pressure persists. The presence of hydrocephalus and RICP is a clear indication for removing CSF (intermittently or continuously via ventriculostomy reservoir), but it is not a clear indication for permanent CSF shunting. CSF shunts should only be inserted because of clinical features, the CT scan appearance, ICP levels, waveforms and amplitude, and sleep pressure recording, together with an estimate of the CBF velocity (resistance index) by pulsed Doppler, which has a significant relationship to CPP level in hydrocephalic infants (Figs. 7.23, 7.24). A high resistance index indicates that the level of ICP is sufficiently high to impair CBF velocity and is therefore liable to produce ischaemia. In conclusion, the dilated ventricles—with a normal baseline pressure—may indicate an arrested or an arresting hydrocephalus (if there are additional intermittent elevations in sleep),

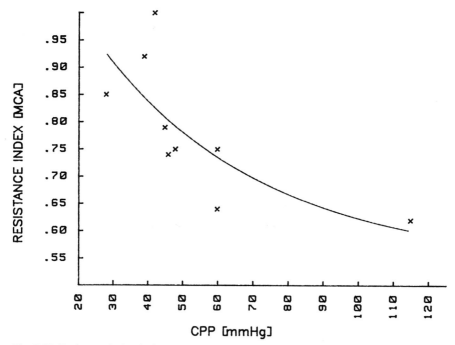

Fig. 7.23. Resistance index (RI) from the middle cerebral artery with concurrent CPP measurements.

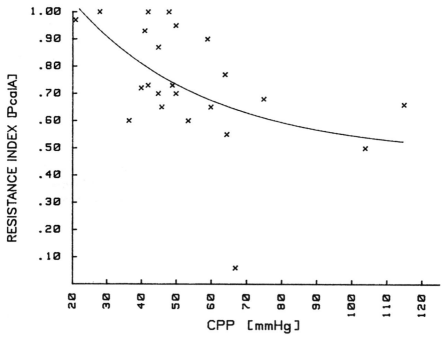

Fig. 7.24. RI from pericallosal artery with simultaneous CPP measurements.

232

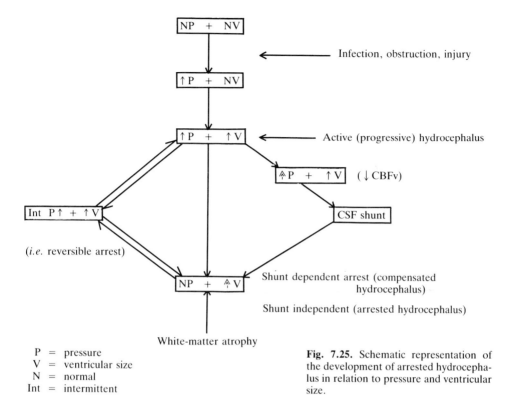

Fig. **7.25.** Schematic representation of the development of arrested hydrocephalus in relation to pressure and ventricular size.

P = pressure
V = ventricular size
N = normal
Int = intermittent

and the presence of a wide pulse-amplitude or interference with the CBF velocity may help differentiate the arresting cases (Fig. 7.25).

ICP/CPP monitoring during sleep in hydrocephalus (original data)
A computer-based ICP monitoring system which automates the data collection, logging and analysis was used in 20 hydrocephalic children who had overnight ICP (and CPP) monitoring. The mathematical ability of the computer was used to process the true mean ICP values, mean CPP values, waveforms and other parameters, such as the percentage of sleep time in which the CPP was compromised.

We identified 20 patients who had overnight ICP monitoring with concurrent blood-pressure monitoring. The mean age at the time of monitoring was 78.9 months, ranging from seven months to 16 years of age. There were 14 males and six females. The duration of ICP monitoring was a mean of 12.47 hours ± 3.93 hours, and ranged from a short two-hour recording to more than 16 hours. Table 7.XVII shows the medical diagnostic background of these 20 children and the indications for overnight monitoring, together with the CT scan appearance and outcome. There were various aetiologies for the hydrocephalus, and no case was due to tuberculous meningitis. The results, however, are still applicable to hydrocephalus regardless of the aetiology.

TABLE 7.XVII

Patient	Age at monitoring (yrs)	Sex	Duration ICPM (hrs)	Sleep ICP									Sleep CPP				
				X̄ mmHg	<9 %	10–19 %	20–29 %	30–39 %	40–49 %	50–59 %	60–69 %	70–79 %	X̄ mmHg	0–9 %	10–19 %	20–29 %	30–39 %
1	7.0	F	12+	7.64	71	24	3	0.5	—	—	—	—	66.5	—	—	—	—
2	6.0	M	15+	15.9	7	67	20	3	—	—	—	—	48.9	0.17	0.18	4	13
3	0.7	M	15	11.2	34	62	2	—	—	—	—	—	62.6	2	0.3	0.4	2
4	0.10	M	15	11.1	51	38	9	—	—	—	—	—	73.4	—	—	—	—
5	8.0	M	15	4.5	93	6	—	—	—	—	—	—	66.6	—	—	—	—
6	15.5	M	11.5	5.7	99	—	—	—	—	—	—	—	60.6	—	—	—	—
7	8.5	M	15+	6.8	80	18	0.6	—	—	—	—	—	74	—	—	—	—
8	16.0	M	9	16	79	20	—	—	—	—	—	—	63.2	—	—	—	—
9	4.0	M	12	11	36	51	11	—	—	—	—	—	62.5	—	—	—	0.3
10	1.2	M	16	21.3	—	50	33	7	4	2	—	—	46.6	—	—	6	4
11	1.2	M	15	18.8	—	67	26	4	1	0.1	—	—	61.8	—	—	—	4
12	3.5	M	2	22.8	—	57	11	21	9	—	—	—	49.8	—	—	7	13
13	5.0	F	16+	8.7	52	46	0.6	—	—	—	—	—	41.6	—	0.5	11	36
14	6.5	F	14	6.4	88	10	—	—	—	—	—	—	56.1	—	—	—	—
15	9.75	M	10+	15.5	23	50	18	7	0.7	—	—	—	58.6	—	—	—	1
16	14.0	M	15	7	99	—	—	—	—	—	—	—	71	—	—	—	—
17	14.0	M	15+	12.5	1.5	98	—	—	—	—	—	—	50	—	—	0.2	5
18	3.0	F	9	23.4	3	33	33	23	4	0.4	—	—	45.5	0.1	1	6	20
19	3.5	F	4	12	100	—	—	—	—	—	—	—	52.8	—	—	—	—
20	3.5	F	14+	-0.6	90	5	1	—	—	—	—	—	70.7	3.5 artifact	—	—	—

(*Table continues opposite.*)

Table 7.XVII, contd.

						Awake ICP									Awake CPP		
40–49 %	50–59 %	60–69 %	70–79 %	80–89 %	90–100+ %	$\bar{X}$ mmHg	<9 %	10–19 %	20–29 %	30–39 %	40–49 %	50–59 %	60–69 %	70–79 %	$\bar{X}$ mmHg	0–9 %	10–19 %
2	6	56	34	0.3	—	13	17	76	5	—	—	—	—	—	67	—	—
24	42	10	2	0.85	0.17	16	—	88	10	—	—	—	—	—	53	—	—
8	24	30	12	5	6	12	8	89	1	—	—	—	—	—	63	—	1
—	1	28	50	14	4	13	7	83	4	3	1	—	—	—	83	—	—
5	14.5	45	26	4	4	0	100	—	—	—	—	—	—	—	85	—	—
—	53	43	1	—	—	7	86	13	—	—	—	—	—	—	65	—	—
0.3	6	24	37	26	4	8	86	13	—	—	—	—	—	—	83	1	—
2	31	36	28	1	0.3	14	—	99	—	—	—	—	—	—	69	—	—
4	29	43	19	1.5	—	18	—	59	40	—	—	—	—	—	62	—	—
63	19	7	—	—	—	19	—	60	34	4	—	—	—	—	62.4	—	—
4	33	45	8	6	—	27	—	13	56	22	4	3	—	—	63.3	—	—
18	38	23	—	—	—	19	3	41	53	1	—	—	—	—	58	—	—
31	14	3	1	—	—	13	5	91	3	—	—	—	—	—	43	2	—
3	71	22	3	—	—	9	51	48	—	—	—	—	—	—	66	—	—
14	36	33	13	—	—	17	5	66	22	3	—	1	—	—	69	—	—
—	1	39	47	9	—	6	99	—	—	—	—	—	—	—	80	—	—
38	43	11	0.3	—	—	12	—	100	—	—	—	—	—	—	53	—	—
37	25	7	1	0.5	—	22	4	30	51	7	4	2	—	3	57	—	1
12	86	—	—	—	—	2	98	1	—	—	—	—	—	—	52	—	—
1	7	16	42	22	3	−1	100	—	—	—	1	—	—	—	71	—	—

(*Table continues over page.*)

20–29 %	30–39 %	40–49 %	50–59 %	60–69 %	70–79 %	80–89 %	90+ %	Cushing Y/N	No. of episodic ICP elevations	$\bar{X}$ max. ICP mmHg	$\bar{X}$ duration	No of pot. ischaemic episodes CPP <50	due RICP	due ↓ SAP	MAP (awake)	MAP (asleep)
—	—	—	13	47	32	6	—	Y	4	24	34′	2	(1)	(1)	81	74
—	2	23	48	23	—	—	—	Y	8	31	26′	5 CPP<25	(5)	—	73	66
1	—	1	34	32	15	11	2	—	4	18	32′	3	—	(3)	82	74
—	—	—	2	8	33	25	28	Y	13	19	32′	0	—	—	95	84
—	—	—	—	—	18	50	31	—	0	—	—	3	—	(3)	88	71
—	—	—	13	68	15	2	—	—	0	—	—	0	—	—	73	68
—	—	—	—	2	20	42	31	—	2	19	23′	2	—	(2)	101	81
—	—	—	2	39	55	1	—	—	1	24	47′	6	(2)	(4)	84	79
—	1	5	31	40	14	3	1	Y	12	20	41′	7	(4) (+2 both)	(1)	82	74
—	—	—	26	48	26	—	—	—	11	41	24′	10+	(10+) lowest CPP 6	—	63	68
—	—	12	14	63	11	—	—	Y	10	38	40′	12	(9) +2 both lowest CPP 16 (16–42)	(1)	90	81
—	5	26	39	9	9	3	6	—	1	38	26′	4	(2)	(2)	84	73
4	30	35	15	7	2	—	—	N	6	21	80′	Almost whole record CPP <50. Lowest about 10mmHg all due to low BP			56	50
—	—	3	17	42	31	4	—	—	0	—	—	2	Lowish BP throughout responsible for both these low CPP (93, 45)		77	63
—	—	—	7	38	45	6	—	—	6	31	17′	Constantly borderline 12+	(12+)		87	74
—	—	—	—	1	44	45	9	—	0	0	0	0	—	—	83	78
—	5	24	57	10	—	—	2	—	0	0	0	Freq. borderline CPP without episodic RICP i.e. all due to low BP. Lowest 36. Flat record			63	63
1	8	23	13	31	12	6	—	N	8	32	58′	Freq. rises one after another. Borderline CPP low throughout (min. 10) with low CPP due both low BP + ↑ ICP			76	69
—	—	10	86	2	—	—	—	?	2	4.5	16′	3 episodes wide P Pressure. CPP range from −30 to −18 ?? cause. Unchanging BP throughout record i.e. 55mmHg. ? vasoparalysis			55	54
—	—	—	1	41	38	18	—		1	22	146′	All low CPP assoc. with 1 complex of RICP. Min CPP of 32 i.e. 1	(1)	(0)	69	70

(Table continues opposite.)

Table 7.XVII, *contd.*

MDB	Indication for OICPM	CT	Outcome
SB, HC noted on CT aged 6, so reservoir only inserted for OICPM	Ventricular dilatation on CT. No symptoms RICP	Vent. dilat. with prominent sulci	No action
Idiopath. HC shunted at 9 mths. Midline facial defect	3 days of swelling over nose + shunt. ↑ squint, scalp veins ↑. Fit 3 wks previously	No increase in ventricular size	No action
↑ OFC noted at 6 mths. CT showed large post. fossa cyst and ↑ all ventricles. Rickham—cysto-P shunt inserted 6 mths.	Assessment post. shunting	Post. fossa cyst + comm. HC	No action
Achondroplasia with large OFC. Non-comm. HC. Rickham inserted for OICPM.	↑ OFC with achrondroplasia. ? shunt needed	Supratentorial HC, 4th vent. N.	No action this time
Severe comm. idiopath. HC, shunted 2 yrs. 1 ventriculitis, 1 distal block. Bilat. hygromata from o' drainage.	6 wks of headache + tinnitus + diplopia. Deterioration in writing for 6 wks	Vents. N., with hygromata	No action
Idiopath. comm. HC. Shunted age 3. Revisions × 8 (blocks)	2 mths history headaches, leg weakness	V. small ventricles	Removal of Cosman, replacement with Ommaya reservoir
Severe comm. idiopath. HC, shunted 2 yrs. 1 ventriculitis, 1 distal block. Bilat. hygromata from O' drainage	Dizziness 5 days. 4 days headache + photophobia, vomit × 1, sore stomach	V. small ventricles	No action
SB-occip. encephalocele. 4 revisions (inc. 1 ventriculitis). Cosman device first shunted at <1 yr	1 yr ↑ behav. problems. 4/12 headaches, ↑ fits, occasional limb tremor	Increase in ventricular size	No action
Large R. temporal subarachnoid cyst, with 1 vent. dilatation, cysto-P shunt at 8 mths	Diplegic signs, early optic atrophy noted at clinic	Cyst + gross vent. dilatation persists	No action
Cong. bilat. temporal cysts: bilat. cysto-P shunt at 7 wks. Visual impairment. Craniosynostosis-sutures split	Swelling on forehead, irritability, known RICP	Pre-suture split—slit vents + fused sutures	Sutures redivided
Cong. bilat. temporal cysts: bilat. cysto-P shunt at 7 wks. Visual impairment. Craniosynostosis-sutures split	Swelling on forehead, irritability, known RICP	Pre-suture split—slit vents + fused sutures	Sutures redivided
Sturge–Webber synd. Comm. HC. Shunted at 8 mths: 2 revisions—1 ventriculitis, 1 block	1 day of headache, vomit, ataxia. RICP, open drainage-o'drainage. IOCPM to assess state for surgery	Slit like ventricles due to o'drawn from	Shunt revision, distal block
Pre-term—IVH. Shut <2 mths 14 revisions CP. Ataxic diplegia, R. hemi., VI palsy	3 mths. of morning headaches + some drowsiness, ↑ ataxia, vomit. 3 wks off food	Slight ↑ in 3rd + lat. ventricles	No action
Idiopath. low pressure HC. Shunted at 2.5 yrs. 6 revisions (3 for choroid bleeds). Visual + motor problems	~4 mths of headaches, morning vomits, drowsiness	N	No action
SB shunted at <1 mth. 1 revision for block. Flaccid legs + bladder	1 day of headache, sticky valve, a fit, vomit × 2	Ventricles slightly dilated	Revision for distal block
SB shunted at 10 days old. Revisions × 3, all blocks	4 mths intermittent headaches (since last revision). Dystonic hand movements	? prox. tubing at basal ganglia	No action taken
5 mths of chronic pneumo-meningitis. 4th vent. syndrome, post. fossa decomp., supresellar abscess. L. hemi., hemianopia, facial asymm	CT results, ↑ 4th + L. lat. ventricle. No symptoms	↑ in size of 4th vent. ↑ L. lateral vent.	No action
SB. HC. Shunted at <2 mths of age. 1 revision for block	2 wks vomiting, drowsiness, irritability	Slight dilatation of ventricles	Revision—distal tubing fractured
SB. HC. Shunted at <2 mths of age. 2 blockages, 2 revisions	2 mths history ↑ fits, sleepiness + spiking temperatures	—	No action
SB. HC. Shunted at <2 mths of age. 2 blocks, 2 revisions. SVS	3 days drowsiness and vomiting, hypotensive	No vent. dilatation	Shunt revision

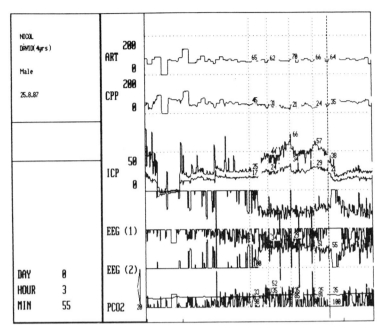

Fig. 7.26. Long-term playback of computerised monitoring during sleep in which the ICP reached a maximum of 66/34mmHg, and despite a modest rise in systemic pressure (Cushing response), potential ischaemia may occur with a CPP of 21mmHg.

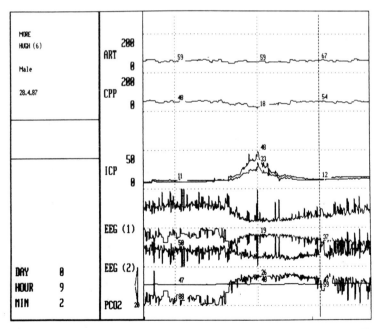

Fig. 7.27. Potential ischaemic episode during sleep with a CPP of 18mmHg as a result of RICP (48/33mmHg) in a child with craniocerebral disproportion.

238

Potential ischaemic episodes, with a CPP less than 50mmHg, have been attributed either to RICP or to a falling systemic arterial pressure wherever possible (Figs. 7.26, 7.27). The MAP has also been recorded for the awake and asleep epochs, and normative ICP and BP data were researched from the literature, for comparison and to establish normative ICP and CPP levels for the different age-groups in this study.

After analysing the recording, proformas were filled out which quantified (i) the absolute time and percentage time spent in ICP and CPP pressure-bands for the whole of sleep; (ii) the absolute time and percentage of time spent in ICP and CPP pressure-bands for a single, quiet episode of awake recording; (iii) the time, duration, maximum ICP and minimum CPP for any intermittent event which caused a pressure rise; and (iv) a mean awake BP reading.

Results

There were three main comparisons in this study. Firstly, the CPP of the whole group awake was compared with the estimated CPP from normative data. The actual CPP was statistically compared to normative CPP data; our sample had an over-all lower mean awake CPP than normal, but this did not reach statistical significance.

There was, however, a significant difference between the awake and the asleep CPP in our sample of 20 patients. Likewise, there was a significant difference between the percentage of time spent with a CPP less than 50mmHg and the percentage of time spent when the CPP was less than 40mmHg between the awake and asleep period.

The patients were also divided into subgroups based on the clinical and physiological data. Six patients had progressive hydrocephalus, seven had evidence of slit-ventricle syndrome (three of whom had high pressure and four of whom had low pressure), a further three patients had intermittently active hydrocephalus, and the remaining four had arrested hydrocephalus. The mean CPP in sleep was T-tested in all permutated pairs of these groups. Patients with slit-ventricle syndrome with associated high pressure had a significantly lower CPP than those with slit-ventricle syndrome and low pressure. The latter, however, had a significantly higher CPP than the group with arrested hydrocephalus.

These subgroups were again T-tested in permutated pairs to examine the percentage of time spent at a CPP of less than 40mmHg and less than 30mmHg. This showed that patients with slit-ventricle syndrome who had low pressure had significantly more time when their CPP was less than 30mmHg than those with active hydrocephalus. Patients with slit-ventricle and high pressure had significantly less time with a CPP less than 40mmHg than the arrested group.

Attempts were made to assess the Cushing response on the proforma, but this could only be estimated in a small group (N = 7), due to the lack of autoregulation challenge. There was a positive Cushing response in five and a negative Cushing response in two.

There was a mean of 4.45 episodic ICP elevations per patient, ranging from 0 to 13 episodes. The mean maximum ICP for these episodic rises for the 15 patients was 25.5mmHg (ranging from 4.5 to 41mmHg).

239

TABLE 7.XVIII

Comparison of awake *vs* asleep CPP in 20 hydrocephalic patients with overnight pressure monitoring showing the mean CPP levels for total sleep and awake recordings plus the percentage of sleep and awake epochs when CPP was less than 50mmHg and less than 40mmHg

| Patient | CPP | | % | | | |
	Asleep Mean (mmHg)	Awake Mean (mmHg)	Asleep <50 (mmHg)	<40	Awake <50 (mmHg)	<40
1	67	67	2	0	0	0
2	49	53	41	17	25	2
3	63	63	13	5	3	2
4	73	83	0	0	0	0
5	67	85	5	0	0	0
6	61	65	0	0	0	0
7	74	83	0	0	0	0
8	63	69	2	0	0	0
9	63	62	4	0	6	1
10	47	62	73	10	0	0
11	62	63	8	4	12	0
12	50	58	38	20	31	5
13	42	43	79	48	71	36
14	56	66	74	3	3	0
15	59	69	15	1	0	0
16	71	80	0	0	0	0
17	50	53	43	5	29	5
18	46	57	64	27	33	10
19	53	52	12	0	10	0
20	71	71	1	0	0	0

The mean duration of these episodic ICP elevations in the 15 patients was 42.8 minutes (ranging from 16 to 146 minutes). Table 7.XVII shows the number of potential ischaemic episodes occurring in each recording (*i.e.* where CPP was below 50mmHg) and from the recording, whether this was due to RICP or low systemic arterial pressure.

Table 7.XVIII shows the results of the CPP study analysis on all 20 patients. The mean asleep CPP was approximately 60mmHg, and the mean awake CPP 65mmHg. For all patients during sleep, the CPP was less than 50mmHg for 23.7 per cent of the sleep recording and less than 40mmHg for 7 per cent of the total recording. In a T-test of the awake CPP versus the asleep CPP for the 20 patients, $\tau = -4.685$ (p < 0.01) and the T-test of asleep CPP less than 50mmHg versus the awake CPP less than 50mmHg for all patients, $\tau = 2.561$ (p < 0.01). In a T-test of asleep CPP less than 40mmHg versus awake CPP less than 40mmHg, again for all 20 patients, $\tau = 2.896$ (p < 0.01).

When considering the amount of time spent during sleep, when the CPP was less than 30mmHg for all 20 patients, only 2 per cent of the total sleep recorded had a CPP as low as this. There was virtually no time less than 30 mmHg for patients with slit-ventricules and high pressure, and virtually no time at this level for patients with intermittent active hydrocephalus. A very small amount (1.7 per cent) occurred in those with arrested hydrocephalus, and 1.7 per cent for those with

240

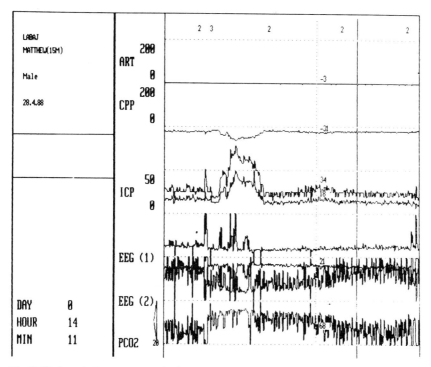

Fig. 7.28. Sample from computerised recording showing ICP elevation during REM sleep.

active hydrocephalus. However, those children with a low ICP from slit-ventricle syndrome spent 6 per cent of their total sleep with a CPP less than 30mmHg.

Phasic pressure changes in sleep (original data)
Cooper and Hulme (1966) continuously monitored the ICP during sleep in 15 adults and found large intermittent increases in pressure occurring most frequently during REM sleep, but occasionally during Stage 2 light sleep. The mechanism for these increases is probably an increase in the regional CBF during sleep; this has been established in cats (Reivich *et al.* 1968). They found a significant increase in flow in all regions, which varied from 62 per cent increase in the cerebellar white matter and sensory motor cortex, to 173 per cent in the cochlea nuclei during REM sleep.

In this series, irregular pressure oscillations have occurred in association with a spiky alpha pattern on the EEG in Stage 2 (and in Stage 3 in one patient) (Fig. 7.28). In other patients the pressure has been elevated in Phase 2 of sleep, very much increased in REM phase, and decreased in slow-wave sleep. A further child had a maximum ventricular pressure measured when drowsy in Stage 1, and although it was slightly raised in REM, it was less than the level occurring in the first stage of sleep. This pressure in Stage 1 in this patient occurred with alpha replacement by theta. In this same patient, the ventricular pressure came down well before the end of REM sleep and a sigh heralded the end of the pressure response. In a further patient, the peak of ventricular pressure oscillation occurred only after 25 minutes of REM sleep at the end of the night, while a focal fit occurred in Stage 2. In summary, therefore, in our patients the pressure was elevated in REM sleep, the second most common elevation was in Stage 2 non-REM sleep, and on one occasion in Stage 1. Gaab *et al.* (1980) described changes in pulse pressure, B waves and slow-tonic D waves which occurred especially during REM sleep in hydrocephalic patients. Hypnograms of our hydrocephalic patients appear to vary considerably from normal children of the same age (Fig. 7.29). When the various sleep stages of these 10 hydrocephalic children were compared with the EEG sleep of healthy children aged six to 12 (Coble *et al.* 1987) by means of T-tests, REM sleep was not significantly different. There was more Stage 1 non-REM sleep in the hydrocephalic patients ($p < 0.01$) and more Stage 3 non-REM sleep in the hydrocephalic patients ($p < 0.001$). There was less Stage 2 ($p < 0.001$) and less Stage 4 non-REM in the hydrocephalic patients ($p < 0.02$). A further problem is the medication hydrocephalic children are often taking as well as the artificial (hospital) environment under which sleep studies are done. Sleep therefore induces pressure changes, and pressure (hydrocephalus) induces a different quality of sleep.

In our sample the CPP of 20 patients during the awake state was not significantly different from calculated normals. There was, however, a significant difference between the awake and sleep CPP in our sample of 20 patients, and, in particular, patients with slit-ventricle syndrome with high pressure had a lower CPP than slit-ventricle syndrome patients with low pressure. The slit-ventricle patients with low pressure had a significantly higher CPP than the arrested hydrocephalic group. Likewise, there was a significant difference between the percentage of time asleep spent with a CPP less than 50mmHg (and CPP less than 40) between the awake and asleep state.

For all of our subjects, therefore, about a quarter of sleep was associated with a CPP less than 50mmHg, but in only 7 per cent of sleep was the CPP less than 40mmHg. Our results suggest that for arrested hydrocephalus as one might expect, there is very little diminution in the CPP during sleep, but in the six patients with active hydrocephalus, approximately 9 per cent of sleep was associated with a CPP less than 40mmHg. For patients with slit ventricle and high pressure 10 per cent of their sleep was spent with a CPP less than 40mmHg, and those with intermittently active hydrocephalus had something approaching 16 per cent of their sleep when the CPP was compromised. The greatest problem of interpretation of ICP records during sleep is not knowing the significance of the intermittent phasic pressure waves. We do not, however, agree with Renier *et al.* (1982) that they are normal.

The critical threshold for CPP in patients with hydrocephalus is different from that in comatose patients, where the CBF will depend on metabolic autoregulation. An index of cerebrovascular compromise has been devised as the transmission ratio of the pulse pressure of the ICP wave to the pulse pressure of the systemic arterial pressure wave.

$$\text{nHB} = \frac{\text{ppICP}}{\text{ppSABP}} \text{ (Ikeyama } et\ al.\ 1976)$$

When the CPP is plotted against this index, a significant bilinear relationship is found

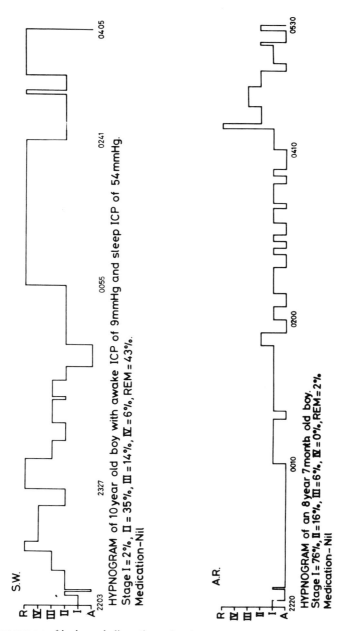

Fig. 7.29. Hypnograms of hydrocephalic patients showing percentage spent in various stages of sleep, levels of ICP and any additional medication. (*Figure continues over page.*)

243

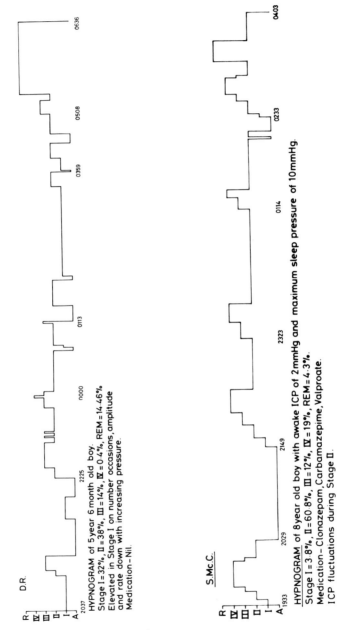

D.R.

HYPNOGRAM of 5 year 6 month old boy.
Stage I = 32%, II = 38%, III = 14%, IV = 0.4%, REM = 14.46%
Elevated in Stage I on number occasions, amplitude
and rate down with increasing pressure.
Medication – Nil.

S.Mc.C.

HYPNOGRAM of 8 year old boy with awake ICP of 2 mmHg and maximum sleep pressure of 10 mmHg.
Stage I = 3.8%, II = 60.8%, III = 12%, IV = 19%, REM = 4.3%.
Medication – Clonazepam, Carbamazepime, Valproate.
ICP fluctuations during Stage II.

Fig. 7.29, *contd. (Figure continues opposite.)*

244

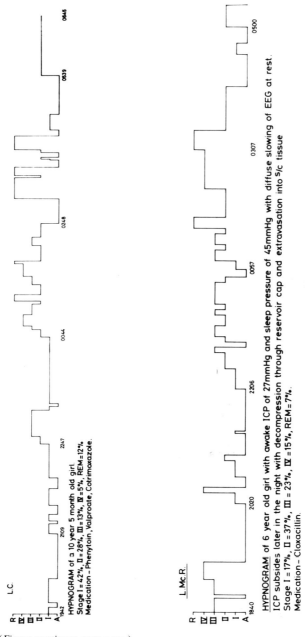

L.C.

HYPNOGRAM of a 10 year 5 month old girl.
Stage I = 42%, II = 28%, III = 13%, IV = 5%, REM = 12%.
Medication - Phenytoin, Valproate, Cotrimoxazole.

L McR

HYPNOGRAM of 6 year old girl with awake ICP of 27mmHg and sleep pressure of 45mmHg with diffuse slowing of EEG at rest.
ICP subsides later in the night with decompression through reservoir cap and extravasation into S/c tissue
Stage I = 17%, II = 37%, III = 23%, IV = 15%, REM = 7%.
Medication - Cloxacillin.

Fig. 7.29, *contd.* (*Figure continues over page.*)

245

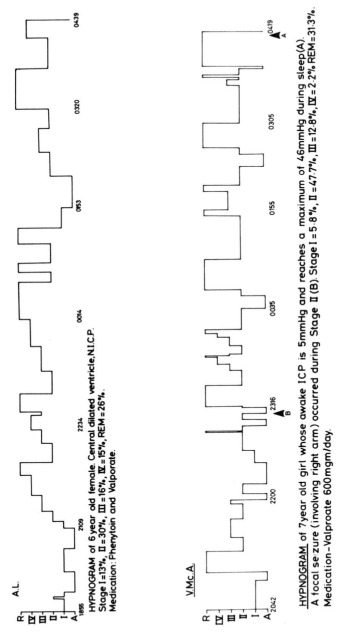

A.L.

HYPNOGRAM of 6 year old female. Central dilated ventricle. N.I.C.P.
Stage I=13%, II=30%, III=16%, IV=15%, REM=26%.
Medication: Phenytoin and Valporate.

V.Mc.A.

HYPNOGRAM of 7 year old girl whose awake ICP is 5mmHg and reaches a maximum of 46mmHg during sleep(A).
A focal seizure (involving right arm) occurred during Stage II (B). Stage I = 5·8%, II = 47·7%, III = 12·8%, IV = 2·2% REM = 31·3%.
Medication–Valproate 600mgm/day.

Fig. 7.29, *contd. (Figure continues opposite.)*

246

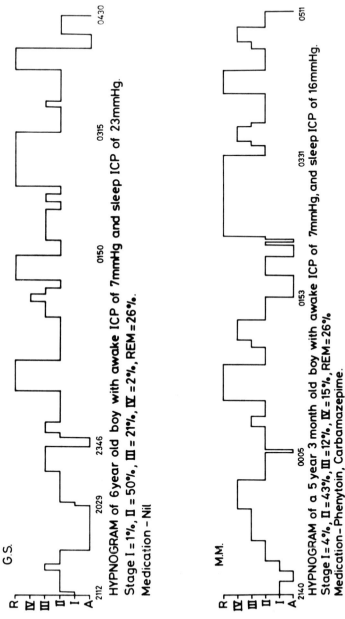

G.S.

HYPNOGRAM of 6year old boy with awake ICP of 7mmHg and sleep ICP of 23mmHg.

Stage I = 1%, II = 50%, III = 21%, IV = 2%, REM = 26%.

Medication – Nil

M.M.

HYPNOGRAM of a 5 year 3 month old boy with awake ICP of 7mmHg, and sleep ICP of 16mmHg.

Stage I = 4%, II = 43%, III = 12%, IV = 15%, REM = 26%.

Medication – Phenytoin, Carbamazepime.

Fig. 7.29, *contd.*

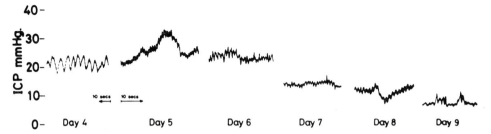

Fig. 7.30. Two-year-old girl with tuberculous meningitis showing sequential samples of ICP tracing from day 4 to day 9, from admission.

from which a 'breakpoint' or critical threshold can be deduced according to developmental age. For preterm babies at birth, this critical value is considered to be 20mmHg, and 18mmHg for a 12-month-old. This changing critical CPP has been assessed in hydrocephalic infants, and 70 per cent of those with a DQ less than 55 had a CPP threshold less than 2SD from the critical breakpoint graph (Sato *et al.* 1988). This index is similar to the Brain Vasomotor Index (Rougemond *et al.* 1976).

Another assessment of critical CPP in hydrocephalus has been deduced from assessments of mean transit time (MTT) which is an index of the ratio between CBV and CBF in patients with measured CPP. A critical CPP of approximately 60mmHg was found (Minns and Merrick 1989), and unpublished data of CBF velocity and CPP (accepting a normal RI of 0.7) show a critical CPP also of 60mmHg (Minns 1990).

Clinical correlates of the RICP showed that there was no significant relationship between the clinical signs for tuberculous meningitis and hydrocephalus generally and the CSF pressure; in fact, they are significantly different (Schoeman *et al.* 1985, Kirkpatrick and Minns 1989). Schoeman *et al.* (1985) commented that children with a 'sunsetting' eye sign made an excellent recovery, while those with an absent oculocephalic reflex did poorly.

Cases illustrative of TBM
The duration of symptoms on admission in all eight of our cases of tuberculous meningitis was a mean of nine ± four days. In all eight cases hydrocephalus was present on imaging and was diagnosed a mean of 16 ± seven days into the illness. The results before routine ICP monitoring showed a morbidity with cortical blindness or hemiplegia, while the latter cases significantly have no mortality or morbidity since raised pressure was attended to early.

CASE A 26-month-old girl was admitted with symptoms for seven days prior to
5 admission. Three days after admission she developed an encephalopathy with coma, with a return of primitive reflexes, and became cortically blind. An urgent CT scan showed a moderately severe, symmetrical, four-ventricle hydrocephalus with basal adhesions and periventricular lucencies about the anterior horns. A Rickham reservoir was inserted as an emergency, and at the time of operation CSF pressure was found to be very high. On return from the operating theatre, continuous pressure monitor-

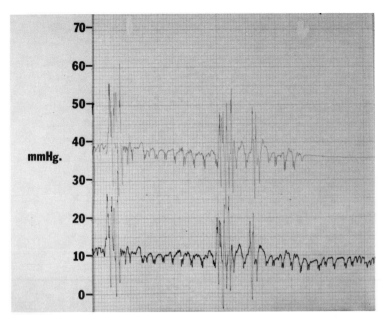

Fig. 7.31. Simultaneous measurement of ventricular and lumbar CSF pressure. Zero for ventricular measurement was at the 30mmHg mark.

ing was instituted and within the next 24 hours her pressure gradually rose to a baseline of 24mmHg, with a CPP of 71mmHg. She had daily ventricular taps in response to the measured levels of ICP. Figure 7.30 shows samples of the ICP tracing from day four after admission to day nine. Apart from the decrease in mean ICP level, there is a fall in the pulse amplitude. The daily ventricular taps were successful in reducing her pressure and her hydrocephalus. Fifteen days after admission, a further CT scan showed a considerable resolution of her hydrocephalus. She had a simultaneous measurement of ventricular pressure and lumbar CSF pressure on several occasions, with good approximation of the CSF pressure levels (Fig. 7.31).

A 20-month-old girl was admitted with symptoms for three days prior to CASE admission. Two days after admission a CT scan was performed, which was 6 within normal limits. She became progressively unconscious, and on the 10th day after admission a further CT scan showed a hydrocephalus with no evidence of tuberculomata or infarcts. A Rickham ventriculostomy reservoir was inserted the same day and the initial pressure measurement, at operation, was grossly elevated. Six hours post-operatively, the pressure recording showed a slow build-up in the mean and pulse pressure. Subsequent pressure measurement from the ventriculostomy reservoir showed a mean resting pressure of 20mmHg and a peak pressure of 55mmHg. The following day the mean peak pressure was 45mmHg. There were intermittent elevations from a baseline pressure of 15mmHg (Fig.

249

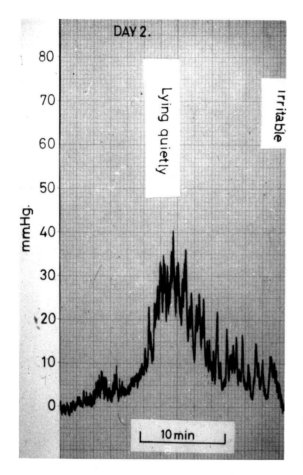

Day 2.

Lying quietly

Irritable

mmHg.

80

70

60

50

40

30

20

10

0

10 min

Fig. 7.32. Intermittent elevations of pressure on day 2 post-reservoir in 20-month-old child with tuberculous meningitis.

7.32). For the next three days she had twice-daily taps of the reservoir to control the pressure. On the third post-ventriculostomy day the lumbar and ventricular fluid pressure levels were similar; and although movement, artefact and other physiological procedures will influence the ICP trace, the intermittent elevations of pressure were associated with irritability. This was followed by seven days of closed ventricular drainage, and a further 10 days of daily ventricular taps. She did not require CSF shunting subsequently, and made a complete recovery with no neurological deficit.

CASE
7

A 9½-year-old boy, who had had symptoms for 14 days, was admitted with a decreasing conscious state. A CT scan showed a four-ventricle hydrocephalus of moderate severity, and two days following admission an Ommaya ventriculostomy reservoir was inserted. The fluid was noted to be under increased pressure at operation. The ICP level was persistently elevated, and continuous closed ventricular drainage was set up.

Within 30 minutes of closure of the drain, the pressure would rise to

24mmHg. Two days post-ventriculostomy reservoir, the pressure elevated to 20mmHg within 20 minutes of drain closure. At all times the pressure was in excess of 20mmHg. Because of the persistent elevation of pressure and the failure of the drainage to produce lasting decrease in the pressure level, a Raimondi shunt was inserted on the ninth day after admission. One month after admission, a repeat CT scan showed total resolution of the hydrocephalus and the patient made a full neurological recovery.

The above cases illustrate the usefulness of an urgent neurosurgical involvement in acute tuberculous meningitis and the normal outcome when measures are taken to monitor and treat the RICP as well as the institution of appropriate anti-tuberculous treatment.

Outcome
The mortality rate and neurological sequelae in tuberculous meningitis are higher (i) with delayed diagnosis, (ii) in younger children, or (iii) if coma or focal neurological signs are present (Idriss *et al.* 1976, Delage and Dusseault 1979, Kennedy and Fallon 1979), although the most important of these is the delayed diagnosis. Neurosurgery with ICP monitoring, ventricular drainage, externally or by CSF shunting, may result in a dramatic improvement in the neurological state and the outcome.

Herpes simplex virus encephalitis
This is the most common form of sporadic, severe encephalitis. Children present with a prodromal 'viral syndrome' with upper respiratory or gastro-intestinal symptoms, and 5 per cent of cases have either herpetic skin lesions or a herpes stomatitis.

A typical presentation is with personality change, seizures and a rapid neurological deterioration to coma, neck stiffness and fever. Illis (1977) described focal neurological signs in order of their frequency, with hemiparesis being the most common, followed by facial weakness, third-nerve palsy, dysphasia, other cranial nerve palsies, nystagmus, hemianopia, squint and dysarthria.

Pathological mechanisms of brain damage
Intranuclear inclusion body encephalitis results in a necrotising and haemorrhagic encephalitis, with a predisposition for involving the medial temporal lobe or the orbital section of the frontal lobe. The congestion and central softening may occur in one temporal lobe more than the other, or both may be affected equally. The overlying meninges become clouded and congested, and deeper areas are also seen to be involved (the unci, amygdaloid nucleus, hippocampi and insulae) affecting the whole of the limbic system.

The intranuclear inclusions are eosinophilic and occur in oligodendroglia and less so in neurons and other glia. These intranuclear inclusions (Cowdry Type A) are not specific for HSV and may also occur in measles, cytomegalovirus and varicella-zoster virus infections.

251

Ischaemic change. The virus-mediated damage is the most important process in the intense necrosis (Esiri 1982), but there is also evidence of secondary vascular pathology, with endothelial damage and fibrin and thrombin in small vessels, and together with neuronal change this is evidence of ischaemic damage. The lytic effect of this virus is therefore followed by an inflammatory reaction with perivascular cuffing in the cortex, white matter, parenchyma and meninges.

RICP with secondary brain shifts, including midbrain compression. Brain oedema is particularly a problem in the first few days, but it may persist and be intractable for several weeks. The tremendous levels of RICP that occur in this condition have seldom been reported in the literature, though in my experience the most intractable and difficult pressure problems have occurred in HSV encephalitis. Following the transtentorial herniations there will be the classical clinical accompaniments of pupillary changes of Charcot's triad and episodes of decerebration.

Inappropriate ADH secretion with hyponatraemia has been reported in HSV encephalitis.

Focal oedema may be seen on CT scan, with decreased density in a temporal lobe. When secondary focal haemorrhagic necrosis occurs, there may be increased or decreased density on the border zones.

Acute haemorrhagic leukoencephalitis and perivenous encephalitis have been described as rare complications of HSV encephalitis.

Other mechanisms include thrombocytopenia, hypoprothrombinaemia and disseminated intravascular coagulation.

Diagnosis

The major differential diagnosis of HSV encephalitis is a tumour or abscess. The CSF shows an increased protein and white-cell count, the latter predominantly mononuclear cells with or without a polymorphonuclear response. A raised CSF IGG will occur in the second week, and occasionally there are red cells in the CSF. A rise in *antibody titre* in the serum usually occurs too late to be of practical benefit in management. *Immunofluorescence of cells* in the CSF, if positive, gives a definite diagnosis, provided there are no primary mucocutaneous infections. The ratio of serum to CSF antibody levels is a normal 200 : 1 because of the intact blood-brain and blood-CSF barrier.

The EEG is perhaps the best of the routine investigations in demonstrating the focal lesions of early HSV encephalitis. This shows slowing of the background, with repetitive slow-wave discharges from one temporal region.

The *brain biopsy* has always been controversial. Kohl and James (1985) reported 12 patients, aged between one day and 11 years, with suspected HSV encephalitis who underwent brain biopsy: five of these proved positive, and their clinical and laboratory results did not help differentiate HSV encephalitis from other causes. It is rare to get complications of a careful brain biopsy, which is performed either by sampling the temporal lobe or by stereotactic biopsy with computerised tomography guidance. The indications for biopsy are clinical, electrophysiological and imaging evidence of focal brain disease in the temporal lobe. While the only certain method of virological diagnosis is isolation of the virus from the brain, electron microscopy (EM) of brain tissue material identifies virus particles and gives a satisfactory definitive diagnosis. Even brain biopsy, which is the most accurate method of demonstrating the presence of the virus, may give a false negative result.

Brain perfusion studies have been carried out in 14 patients with acute encephalopathy by the use of iodinated amphetamine or technetium hexamethyl-propyleneamine and SPECT. Six of the patients who had HSV encephalitis had a strong increased accumulation of radiotracer in the affected temporal lobes. The other eight cases were normal. The CT scan, at the time, was normal. There was a gradual change to subnormal accumulation over the next four to 10 weeks (Launes *et al.* 1988). HSV encephalitis is the only condition associated with such hyper-perfusion other than the ictal changes in focal epilepsy and the 'luxury perfusion' phase of stroke. This accumulation of radiotracer reflects brain bloodflow, and is not due to destruction of the blood-brain barrier, since brain scintigraphy at the same time was normal. The later subnormal accumulation represents neuronal death and a fall-off in metabolism and regional CBF.

Steroids

The use of steroids has been controversial, although convincing results were reported by Illis and Merry (1972), in which they lowered the mortality in HSV encephalitis from 70 per cent to 44 per cent by the use of steroids, or ACTH. Since that time, however, there has been a tendency to withhold steroids and to treat the brain-swelling with other measures, while using acyclovir. If brain biopsy has not been done to confirm the diagnosis, then empiric antiviral treatment is begun. Acyclovir inhibits DNA polymerase of HSV and terminates the DNA chain production by competing with guanosine triphosphate. The dosage is 10mg/kg, three times a day, intravenously, for a full 10-day course. Side effects are negligible, but include reversible tremor (Skoldenberg *et al.* 1984, Whitley *et al.* 1985).

RICP is part of the secondary injury (along with seizures and inappropriate ADH secretion), and while the single most important determinant of outcome is the extent of the viral damage and secondary vascular pathology, the raised pressure is a treatable secondary injury and vigorous attempts should be made to control it. An ICP transducer or, in our practice, a Cordis nondistensible catheter can be inserted in the subarachnoid space, at the same time as the brain biopsy is performed. The catheter is then primed and connected to an external pressure transducer, and full intensive monitoring undertaken with continuous blood pressure, ICP and jugular bulb oxygen. The general principles of management are similar to management of other encephalopathies as outlined in the section on Reye's syndrome, but additional measures may be necessary to treat any hyperthermia. In some units, brain decompression is used for this condition if repeated mannitol is insufficient to control the RICP, and then only when there is imaging evidence of a marked unilateral temporal lobe swelling causing significant midline shift.

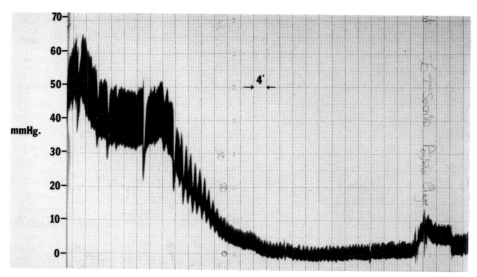

Fig. 7.33. Plateau wave was unresponsive to 'hand-bagging', and mannitol (80ml of 20 per cent solution) together with 1mg of frusemide resulted in decrease in ICP and improvement in CPP from 30mmHg to 60mmHg. Note the gradation from A waves to B waves before a normal mean ICP level is attained, but still with a wide pulse pressure.

CASE 8 This 15-month-old girl was admitted with a three-day history of pyrexia and being generally unwell. The day before admission she was noted to be sleepy, and immediately prior to admission had an episode in which all four limbs became rigid.

She had been born by elective Caesarean section for cephalopelvic disproportion, but had no neonatal problems nor other previous illnesses, and was fully immunised.

At the time of admission she was febrile and alert, but disliked handling. On the first evening of admission she developed focal left-sided convulsions, which were responsive to rectal valium. At this stage there were no focal neurological signs.

Treatment was continued with intravenous diazepam and mannitol, and lumbar puncture showed normal CSF pressure, at 7 to 8mmHg, with 50 WBC/mm³, of which 89 per cent were neutrophils, 9 per cent were lymphocytes and 1 per cent monocytes. Serum sodium was 129mmol/l and the CSF glucose was normal. She was commenced treatment on penicillin, chloramphenicol and phenytoin. Despite this she continued to have fits, and an urgent CT scan revealed no abnormal density patterns nor any evidence of subdural fluid collection. The ventricular system and basal cisterns were all normal in size and shape, and there was no shift of the midline.

She then developed episodic cycling movements of her arms and legs, and tonic eye deviation. An EEG revealed bilateral but asymmetrical PLEDS.

With a presumptive diagnosis of meningo-encephalitis, she proceeded

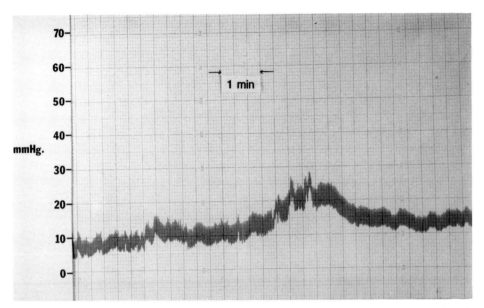

Fig. 7.34. ICP tracing prior to thiopentone infusion. Frequent generalised and focal seizures responded to paraldehyde with a fall in ICP level but with persistently wide pulse pressure.

on the day after admission to a right frontal burr-hole and a subdural catheter for ICP monitoring, and supported ventilation. Her raised pressure was treated with mannitol, hyperventilation, sedation with intravenous diamorphine, fluid restriction and diazepam infusion. Intravenous acyclovir was commenced.

Blood, sent for viral studies, subsequently revealed very firm evidence of recent infection with HSV, with a rise in titre from less than 16 to more than 256. Her continued fits and raised pressure necessitated pancuronium for paralysis, and ultimately a thiopentone infusion to control her RICP (Figs. 7.33 to 7.37).

She remained on a ventilator for three weeks, by which time a repeat CT scan revealed multiple areas of cortical low-density, extending in some areas into the white matter (Fig. 7.38). The ventricles were all also slightly prominent and the appearances suggested multiple cortical infarcts.

There was evidence of significant disability one month after, with phasic spasticity and asymmetry of the temporal EEG, with the right temporal leads being flat in comparison with more activity on the left. Visual evoked responses were also abnormal, and she remained grossly developmentally delayed. At the age of four years she is profoundly mentally and physically handicapped, with epilepsy, an intermittent extensor dystonic pattern of tetraplegia, hyperexplexia, and a secondary microcephaly.

A series of figures depicts the course of the protracted pressure problems that occurred over a three-week period in this child.

255

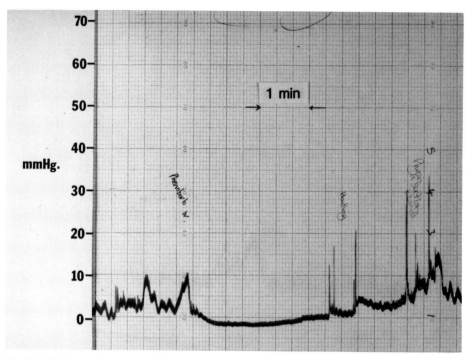

Fig. 7.35. Following thiopentone infusion there is a significant fall in mean ICP level with an associated decrease in pulse pressure.

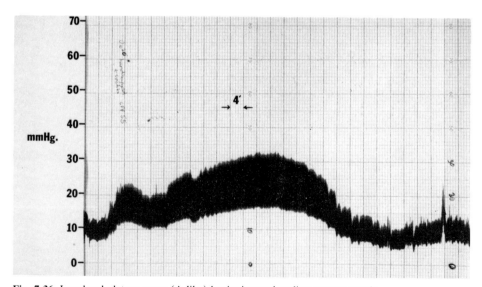

Fig. 7.36. Low-level plateau wave (A-like) beginning and ending spontaneously.

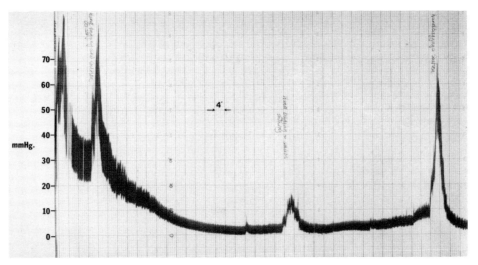

Fig. 7.37. From initial high mean ICP with frequent B and Awaves, the latter part of the recording in this girl was dominated by exceedingly high-pressure waves to levels of 80mmHg and over, frequently aborting spontaneously.

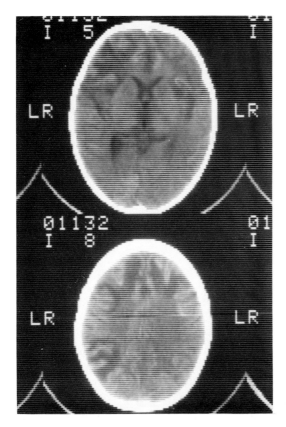

Fig. 7.38. CT scan showing multiple areas of low density in cortex and extending into white matter, consistent with multiple cortical venous infarcts.

257

TABLE 7.XIX

Differential diagnosis in Reye's syndrome

Liver failure—hepatitis or drugs (halothane or paracetamol)
Herpes simplex encephalitis
Toxic shock encephalopathy
Other infections encephalopathies
Salicylate ingestion
Valproate encephalopathy

Metabolic defects
Fructosaemia

Urea cycle enzyme defects
Arginase deficiency
N-acetyl glutamate synthetase deficiency
Ornithine transcarbamylase deficiency (OTC)
Carbamyl phosphate synthetase deficiency (CPS)
Citrullinaemia (ASS'ase deficiency)
Arginosuccinic acid lyase deficiency
Triple-H syndrome (hyperammonaemia, hyperornithinaemia,
hypercitrullinaemia)

Organic acidurias
Isovaleric acidaemia
Glutaric aciduria type I
Multiple acyl-CoA (glutaric aciduria type II)
Acyl-CoA dehydrogenase deficiencies (long/medium/short chain)
Systemic carnitine deficiency
Propionic acidaemia and methylmalonic acidaemia
Multiple carboxylase deficiency (biotinidase deficiency)
Maple syrup urine disease (branched chain ketoacid)
3-hydroxy-3-methylglutaric aciduria (HMG-CoA lyase deficiency)

Outcome

Acyclovir has been demonstrated to be the drug of choice in HSV encephalitis (Skoldenberg *et al.* 1984, Whitley *et al.* 1985). It is given in a dose of 10mg/kg bodyweight, three times a day for 10 days, and because of the negligible side-effects associated with acyclovir and the fact that the diagnosis of HSV encephalitis is not always made within a five-day period, then for those cases where HSV is not specifically identified it is still reasonable to give a full 10-day course of this antiviral therapy.

The course of HSV encephalitis is variable, but the first two weeks are crucial for subsequent outcome. Significant clinical recovery may go on for many months. Mortality in a Swedish collaborative study was 19 per cent in an acyclovir-treated group (Skoldenberg *et al.* 1984), and 56 per cent of the acyclovir-treated patients had resumed normal life at six months. Furthermore, four of 10 patients in coma or semi-coma treated with acyclovir returned to normal. In a US collaborative study at one year, 69 per cent of acyclovir-treated patients survived, and at six months 32 per cent had returned to normal life.

In the age-group less than two years the mortality is high and death occurs in the second week, usually from respiratory, cardiac and RICP problems.

The continuing neurological problems in the survivors include a gross memory

memory impairment due to bilateral temporal pole destruction, with thickened, necrotic leptomeninges overlying them. There may also be a resultant aphasia, motor and other cognitive problems, seizures, hemiparesis, and speech problems. The outcome from one neonatal case of HSV encephalitis was a multicystic cerebral degeneration and microcephaly (Smith *et al.* 1977).

Reye's syndrome
Clinico-pathological description
Reye's syndrome is an acute and generalised disorder of mitochondrial function, *i.e.* a mitochondriopathy with a decreased mitochondrial enzyme activity but normal cytoplasmic enzyme activity. There is a resultant intense catabolic state with a tremendous ammonia load requiring detoxification by the liver. At the same time ammonia disposal via urea synthesis is impaired due to decreased activity of the two intramitochondrial enzymes of urea cycle (CPS and OTC). The ammonia is taken up by the brain in patients with Reye's syndrome and CSF levels of ammonia rise, as do blood and CSF glutamine levels, the latter indicating a degree of buffering of ammonia load. Abnormalities of carbohydrate, nitrogen and lipid metabolism result from this mitochondrial dysfunction. Mitochondrial dysfunction may result, in susceptible individuals, from mitochondriopathies due to viral infections, toxins such as aflatoxin, drugs such as sodium valproate and salicylates, Jamaican vomiting sickness (a response to eating unripe Ake fruit), or they may be consequent on hypoxia, inborn errors of metabolism or even a substrate deprivation (*e.g.* starvation). If there is no primary underlying metabolic defect, the syndrome could be called 'primary Reye's syndrome', while if there is an underlying inborn error of metabolism it could be called 'secondary Reye's syndrome'. The differential diagnosis of Reye's syndrome is seen in Table 7.XIX based on a comprehensive review (Robinson 1987).

The condition of primary Reye's syndrome is a sporadic disorder, with an incidence in the UK of 0.3 to 0.6 per 100,000 children under 16 years of age. While there have been cases in adults, it primarily affects children. In the UK the median age for presentation was 14 months, with a range of eight days to 14 years. It has always been associated with a high mortality, previously a mortality as high as 66 per cent, especially in older children in the UK, although the more recent mortality figures have been reduced to approximately 22 per cent. A significant morbidity results from the cerebral oedema.

The clinical presentation of primary Reye's syndrome is of a biphasic illness. The prodrome consists of a trivial upper-respiratory infection (in 75 per cent of cases), gastro-intestinal upset (in 15 per cent of cases), or chicken pox (in 15 per cent of cases). The viral trigger may be Influenza B virus, varicella-zoster virus, or less frequently Influenza A virus. The typical clinical presentation is an abrupt onset of repeated vomiting a couple of days after a trivial upper-respiratory infection or chicken pox in a child whose behavioural responses are altered. The presentation may be more subtle in infants, when the first indication may be sudden respiratory disturbances, including apnoea.

The second phase of the illness occurs three or four days later, with vomiting

TABLE 7.XX

Lovejoy staging

Stage	Consciousness	Response	Response pain	Other CNS
1	Lethargic/drowsy	None	Appropriate	N. pupils
2	Disoriented delirium, restless agitated	Hyperventilation	Appropriate	N. pupils
3	Obtunded/comatose light coma	Hyperventilation	Decorticate	N. pupils
4	Coma	Hyperventilation or C. Stokes	Decerebrate	Fixed dilated pupils
5	Deep coma, seizures	CS or apnoea	Flaccid	Fixed dilated pupils

(Reprinted by permission of the *American Journal of Disease in Childhood*)

old blood, a progressive diminution in conscious state into a toxic delirium, and sometimes seizures. Examination shows an increase in muscle tone with either decorticate or decerebrate posturing, possibly alternating with episodes of hypotonia. There are usually no focal neurological signs, but hyperventilation occurs in response to the hyperammonemia, which is also responsible for the vomiting, confusion and ataxia. The hyperpnoea occurs with a tachycardia, and apart from being due to hyperammonaemia, may also be due to a central neurogenic hyperventilation if the cerebral oedema is causing herniation. Pupillary abnormalities may also reflect coning. Hypoglycaemia may be variable in extent. Hepatomegaly is evident in 50 to 75 per cent of cases, and the hyperammonaemia is usually elevated two or three times normal. Anicteric hepatic dysfunction occurs with normal bilirubin, but alanine and aspartate transaminases are more than two or three times normal. Blood-gas analysis reveals a metabolic acidosis co-existing with a respiratory alkalosis. The prothrombin time is increased. There is no evidence of papilloedema, but there is usually engorgement of the retinal veins and a loss of venous pulsations on the optic disc. The increased prothrombin time may result in haematemesis and melaena, while a secondary cerebral hypoxia and ischaemia results if a respiratory or circulatory collapse occurs. Seizures occur infrequently (mostly multifocal and clonic), but tend to be later on in the illness, and when the prognosis is likely to be worse. There are low levels of all the clotting factors synthesised by the liver (*i.e.* Factors I, II, V, VII, IX, X), and the white-cell count frequently shows a neutrophil leucocytosis. The Communicable Disease Surveillance Unit criteria have included (i) an unexplained encephalopathy, (ii) hepatomegaly with fatty change of a microvesicular type or an increase in the transaminases more than 100iu/l, without hyperbilirubinaemia, and (iii) a marked dicarboxylic aciduria in the acute phase. The original description of Reye from Australia was of coma, hypoglycaemia, hepatic dysfunction with increased transaminases and normal bilirubin, prolonged prothrombin, cerebral oedema and a fatty liver. Clinical staging in Reye's syndrome was described by Lovejoy *et al.* (1974) in five stages (Table 7.XX). The critical stage in intensive care management is Stage two, where there is extreme restlessness or delirium associated with

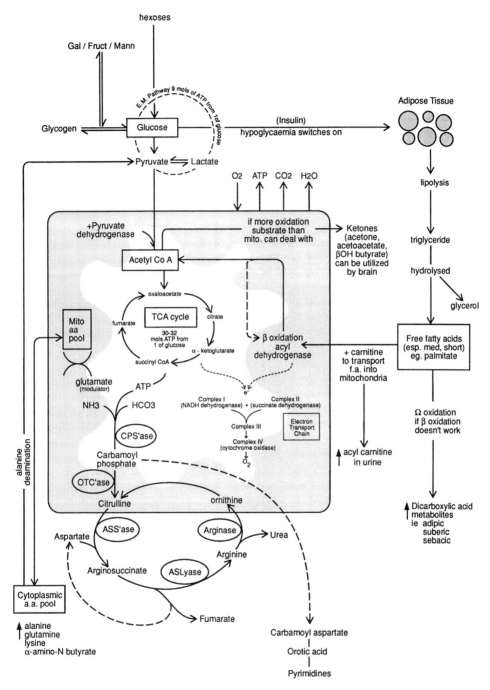

Fig. 7.39. Cytosolic and mitochondrial biochemical pathways in Reye's syndrome.

tachypnoea or inco-ordinated respiration (*i.e.* the patient is unresponsive to verbal commands.

Biochemical defects in Reye's syndrome
Figure 7.39 shows the cytosolic and mitochondrial biochemical pathways, abnormalities of which result in the biochemical and clinical features of Reye's syndrome.

The most striking pathological features are of an enlarged and pale yellow liver, and on biopsy there is fat deposition in the form of panlobular microvesicular droplets of triglyceride in the cells, without necrosis or inflammation, but with gross diminution of glycogen stores. The fat deposition is initially seen in the periphery of the lobule and eventually throughout the liver. There is also infiltration with lipid droplets in the kidney, myocardium and other organs. On liver biopsy there is a decreased succinate dehydrogenase activity, and abnormalities of mitochondria.

Electron microscopy of mitochondria shows evidence of reversible mitochondrial injury with loss of cristae and flocculant matrix. There is a good deal of mitochondrial pleomorphism and finally gross swelling and outer membrane rupture. The mitochondria in the body are most numerous in the liver and at the blood-brain barrier, that is at the endothelial cells of the brain capillaries. Brain pathology seen at post-mortem examination shows an increase in brain weight, flattening of the gyri, diminution of the ventricular dimensions, and tonsillar coning, and microscopy shows swollen astrocytes; however, the mitochondria in the brain appear to be normal, as do the capillary endothelial cell mitochondria. Myelin blebs are evident; in a study from Thailand, Evans *et al*. (1970) found significant deep white-matter swelling, although the cortico-medullary junction was clear. On top of these findings were the typical axonal neuronal changes, possibly due to the hypoglycaemia, the seizures and the acidosis.

The mechanism of cerebral oedema has been much argued, and while a number of possible mechanisms have been raised, the first of these would be the possibility of a straight vasogenic oedema from mitochondrial injury within the blood-brain barrier. Since the mitochondria have not been found to be abnormal, it is unlikely that this is responsible—although some investigators have found lipid droplets in the endothelial cells of the brain capillaries. A second postulated mechanism for the cerebral oedema has been that the elevated free fatty acids might produce a toxic encephalopathy with brain-swelling. This also seems unlikely since children fasted for 20 hours develop free fatty acid levels which are as high as those encountered in Reye's syndrome but without any accompanying cerebral oedema.

Thirdly, lactic acidaemia, which is usually moderate or high, may produce a chronic encephalopathy, but this tends to be much milder than in Reye's syndrome.

The fourth possibility is hyperammonaemia. In rat studies after ammonia infusion, the animals developed RICP. No increase in tissue water was found and the suggested rise in pressure was thought to be due to an increase in CBV caused by impairment of vascular autoregulation. It is also thought that the hyperammonaemia, together with the elevated free fatty acids, may act synergistically to produce coma in Reye's syndrome.

In summary, therefore, many of the brain pathological findings are of a non-specific nature. The oedema is largely cytotoxic, possibly due to the hyperammon-aemia and the lactic acidaemia, and there is preservation of the microcirculation with a lot of anoxic neuronal changes which have been noted in the form of a shrunken cell bodies, eccentric pyknotic nuclei and eosinophilic cytoplasms, no doubt due to the secondary anoxic-ischaemic injury. White-matter swelling is predominant, with an increase in CBV and defective cerebrovascular autoregulation.

The other source of glycogen is muscle. EM muscle has shown a slight or moderate alteration of the matrix density of mitochondria in most of those examined, while a few show more severe changes similar to that occurring in the liver and the pancreas, with gross mitochondrial disruption. The serum creatinine phosphokinase is often elevated to the order of 7000 units/l, although a level of 47,000 units/l has been reported. The isoenzymes of creatinine phosphokinase showed that skeletal and cardiac CK was responsible, not the brain isoenzyme, and the CSF glutamine is elevated—evidence of the mopping up of ammonia not utilised by the brain. Examination of the muscles shows pronounced infiltration of the myo-fibres with fat micro-droplets and it may be that a muscle biopsy would suffice to demonstrate the micro-fat droplets on oil red O stains, instead of liver biopsy in acute Reye's syndrome, where the prothrombin time may be prolonged with other coagulation disorders. The histological hallmarks of Reye's syndrome on liver biopsy include fat distribution, as mentioned above, depressed succinate dehydro-genase activity, and evidence of mitochondrial change from electron microscopy.

Rationale of management

1. CLINICAL STATUS AT PRESENTATION

Evaluating clinical status is only possible before intensive-care unit procedures are undertaken. The commonest one is that of Lovejoy, Stages 1 to 5, which is really a staging of the development of tentorial herniation. Its main purpose is to compare results from one centre with another (Table 7.XX).

2. CT SCAN

No lumbar puncture should ever be done in a comatose child without evidence from a CT scan of open cisterns, particularly ambiens cistern, as well as evidence of no intracranial mass or shift. If the third ventricle is seen on CT scan in adults, then 95 per cent of the patients are said to have a normal ICP.

3. GLUCOSE INFUSION

A 10 to 15 per cent solution of dextrose is infused to keep the blood glucose in a hyperglycaemic range, i.e. 11 to 16mmol/l (200 to 300mg/100ml). If concentrated glucose is required for precipitate falls in blood sugar, then a 20 per cent solution given in a bolus should be administered, not a 5 per cent solution which would make water intoxication a possibility. The glucose infusion has a further effect of keeping the osmolality elevated to an ideal 310 to 330mosmols/kg. Glucose homeostasis may be upset by RICP, so that the glucose tolerance curve resembles a diabetic curve, which will return to normal after the raised pressure has been relieved. Hypoglycaemia may cause brain damage with an encephalopathy, as well as being a possible result of brain damage.

4. ELECTIVE PARALYSIS AND VENTILATION

The indications for paralysis and ventilation are the same as the indications for ICP monitoring, because paralysis means that only physiological monitoring can be achieved. The indications are (i) all but the mildest cases, (ii) Stage 2 Lovejoy or a modified Glasgow coma scale of 8 or less, that is extreme restlessness or delirium together with tachypnoea or inco-ordinate respiration, or (iii) a blood ammonia greater than 300µg/100ml (normal range up to 50).

Pancuronium is the muscle paralysing agent of choice 0.05mg/kg/hour (*i.e.* 50µg, although up to 100µg could be used). Unfortunately, 30 per cent of this is metabolised in the liver and it may be more logical to use vecuronium bromide, which is hydrolysed totally in the blood (dosage is 0.1mg/kg/hour). Unfortunately other paralysing agents, such as atracurium besylate, wear off abruptly and cause tachyphylaxis.

Ventilation is via a naso-tracheal tube, 15 to 20 breaths per minute, and the minute volume (that is, tidal volume by rate) is adjusted to keep the $PaCO_2$ in the normal range (4.4 to 6.1 kPa). The patient is *hyperventilated* only during episodes of RICP to a $PaCO_2$ level of 3.0 to 3.5kPa, and hyperventilation should not be used preventatively. The PaO_2 is maintained at approximately 20kPa. Cerebral vessels are very sensitive to changes in CO_2 tension, and 'blowing off' the CO_2 leads to a global reduction of CBF (10 per cent CBV reduction in vessel diameter) and CBV, but the cerebral vasoconstriction, changes in pH, bicarbonate, and CO_2 reactivity are not maintained if hyperventilation is continued for longer than 24 hours. Hyperventilation will result in an ischaemia as evidenced by an increased $AVDO_2$ and a PCr : pi ratio on MRS. Prolonged or excessive hyperventilation (megaventilation) can lead to a diffuse cerebral hypoxia and increased parenchymal tissue lactic acid, *i.e.* a Posner encephalopathy (Posner and Plum 1967). The problem of vascular reactivity to CO_2, and whether it may be regionally or only globally lost, is discussed in Chapter 8. Apart from the ventilated child, respiratory homeostasis may be upset with bradypnoea from foramen magnum impaction, tachypnoea, Cheyne Stokes respiration, or epileptic respiratory arrhythmias. Central neurogenic hyperventilation with tachypnoea, a low $PaCO_2$ and alkalosis is seen if there is hepatic failure or blood or micro-organisms in the CSF. Pulmonary oedema mediated by the sympathetic nervous system may occur in response to RICP.

5. SEDATION

Our sedation of choice is fentanyl at a constant infusion rate of 5µg/kg/hr. This is a short-acting opiate, and its use in a non-phasic fashion means that unlike long-acting sedatives, such as morphine, there is no need to monitor the pupil size or restlessness in order to assess whether it is wearing off. Nor does it mean that action is taken after the physiological stress has occurred. An alternative sedation would be phenoperidine hydrochloride.

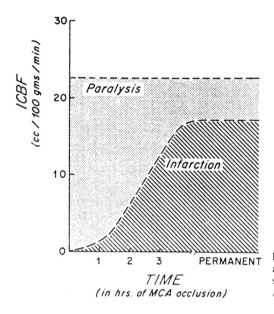

Fig. 7.40. Relation between minimum CPP and outcome in 39 patients with Reye's syndrome. (Reprinted by permission of the *British Medical Journal.*)

ICBF (cc / 100 gms / min)

Paralysis

Infarction

1   2   3   PERMANENT

TIME
(in hrs. of MCA occlusion)

6. HEAD ELEVATION

Nurse the patient head up, 10° to 15° (with the head in neutral). It is common practice to elevate the head of the bed in order to enhance the cerebrovenous drainage. It has been found, however, that the maximum CPP occurs with the patient horizontal. A reduction in the hydrostatic force of the systemic circulation occurs when the head is elevated above the heart. Therefore the effect of 'filtration oedema' may be offset by a drop in the CPP and a drop in the CBF if autoregulation is defective. This will give rise to cerebral vasodilatation and an increase in ICP. Whenever changes are therefore made to the patient's position, it is important to assess the ICP and any neurological change resulting (Rosner and Becker 1984).

7. ICP AND CPP MONITORING

It is our routine practice to insert a Cordis catheter in the subdural or subarachnoid space via a burr-hole. In other centres a Ladd epidural transducer or subarachnoid bolt have been used, although these methods are less accurate. In some centres a twist drill-hole is performed at the bedside, and a ventricular puncture attempted. This is likely to be more problematic with small and shifted ventricles.

Continuous ICP monitoring, together with computer-calculated CPP monitoring, is performed at the bedside. With a computerised process, the recordings can be analysed later and continual display of trends obtained. The CPP is probably a better guide to prognosis than the ICP alone and the aim is to keep the CPP above 60mmHg.

Jenkins (1987) found the outcome in Reye's syndrome related to the minimal CPP (48.5mmHg), and this was significant at the 1 per cent level. Patients with a good outcome had a mean CPP of 56mmHg and those with a bad outcome 31mmHg. They considered 40mmHg the critical cut-off point for full recovery (Fig. 7.40).

In Reye's syndrome, there are rapid and unpredictable rises of ICP, particularly with A waves which presage transtentorial herniation. Often these periodic A waves or B waves occur on a background of a normal baseline of ICP. They can occur up to 10 days after the onset of the coma, but the ICP is most difficult to control in the first few days. ICP monitoring is now standard practice for the management of Reye's syndrome.

On multiple regression analyses, Shaywitz *et al.* (1980) found in 29 patients that the maximum concentration of blood ammonia significantly correlated with the duration of ICP monitoring and the amount of mannitol required. Those with a high ammonia level required a mean of 25 boluses, those with a low ammonia required a mean of zero boluses.

Shaywitz found levels of ICP greater than 20mmHg in 83 per cent of cases; in two cases the ICP was uncontrollable and required decompressive craniectomy. ICP levels are difficult to establish because measures are taken to control the pressure.

With a pressure level of 20 to 25mmHg, the blood gases should be checked and the patient manually hyperventilated with an Ambu bag.

In the case of continued increase in ICP, use a combination of osmotic and loop diuretic, *i.e.* mannitol and frusemide together. The reduction of ICP is most effective with this combination. Mannitol itself is effective within five minutes of administration, and the pressure usually remains low for approximately 1½ to 2½ hours. The advantage of pressure-monitoring at the same time means that only enough mannitol is administered in order to bring the pressure to the normal range. Excessive use of mannitol may not only result in rebound pressure, but the hyperosmolality may also cause metabolic acidosis, hypokalaemia, oliguria, permanent renal damage and subdural haematomata (Becker and Vries 1972, Langfitt 1982). The most successful treatment of raised pressure in Reye's syndrome is intermittent mannitol and hyperventilation. The osmolality alone, even if it goes above 400mmol/kg, will be insufficient to control elevations of ICP, and it is suggested that the optimum combination of efficacy and safety is at 320mmol/kg. Other treatments, such as glycerol (1g/kg/3-hourly by naso-gastric tube), are less effective and only for short periods; they have a delayed action of some 30 to 60 minutes, and may cause significant gastro-intestinal irritation.

The mannitol is given as 7ml/kg of a 20 per cent solution, or 0.21g/kg/dose, together with frusemide at the end of the mannitol infusion in a dose of 0.5mg/kg. Hypertonic drugs (osmotherapy) have several possible modes of action:
(1) They cause controlled hyperosmolar dehydration by reducing brain-water content (Katzman and Pappius 1973) by osmotically withdrawing water from normal brain tissue (Langfitt 1982) and not due to the diuretic effect (Javid and Anderson 1959). The action of osmotherapy can be prolonged by the use of loop diuretics, such as frusemide or ethacrynic acid, which preferentially excrete water compared to solute (Pollay 1985). Some efflux may occur from oedematous tissue provided there is an intact capillary membrane across which osmotic gradients may be operative—Starling's hypothesis (Milhorat 1987). Mannitol induces a diuresis within 20 minutes in normal children and this is accompanied by an increased excretion of sodium, potassium, chloride and calcium; it is important to avoid possible urinary retention.

A mannitol and frusemide combination shrinks the circulating volume, and therefore there is a need to increase the volume depending on the CVP and blood pressure by administering PPS in a dose 2 to 5ml/kg.

(2) Mannitol reduces blood viscosity and increases local CBF (Muizelaar *et al.* 1985). This increased CBF locally will then cause vasoconstriction if autoregulation is intact with a reduced CBV but preserved CBF. When there has been considerable membrane damage, mannitol will be ineffective in osmotically withdrawing water and this is seen clinically in severe cases where mannitol is ineffective, indicating a bad prognosis. Mannitol will, however, withdraw brain water whether cerebrovascular autoregulation is intact or not. Further evidence for mannitol's vascular effect is seen in the circumference of infarcts where local CBF is improved and cellular swelling reduced (Meyer *et al.* 1987).

(3) A third suggested mode of action for mannitol has been 'mopping up' free radicals which cause cellular death. While liver and pancreas cells seem to undergo necrosis via this mechanism (based on glutathione reductase), in other organs such as the brain, early post-mortem investigations of post-hypoxic ishaemic cases do not show the expected glutathione reactions. This makes the use of superoxide dismutase more problematic in traumatic and non-traumatic encephalopathies.

A combination of dexamethasone with mannitol is often used in an attempt to minimise the risk of exacerbating the oedema due to the unwanted escape of mannitol across the blood-brain barrier, for example into an infarcted area of brain.

At the end of monitoring, when the ICP and clinical state is stable, the osmolality should be reduced gradually at a rate not greater than one milliosmol per hour. There is normally a six-hour gap in equilibrium between the blood and CSF, so that an osmolar gap exceeding six milliosmols is likely to be associated with an osmotic disequilibrium and rebound oedema (Habel and Simpson 1976).

If there is still a continued increase in ICP, then start a bolus of thiopentone sodium in a dose of 1 to 2mg/kg, and increase this dosage if necessary to an anaesthetic induction dose of 5mg/kg, given slowly.

The thiopentone sodium is used only if the blood-pressure and CVP are satisfactory at the outset. Be prepared to increase the blood-pressure with inotropic drugs, *e.g.* dopamine hydrochloride 5 to 10mg/kg/min in an infusion.

Barbiturates reduce the metabolic needs and hence the CBF requirements of the brain (Goldstein *et al.* 1966, Shapiro *et al.* 1974, Hoff *et al.* 1975). Their usefulness in vasogenic oedema may be related to their effect on the systemic arterial pressure and hence a reduction of filtered fluid across leaky capillaries. Their disadvantage is the effect of precipitous hypotension. It is important to keep the EEG at burst-suppression level, with close monitoring of the serum levels to be kept between 20 and 40mg/l (Marshall *et al.* 1977, Shaywitz *et al.* 1980). It is good practice to do a sensitivity test of 4mg/kg before embarking on a full dosage range of barbiturates.

For persistent increases in RICP the treatments are thiopentone sodium in a dose to cause barbiturate coma, or a decompressive (*e.g.* bifrontal craniectomy), although our current practice suggests that by this stage most measures will be

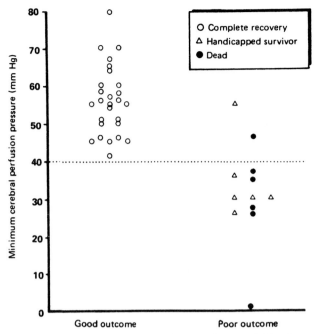

Fig. 7.41. Ischaemic thresholds. When local cerebral bloodflow (lCBF) falls below 23cc/100g/min, reversible paralysis occurs. Even profound ischaemia is reversible for a brief time. When lCBF falls below 10cc/100g/min for two hours, or below 18cc/100g/min during permanent occlusion, irreversible infarction occurs. (Reproduced by permission of the *Journal of Neurosurgery.*)

ineffective. Even radical decompression with bilateral hemicalvarectomy or circumferential craniotomy is less effective. A possible exception is a subtemporal decompression with dural opening for unilateral hemispheric swelling and progressive tentorial herniation (Milhorat 1987). There is approximately 26 per cent increase in the space available within the skull following subtemporal decompression and a consequent 30 per cent reduction in the ICP level. If ventricular cannulation has been possible for monitoring the ICP, then external ventricular drainage is a way of assisting transventricular clearance of interstitial oedema. Other experimentally effective measures, such as hypothermia, the use of drugs and water-cooled blankets, and hyperbaric oxygen, are not really practical.

An estimation of CSF hydrodynamics is undertaken routinely and at the time of any acute change in the neurological or physiological state. It may also be useful to measure PVI, volume pressure response, CSF production, outflow resistance and absorptive capacity.

8. AVDO₂ OR JUGULAR VENOUS OXYGEN SATURATION

The jugular venous oxygen difference, sampled from the jugular bulb catheter and from the radial artery, can be done daily if the ICP is stable and the CPP satisfactory. The normal AVDO₂ is four to eight volumes per cent in children, and a value of three to seven in adults. If metabolic coupling is present (*i.e.* if there is metabolic autoregulation), then the flow and metabolic demands are equal, whether increased or decreased, and the $AVDO_2$ is in the normal range.

If the $AVDO_2$ is increased, there is metabolic uncoupling and maximum extraction of oxygen, so the flow is low. Most ischaemic events tend to be iatrogenic, *e.g.* suction and fits.

If the $AVDO_2$ is decreased, then there is uncoupling due to hyperaemia or luxury perfusion. Barbiturates or mannitol are used to combat ischaemia but hyperventilation is required for hyperaemic states.

The oxygen content is calculated by multiplication of the haemoglobin by 1.39. However, if the patient is eight years of age or older, it may be possible to put a continuous catheter into the jugular bulb with a fibre-optic determination of continuous jugular haemoglobin saturation. This assumes that the haemoglobin and the arterial oxygen concentration are quite normal, and continuous monitoring of the jugular venous saturation on a monitor will normally read about 75 per cent. However, precipitous falls and rises indicate ischaemia and hyperaemia respectively.

9. CBF

Ordinarily this can only be sampled using xenon-iodinated amphetamines, which limits its usefulness in routine management of the intracranial dynamics. But if continual estimates were possible, then it would be important to know the cerebral perfusion in ml/100g of brain/min, since the critical level for ischaemia is 20ml/100g of brain tissue/min (Jones *et al.* 1981) (Fig. 7.41). It would also be important to know if the cerebrovascular autoregulation was intact. The cerebrovascular autoregulation is the restoration of normal brain bloodflow by changing the cerebrovascular resistance in the presence of a changing blood pressure or CPP (*i.e.* if autoregulation is intact, a falling blood pressure will be associated with a maintained CBF and an increased CBV). Ordinarily, with a mean arterial pressure between 60 and 150mmHg, there is adequate CBF. However, below a mean arterial pressure of 60mmHg the CBF is pressure passive from the systemic blood pressure, and above 150mmHg mean arterial pressure there is a breakthrough in the cerebral circulation. It would also be important to know whether CO_2 responsiveness was present. This is indicated by the response of the ICP to ventilation. Normally, there is a 4 per cent increase in CBF in response to 1mmHg change in $PaCO_2$ (vasodilatation). Similarly, a decreased $PaCO_2$ results in a decreased CBF, and significant drop in $PaCO_2$ results in ischaemia due to lactic acidosis. Hypoxia itself results in a post-hypoxic vasodilatation with an increase in CBF. The CO_2 responsiveness may be lost independently of autoregulation.

Ordinarily the CPP is a good guide to the adequacy of CBF when the patient is awake. This is not the case in coma states, however, and if continuous CBF estimate could be obtained and the state of cerebrovascular autoregulation known this would enable the CBF to be matched to the metabolic needs by adjusting peripheral blood pressure up or down by using drugs which add directly. With the possibility of continuous Doppler waveform and continuous RI estimates of CBF velocity by transcranial monitoring through the squamous temporal bone insonating the MCA, this may be a useful measure of CBF adequacy, although not of perfusion.

10. FLUIDS AND ELECTROLYTES

Fluid is restricted to 60 per cent maintenance by the use of 1/5 normal saline and 4 per cent dextrose, together with added potassium to keep the electrolytes normal. Although the patients are fluid-restricted, they must not be allowed to become hypovolaemic, and intravascular expanders (colloid), either albumin or PPS, are used depending on the CVP and blood pressure. It may be difficult to strike a balance between overhydration (risking cerebral oedema), and underhydration (risking hyperviscosity and 'sludging'). Blood pressure and haematocrit must be routine, and it is ideal to keep the haematocrit low at 35.

11. ANTIBIOTICS

These should probably be used while an intracranial catheter is in place, although literature reports indicate that there have been no infectious problems despite ICP monitoring up to 16 days. It is our practice to use a cephalosporin prophylactically (cefotaxime 200 to 300mg/kg/day).

12. STEROIDS

Dexamethasone has little effect on the ICP in Reye's syndrome, except to stabilise membranes and lysosomes. The earlier studies of Reye's syndrome indicated that patients had an improved chance of survival if given dexamethasone. Offsetting any advantage to the microcirculation and membranes is the possibly deleterious effect of enhanced protein catabolism.

Steroids are of no use in reducing brain bulk secondary to an increased vascular volume, or secondary to cytotoxic swelling or interstitial oedema, apart from vasogenic oedema where autoregulation is intact (Milhorat 1987). Most intracranial conditions produce a mixed oedema. Steroids have some effect in ischaemic strokes (Patten *et al.* 1971) and Reye's syndrome (Pollay 1985), which probably has a vasogenic component. They are, however, most useful in perifocal oedema surrounding mass lesions, such as tumours and abscesses. At the same time there is decreased CT enhancement, suggesting some restoration of the blood-brain barrier (Pollay 1985). Steroids may be positively harmful in hypoxic ischaemic brain damage owing to an augmentation of the metabolic needs and induction of hypoglycaemia and increased brain lactate levels. Dexamethasone is the steroid most commonly used in a dose of 0.5 to 1mg/kg, and a suggested dosage regime is 2mg six-hourly for an infant, 4mg six-hourly for a young child and 10mg six-hourly for a child aged 12 or older. It should be withdrawn over several days.

Apart from the immune suppressant, the anti-inflammatory effects and the effect on leukocyte diapedesis and the reduction of CSF formation, the main steroidal actions are: (i) stabilisation of and tightening of endothelial junctions of the blood-brain barrier; lysosomal activity increase; and a restoration of the microcirculation. In very large doses, that is 10 times normal in the shock state, there is considerable vasodilatation and opening of the microcirculation; (ii) inhibition of release of free radicals, fatty acids, prostaglandins from arachidonic acid, and products of catecholamine metabolism; (iii) glial uptake and transcapillary efflux causing resolution of oedema. The steroid molecule easily crosses the

270

blood-brain barrier to reach receptor sites. The receptor sites are intracellular binding proteins. This receptor steroid complex is attached to the chromatin of the cell nucleus leading to *de novo* synthesis of RNA and subsequent proteins and enzymes, such as sodium, potassium ATPase, glycerol phosphate dehydrogenase, glutamate synthetase, TCA enzymes; and (iv) a direct effect on cerebral metabolism, with increased neuronal function and stimulation of oxygen and glucose consumption.

13. NON-STEROIDAL ANTI-INFLAMMATORY DRUGS (INDOMETHACIN, IBUPROFEN, PROBENECID)

These are safe and effective in the treatment of systemic inflammation. In experimentally induced gliomas and experimental brain inflammation, they have been found to reduce the vascular permeability (Gamache and Ellis 1986, Reichman *et al.* 1986). They inhibit arachidonic acid-prostaglandin cascade, but have not been evaluated in childhood encephalopathy as yet.

14. URINE OUTPUT

Urine output is monitored continuously with a Foley indwelling catheter.

15. CVP CONTINUOUS MONITOR

CVP continuous monitoring is a measure of right heart output, which is normally 2 to 6mmHg. An inotrope is required if this increases to 10mmHg at the same time as a high ICP or low CPP. This is routinely used as a guide to fluid volume.

16. PULMONARY WEDGE PRESSURE

Pulmonary wedge pressure is a guide to left heart output, and a Swan-Ganz catheter is used via the femoral or antecubital vessel using a thermal dilution technique. This technique is probably useful only if there is pulmonary oedema or poor pulmonary function, myocardial disease with a discrepancy between the right and left heart output, or multi-organ failure. I do not routinely use it in Reye's syndrome.

17. ARTERIAL BLOOD PRESSURE

Arterial blood pressure is continuously monitored from the radial artery in order to maintain an adequate blood pressure, which is the main determinant of CPP. The cerebro-vasodilatation is a compensatory response to RICP, increasing the CBF. It does not have any effect on the systemic arterial pressure, but if the ICP continues to rise and approaches the systemic diastolic pressure, then the Cushing response comes into play. Systemic arterial blood pressure is increased by efferents from the vasomotor centre, resulting in a sympathetic discharge and an increase in peripheral resistance. The Cushing response is lost if the ICP continues to rise to very high limits. The response may be very marked in children with acute brain-swelling, and we have recorded blood pressures of the order of 260/160mmHg in several children below four years of age. However, in six infants Kaiser and Whitelaw (1988) found rather less marked increases in systemic arterial pressure in predominantly anoxic ischaemic damaged children, and for every 1mmHg increase in ICP there was a 0.2mmHg increase in systemic arterial pressure (*i.e.* a net drop in CPP of 0.8mmHg). Paroxysmal hypertension unrelated to the RICP may also occur and persist for days or weeks. It is also unrelated to the Cushing response, which is a compensatory hypertension from a primary intracranial cause.

Controlled hypotension may have a beneficial effect in cerebral oedema. Any elevation of blood pressure above the physiological range can be reduced by an intravenous infusion of sodium nitroprusside 0.1µg/kg/min. If this is undertaken, it is essential that careful monitoring is maintained in order to ensure an adequate CPP if the blood pressure is to be allowed below the physiological range. Systemic hypertension occurs in other acute encephalopathies, such as acute nephritis, tricyclic poisoning, haemolytic-uraemic syndrome and fluid overload. If pressure agents are being considered for hypotension, then it is essential to ensure that hypovolaemia is corrected first.

18. EEG

EEG continuous monitoring (CFAM) as soon as the paralysis is undertaken, and particularly if barbiturate is used. Fits are infrequent in early Reye's syndrome, but occur later when the prognosis is poor. They are multifocal and clonic, and Aoki and Lombroso (1973) found that there was sometimes a lack of EEG evidence of a seizure, despite the clinical observation of one. The background EEG is of high-voltage delta waves, with or without superimposed spike discharges (*i.e.* a nonspecific encephalopathy picture). The possibility of evoked potential monitoring should also be entertained. Early seizures are a bad indicator for outcome, although hypoglycaemic seizures may occur. If an anticonvulsant is required, phenytoin, ± paraldehyde are the drugs of choice. Seizures (along with hypoxia, raised pressure and hypothermia) form part of the secondary injury in Reye's syndrome because of the increased oxygen demands of the convulsing brain, as well as the significant compounding RICP they induce themselves (Minns and Brown 1978).

If rapid 'epanutinisation' is required, then 10mg/kg/IV Stat is given slowly at 50ml/min. Five mg/kg/IV is given one hour later, and then 10mg/kg in divided doses over the next 24 hours (four-, six- and eight-hourly). The blood level is measured daily, because if the child becomes toxic, this may induce seizures at levels above 150µmol/l. A maintenance regime of 2 to 8mg/kg/day is necessary to maintain a therapeutic range of 40 to 80 µmol/l. Higher doses may be necessary if there is enzyme induction from barbiturates or chlormethiozole, but again it is important to monitor the blood levels carefully. For the newborn there is a wider range of dosage, from 2 to 25mg/kg, but the requirements usually change significantly in the second week of life.

19. PERIPHERAL PERFUSION

Peripheral perfusion is monitored by the core-peripheral temperature gradient which gives an idea of the adequacy of cardiac output. A gradient steeper than two degrees is indicative of increased peripheral resistance and inadequate perfusion. In a child presenting with poor peripheral perfusion with cold peripheries, and sluggish capillary return with mottled skin, it is safer initially to use normal saline 10ml/kg with 5 per cent dextrose, although endotoxaemia with abnormal vasoreactivity may be responsible rather than hypovolaemia (from toxic cardio-myopathy, trauma or excessive use of diuretics). If drugs (*e.g.* sodium nitro-prusside) are used immediately to open the peripheral circulation the CPP might be lowered below the critical level for cerebral ischaemia.

20. DRUGS AND SUBSTANCES TO BE AVOIDED

These include amino acids, intravenous fat solutions, sodium valproate, salicylates, fructose and steroids.

21. NEOMYCIN, ± LACTULOSE

Neomycin, ± Lactulose by naso-gastric tube, is a gentle cleansing enema which will minimise ammonia production by the gut. Autonomic imbalance with vagal overactivity may result in acute erosions with GI haemorrhage. If there is evidence of GI bleeding then cimetidine 3mg/kg six-hourly is considered together with alkali on a regular basis.

22. VITAMIN K

Vitamin K is routinely given on diagnosis.

23. OTHER MONITORING ARRANGEMENTS

(1) A pulse oximeter for oxygen saturation.

(2) ECG because the pulse-rate may change from bradycardia to sinus tachycardia, sinus arrest and cardiac arrest. If there is sympathetic overactivity with heart-rates over 200/min, there may be impaired diastolic filling. Myocardial necrosis and ECG changes may also complicate the management.

(3) Blood gases four-hourly: the internal control for pH is in chemoreceptors in the carotid body and in the area postrema of the fourth ventricle. The body regulates acid base status by regulating ventilation. Many non-comatose children with raised pressure will hyperventilate automatically. A metabolic acidaemia as in Reye's syndrome may occur and is usually associated with a normal pH in the CSF. CO_2 passes freely into and out of CSF while bicarbonate does not, and there is loss of consciousness if the CSF pH falls below 7.2. A blood pH of less than 7.25 should be corrected with sodium bicarbonate.

(4) Urea and electrolytes twice daily—hyponatraemia is common in all enceph-alopathies with raised pressure, commonly due to inappropriate ADH. These patients are water-intoxicated, not salt-depleted, and therefore require fluid restriction. This is now done prophylactically. True sodium loss, however, may occur from mannitol and from sympathetic overactivity, with the signs of weight loss and dehydration. In such situations the sodium is usually below 120mmol/l and osmolality below 260/mosmol/kg, with fits and enhanced oedema. These children require normal saline. Hypernatraemia, the loss of body water, acidosis and high haematocrit result in a hyperviscose syndrome and the possibility of thrombosis. Therefore it is necessary to restore circulating volume with normal saline and

plasma expanders. The osmolality should be reduced slowly as previously mentioned.

(5) Calcium and phosphate daily.

(6) Glucose/dextrostix hourly.

(7) Initial coagulation study. A profoundly prolonged prothrombin time is an indicator of bad prognosis, and if the prothrombin ratio (PTR) is not greater than 2:1, then neurosurgery is possible for the insertion of monitors; osmolality of blood and urine twice daily; initial salicylate levels; daily blood ammonia estimation; daily serum transaminases estimations.

(8) Temperature should be measured twice daily, since hyperthermia, even in the absence of infection, may be a management problem.

These patients are prone to develop thick mucous plugs that may obstruct bronchioles and further complicate RICP by increasing the intrathoracic pressure. They therefore require regular chest therapy to remove plugs and minimise the intrathoracic resistance.

24. END OF MONITORING

If the ICP is less than 20 to 25mmHg for one day, CO_2 should be allowed to rise slowly over an eight-hour period by changing the ventilator settings.

If the ICP stays down with a normal CO_2, the physician should stop paralysis and sedation, although some children will require continuous positive airway pressure up to a week later.

Dexamethasone should be reduced if the ICP stays down with the patient breathing air.

If the ICP remains down 24 hours later, the ICP monitoring catheter should be removed.

REFERENCES

Adams, R. D., Kubik, C. S., Bonner, F. J. (1948) 'The clinical and pathological aspects of influenzal meningitis.' *Archives of Pediatrics*, **65**, 345–380, 408–459.

Addy, D. P. (1987) 'When not to do a lumbar puncture.' *Archives of Disease in Childhood*, **62**, 873–875.

American Trudeau Society (1954) 'A statement by the Committee on therapy concerning treatment of tuberculous meningitis.' *American Review of Tuberculosis*, **70**, 756–758.

Angonese, I., Żórzi, C. (1986) 'Transfontanelle cerebral sonography utilization in bacterial meningitis of the neonate and nursing baby.' *Journal of Pediatric Neurosciences*, **2**, 174–180.

Aoki, Y., Lombroso, C. T. (1973) 'Prognostic value of electroencephalography in Reye's syndrome.' *Neurology*, **23**, 333.

Auer, L. M., Sayama, I. (1983) 'Intracranial pressure oscillations (B-waves) caused by oscillations in cerebrovascular volume.' *Acta Neurochirurgica*, **68**, 93–100.

Auerbach, O. (1951) 'Tuberculous meningitis: correlation of therapeutic results with pathogenesis and pathologic changes—pathologic changes in untreated and treated cases.' *American Review of Tuberculosis*, **64**, 419.

Bayston, R., Penny, S. R. (1972) 'Excessive production of mucoid substance in Staphylococcus SIIA: a possible factor in colonization of Holter shunts.' *Developmental Medicine and Child Neurology* (Suppl. 27), 25–28.

Becker, D. P., Vries, J. K. (1972) 'The alleviation of increased ICP by the chronic administration of osmotic agents.' *In* Brock, M., Dietz, H. (Eds.) *Intracranial Pressure*. Berlin: Springer.

Bell, W. E., McCormick, W. F. (1981) *Neurologic Infections in Children, Vol. XII: Major Problems in Clinical Pediatrics (2nd Edn.)* Philadelphia: W. B. Saunders.

Belloni, G., DiRocco, C. (1975) 'A practical approach to the phlebographic study of the lateral cerebral ventricles.' *Neuroradiology*, **10**, 111–119.

Benjamin, C. M., Newton, R. W. Clarke, M. A. (1988) 'Risk factors for death from meningitis.' *British Medical Journal*, **296**, 20.

Berman, P. H., Banker, B. Q. (1966) 'Neonatal meningitis: a clinical and pathological study of 29 cases.' *Pediatrics*, **38**, 6–24.

Bhagwati, S. N., George, K. (1986) 'Use of intrathecal hyaluronidase in the management of tuberculosis meningitis with hydrocephalus.' *Child's Nervous System*, **2**, 20–25.

Bhargava, S., Gupta, A. K., Tandon, P. N. (1982) 'Tuberculous meningitis—a CT study.' *British Journal of Radiology*, **55**, 189–196.

Bird, M. T., Ratcheson, R. A., Siegel, B. A., Fishman, M. A. (1973) 'The evaluation of arrested communicating hydrocephalus utilizing cerebrospinal fluid dynamics: a preliminary report.' *Developmental Medicine and Child Neurology*, **15**, 474–482.

Blacklock, J. W. S., Griffin, M. A. (1935) 'Tuberculous meningitis in children.' *Journal of Pathology and Bacteriology*, **40**, 489–502.

Bodino, J., Lylyk, P., Del Valle, M., Wasserman, J. P., Leiguarda, R., Monges, J., Lopez, E. L. (1982) 'Computed tomography in purulent meningitis.' *American Journal of Diseases of Children*, **136**, 495–501.

Brandtzeac, P., Skulberg, A. (1987) 'Prognosis of meningococcal septicaemia.' *Lancet*, **2**, 862.

Brown, J. K., Ingram, T. T. S., Seshia, S. S. (1973) 'Patterns of decerebration in infants and children: Defects in homeostasis and sequelae.' *Journal of Neurology, Neurosurgery and Psychiatry*, **36**, 431–444.

Bruce, D. A., Langfitt, T. W., Miller, J. D. (1973) 'Regional cerebral blood flow, intracranial pressure and brain metabolism in comatose patients.' *Journal of Neurosurgery*, **38**, 131.

—— Alavi, A., Bilaniuk, L., Dolinskas, C., Obrist, W., Uzzell, B. (1981) 'Diffuse cerebral swelling following head injuries in children: the syndrome of malignant brain edema.' *Journal of Neurosurgery*, **54**, 170–178.

—— Raphaely, R. C., Goldberg, A. I. (1979) 'Pathophysiology, treatment and outcome following severe head injury in children.' *Child's Brain*, **5**, 174–191.

Bullock, M. R. R., Van Dellen, J. R. (1982) 'The role of cerbrospinal fluid shunting in tuberculous meningitis.' *Surgical Neurology*, **18**, 274–277.

Cathie, I. A. B., McFarlane, J. C. W. (1950) 'Adjuvants to streptomycin in treating tuberculous meningitis in children.' *Lancet*, **2**, 784–789.

Christie, A. B. (1980) *Infectious Diseases: Epidemiology and Clinical Practice, 3rd Edn.* London: Churchill Livingstone. pp. 607–610.

Choremis, C., Economos, D., Papadatos, D. (1956) 'Intraspinal epidermoid tumours (cholesteatomas) in patients treated for tuberculous meningitis.' *Lancet*, **2**, 437–439.

Coble, P. A., Kupfer, D. J., Reynolds, C. F., Houck, P. (1987) 'EEG sleep of healthy children 6 to 12 years of age.' *In* Guilliminault, C. (Ed.) *Sleep and its Disorders in Children.* New York: Raven Press. pp. 29–41.

Conner, W. T., Minielly, J. A. (1980) 'Cerebral oedema in fatal meningococcaemia.' *Lancet*, **2**, 967.

Cooper, R., Hulme, A. (1966) 'Intracranial pressure and related phenomena during sleep.' *Journal of Neurosurgery and Psychiatry*, **29**, 564–570.

Coovadia, Y. M., Dawood, A., Ellis, M. E., Coovadia, H. M., Daniel, T. M. (1986) 'Evaluation of adenosine deaminase activity and antibody to *Mycobacterium tuberculosis* antigen 5 in cerebro-spinal fluid and the radioactive bromide partition test for the early diagnosis of tuberculous meningitis.' *Archives of Disease in Childhood*, **61**, 428–435.

Cutler, R. W. P., Page, L., Galwich, F. (1968) 'Formation and absorption of cerebrospinal fluid in man.' *Brain*, **91**, 707–720.

Dacey, R. G. J. R., Scheld, W. M., Winn, H. R. (1983) 'Bacterial meningitis: selected aspects of cerebrospinal fluid pathophysiology.' *In* Wood, J. J. (Ed.) *Neurology of Cerebrospinal Fluid.* New York: Plenum. pp. 727–738.

Danziger, J., Bloch, S. (1975) 'Tapeworm cyst infestations of brain.' *Clinical Radiology*, **26**, 141–148.

—— —— Cremin, B. J., Goldblatt, M. (1976) 'Cranial and intracranial tuberculosis.' *South African Medical Journal*, **50**, 1403–1405.

Dastur, D. K., Udani, P. M. (1966) 'The pathology and pathogenesis of tuberculous encephalopathy.' *Acta Neuropathologica*, **6**, 311–326.

—— Lalitha, V. S., Udani, P. M., Parekh, U. (1970) 'The brain and meninges in TBM. Gross pathology in 100 cases and pathogenesis.' *Neurology, India*, **18**, 86–100.

Davies, P. A. (1977) 'Neonatal bacterial meningitis.' *British Journal of Hospital Medicine*, **18**, 425–434.

Davson, H. (1976) *Physiology of the Cerebrospinal Fluid*. London: Churchill Livingstone.

Delage, G., Dusseault, M. (1979) 'Tuberculous meningitis in children: retrospective study of 79 patients with an analysis of prognostic factors.' *Canadian Medical Association Journal*, **120**, 305–309.

DiRocco, C., Caldarelli, M., Maira, G., Rossi, G. F. (1977) 'The study of cerebrospinal fluid dynamics in apparently "arrested" hydrocephalus in children.' *Child's Brain*, **3**, 359–374.

—— Pettorossi, V. E., Caldarelli, M., Mancinelli, R., Velardi, F. (1978) 'Communicating hydrocephalus induced by mechanically increased amplitude of the intraventricular cerebrospinal fluid pressure: experimental studies.' *Experimental Neurology*, **18**, 40–52.

Dodge, P. R., Swartz, M. N. (1965) 'Bacterial meningitis—a review of selected aspects.' *New England Journal of Medicine*, **272**, 1003–1010.

Drapkin, A. J., Sahar, A. (1978) 'Experimental hydrocephalus: cerebrospinal fluid dynamics and ventricular distensibility during early stages.' *Child's Brain*, **4**, 278–288.

Ekstedt, J. (1978) 'CSF hydrodynamic studies in man. 2: normal hydrodynamic variables related to CSF pressure and flow.' *Journal of Neurology, Neurosurgery and Psychiatry*, **41**, 345–353.

Enzmann, D. R., Britt, R. H., Yeager, A. S. (1979) 'Experimental brain abscess evolution: CT and nemopathologic correlation.' *Radiology*, **133**, 113–120.

Escobar, J. A., Belsey, M. A., Duenas, A., Medina, P. (1975) 'Mortality from tuberculous meningitis reduced by steroid therapy.' *Pediatrics*, **56**, 1050–1055.

Esiri, M. M. (1982) 'Herpes simplex encephalitis: an immunohistological study of the distribution of viral antigen within the brain.' *Journal of the Neurological Sciences*, **54**, 209–226.

Evans, H., Bourgeois, C. H., Comer, D. S., Keschamras, N. (1970) 'Brain lesions in Reye's syndrome.' *Archives of Pathology*, **90**, 543.

Ferris, E. B. (1941) 'Objective measurement of relative intracranial blood flow in man with observations concerning hydrodynamics of the craniovertebral system.' *Archives of Neurology and Psychiatry*, **46**, 377–401.

Findlay, L., Kemp, F. H. (1943) 'Osteomyelitis of the spine following lumbar puncture.' *Archives of Diseases in Childhood*, **18**, 102–105.

Fischer, G. W., Brenz, R. W., Alden, E. R., Beckwith, J.B. (1975) 'Lumbar punctures and meningitis.' *American Journal of Diseases of Children*, **129**, 590–592.

Fisher, R. M., Lipinski, J. K., Cremin, B. J. (1984) 'Ultrasonic assessment of infectious meningitis.' *Clinical Radiology*, **35**, 267–273.

Foltz, E. L., Aine, C. (1981) 'Diagnosis of hydrocephalus by CSF pulse-wave analysis: a clinical study.' *Surgical Neurology*, **15**, 283–293.

French, G. L., Chan, C. Y., Cheung, S. W., Teoh, R., Humphriews, M. J., O'Mahony, G. (1987) 'Diagnosis of tuberculous meningitis by detection of tuberculostearic acid in cerebrospinal fluid.' *Lancet*, **2**, 117–119.

Gaab, M. R., Sorenson, N., Brawanski, A., Bushe, K. A., Wodarz, R. (1980) 'Non-invasive intracranial pressure monitoring by fontanometry.' *Zeitschrift für Kinderchirurgie*, **31**, 339–347.

Gamache, D. A., Ellis, E. F. (1986) 'Effect of dexamethasone, indomethacin, ibuprofen, and probenecid on carrageenan-induced brain inflammation.' *Journal of Neurosurgery*, **65**, 686.

Gelabert, M., Castro-Gago, M. (1988) 'Hydrocephalus and tuberculous meningitis in children. Report on 26 cases.' *Child's Nervous System*, **4**, 268–270.

Gordon, N. S., Fois, A., Jacobi, G., Minns, R. A., Seshia, S. S. (1983) 'Consensus statement: the management of the comatose child.' *Neuropediatrics*, **14**, 3–5.

Gerlach, J., Jenson, H. P., Koos, W., Kraus, H. (1967) *Pediatrische Neurochirurgie mit klinisch Diagnostik and Differentialdiagnostik in Pediatrie und Neurologie*. Stuttgart: Georg Thieme. p. 139.

Gibson, N. F., Ball, M. M., Kelsey, D. S., Morrison, L. (1975) 'Anterior fontanelle herniation.' *Pediatrics*, **56**, 466–468.

Gilland, O., Tourtellotte, W. W., O'Tauma, L., Henderson, W. G. (1974) 'Normal cerebrospinal fluid pressure.' *Journal of Neurosurgery*, **40**, 587–593.

Goitein, K. J., Amit, Y. (1982) 'Percutaneous placement of subdural catheter for measurement of intracranial pressure in small children.' *Critical Care Medicine*, **10**, 46–48.

—— —— Mussaffi, H. (1983) 'Intracranial pressure in central nervous system infections and cerebral ischaemia of infancy.' *Archives of Disease in Childhood*, **58**, 184–186.

Goldstein, A. Jr., Wells, B. A., Keats, A. S. (1966) 'Increased tolerance to cerebral anoxia by pentobarbital.' *Archives Internationales de Pharmacodynamie et de Thérapie*, **161**, 138.

Goodman, S. J., Becker, D. P. (1973) 'Vascular pathology of the brain stem due to experimentally increased intracranial pressure: changes noted in the micro- and macrocirculation.' *Journal of*

Neurosurgery, **39**, 601–609.

Gordon, N. S., Fois, A., Jacobi, G., Minns, R. A., Seshia, S. S. (1983) 'The management of the comatose child.' *Neuropediatrics, Journal of Pediatric Neurobiology, Neurology and Neurosurgery*, **14**, 3–5.

Grant, R., Condon, B., Lawrence, A., Hadley, D., Patterson, J., Bone, I., Teasdale, G. M. (1984) *Normal and Physiological Variations in Cranial CSF Volume Measured by Magnetic Resonance Imaging*. Newcastle: Association of British Neurologists.

Gray, E. D., Peters, G., Verstegen, M., Regelmann, W. E. (1984) 'The effects of extracellular slime substance from *Staphylococcus epidermidis* on the human cellular immune response.' *Lancet*, **1**, 365–367.

Habel, A. H., Simpson, H. (1976) 'Osmolar relation between cerebrospinal fluid and serum in hyperosmolar hypernatraemic dehydration.' *Archives of Disease in Childhood*, **51**, 660–666.

Habib, M., Fosse, T., Pellissier, J. F., Khalil, R. (1984) 'Metastatic cerebral abscesses due to *Hemophilus paraphrophilus*.' *Archives of Neurology*, **41**, 1290–1291.

Hass, W. K. (1977) 'Prognostic value of cerebral oxidative metabolism in head trauma.' *In* McLaurin, R. (Ed.) *Head Injuries*. New York: Grune and Stratton. pp. 35–37.

Hayden, P. W., Shurtleff, D. B., Foltz, E. L. (1970) 'Ventricular fluid pressure recordings in hydrocephalic patients.' *Archives of Neurology*, **23**, 147–154.

Heinz, E. R., Ward, A., Drayer, B. P., Dubois, P. J. (1980) 'Distinction between obstructive and atrophic dilatation of ventricles in children.' *Journal of Computer Assisted Tomography*, **4 (3)**, 320–325.

Hoff, J. T., Smith, A. L., Hankinson, H. L., Nielsen, S. L. (1975) 'Barbiturate protection from cerebral infarction in primates.' *Stroke*, **12**, 211–215.

Horne, N. W. (1951) 'Tuberculous meningitis: problems in pathogenesis and treatment.' *Edinburgh Medical Journal*, **58**, 413–417.

Horwitz, S. J., Boxerbaum, B., O'Bell, J. (1980) 'Cerebral herniation in bacterial meningitis in childhood.' *Annals of Neurology*, **7**, 524–528.

Huttenlocher, P. R. (1972) 'Relation of outcome to therapy.' *Journal of Pediatrics*, **80**, 845–850.

Idriss, Z. H., Sinno, A. A., Kronfol, N. M. (1976) 'Tuberculous meningitis in children. Forty-three cases.' *American Journal of Diseases of Childhood*, **130**, 364–367.

Ikeyama, J., Maeda, S., Banno, K., Ito, A., Wagai, H., Kageyama, N. (1976) 'Normal intracranial circumstances—the theory of "the open and the closed cavities."' *Brain Nerve*, **28**, 539–547.

Illis, L. S. (1977) 'Encephalitis.' *British Journal of Hospital Medicine*, **18**, 412–422.

—— Merry, R. T. G. (1972) 'Herpes simplex encephalitis.' *Journal of the Royal College of Physicians of London*, **7**, 34.

Javid, M., Anderson, J. (1959) 'The effect of urea on cerebrospinal fluid pressure in monkeys before and after bilateral nephrectomy.' *Journal of Laboratory and Clinical Medicine*, **53**, 484.

Jennett, B., Bond, M. R. (1975) 'Assessment of outcome after severe brain damage.' *Lancet*, **1**, 480.

—— Teasdale, G. (1977) 'Aspect of coma after severe head injury.' *Lancet*, **1**, 878–881.

Jones, H. C. (1987) 'The pathophysiology of congenital hydrocephalus.' *Journal of Pediatric Neurosciences*, **3**, 9–20.

Jones, T. H., Morawetz, R. B., Crowell, R. M., Marcous, F. W., FitzGibbon, S. J., DeGirolami, U., Ojemann, R. G. (1981) 'Thresholds of focal cerebral ischemia in awake monkeys.' *Journal of Neurosurgery*, **54**, 773–782.

Juncos, J., Epstein, F., Hunnicupp, E., Nathanson, J. (1982) 'Pharmacologic characterisation of hormone receptors in vitro.' *Neurology*, **32**, 4.

Kaiser, A. M., Whitelaw, A. G. L. (1986) 'Normal cerebrospinal fluid pressure in the newborn.' *Neuropediatrics*, **17**, 100–102.

—— —— (1988) 'Hypertensive response to raised intracranial pressure in infancy.' *Archives of Disease in Childhood*, **63**, 1461–1465.

Kalra, V., Paul, V. K., Marwah, R. K., Kochhar, G. S., Bhargava, S. (1987) 'Neurocysticercosis in childhood.' *Transactions of the Royal Society of Tropical Medicine and Hygiene*, **81**, 371–373.

Katzman, M. D., Hussey, F. (1970) 'A simple constant-infusion manometric test for measurement of CSF absorption.' *Neurology*, **20**, 534–544.

—— Pappius, H. M. (1973) *Brain Electrolytes and Fluid Metabolism*. Baltimore: Williams and Wilkins.

Kennedy, D. H., Fallon, R. J. (1979) 'Tuberculous meningitis.' *Journal of the American Medical Association*, **241**, 264–268.

Kirkpatrick, M., Engleman, H., Minns, R. A. (1989) 'Symptoms and signs of progressive hydrocephalus.' *Archives of Disease in Childhood*, **64**. 124–128.

Kishore, P. R. S., Lipper, M. H., Miller, J. D., Girevendulis, A. K., Becker, D. P., Vines, F. S. (1978)

277

'Post-traumatic hydrocephalus in patients with severe head injury.' *Neuroradiology*, **16**, 261–265.

Klein, J. O., Geigin, R. D., McCracken, G. H. (1986) 'Report of the task force on diagnosis and management of meningitis.' *Pediatrics*, **75** (Suppl. 5), 959–982.

Kocen, R. S. (1977) 'Tuberculous meningitis.' *British Journal of Hospital Medicine*, **18**, 436–445.

Kohl, S., James, A. R. (1985) 'Herpes simplex virus encephalitis during childhood: importance of brain biopsy diagnosis.' *Journal of Pediatrics*, **107**, 212–215.

Kontopolous, E., Minns, R. A., O'Hare, A. E., Eden, O. B. (1986) 'Sedimentation cytomorphology of the CSF in ventriculitis.' *Developmental Medicine and Child Neurology*, **28**, 213–219.

Langfitt, T. W. (1982) 'Increased intracranial pressure and the cerebral circulation.' *In* Youmans, J. R. (Ed.) *Neurological Surgery, 2nd Edn.* Philadelphia: W. B. Saunders.

Launes, J., Lindroth, L., Liewendahl, K., Nikkinen, P., Brownell, A. L., Iivanainen, M. (1988) 'Diagnosis of acute herpes simplex encephalitis by brain perfusion single photon emission computed tomography.' *Lancet*, **2**, 1188–1191.

Lees, A. J., MacLeod, A. F., Marshall, J. (1980) 'Cerebral tuberculomas developing during treatment of tuberculous meningitis.' *Lancet*, **1**, 1208–1211.

Levin, B. E. (1978) 'The clinical significance of spontaneous pulsations of the retinal vein.' *Archives of Neurology*, **35**, 37–40.

Levinson, A. (1923) *Cerebrospinal Fluid in Health and in Disease, 2nd Edn.* St Louis: C. V. Mosby. pp. 87–90.

—— (1928) 'Cerebrospinal fluid in infants and in children.' *American Journal of Diseases of Children*, **36**, 799–818.

Levison, A., Luhan, J., Maurelis, W. P., Herzon, H. (1950) 'The effect of streptomycin on tuberculous meningitis. A pathologic study.' *Journal of Neuropathology and Experimental Neurology*, **9**, 406.

Levy, D. E., Bates, D., Caronna, J. J. (1981) 'Prognosis in non-traumatic coma.' *Annals of Internal Medicine*, **94**, 293–301.

Lewelt, W., Jenkins, L. W., Miller, J. D. (1980) 'Autoregulation of cerebral blood flow after experimental fluid percussion injury of the brain.' *Journal of Neurosurgery*, **53**, 500–511.

Liechty, E. A., Gilmor, R. L., Bryson, C. Q., Bull, M. J. (1983) 'Outcome of high-risk neonates with ventriculomegaly.' *Developmental Medicine and Child Neurology*, **25**, 162–168.

Lincoln, E. M., Sordillo, S. V. R., Davies, P. A. (1960) 'Tuberculous meningitis in children.' *Journal of Pediatrics*, **57**, 807–823.

Lorber, J. (1951) 'Sexual precocity following recovery from tuberculous meningitis with hydrocephalus.' *Proceedings of the Royal Society of Medicine*, **44**, 726–727.

—— (1961) 'Long-term follow-up of 100 children who recovered from tuberculous meningitis.' *Pediatrics*, **28**, 778–791.

—— (1980) *Personal communication*.

—— Sunderland, R. (1980) 'Lumbar puncture in children with convulsions associated with fever.' *Lancet*, **1**, 785–786.

Lorenzo, A. V., Page, L. K., Watters, G. V. (1970) 'Relationship between cerebrospinal fluid formation, absorption, and pressure in human hydrocephalus.' *Brain*, **93**, 679–692.

Lovejoy, F. R., Smith, A. L., Bresnan, M. J., Word, J. N., Victor, D. I., Adams, P. C. (1974) 'Clinical staging in Reye's syndrome.' *American Journal of Diseases of Children*, **128**, 36–41.

Lups, S., Haan, A. M. F. H. (1954) *The Cerebrospinal Fluid*. Amsterdam: Elsevier. p. 31.

McCarthy, K. D., Reed, D. J. (1974) 'The effect of acetazolamide and frusemide on cerebrospinal fluid protection and choroid plexus carbonic anhydrase activity.' *Journal of Pharmacological and Experimental Therapy*, **180**, 194–201.

McComb, J. G. (1983) 'Recent research into the nature of cerebrospinal fluid formation and absorption.' *Journal of Neurosurgery*, **59**, 369–383.

McCracken, G. H. Jr. (1984) 'Management of bacterial meningitis in infants and children. Current status and future prospects.' *American Journal of Medicine*, **76**, 215–223.

—— Sarff, L. D. (1976) 'Endotoxin in cerebrospinal fluid: detection in neonates with bacterial meningitis.' *Journal of the American Medical Association*, **235**, 617–620.

McCullough, D. C. (1980) 'A critical evaluation of continuous intracranial pressure monitoring in pediatric hydrocephalus.' *Child's Brain*, **6**, 225–241.

McLaurin, R. L. (1973) 'Infected cerebrospinal fluid shunts.' *Surgical Neurology*, **1**, 191–195.

McMenamin, B., Volpe, J. J. (1984) 'Bacterial meningitis in infancy: effects on intracranial pressure and cerebral blood flow velocity.' *Neurology*, **34**, 500–504.

MacVicar, D., Symon, D. N. K. (1985) 'Timing of lumbar puncture in severe childhood meningitis.' *British Medical Journal*, **291**, 898.

Mace, J. W., Peters, E. R., Mathies, A. W. Jr. (1968) 'Cranial bruits in purulent meningitis in childhood.' *New England Journal of Medicine*, **278**, 1420–1422.

Maira, G., Anile, C., Mangiola, A., Proietti, R., Zanghi, F., Della Corte, F. (1987) 'Intracranial elastance and CSF pulse waveform. Experimental study and clinical applications in comatose patients.' *Journal of Pediatric Neurosciences*, **3**, 92–100.

Margolis, C. Z., Cook, C. D. (1973) 'Risk of lumbar puncture in pediatric patients with cardiac and/or pulmonary disease.' *Pediatrics*, **51**, 562–564.

Margolis, L. H., Shaywitz, B. A. (1980) 'The outcome of prolonged coma in childhood.' *Pediatrics*, **65**, 477–483.

Marshall, L. F., Bruce, D. A., Bruno, L. A., Schut, L. (1977) 'Role of intracranial pressure monitoring and barbiturate therapy in malignant intracranial hypertension.' *Journal of Neurosurgery*, **47**, 481.

Masserman, J. H. (1934) 'Cerebrospinal hydrodynamics IV: clinical experimental studies.' *Archives of Neurology and Psychiatry*, **32**, 523–553.

—— (1935) 'Cerebrospinal hydrodynamics IV: correlation of the pressure of the cerebrospinal fluid with age, blood pressure and the pressure index.' *Archives of Neurology and Psychiatry*, **34**, 564–566.

Mendoza, S. A. (1976) 'Syndrome of inappropriate antidiuretic hormone secretion (SIADH).' *Symposium on Pediatric Nephrology, Pediatric Clinics of North America*, **23**, 681–690.

Merritt, H. H., Fremont-Smith, F. (1937) *The Cerebrospinal Fluid*. Philadelphia: W. B. Saunders. p. 333.

Mervis, B., Lotz, J. W. (1980) 'Computed tomography (CT) in parenchymatous cysticercosis.' *Clinical Radiology*, **31**, 521–528.

Meyer, F. B., Anderson, R. E., Sundt, T. M., Yaksh, T. L. (1987) 'Treatment of experimental focal cerebral ischemia with mannitol. Assessment by intracellular brain pH, cortical blood flow, and electroencephalography.' *Journal of Neurosurgery*, **66**, 109.

Milhorat, T. J. H. (1975) 'The third circulation revisited.' *Journal of Neurosurgery*, **42**, 628–645.

—— (1987) *Cerebrospinal Fluid and the Brain Edemas*. New York: Neuroscience Society of New York.

Miller, J. D., Stanck, A., Langfitt, T. W. (1972) 'Concept of cerebral perfusion pressure and vascular compression during intracranial hypertension.' *Progress in Brain Research*, **35**, 411–432.

—— Becker, D. P., Ward, J. D., Sullivan, H. G., Adams, W. E., Rosner, M. J. (1977) 'Significance of intracranial hypertension in severe head injury.' *Journal of Neurosurgery*, **47**, 503–510.

Minns, R. A. (1977) 'Clinical application of ventricular pressure monitoring in children.' *Zeitschrift für Kinderchirurgie und Grenzgebiete*, **224**, 430–443.

—— (1979) *Monitoring of Intracranial Pressure in Infants and Children*, PhD Thesis, University of Edinburgh.

—— (1984) 'Intracranial pressure monitoring.' *Archives of Disease in Childhood*, **59**, 486–488.

—— (1990) 'The correlation of Resistance Index and ICP before and after CSF drainage in infantile hydrocephalus.' (*In preparation.*)

—— Brown, J. K. (1978) 'Intracranial pressure changes associated with childhood seizures.' *Developmental Medicine and Child Neurology*, **20**, 561–569.

—— —— Engleman, H. M. (1987) 'CSF production rate: "real time" estimation.' *Zeitschrift für Kinderchirurgie*, **42**, (Suppl. I), 36–40.

—— Engleman, H. M. (1988) 'The use of CSF pressure recordings in acute purulent meningitis.' *Zeischrift für Kinderchirurgie*, **43**, (Suppl. 2), 28–29.

—— Merrick, M. V. (1989) 'Cerebral perfusion pressure and nett cerebral mean transit time in childhood hydrocephalus.' *Journal of Pediatric Neurosciences*, **5**, 69–77.

—— Engleman, H. M., Stirling, H. (1989) 'Cerebrospinal fluid pressure in pyogenic meningitis.' *Archives of Disease in Childhood*, **64**, 814–820.

Mori, K., Kamisura, Y., Kurisaka, M., Uchida, Y., Eguchi, S. (1986) 'ICP monitoring in long-standing hydrocephalus associated with myelomeningocele.' *Journal of Pediatric Neurosciences*, **2**, 195–204.

Morray, J. P., Tyler, D. C., Jones, T. K., Stuntz, J. T., Lemire, R. J. (1984) 'Coma scale for use in brain-injured children.' *Critical Care Medicine*, **12**, 1018–1020.

Moxon, E. R., Smith, A. L., Averill, D. R., Smith, D. H. (1974) *Journal of Infectious Diseases*, **129**, 154.

MRC Brain Injuries Committee (1941) *War Memorandum No. 4*, London: HMSO.

Muizelaar, J. P., Wei, E. P., Kontos, H. A. (1983) 'Mannitol causes compensatory vasoconstriction and vasodilatation in response to blood viscosity changes.' *Journal of Neurosurgery*, **59**, 822–828.

—— Becker, D. P., Lutz, H. A. (1985) 'Present application and future promise of CBF monitoring in head injury.' *In* Dacey, R. G., Winn, H. R., Rimel, R., Jane, J. A. (Eds.) *Trauma of the Central Nervous System*. New York: Raven.

—— Obrist, W. D. (1985) 'Cerebral blood flow metabolism with brain injury.' *In* Becker, D. P., Povlishock, J. T. (Eds.) *Central Nervous System Trauma Status Report*, NINCDS, NIH. pp.

279

123–137.

—— Marmarou, A., DeSalles, A. A. F., Ward, J. D., Zimmerman, R. S., Li, Z., Young, H. F (1989*a*) 'Cerebral blood flow and metabolism in severely head-injured children. Part 1: Relationship with GCS score, outcome, ICP, and PVI.' *Journal of Neurosurgery*, **71**, 63–71.

—— Ward, J. D., Marmarou, A., Newlon, P. G., Wachi, A. (1989*b*) 'Cerebral blood flow and metabolism in severely head-injured children. Part 2: Autoregulation.' *Journal of Neurosurgery*, **71**, 72–76.

Munro, D. (1928) 'Cerebrospinal fluid pressure in the newborn.' *Journal of the American Medical Association*, **90**, 1688–1689.

Myint, P. T. (1980) 'Tuberculous meningitis and BCG vaccination in Burmese children.' *Journal of Tropical Paediatrics*, **26**, 227–231.

Naughten, E., Newton, R., Weindling, A. M., Bower, B. D. (1981) 'Tuberculous meningitis in children—recent experience in two English centres.' *Lancet*, **2**, 973–975.

Obrist, W. D., Langfitt, T. W., Jaggi, J. L., Cruz, J., Gennarelli, T. A. (1984) 'Cerebral blood flow and metabolism in comatose patients with acute head injury. Relationship to intracranial hypertension.' *Journal of Neurosurgery*, **61**, 241–253.

Patten, B. M., Mandel, J., Bruun, B., Curtin, W., Carter, S. (1971) 'Double-blind study of the effect of dexamethasone on acute stroke.' *Neurology*, **21**, 402.

Paul, F. M. (1961) 'Tuberculosis in BCG vaccinated children in Singapore.' *Archives of Disease in Childhood*, **36**, 530–536.

Petersdorf, R. G., Swarner, D. R., Garcia, M. (1962) 'Studies on the pathogenesis of meningitis: II. Development of meningitis during pneumococcal bacteremia.' *Journal of Clinical Investigation*, **41**, 320–327.

Pollay, M. (1985) 'Blood-brain barrier; cerebral edema.' *In* Wilkins, R. H., Rengachary, S. S. (Eds.) *Neurosurgery*. New York: McGraw-Hill. pp. 70–116.

—— Curl, F. (1967) 'Secretion of cerebrospinal fluid by the ventricular ependyma of the rabbit.' *American Journal of Physiology*, **213**, 1031–1038.

Poser, C. M., Kuiken, B. C. (1968) 'Acute hydrocephalus following *H. influenzae* meningitis.' *Diseases of the Nervous System*, **29**, 823–826.

Posner, J. B., Plum, F. (1967) 'Spinal fluid pH and neurologic symptoms in systemic acidosis.' *New England Journal of Medicine*, **277**, 605–613.

Quincke, H. (1891) 'Über Hydrocephalus.' *Verhandlungen Congresses Innere Medizin*, **10**, 321–340.

Raimondi, A. J., DiRocco, C. (1979) 'The physiopathogenetic basis for the angiographic diagnosis of bacterial infections of the brain and its coverings in children: (i) hepatomeningitis, (ii) cerebritis and brain.' *Child's Brain*, **5**, 1–13; 398–407.

—— Hirschauer, J. (1984) 'Head injury in the infant and toddler: coma scoring and outcome scale.' *Child's Brain*, **11**, 12–35.

Raju, T. N. K., Vidyasagar, D., Torres, C., Grundy, D., Bennett, E. J. (1980) 'Intracranial pressure during intubation and anesthesia.' *Journal of Pediatrics*, **96**, 860–862.

—— Doshi, U. V., Vidyasagar, D. (1982) 'Cerebral perfusion pressure studies in healthy pre-term and term newborn infants.' *Journal of Paediatrics*, **100**, 139–142.

Rao, P. S., Dahm, C. H., Ritter, H. A. (1978) 'Impairment of myocardial performance in endotoxic shock.' *Journal of Molecular Cell Cardiology*, **10**, (Suppl. 1), 8.

Reichman, H. R., Farrell, C. L., Del Maestro, R. F. (1986) 'Effects of steroids and nonsteroid anti-inflammatory agents on vascular permeability in a rat glioma model.' *Journal of Neurosurgery*, **65**, 233.

Reivich, M., Usaacs, G., Evarts, E., Kety, S. (1968) 'The effect of slow wave sleep and REM sleep on regional cerebral blood flow in cats.' *Journal of Neurochemistry*, **15**, 301–306.

Renier, D., Sainte-Rose, C., Marchac, D., Hirsch, J. F. (1982) 'Intracranial pressure in craniostenosis.' *Journal of Neurosurgery*, **57**, 370–377.

Reynolds, D. W., Dweck, H. S., Cassidy, G. (1972) 'Inappropriate antidiuretic hormone secretion in a neonate with meningitis.' *American Journal of Diseases of Children*, **123**, 251–253.

Rich, A. R., McCordock, H. A. (1933) 'The pathogenesis of tuberculous meningitis.' *Johns Hopkins Medical Journal*, **52**, 5–38.

Robinson, J. S. Jr. (1986) 'Failure of glucocorticoids to significantly affect aramine-induced hypertensive opening of the blood-brain barrier.' *Journal of Pediatric Neurosciences*, **2**, 262–268.

Robinson, R. O. (1987) 'Differential diagnosis of Reye's syndrome.' *Developmental Medicine and Child Neurology*, **29**, 110–116.

Rosner, M. J., Becker, D. P. (1984) 'Origin and evolution of plateau waves. Experimental observations and a theoretical model.' *Journal of Neurology*, **60**, 312–324.

Rougemond, J. de, Benabid, A. L., Chirossel, J. P., Barge, M. (1976) 'The brain vasomotor tone index as a prognostic leader in severe head injuries.' *In* Becks, J. W. F., Bosch, D. A., Brock, M. (Eds.) *Intracranial Pressure, III.* Berlin: Springer.

Rougemont, J. D., Ames, A., Nesbitt, F. B., Hoffmann, H. E. (1960) 'Fluid formed by choroid plexus.' *Journal of Neurophysiology*, **23**, 485–495.

Rubin, R. C., Henderson, E. S., Ommaya, A. K., Walker, M. D., Rall, D. P. (1966) 'The production of cerebrospinal fluid in man and its modification by acetazolamide.' *Journal of Neurosurgery*, **25**, 430–436.

Sato, H. (1986) 'Experimental congenital hydrocephalus. Pathogenetic processes in differentiating brain.' *Neurol. I Med. Chir. (Tokyo)*, **26**, 11–18.

—— Sato, N., Tamaki, N., Matsumoto, S. (1988) 'Threshold of cerebral perfusion pressure as a prognostic factor in hydrocephalus during infancy.' *Child's Nervous System*, **4**, 274–278.

Scheidemantel, J., Weis, K. H. (1983) 'Tuberculous meningitis in intensive care.' *Anasthesie, Intensivtherapie, Notfallmedizin*, **18**, 273–275.

Schoeman, J. F., le Roux, D., Bezuidenhout, P. B., Donald, P. R. (1985) 'Intracranial pressure monitoring in tuberculous meningitis: clinical and computerized tomographic correlation.' *Developmental Medicine and Child Neurology*, **27**, 644–654.

Seshia, S. S., Johnston, B., Kasian, G. (1983) 'Non-traumatic coma in childhood: clinical variables in prediction of outcome.' *Developmental Medicine and Child Neurology*, **25**, 493–501.

——Seshia, M. M. K., Sachdeva, R. K. (1977) 'Coma in childhood.' *Developmental Medicine and Child Neurology*, **19**, 614–628.

Shapiro, H. M., Wyte, S. R., Loeser, J. (1974) 'Barbiturate-augmented hypothermia for reduction of persistent intracranial hypertension.' *Journal of Neurosurgery*, **40**, 90.

Shapiro, K., Marmarou, A., Shulman, K. (1979) 'Characterization of clinical CSF dynamics and neural axis compliance using the pressure-volume index: I. The normal pressure-volume index.' *Annals of Neurology*, **7**, 508–514.

—— Takei, F., Fried, A., Kohn, I. (1985) 'Experimental feline hydrocephalus. The role of biomechanical changes in ventricular enlargement in cats.' *Journal of Neurosurgery*, **63**, 82–87.

—— Fried, A. (1986) 'Changing biomechanical properties of the hydrocephalic brain in childhood.' *Journal of pediatric Neurosciences*, **2**, 105–115.

Shaywitz, B. A., Rothstein, P., Venes, J. L. (1980) 'Monitoring and management of increased intracranial pressure in Reye syndrome: results in 29 children.' *Pediatrics*, **66**, 198–204.

Shortland-Webb, W. R. (1968) 'Proteus and coliform meningoencephalitis in neonates.' *Journal of Clinical Pathology*, **21**, 422–431.

Sidbury, J. B. (1920) 'The importance of lumbar puncture haemorrhage of the newborn.' *Archives of Pediatrics*, **37**, 545–553.

Simpson, D., Reilly, P. (1982) 'Paediatric coma scale.' *Lancet*, **2**, 450.

Sinclair, J. F., (1988) 'The management of fulminant meningococcal septicaemia in children.' *Intensive Care World*, **5**, 89–91.

—— Skeach, C. H., Halworth, D. (1987) 'Progress of meningococcal septicaemia.' *Lancet*, **2**, 38.

Sklar, F. H., Reisch, J., Elashvilli, T., Smith, T., Long, D. M. (1980) 'Effects of pressure on cerebrospinal fluid formation: non-steady state measurements in dogs.' *American Journal of Physiology*, **2394**, 277–284.

Skjodt, T., Svendsen, J., Jacobsen, E. B., Torfing, K. F. (1987) 'Cerebral atrophy in younger persons: a comparative study between clinical examinations and computed tomography.' *Clinical Radiology*, **38**, 367–370.

Skoldenberg, B., Forsgren, M., Alestig, K., Bergstrom, T., Burman, L., Forkman, A., Lövgren, K., Norrby, R., Stiernstedt, G., Forsgren, M., Bergstrom, T., Dahlqvist, E., Fryden, A., Norlin, K., Olding-Stenkvist, E., Uhnoo, I., De Vahl, K. (1984) 'Acyclovir versus vidarabine in herpes simplex encephalitis. Randomized multi-center study in consecutive Swedish patients.' *Lancet*, **2**, 707–711.

Slack, J. (1980) 'Coning and lumbar puncture.' *Lancet*, **2**, 474–475.

Smith, A. L. (1975) 'Tuberculous meningitis in childhood.' *Medical Journal of Australia*, **1**, 57–60.

Smith, H. V., Vollum, R. L. (1954) 'The diagnosis of tuberculous meningitis.' *British Medical Bulletin*, **10**, 140–144.

Smith, J. B., Groover, R. V., Klass, D. W., Houser, O. W. (1977) 'Multicystic cerebral degeneration in neonatal herpes simplex virus encephalitis.' *American Journal of Diseases of Children*, **131**, 568–572.

Smith, J. D., Landing, B. H. (1960) 'Mechanism of brain damage in *H. influenzae* meningitis.' *Journal of Neuropathology and Experimental Neurology*, **19**, 248–265.

Snodgrass, S. R., Lorenzo, A. V. (1972) 'Temperature and cerebrospinal fluid production rate.'

American Journal of Physiology, **222**, 1524–1527.

Snyder, R. D. (1984) 'Ventriculomegaly in childhood bacterial meningitis.' *Neuropediatrics, Journal of Pediatric Neurobiology, Neurology and Neurosurgery*, **15**, 136–138.

Spina-Franca, A. (1963) 'Variacoes fisiologicas de pressao do liquido cefalorraqueano na cisterna magna.' *Arquivos de Neuro-psiquiatria*, **21**, 19–24.

Starmark, J. E., Holmgren, E., Stalhammar, D. (1988) 'Current reporting of responsiveness in acute cerebral disorders.' *Journal of Neurosurgery*, **69**, 692–698.

Stephenson, J. B. P. (1985) 'Timing of lumbar puncture in severe childhood meningitis.' *British Medical Journal*, **291**, 1123.

Stovring, J., Snyder, R. D. (1980) 'Computed tomography in childhood bacterial meningitis.' *Journal of Pediatrics*, **96**, 820–823.

Tandon, P. N., Rao, M. A. P., Pathak, S. N., Dhar, J. (1973) 'RHISA cisternography in the management of tuberculous meningitis.' *In Tuberculosis of the Nervous System*. Indian Academy of Medical Science. p. 55.

—— Rao, M. A. P., Banerju, A. K., Pathak, S. N., Dhar, J. (1975) 'Isotope scanning of the cerebrospinal fluid pathways in tuberculous meningitis.' *Journal of the Neurological Sciences*, **25**, 401–413.

—— Tandon, H. D. (1975) 'Tuberculous meningitis. A continuing challenge.' *Journal of All India Institute of Medical Sciences*, **2**, 99–103.

Tasker, R. C., Matthew, D. J., Helms, P., Dinwiddie, R., Boyd, S. (1988) 'Monitoring in non-traumatic coma. Part I: invasive intracranial measurements.' *Archives of Disease in Childhood*, **63**, 888–894.

Taylor, R. D., Corcosan, A. C., Page, I. H. (1954) 'Increased cerebrospinal fluid pressure and papilledema in malignant hypertension.' *Archives of Internal Medicine*, **93**, 818–820.

Teasdale, G., Jennett, B. (1974) 'Assessment of coma and impaired consciousness. A practical scale.' *Lancet*, **1**, 290–291.

—— Murray, G., Parker, L., Jennett, B. (1979) 'Adding up the Glasgow Coma Score.' *Acta Neurochirugica*, **28**, 13–16.

—— Jennett, B., Murray, L., Murray, G. (1983) 'Glasgow Coma Scale. To sum or not to sum?' *Lancet*, **2**, 678.

Tourtellotte, W. W., Haerer, A. F., Heller, G. L., Somers, J. E. (1964) *Post Lumbar Puncture Headaches*. Springfield: Thomas.

van Vught, A. J., Troost, J., Willemse, J. (1976) 'Hypertensive encephalopathy in childhood.' *Neuropädiatrie*, **7**, 92–100.

Visudhiphan, P., Chiemchanya, S. (1979) 'Hydrocephalus in tuberculous meningitis in children: Treatment with acetazolamide and repeated lumbar puncture.' *Journal of Pediatirics*, **95**, 657–660.

Waters, K., Gillis, J. (1987) 'Meningitis presenting as hypertension.' *Archives of Disease in Childhood*, **62**, 191–193.

Weiss, M. H., Werlman, N. (1978) 'Modulation of CSF production by alterations in cerebral perfusion pressure.' *Archives of Neurology*, **35**, 527–529.

Welch, K. (1975) 'The principles of physiology of the cerebrospinal fluid in relation to hydrocephalus including normal pressure hydrocephalus.' *In* Friedlander, W. J. (Ed.) *Current Reviews, Advances in Neurology, Vol 13*. New York: Raven. pp. 247–332.

—— (1978) 'Normal pressure hydrocephalus in infants and children: a re-appraisal.' *Zeitschrift für Kinderchirurgie*, **25**, 319–324.

—— (1980) 'The intracranial pressure in infants.' *Journal of Neurosurgery*, **52**, 693–699.

—— Friedman, V. (1960) 'The cerebrospinal fluid valves.' *Brain*, **83**, 454–469.

Whitley, R. W., Soong, S. J., Alford, C. A., Hirsch, M. S., Schooley, R. (1985) 'Treatment of biopsy proven herpes simplex encephalitis: vidarabine versus acyclovir.' *Clinical Research*, **33**, 422A (Abstract).

von Wild, K., Porksen, C. (1980) 'Non-invasive technique for monitoring intracranial pressure via the fontanelle in premature infants and newborns with hydrocephalus.' *Zeitschrift für Kinderchirurgie*, **31**, 348–353.

Williams, C. P. S., Swanson, A. G., Chapman, J. T. (1964) 'Brain swelling with acute purulent meningitis.' *Pediatrics*, **49**, 220–227.

Yager, J. Y., Johnston, B., Seshia, S. S. (1990) 'Coma scales in pediatric practice.' *American Journal of Diseases in Childhood (in press)*.

8

INTRACRANIAL PRESSURE AND CEREBRAL BLOODFLOW IN NON-TRAUMATIC COMA IN CHILDHOOD

F. J. Kirkham

The prognosis for many serious childhood diseases has improved in recent years with the advent of antibiotics for serious infections, surgery for congenital heart disease, and dialysis and transplant for chronic renal failure. Paediatric intensive care is now commonplace, and the outcome is often determined by the neurological condition of the child rather than by the degree of systemic upset. Considerable interest has therefore been generated in cerebrally orientated intensive care directed towards maintaining an adequate level of cerebral bloodflow to prevent secondary ischaemic damage, preventing herniation of the brain due to intracranial hypertension, and preventing other poorly understood secondary insults to the brain of the comatose child. Once the patient is unconscious, few neurological signs may be elicited (Plum and Posner 1980), and although careful clinical assessment may be of some prognostic use (Levy *et al*. 1981, Seshia *et al*. 1983, Mullie *et al*. 1988), it is rarely possible to predict outcome with a sufficient degree of accuracy within 72 hours of admission (Reinmuth *et al*. 1988), or to assess the response to treatment precisely. Methods of monitoring the patient have therefore been developed, which may offer more accurate early prognosis, some insight into the pathophysiology of brain insults and their secondary consequences, and may allow more rational minute-to-minute management of the individual patient, although outcome has yet to be shown to be improved. There is much more clinical experience with ICP monitoring, and therefore the role of this technique in managing the individual patient in non-traumatic coma will be discussed. The measurement of CBF is technically difficult and is liable to serious errors which make results difficult to interpret. CBF measurement has not found a major role in intensive care, but an understanding of the pathophysiology of the cerebral circulation in coma is essential if management is to be improved.

Intracranial pressure
Measurement of ICP has been performed in intensive care units for over 30 years, most widely in the management of head injury, but also in non-traumatic coma in children and adults. Most published work has been from retrospective series in individual centres and must therefore be interpreted with some caution, particularly as management protocols may change frequently. More recently, authors have quoted data on CPP, the difference between MAP and ICP.

Conditions associated with intracranial hypertension
(1) PRIMARY INTRACRANIAL DISEASE
CNS infections. Intracranial hypertension certainly occurs in childhood CNS infections. There is still a significant morbidity and mortality in meningitis (Feigin and Dodge 1976, Herson and Todd 1977), particularly in those children whose level of consciousness deteriorates. Evidence of brain herniation may be found at post-mortem examination (Adams *et al.* 1948, Dodge and Swartz 1965), and may be apparent clinically in some cases of meningitis due to *Haemophilus influenzae* and *Streptococcus pneumoniae* (Horwitz *et al.* 1980). This is thought to be due to ventricular dilatation (Stovring and Snyder 1980) secondary to obstruction of CSF absorption pathways and to cerebral oedema and vasomotor disturbance (Fuhrmeister *et al.* 1980). When measured by the lumbar route, mean resting CSF pressure has been shown to be increased in the acute phase of the illness in most patients (Dodge and Swartz 1965, Belsey *et al.* 1969, Minns *et al.* 1989), decreasing over the following few weeks (Fuhrmeister *et al.* 1980). ICP is high in unconscious children with meningitis (Nugent *et al.* 1979, Goitein *et al.* 1983b, Rebaud *et al.* 1988, Pesso *et al.* 1988). Although often amenable to treatment with intravenous hypertonic solutions (Williams *et al.* 1964, Horwitz *et al.* 1980) or CSF drainage from the ventricles (Goitein and Tamir 1983), intracranial hypertension appears to be a significant cause of death and brain damage (Horwitz *et al.* 1980). It is more important to be aware of the possibility of cerebral herniation, particularly after the diagnostic lumbar puncture and probably after seizures, rather than to monitor ICP, as in most cases this complication occurs soon after admission (Horwitz *et al.* 1980). It is not certain whether prolonged monitoring of the unconscious patient with meningitis is of any benefit, although if performed by the intraventricular method, it allows rapid drainage of CSF in response to ICP spikes (Goitein and Tamir 1983). There is a risk that the inflamed brain may bleed, however. With due care, CSF drainage may also be achieved by the lumbar route, as the hydrocephalus is usually communicating, although many clinicians would prefer to treat with regular small doses of mannitol, occasionally measuring the lumbar CSF pressure.

Coma is a poor prognostic sign in all forms of encephalitis (Kennard and Swash 1981) including that due to herpes simplex virus infection, for which the prognosis has undoubtedly improved since the introduction of effective antiviral agents (Whitley *et al.* 1986). Of 25 children with a diagnosis of encephalitis in a recent series, intracranial hypertension was suspected in five on clinical grounds (decerebrate posturing, papilloedema) and was measured as greater than 20mmHg in three, including one infant in whom there were no clinical signs (Kennedy *et al.* 1987). Chandler and Kindt (1976) found only mild intracranial hypertension (less than 23mmHg) with no evidence of plateau waves in two adults with encephalitis (one due to HSV) who both did well. More recently, sustained intracranial hypertension has been shown to be associated with deteriorating level of consciousness in some adults with encephalitis (mainly HSV), and was maximal late in the illness with the peak ICP occurring on the 12th day of illness on average (Barnett *et al.* 1988a). In a paediatric series, raised ICP was universal in acute primary encephalitis and was common in post-infectious encephalitis (Rebaud *et al.* 1988).

When measured directly in CNS infections in children, opening ICP was often high, but was a poor indicator of the maximal ICP sustained (Goitein *et al.* 1983*b*). There is a good case for monitoring ICP in children with CNS infections whose Glasgow coma score, modified for paediatric use (Gordon *et al.* 1983) is less than 9, and for continuing to monitor until full consciousness is regained. Encephalopathy may also be a feature of systemic infections, such as *Shigella flexneri* gastro-enteritis (Sandyk and Brennan 1983), and the criteria for monitoring should be the same.

Cerebrovascular disease. Intracerebral haematoma in childhood is associated with a high mortality and morbidity (Livingston and Brown 1986), particularly if haemorrhage is intracerebellar or purely intraventricular, or is associated with a tumour or bleeding diathesis. The prognosis for supratentorial bleeds secondary to angiomatous malformations or aneurysms appeared to be good in this series. ICP has been shown to be raised in comatose adults with intracerebral haematomata (Ropper and King 1984, 1985), and although the pathology is different in children and published data are not available, ICP monitoring is advisable in those with a deteriorating level of consciousness and after operation for removal of arterio-venous malformations when severe brain-swelling may occur (Batjer *et al.* 1988). RICP is also a feature of stroke patients with deteriorating levels of consciousness (Ropper and Shafran 1984) and may be worth monitoring in paediatric cases, at least as part of a research protocol. The ICP may also be raised after subarachnoid haemorrhage (Mullan *et al.* 1978), but monitoring and management may both be associated with a high risk of rebleeding. The evidence suggests that the main aetiological association with delayed neurological deficit in patients who would otherwise be predicted to do well is vasospasm of the large cerebral arteries (Wilkins 1980).

Status epilepticus ICP rises during generalised seizures in childhood (tonic-clonic, absence, adversive and myoclonic), and may remain high for some time after the electrical activity has ceased (Minns and Brown 1978). The time course of the ICP wave appears to be dependent on the frequency of the epileptogenic spikes and the brain compliance and it is likely that prolonged seizures in coma are associated with significant intracranial hypertension (Gabor *et al.* 1984) although there is little direct evidence for this in humans. Children who do not recover consciousness within an hour of the termination of a prolonged seizure should receive a single dose of mannitol and most then wake up. If this does not happen or status is continuing, the child should be ventilated and carefully monitored (blood pressure, EEG and sometimes ICP).

(2) SYSTEMIC DISEASE ASSOCIATED WITH COMA

Hepatic encephalopathy. Cerebral oedema has been found at post-mortem examination in a large number of patients dying from fulminant hepatic failure, especially in patients less than 30 years old and in those who were in stage IV coma (Ware *et al.* 1971). In an animal model, ICP was found to rise progressively after surgical devascularisation (Hanid *et al.* 1979), whereas in humans, ICP monitored extradurally rose intermittently and appeared amenable to treatment (Hanid *et al.* 1980, Canalese *et al.* 1982, Ede and Williams 1986).

Renal disease. Encephalopathy which is probably due to cerebral oedema (Winney *et al.* 1986) may also occur as a complication of haemodialysis, either for acute renal failure or in patients with chronic renal failure commencing dialysis. Coma occurring as a complication of haemolytic-uraemic syndrome is of grave prognostic significance (Bale *et al.* 1980), particularly if the patient's respiratory pattern is abnormal (Bos *et al.* 1985). The following pathologies have been described: hypoxic-ischaemic damage and cerebral oedema (Rooney *et al.* 1971), multiple microvascular thrombi (Upadhyaya *et al.* 1980) and major cerebral vessel thrombosis (Trevathan and Dooling 1987). ICP was raised in the three children with the latter pathology, and is probably worth monitoring in all deeply unconscious children with the condition, as the prognosis is not necessarily poor (Steele *et al.* 1983) even for those with focal infarction demonstrated on CT scan (Crisp *et al.* 1981, Steinberg *et al.* 1986) and some morbidity and mortality may be prevented by careful attention to fluid and electrolyte balance, guided by ICP measurement. RICP may also be a feature of hypertensive encephalopathy (with or without superimposed ischaemic encephalopathy from over-rapid reduction of blood pressure) and may lead to brain herniation (Griswold *et al.* 1981).

Diabetic ketoacidosis. Deterioration of conscious level during treatment for diabetic ketoacidosis is a well recognised phenomenon, and appears to be associated with raised CSF pressure (Clements *et al.* 1971) and with cerebral oedema at post-mortem examination (Young and Bradley 1967). Subclinical cerebral oedema may be quite common (Krane *et al.* 1985), and paradoxically brain-swelling is maximal when the patient's biochemistry is improving, possibly because conditions favour Na^+/H^+ exchange and therefore Na^+ entry into the cell (Van der Meulen *et al.* 1987). The role of rapid fluid administration in precipitating brain herniation is controversial, but a recent paper pointed out a significant inverse relationship between the timing of herniation and the rate of fluid administration in the published cases, with excessive secretion of antidiuretic hormone as a probable additional factor (Duck and Wyatt 1988). Harris *et al.* (1988) recommended careful calculation of the rate of rehydration, with an emphasis on slow, steady correction of fluid and electrolyte imbalance. Failure to regain consciousness in parallel with biochemical improvement or clinical signs of incipient brain herniation are indications for urgent management of presumed cerebral oedema with mannitol (Franklin *et al.* 1982) and a reduction in the rate of fluid administration. ICP monitoring might be worthwhile in those at greatest risk of this complication (Harris *et al.* 1988). Cerebral oedema is also a feature of other metabolic encephalopathies which are discussed elsewhere in this volume.

Burns. Encephalopathy, with seizures and/or coma, is well recognised after major and relatively minor burns and scalds in children, with a reported incidence of 5 to 14 per cent in published series (Antoon *et al.* 1972, Mohnot *et al.* 1982). Cerebral oedema with cerebellar herniation has been described at post-mortem examination (Emery and Campbell-Reid 1962), and the condition may also be associated with significant neurological morbidity. The aetiology appears to be multifactorial, with hyponatraemia, hypocalcaemia and sepsis often implicated. It is possible that the incidence and severity may be decreasing with improved management of fluid and electrolyte balance (Mohnot *et al.* 1982), although encephalopathy is still a significant problem in children with major burns, particularly if exacerbated by hypoxia due to smoke inhalation. ICP was monitored in one child in Mohnot's series and in three by Kay *et al.* (1986), and was found to be significantly elevated in one. As Kay pointed out, rational management of fluid balance was very much easier when ICP was monitored. This may be important in preventing other serious neurological complications of burns, such as central pontine myelinolysis, which may be associated with high serum osmolality (McKee *et al.* 1988). ICP should therefore be monitored in those who are unconscious.

(3) ISCHAEMIA
Cardiac arrest. Hypoxic ischaemic encephalopathy is not uncommon in childhood and prognosis is poor (Seshia *et al.* 1979, Torphy *et al.* 1984). An additional ischaemic insult worsens the prognosis for other encephalopathies, such as that occurring after head injury (Graham *et al.* 1989). In our series of 89 patients studied after cardiac arrest in three London centres between 1982 and 1985, only 39 per cent recovered consciousness within one month. Twenty-seven per cent died a cardiac death whilst in coma, and the others suffered either brain death or remained in a vegetative state.

In animal experiments, where ICP has been monitored for a few hours after global ischaemia, the ICP (measured subdurally) was found to be high for the first few minutes and then to fall for the next few hours, subsequently rising slowly (Snyder *et al.* 1975). EEG recovery was not usually monitored, and it is noteworthy that ventricular pressure was higher than subdural. Clinical experience is rather different. Intracranial hypertension was a feature of all the patients with hypoxic-ischaemic encephalopathy studied by Langfitt *et al.* (1971). Senter *et al.* (1981) found that intracranial hypertension was a feature of ischaemic, but not of hypoxic, insults. Neither of these authors monitored CPP.

There is some experimental (Raichle 1983) and clinical (Seshia *et al.* 1979, 1983; Constantinou *et al.* 1989) evidence of secondary deterioration after ischaemia. In our series, 23 patients showed partial recovery of consciousness, recovery of brainstem function, and recovery of the EEG to diffuse slowing or better, and then deteriorated wtih poor eventual neurological outcome. Factors associated with this secondary deterioration included prolonged seizures (longer than 20 minutes), a positive fluid balance of more than 7 per cent and a mean arterial pressure, averaged over 24 hours, of less than 50mmHg. ICP was monitored in 18 and was persistently raised (mean ICP greater than 10mmHg) in 10 of these. The two children with good outcome, and the child who made a cognitive recovery but was left with a spastic quadriparesis (probably due to a posterior fossa haematoma), all had mean ICP between 9 and 15mmHg and maximum ICP up to 35mmHg (*i.e.* above the normal range—Minns *et al.* 1989) but mean CPP was maintained above 60mmHg and CPP never fell below 37mmHg. In the other 15 children, either the EEG prior to ICP monitoring suggested a poor outcome (Tasker *et al.* 1988*b*) or mean CPP could not be maintained above 60mmHg and minimum CPP above 40mmHg because of poor cardiac function or persistent intracranial hypertension.

Whether or not intracranial hypertension is a preventable cause of secondary deterioration is, however, much more controversial. There is very little data available, but many groups have given up monitoring and aggressively managing intracranial hypertension in children with hypoxic-ischaemic encephalopathy for fear of increasing the number of children left severely handicapped or in a persistent vegetative state. There are other possible candidates for a role in secondary deterioration *e.g.* excitotoxins (Rothman and Olney 1986) and calcium (Cheung *et al.* 1986), but these may have an effect on CPP, and it may be important to measure this parameter when giving putative brain resuscitative agents within the 'therapeutic window'. There is a good case for monitoring ICP as part of research protocols designed to improve outcome in this important group of patients. Monitoring should also be considered for the individual child who has been well resuscitated using modern cardiopulmonary resuscitation techniques, in whom the EEG has recovered to diffuse slowing or better, but who remains unconscious or sedated for ventilation, providing that CPP is also frequently recorded and is managed appropriately. As adequate CBF is very likely to have been restored in this group and may even be high, thereby increasing CBV, ICP is likely to be increased. The pathophysiology of hypoxic-ischaemic injury is complex and may be variable from patient to patient, necessitating individually tailored treatment which is impossible to manage without full systemic and cerebral monitoring. Very small changes in MAP and ICP may be critical if CPP and therefore CBF is only just adequate for metabolic demand, as is commonly the case in these children.

Near-drowning is a specialised case of hypoxic-ischaemic encephalopathy. The prognosis for the child pulled from the water apparently dead is excellent (Pearn 1985), provided that CPR is commenced immediately, that the child gasps within 40 minutes of rescue and regains consciousness soon afterwards. The prognosis is much worse for the child admitted to casualty or the emergency room deeply unconscious with fixed dilated pupils, requiring continuing cardiopulmonary resuscitation and with an arterial pH of less than 7.00 (Peterson 1977, Kruus *et al.* 1979, Frates 1981, Dean and Kaufman 1981, Oakes *et al.* 1982, Orlowski 1987) especially if there is little recovery by the time of admission to the intensive care unit (Turner and Levin 1985). However, none of these poor prognostic indicators precludes a good outcome (Nussbaum 1985), and apparently miraculous recoveries have occurred, mainly of children who have drowned in very cold water (Conn *et al.* 1980, Montes and Conn 1980, Nugent and Rogers 1980, Young *et al.* 1980).

Intracranial hypertension is certainly a common but not universal feature of the encephalopathy which follows serious near-drowning incidents (Dean and McComb 1981, Nussbaum and Galant 1983), although again, whether or not measurement is of prognostic use (Nussbaum 1985, Frewen *et al.* 1985*b*, Bell *et al.* 1985) or treatment prevents secondary deterioration (Conn *et al.* 1979, Bruce *et al.* 1983, Sarnaik *et al.* 1985) is much more controversial. Some units previously recommending the routine monitoring and aggressive treatment of ICP after near-drowning have recently become more conservative in their approach (Bohn *et al.* 1986). It must be remembered, however, that the prognosis for those admitted unconscious to emergency rooms has apparently improved over the past decade,

TABLE 8.I

Early signs of cerebral herniation

Level of consciousness (Use modified coma scale)	Loss of $\left\{\begin{array}{l}\text{comprehensive}\\\text{expressive}\end{array}\right\}$ language Agitation Drowsiness Coma (eyes closed)
Posture/tone	Bilateral/unilateral hypertonia Decorticate posturing Decerebrate posturing
Plantar response	Bilaterally/unilaterally extensor
Eye movements	Unilateral III palsy (eye down and out, severe ptosis, pupil dilated) Unilateral/bilateral VI palsy
Oculocephalic/oculovestibular responses	Conjugate Dysconjugate
Pupil size	Small Asymmetrical
Pupil reaction to light	Bilaterally/unilaterally sluggish
Respiration	Deep sighs or yawns Cheyne-Stokes Spontaneous hyperventilation Shallow or irregular respiration

N.B. Papilloedema is rare in acute intracranial hypertension.

particularly in cold water near-drowning, and although much of this may be due to improved CPR by casualty officers, some may be attributable to improved management of the cerebral insult. Adequate controlled trials are required before aggressive management is abandoned too hastily (Nussbaum and Maggi 1988). Criteria for ICP monitoring should be the same as for hypoxic-ischaemic encephalopathy.

Indications for and methods of monitoring ICP
Monitoring of ICP in non-traumatic coma is controversial; it is certainly more important to treat urgently any underlying cause, such as meningitis, than to insert an ICP monitor. Increased awareness of potential cerebral problems complicating life-threatening diseases in children may mean that intracranial hypertension can be prevented by careful management of fluid and electrolyte balance and ventilation. Many patients on paediatric wards and ITUS become unconscious during the management of their underlying disease. It is essential that paediatricians are able to recognise deterioration in level of consciousness and are familiar with the clinical signs of early brain herniation (Plum and Posner 1980) (Table 8.I) so that appropriate emergency management (Table 8.II) is instituted. The most important priority in this situation is maintenance of the systemic circulation with plasma (20ml/kg) and inotropic agents (*e.g.* dobutamine 10 to 20µg/kg/min), particularly in children who have had a cardiac arrest or who are shocked. Treatment of presumed intracranial hypertension, with hyperventilation to a PCO_2 of 25 to 30mmHg (3.3 to 4.0kPa), fluid restriction to 60 per cent of requirements (*no* hypo-osmolar fluids) and a bolus dose of mannitol (1g/kg, provided that there is not established renal

TABLE 8.II

Resuscitation prior to ICP monitoring (essential for transfer)

1. Maintenance of systemic circulation with plasma (20ml/kg) and inotropes (*e.g.* dobutamine 20μg/kg/min)
2. Ventilation to PCO_2 3.5kPa with adequate oxygenation
3. Fluid restriction to 60 per cent of requirements (no hypo-osmolar fluids)
4. Bolus dose of 20 per cent mannitol (1g/kg) if circulation allows
5. Aggressive management of seizures
   —intravenous diazepam (0.2 to 0.3mg/kg dose never to be exceeded in an unventilated patient)
   —rectal paraldehyde (0.3ml/kg in an equal volume of arachic oil)
   —phenytoin (loading 20mg/kg given over 30 minutes
6. Maintenance of normothermia
7. Preliminary management of presumed cause (*e.g.* antibiotics, acyclovir)

TABLE 8.III

ICP monitoring in non-traumatic coma

Indications
Glasgow coma score <9
Deteriorating conscious level
EEG/evoked potentials present

Contra-indications
Very unstable circulation
Bleeding diathesis (especially if platelets $<1 \times 10^9/L$)

failure) should be instituted. Clinical seizures should be controlled with bolus doses of intravenous diazepam (0.2 to 0.3mg/kg; this dose never to be exceeded in an unventilated patient) and/or paraldehyde and by loading with a slow infusion of intravenous phenytoin (20mg/kg over 30 minutes, then 5 to 10mg/kg/day with dosage guided by daily plasma levels).

There is usually a delay before an ICP monitor can be inserted, during which time the patient can be assessed clinically, as monitoring can be avoided in the patient who wakes up completely (GCS greater than 12) with at least some form of verbal response such as crying (Simpson and Reilly 1982) or recognition of surroundings and/or parents (Gordon *et al.* 1983). Ideally an EEG should also be performed after treatment has continued for a few hours, so that patients in whom the prognosis is hopeless are not monitored. If the patient has become unconscious in a peripheral unit, he should be transferred with preliminary treatment in progress to a centre with full facilities for neurological intensive care. With these provisos, ICP monitoring should certainly be considered in all children in deep coma (GCS less than 9) for more than six hours (Table 8.III). As the child's condition may be very unstable when the decision to monitor ICP is made, it is probably best to insert the monitor on the intensive care unit. The method of McWilliam and Stephenson (1984) may be used, as it is reliable, is subject to few complications in experienced hands, may be inserted in any age of child, allows CSF drainage and is inexpensive. If the ventricles cannot be located after two attempts, as is sometimes the case in non-traumatic coma if they are compressed by brain-swelling, an intraparenchymal fibre-optic monitor (Ostrup *et al.* 1987) may be passed along the same track. There is often an associated coagulation disorder, particularly in hepatic failure and sometimes in severe infections, so that the potential benefits of monitoring must be weighed against the additional risks. In fact, epidural monitoring of ICP appears to be reasonably safe (Hanid *et al.* 1980, Canalese *et al.* 1982, Ede *et al.* 1986), and should therefore be the method of choice in this situation.

Pathophysiology of intracranial hypertension in non-traumatic coma
Intracranial hypertension may lead either to brain shift if there is a pressure gradient between different areas of the CNS or to ischaemia if CPP is inadequate for metabolic demand (Miller *et al.* 1972). The consequence of the former is damage to the brainstem (Plum and Posner 1980), and brainstem death if the situation is not reversed within minutes. Inadequate cerebral perfusion usually leads to neocortical cerebral damage (Brierley *et al.* 1971) which, if severe, may result in the vegetative state (Jennett and Plum 1972). The aim of management is to prevent both these outcomes, but particularly the latter, which has appalling consequences for the patient and his family.

Cerebral haemodynamics in non-traumatic coma
Measurement of CBF
1. DIRECT CEREBRAL BLOODFLOW AND METABOLISM TECHNIQUES
Since much of the secondary damage occurring in these situations is probably due to ischaemia, it would be preferable to monitor CBF and metabolism in addition to, or even instead of, ICP and CPP. The difficulty is that although there are several techniques for measuring CBF, there are problems with methodology (Kirsch *et al.* 1985) and none is suitable for routine use in the intensive care unit. Most rely on the use of radioactive isotopes, and the techniques cannot be repeated frequently because of the cumulative dosage and because the isotope must be cleared from the body before the next dose is given. There is very little data available in normal children (Kennedy and Sokoloff 1957, Settergren *et al.* 1980, Chugani *et al.* 1987) because of the ethical difficulties. There are serious doubts about the validity of techniques which rely upon the equilibration of a tracer between blood and brain, as the partition coefficient for damaged brain may well be different from that for normal brain and may change during the course of the illness. Very interesting information is beginning to emerge from studies of cerebral metabolism using PET (Powers and Raichle 1985), for example in patients in the recovery phase of head injury (Langfitt *et al.* 1986) or those remaining in a persistent vegetative state (Levy *et al.* 1987) and from magnetic resonance spectroscopy in animals (Crockard *et al.* 1987, Gutierrez and Andry 1989), but there are practical difficulties (Frackowiak 1986, Barnett *et al.* 1988*b*) in maintaining support for the unconscious child in an unstable condition for the duration of such a scan. It may also be possible to monitor cerebral metabolism by combining measurement of $CMRO_2$ and cerebral lactate production (Robertson *et al.* 1987, 1989) or using near infra-red spectroscopy (Brazy and Lewis 1986, Wyatt *et al.* 1986, Brazy 1988), but these methods are in the very early stages of development. At present the most practical

techniques are those which give indirect information about the cerebral circulation such as Doppler ultrasound of the intracranial arteries and continous · EEG monitoring.

2. INDIRECT TECHNIQUES FOR OBTAINING INFORMATION ABOUT THE CEREBRAL CIRCULATION

The *transcranial Doppler (*TCD) ultrasound technique was described by Aaslid and his colleagues (1982). The middle cerebral artery (MCA) is insonated from the temporal bone and the backscattered Doppler signals are displayed in sonogram format with time on the abscissa, frequency on the ordinate and the trace darkness proportional to signal amplitude. Velocity may be reliably (Gillard *et al.* 1986) and reproducibly (Padayachee *et al.* 1986) measured from the MCA sonogram outline of maximum frequency over the cardiac cycle, as the angle between vessel and probe is small. Difficulty may be experienced in obtaining signals in elderly adults (Ringelstein 1988), but this does not appear to be a problem in young children (Bode and Wais 1988). Flow varies directly with the square of the radius of the artery, which cannot be measured at the present time. Under controlled conditions Lindegaard *et al.* (1987) showed in selected patients that velocity is directly related to flow measured with an electromagnetic flowmeter, but with a slope significantly different from 1 and an intercept significantly different from 0. In the unconscious patient, the diameter of the MCA may well be different from normal, particularly after subarachnoid haemorrhage and head injury where vasospasm is likely. Velocity is no longer proportional to flow, but TCD may be used to monitor the time course of vasospasm as blood velocity increases when flowing through narrowed vessels (Seiler *et al.* 1986, Compton *et al.* 1987).

When ICP is very high, there are obvious changes in the shape of the sonogram; indeed when CPP is close to zero, a characteristic waveform with reverse flow throughout diastole, is usually seen (Kirkham *et al.* 1987*a*, Hassler *et al.* 1988). Attempts to monitor ICP or CPP by following changes in sonogram shape, expressed either as the resistance index, s-D/s where s is the systolic peak and D the diastolic peak (Klingelhofer *et al.* 1988) or Fourier analysis of the sonogram outline and of the arterial pressure waveform (Aaslid *et al.* 1986) have met with limited success. Reider and his colleagues from Tubingen (data presented at the second international conference on TCD—Salzburg 1988) showed that ICP measured using an index derived from the latter method of analysis correlated poorly ($r = 0.51$ using linear regression analysis) with ICP measured directly in head-injured patients. The monitoring of dynamic changes in MCA velocity, in response to changes in PCO_2, ICP or CPP is more likely to offer clinically useful information (Giulioni *et al.* 1988).

There is evidence that changes in CBF produced by changing carbon dioxide may be measured in normal patients using the transcranial technique (Markwalder *et al.* 1984, Kirkham *et al.* 1986). Most of the resistance changes due to altering carbon dioxide take place in the small vessels, not the large basal arteries, which probably explains the finding that values for carbon dioxide reactivity measured using TCD are very similar to those obtained using CBF techniques. Carbon dioxide reactivity may be very abnormal in coma, and it has proved possible to use the abnormalities demonstrated using TCD to predict outcome and possibly to guide management (see below). Despite the limitations of the technique, there is preliminary evidence that it is clinically useful.

EEG and cerebral function monitoring. Another approach to obtaining information about the cerebral microcirculation indirectly is to monitor the EEG (Talwar and Torres 1988). The new model of cerebral function analysing monitor (CFAM, Medaid Ltd) which analyses amplitude and frequency of the EEG (Maynard and Jenkinson 1984, Prior and Maynard 1986) provides a substantial amount of information immediately available at the bedside, but it is essential that the trace is interpreted by someone with experience who is able to recognise artefacts and technical problems. Abnormal patterns of EEG activity with prognostic significance may be recognised on single- or dual-channel monitors, but the findings should be confirmed by conventional EEG whenever possible, although this requires the provision of a round-the-clock service.

Pathophysiology of the cerebral circulation and possible mechanisms of secondary deterioration in non-traumatic coma
Very few studies of CBF and metabolism have been performed in the unconscious patient, and the data from animals are conflicting and controversial. The main interest from the clinical point of view lies in possible mechanisms underlying secondary deterioration; those related to changes in CBF and metabolism in pathological situations will be briefly reviewed here.

1. ISCHAEMIA
CBF changes on reperfusion after ischaemia in animal experiments. In a model of reperfusion after global ischaemia, Ames et al. (1968) described the no-reflow phenomenon, in part at least related to hypotension (Cantu et al. 1969) and probably also to increased blood viscosity (Fischer 1973). If hypotension is prevented, most animal data suggest that after ischaemia there is an initial brief period of hyperperfusion when if global CBF is greater than 40ml/100g/min, EEG recovery is likely (Hossmann 1988). This is followed by a period of hypoperfusion (Snyder et al. 1975) when global CBF and metabolism are reduced. This appears to be secondary to an increase in vascular tone rather than to intracranial hypertension (Snyder et al. 1975; Miller et al. 1980a,b; Schmidt-Kastner et al. 1987). Recent evidence suggests that during this period, there may be focal areas of low, normal and high flow adjacent to one another, changing temporally and spatially, but the relationship between flow and metabolism (and in particular, whether the former is adequate for the latter) is ill understood (Moossy et al. 1988). In interpreting the animal literature, it is important to distinguish between experiments examining the selectively vulnerable areas (*e.g.* parts of the hippocampus) and experiments designed to provide information on the survival of the whole brain. In the former, there is little evidence for continuing ischaemia as a mechanism of reperfusion injury, but in the latter, where the severity of the ischaemia is more profound, low global CBF is associated with failure of EEG recovery (Hossmann 1988) and brain death.

Thresholds for ischaemic brain damage. In animal studies of focal ischaemia, the threshold for failure of electrical activity was found to be 18 to 20ml/100g/min, (Branston *et al.* 1974), close to the threshold for energy failure (*i.e.* the depletion of high-energy phosphate compounds—Crockard *et al.* 1987). The threshold for neuronal death was lower, approximately 10 to 12ml/100/min in grey matter and 5 to 8ml/100g/min in white matter (Jones *et al.* 1981, Astrup 1982). In adult humans with and without focal ischaemia, a similar threshold of 19ml/100g/min for normal neurological function was observed, but the threshold for tissue viability of 15ml/100g/min appeared to be higher than that found in the animal experiments, probably because of the methodological differences and difficulties (Powers *et al.* 1985). There are few data on the thresholds for energy failure and infarction after global ischaemia in adult or young animals or humans, but normal outcome has been reported after global insults in preterm and term infants in whom CBF has been measured using PET as being as low as 4.9ml/100g/min (Altman *et al.* 1988). Whether or not brain infarcts when perfused at low rates of CBF also seems to depend on the duration of relative ischaemia (Jones *et al.* 1981).

CBF after cerebral insults in humans. There is no evidence that global CBF is reduced below that required for neuronal function in human studies performed at various intervals after the onset of non-traumatic coma (Fazekas *et al.* 1956, Shapiro and Eisenberg 1969, Brodersen and Jorgensen 1974, Paulson *et al.* 1974, Beckstead *et al.* 1978, Frewen *et al.* 1985a, Bowton *et al.* 1989) although technical difficulties have prevented high-resolution regional examinations and, more importantly, studies when patients have deteriorated secondarily to brain death or vegetative state.

2. LUXURY PERFUSION

This phenomenon was first described by Lassen (1966), and refers to pathological situations where CBF is greater than that required for the metabolic demands of the tissue. It has been demonstrated after human head injury (Obrist *et al.* 1979) in those recovering from systemic shock or with the CT appearance of diffuse cerebral swelling which is common in children (Bruce *et al.* 1981). Luxury perfusion has been observed more frequently in young patients (Muizelaar *et al.* 1989a) and appears to be associated with the development of intracranial hypertension (Obrist *et al.* 1984). This is probably because CBV is also increased (Grubb *et al.* 1975), although this has proved difficult to show conclusively in humans (Kuhl *et al.* 1980).

In non-traumatic coma, CBF is usually higher than would be expected for the metabolic demand, but is not above the normal range. Paulson *et al.* (1974) found that CBF, measured using the intra-arterial [133]xenon technique, was reduced by 30 to 40 per cent from normal values in pneumococcal meningitis and in encephalitis, while hemispheric CBF was within the normal range in meningococcal meningitis. They found an even greater reduction of cerebral metabolism in all three forms of CNS infection, and in meningitis there was an increase in jugular venous PO_2, evidence of luxury perfusion. Shapiro and Eisenberg (1969) found a significant reduction in cerebral metabolic rate for oxygen ($CMRO_2$) but normal CBF in a deeply unconscious patient with St Louis encephalitis, but in patients who were co-operative, CMRO$_2$ was usually normal or increased, with normal CBF. In 12 patients unconscious from cerebral malaria, CBF was within the normal range but CMRO$_2$ and oxygen extraction ratio was reduced (Warrell *et al.* 1988). There is also evidence for luxury perfusion in adults with hepatic encephalopathy (Fazekas *et al.* 1956) and in patients studied more than six hours post cardiac arrest (Brodersen and Jorgensen 1974, Beckstead *et al.* 1978); in the latter situation, high CBF is associated with a poor prognosis (Cohan *et al.* 1989).

The mechanism for this uncoupling of CBF and metabolism is ill understood. Lassen (1966) originally proposed that tissue lactic acidosis might cause vasodilatation, but it is also possible that the increase of CBF is a direct brainstem effect, mediated neurogenically (Langfitt and Kassell 1968).

3. AUTOREGULATION

CBF is known to be autoregulated over a wide range of arterial blood pressure in normal patients (Lassen 1959, Strandgaard and Paulson 1984). In a dog model, Miller *et al.* (1972) showed that CBF was autoregulated to CPP, altered by decreasing MAP to a CPP of 40mmHg, or increasing ICP to a CPP of 50mmHg. Below these levels, CBF was directly dependent on CPP. The lower limit of autoregulation may be higher if hypotension is accompanied by excessive sympathetic drive, as occurs during haemorrhage (Fitch *et al.* 1976), than if the decrease in blood pressure is drug-induced (Fitch *et al.* 1975). At very high blood pressure, CBF is also directly dependent on BP or CPP (Strandgaard *et al.* 1974), but the upper limit of autoregulation is higher in chronic hypertension (Strandgaard *et al.* 1975), probably because of structural changes in blood vessel walls (Johansson and Fredriksson 1985). There is animal evidence that autoregulation may be abolished over the whole range of MAP by hypercapnia (Harper 1965) and by insults such as hypoxia (Freeman and Ingvar 1968) or ICP waves (Johnston *et al.* 1972). In human head injury, the most severe cases were found to be exhibiting false autoregulation (Enevoldsen *et al.* 1976), possibly due to increased tissue pressure.

There are few data on autoregulation in non-traumatic coma. Trewby *et al.* (1978) showed lower CBF in pigs with hepatic encephalopathy than in controls, and this was true at three different levels of blood pressure: 30 to 60, 60 to 90, and 90 to 120mmHg, although not at blood pressures of between 120 to 150mmHg, suggesting a possible loss of autoregulation. Paulson *et al.* (1974) found that autoregulation was globally impaired at normocapnia in several patients with CNS infections, and was restored by hypocapnia.

It is not likely that autoregulation is totally abolished (Miller *et al.* 1972). Rosner (1987) has suggested that it is at least partially preserved, over a narrower range than normal, in most unconscious patients. The precise range of CPP over which CBF is autoregulated may depend on several variables, such as the peripheral vessel from which blood pressure is measured, whether or not the patient is chronically hypertensive, the cause of blood pressure change, the baseline CBF, the PCO$_2$ and PO$_2$ and the presence of vasodilating drugs (*e.g.* hydralazine hydrochloride) or naturally occurring vasodilating substances (*e.g.* lactate and adenosine)

(Barry and Lassen 1984). There are ethical difficulties in testing autoregulation in unconscious patients, and also problems in quantification, as the range as well as the slope must be defined. Muizelaar *et al.* (1984) have suggested that the presence or absence of autoregulation should be defined in terms of cerebrovascular resistance. There is, however, little evidence that testing autoregulation is of use in prognosis or management (Muizelaar *et al.* 1989*b*).

4. CARBON DIOXIDE REACTIVITY

Over the physiological range of arterial PCO_2, CBF is directly dependent on PCO_2, but the relationship is actually sigmoid when taken to extremes (Reivich 1964). There is still controversy as to whether normal CO_2 reactivity is regulated by pH changes or directly by CO_2 (Severinghaus and Lassen 1967, Skinhoj and Paulson 1969, Koehler and Traystman 1982) in the vascular endothelium or whether there is some control at brainstem level (Shalit *et al.* 1967, Reddy *et al.* 1986). It is probable that both mechanisms are important (Kogure *et al.* 1970, Greenberg *et al.* 1978).

The relationship between PCO_2 and CBF is attenuated and may even be abolished at low blood pressure (Harper and Glass 1965) and falls during stage III of vasoparalysis, caused by rising ICP, when slowing and flattening of the EEG occurs (Langfitt 1965*a*,*b*). Attenuation of the cerebrovascular response to carbon dioxide also occurs after global ischaemic insults (Nemoto 1978, Koch *et al.* 1984, Schmidt-Kastner *et al.* 1986), and in models of traumatic coma (Saunders *et al.* 1979, Lewelt *et al.* 1982), hepatic coma (Stanley *et al.* 1975), subarachnoid haemorrhage (Hashi *et al.* 1972, Boisvert *et al.* 1979), stroke (Seki *et al.* 1984) and hyperammonaemia (Chodobski *et al.* 1986) in animals. Abolition of CO_2 reactivity has been shown to be associated with poor outcome in patients after head injury (Obrist *et al.* 1984, Messeter *et al.* 1986). There are few data in non-traumatic coma in humans, but carbon dioxide is known to be toxic in hepatic encephalopathy (Posner and Plum 1960) and CO_2 reactivity is impaired after subarachnoid haemorrhage (Voldby *et al.* 1985, Dernbach *et al.* 1988). Globally impaired CO_2 responsiveness was not seen in the study of encephalitis by Paulson *et al.* (1974), but the outcome was good in these patients. Brodersen and Jorgensen (1974) found no correlation between CBF and PCO_2 in adults in coma with over-all poor outcome, including several studied after ischaemic or hypoglycaemic insults, but they did not study CO_2 reactivity in individual subjects.

Various mechanisms have been proposed to explain this phenomenon. The small vessels may be capable of little further vasodilatation at tissue perfusion pressures at the lower end of the autoregulatory range, produced by low systemic arterial pressure (Harper and Glass 1965), high ICP (Grubb *et al.* 1975) or narrowing of the large cerebral arteries (Harper *et al.* 1972) as occurs in vasospasm. Lactic acid (which is a by-product of glycolysis and is therefore produced whenever oxygen supply is insufficient for the respiratory chain to supply metabolic demand) is a potent vasodilator and may interfere with the regulation of the vascular endothelium. Damage to brainstem regulatory mechanisms (Shalit *et al.* 1967) may also be important. Although the underlying pathological mechanisms may be different in the various conditions in which abnormal CO_2 reactivity has been described, there is no doubt about the ominous prognostic significance of an abolished response.

In patients at risk of stroke on haemodynamic grounds (*e.g.* internal carotid occlusion), the cerebrovascular response to carbon dioxide correlated with the ratio CBF/CBV and with an increase in the oxygen extraction ratio (Herold *et al.* 1988), which are indices measured by PET, suggesting that CBF is inadequate for metabolic demand (Gibbs *et al.* 1984). Such a failure of the reserve capacity of the cerebral circulation is a possible mechanism for cerebral ischaemia causing secondary deterioration in coma. Measurement of CO_2 reactivity might therefore be clinically useful.

5. CHEMICAL MEDIATORS OF DELAYED NEURONAL DEATH

There is little evidence that energy failure, *i.e.* depletion of high-energy phosphate compounds at the time of ischaemia, is directly responsible for neuronal cell-death (Raichle 1983) although irreversible breakdown of neurofilament protein may occur very early (Ogata *et al.* 1989). Much animal research is continuing at the present time into putative neurotoxins, such as calcium, free fatty acids, oxygen-free radicals and excitatory amino acids (Siesjo 1988). These substances are released at the time of ischaemia and may be responsible for a cascade of events leading to neuronal death after an interval. There may be a therapeutic window during which these events might be arrested by the use of a combination of appropriate drugs, but there is still much debate about the relative importance of these mechanisms (Moossy *et al.* 1988, Stephenson *et al.* 1988), and clinicians should remain cautious about introducing potentially dangerous drugs into their practice until their efficacy is proven in animal experiments and carefully conducted clinical trials (Safar 1986, Rolfsen and Davis 1989).

6. THE ROLE OF LACTIC ACIDOSIS

During ischaemia, there is a switch from aerobic to anaerobic metabolism and lactate is produced by the anaerobic metabolism of glucose. High levels of tissue lactate (above 20mmol/kg) appear to be associated with failure of recovery of energy stores (Rehncrona *et al.* 1980), cytotoxic oedema (Plum 1983, Siesjo 1984), cell death (Pulsinelli *et al.* 1987), seizures (Siesjo 1988) and poor outcome (Myers 1979) in adult animal models. There is some evidence that the brain of the immature animal is better able to handle lactate (Raichle 1983), but very few data are available.

Cerebral-tissue lactate may now be measured using MRS in animals, and this probably reflects intracellular lactate (Gadian *et al.* 1987). Measurement of CSF lactate can only give a very indirect reflection of intracellular acid-base balance and certainly cannot be used to monitor acute changes (Javaheri *et al.* 1984). It is, however, of interest that CSF lactate is raised in CNS infections, such as meningitis (Paulson *et al.* 1974, Pavlakis *et al.* 1980, Eross *et al.* 1981), malaria (White *et al.* 1985) and encephalitis (Paulson *et al.* 1974), hepatic encephalopathy (Yao *et al.* 1987), and after cardiac arrest, cerebrovascular accidents and hypoglycaemic insults (Brodersen and Jorgensen 1974, Yao *et al.* 1989).

TABLE 8.IV

Guy's Hospital study 1982–1986.
Diagnosis, ICP, CPP and outcome

Age (yrs)	Diagnosis	On admission GCS	On admission EEG	Outcome Doppler study
10	Cystinosis, HIE	3	II → I	CD
8	Head injury, HIE	3	I	BD
2	Head injury, HIE	3	II → I	CD
4	Myocarditis, HIE*	3	I	SLD and SQ
0.8	Fallot's tetralogy, HIE*	3	II	SLD and SQ
11	Transposition, HIE	3	II → I	BD
4	Near-drowning, HIE	3	N → I	CD
15	Nephronopthisis, HIE	5	I	CD
1	Ventricular septal defect, HIE*	3	II → I	SLD and SQ
1	Intussusception, HIE*	3	II → I	CD
1	Ventricular septal defect, HIE*	5	II → I	CD
7	Cyanotic heart disease, HIE*	8	II → I	VS
0.3	Gastroenteritis, HIE	3	I	BD
0.6	Fallot's tetralogy, HIE*	8	II → I	BD (D)
11	Toxic shock syndrome, HIE*	8	I	CD
6	Posterior fossa haematoma, HIE	3	N	MLD and SQ
2	Epiglottitis, HIE*	5	II → I	N (D)
4	Muscular dystrophy, HIE	7	I	MLD
6	Encephalitis*	11	I	BD
2	Encephalitis	3	II(S)	SLD and SQ
7	Encephalitis*	5	I	MLD (D)
3	Encephalitis*	5	I	MLD and DP
5	Encephalitis*	4	I	N (D)
12	Encephalitis*	8	I	N
11	Encephalitis*	6	I	N
7	Encephalitis	5	I(S)	MLD
8	Encephalitis	5	I(S)	MLD and HP
4	Encephalitis	4	I	N but DP
0.6	Meningitis*	3	II → I	SLD and SQ
1	Sickle cell disease, meningitis*	5	I	SLD and HP
6	Head injury*	5	I	MLD and HP
4	Head injury, cerebellar haematoma*	4	I	MLD and SQ
4	Head injury*	5	I	BD
1	Haemolytic-uraemic syndrome*	10	I	CD (EEG III)
12	Thrombotic-thrombocytopenic purpura*	3	I(S)	BD
0.3	Reye's syndrome*	3	I	SLD, SQ, PV
6	Reye's syndrome	5	I	SLD and SQ (D)
7	Ornithine transcarbamylase deficiency*	5	I	BD
8	Diabetic + ?toluene ingestion*	6	II	N
9	Hypertensive encephalopathy*	3	I	MLD and PV
13	Intracerebral haematoma	4	I	VS

HIE = hypoxic-ischaemic encephalopathy, N = normal, MLD = moderate learning difficulties, SLD = severe learning difficulties, VS = vegetative state, PV = poor vision, SQ = spastic quadriparesis, HP = hemiplegia, DP = diplegia, BD = brain death, CD = cardiac death, GCS = Glasgow coma score, EEG graded according to Tasker *et al.* 1988*b*: N = normal or borderline for age and state, I = slow activity (0.5 to 3 cycles/second), II = generalised low-voltage activity (<50μV), III = electrocerebral silence (isoelectric), S = seizure. * = Doppler study. D = decompressed.

Lassen (1966) proposed that the luxury perfusion and vasoparalysis seen after brain insults might be a consequence of tissue lactic acidosis. This has not been demonstrated directly in humans because of the difficulties in measuring intracellular lactate, but it is noteworthy that Paulson *et al.* (1974) demonstrated a significant negative linear correlation between CSF pH and log CBF in CNS infections and that Brodersen and Jorgensen (1974) showed an indirect linear relationship between CSF bicarbonate and log CBF.

Value of monitoring CBF and ICP in non-traumatic coma

There are at least three possible benefits of ICU monitoring. It may be possible to give a more accurate early prognosis, management may be planned more rationally with improved understanding of the pathophysiology, and outcome may be improved.

TABLE 8.IV

continued

	ICP (mmHg)			Pre EEG deterioration			CPP (mmHg)			Pre EEG deterioration		
Opening	Maximum	Mean	SD	Maximum	Mean	SD	Minimum	Mean	SD	Minimum	Mean	SD
14	18	10.1	5.0	18	10.6	4.8	26	77.0	22.8	48	80.0	20.1
14	54	13.8	7.1	50	14.1	6.5	26	55.4	9.7	33	58.9	9.9
4	38	9.9	6.3	38	9.9	6.3	27	67.2	14.3	27	67.2	14.3
19	45	15.9	4.9	40	15.7	6.4	15	70.5	10.2	15	63.7	11.3
9	14	7.1	4.2	12	11.0	1.7	35	51.6	9.7	44	49.3	5.0
6	70	25.1	10.9	28	15.6	3.9	−7	38.1	11.7	24	41.3	10.9
9	24	6.1	4.8	24	5.9	4.7	−3	51.6	11.7	−3	49.0	10.4
21	65	36.1	14.8	65	36.1	14.8	15	51.6	19.9	15	51.6	19.9
5	18	7.6	6.8	18	6.2	5.7	26	55.7	7.8	38	55.2	6.6
8	10	7.9	1.1	10	7.9	1.1	38	62.6	11.5	38	62.6	11.5
10	16	7.5	3.4	16	11.8	2.6	30	44.6	8.8	33	40.4	5.2
18	48	17.5	7.5	28	17.6	4.1	15	44.6	9.3	28	38.6	6.3
20	36	28.5	4.9	36	26.8	6.0	−5	5.0	7.9	−1	9.4	7.8
28	31	22.1	4.5	31	24.1	5.2	29	36.6	4.8	29	37.1	5.6
8	15	9.2	3.0	12	9.5	1.9	35	47.6	12.7	50	66.0	11.4
7	33	14.4	4.9	—	—	—	37	67.1	12.0	—	—	—
12	14	9.3	3.5	—	—	—	51	67.7	7.7	—	—	—
12	22	14.2	4.0	—	—	—	50	103.1	18.6	—	—	—
12	45	12.4	4.6	45	12.3	4.5	27	59.5	9.2	34	59.8	9.8
11	41	14.6	6.9	11	10.7	0.6	9	67.5	15.5	36	36.7	0.6
45	46	30.3	5.7	—	—	—	34	46.9	6.6	—	—	—
8	34	5.0	5.9	—	—	—	47	75.7	11.2	—	—	—
9	38	13.9	7.0	—	—	—	66	80.0	7.1	—	—	—
7	17	6.6	2.8	—	—	—	59	74.4	7.8	—	—	—
6	17	9.7	3.8	—	—	—	64	81.1	7.9	—	—	—
11	40	8.5	5.6	—	—	—	55	76.7	11.6	—	—	—
7	12	6.6	2.2	—	—	—	64	80.8	7.3	—	—	—
8	29	6.2	3.1	—	—	—	45	75.5	9.6	—	—	—
25	40	16.6	6.4	25	25.0	0	23	54.0	8.8	48	48.0	0
7	11	5.9	2.5	11	7.5	1.4	62	74.0	6.0	65	73.9	6.3
14	58	10.2	6.9	—	—	—	48	76.6	12.2	—	—	—
2	24	8.7	5.6	—	—	—	45	83.3	15.2	—	—	—
14	89	22.2	26.1	94	13.6	8.0	−14	61.7	21.9	1	67.8	11.1
9	19	11.9	4.6	19	11.9	4.6	35	59.7	12.4	35	59.7	12.4
11	68	16.8	10.7	27	16.1	5.1	2	46.3	14.2	9	46.4	12.1
11	26	4.9	3.5	16	5.5	3.7	38	70.3	9.6	38	61.1	8.2
17	70	23.4	12.8	17	17.0	0	39	72.8	11.9	68	68.0	0
10	24	7.4	4.0	21	10.0	5.6	57	85.4	16.5	73	96.9	13.8
12	29	9.8	6.4	25	10.9	4.2	59	82.2	12.6	63	73.5	4.6
40	77	23.2	10.7	—	—	—	35	77.4	15.0	—	—	—
12	36	11.5	6.3	36	11.5	6.4	36	66.6	9.2	36	65.4	9.4

Prognosis

ICP AND CPP

Clinical experience. Authors have attempted to relate ICP, CPP, and CBF measurements to prognosis. Mean ICP, recorded half-hourly over 24-hour periods, appeared to be related to outcome in a series of adults, unconscious from encephalitis (Barnett *et al.* 1988a). The same authors also found that opening ICP was a useful prognostic indicator, but emphasised that transient increases of ICP up to 80mmHg did not preclude a good outcome. In children with ischaemia and with CNS infections, the opening ICP was not found to be a useful guide to the subsequent development of intracranial hypertension but was a guide to prognosis in the group with CNS infections and not in those with ischaemia (Goitein *et al.* 1983a,b). The same was true for the maximum ICP developing during the course of the illness, but a minimum CPP of less than 30mmHg was always associated with death in both groups of patients, while a minimum CPP above this value was always associated

299

with survival (Goitein and Tamir 1983, Goitein *et al.* 1983*a*). More recently, in a group of children unconscious from a variety of aetiologies, Tasker *et al.* (1988*a*) found that those with a minimum CPP of less than 38mmHg all did very badly, but that there were some with poor outcome in whom a CPP below this value was not measured. There is evidence that high ICP and low CPP is also associated with poor prognosis in near-drowning (Nussbaum and Galant 1983), although some patients who do badly do not have intracranial hypertension (Frewen *et al.* 1985*b*). Intracranial hypertension is common in patients in Grade IV hepatic coma, but although trials of treatment have been reported (Ede and Williams 1986), the prognostic significance of this finding in relation to the other important systemic derangements (Fraser and Arieff 1985) has not been defined and CPP does not appear to have been measured.

Intracranial and cerebral perfusion pressures were monitored in 41 children in coma (36 non-traumatic) in a study based at Guy's Hospital between January 1983 and January 1988. Eighteen had suffered a hypoxic-ischaemic event (including two out of the five head injuries), 12 had CNS infections (10 encephalitis and two meningitis), and the remainder were in coma from a variety of causes (Table 8.IV). Outcome was assessed by a paediatric neurologist and a psychologist at least two years after the insult. Full details are given in Table 8.IV. For the statistical analysis, the outcome groups have been divided into *good* (*i.e.* normal or moderately disabled), and *poor* (*i.e.* severely disabled, vegetative or dead). There was no significant difference in opening ICP, maximum ICP or mean ICP between good and poor outcome groups, but minimum and mean CPPs were significantly lower in the poor outcome group (both p<0.01, Mann-Whitney) and all patients with a minimum CPP of 34mmHg or less did badly, as did all those with a mean CPP of 70mmHg or less (except for two who were surgically decompressed) (Fig. 8.1). Mean or minimum CPPs above these values did not preclude a poor outcome. The same findings held when the outcomes compared were death and survival (Fig. 8.2) and when data for patients with CNS infections (Fig. 8.3) and hypoxic-ischaemic encephalopathy (Fig. 8.4) were examined separately.

However, these data do not allow outcome to be predicted in the individual patient, for two reasons. Firstly, the demonstration of a statistically significant difference between two groups does not describe the overlap between them, nor the number of false positives and negatives when using the parameter to predict outcome. This may be overcome by using discriminant analysis (Day and Kerridge 1967). Secondly, when a model has been developed which appears to discriminate between good and poor outcome groups in a retrospective series, it must be tested prospectively. The data from our series has been subjected to discriminant analysis, but has not been tested prospectively.

Minimum CPP successfully discriminated between good and poor outcome in 37 patients, but two patients who were predicted to do badly did well, and two patients predicted to do well did badly. Minimum CPP was much less successful at predicting survival (11 false positives and two false negatives). Mean CPP successfully discriminated between good and poor outcome in 36 patients, but two patients predicted to do badly did well, and three patients predicted to do well did badly.

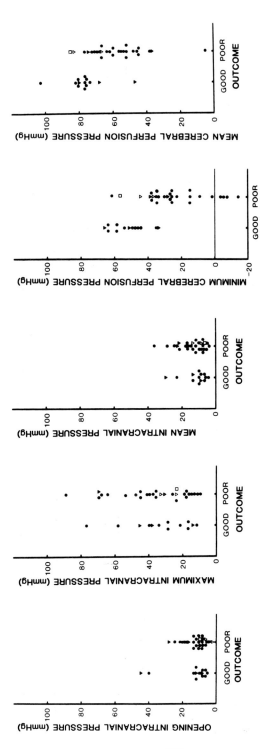

Fig. 8.1. Comparison of opening ICP (NS), maximum ICP (NS), mean ICP (NS), minimum CPP (p<0.01) and mean CPP (p<0.01) with outcome of coma in childhood (Mann-Whitney U test: NS = not significant at 5 per cent level). For discriminant analysis, see text. Open triangles represent two children with posterior fossa haematcmata who both made a cognitive recovery but were left with spastic quadriparesis; open square represents patient in whom ICP monitor was thought to have failed; filled triangles represent five patients who were surgically decompressed; filled circles represent all other patients.

301

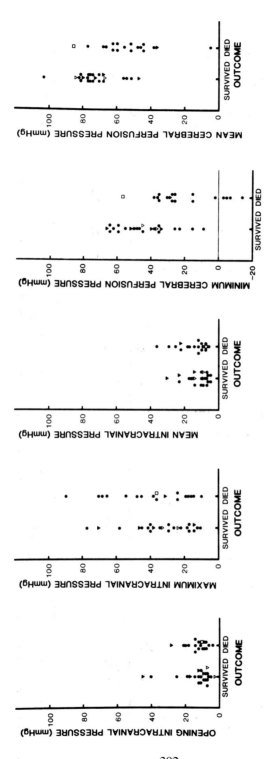

Fig. 8.2. Comparison of opening ICP (NS), maximum ICP (NS), mean ICP (NS), minimum CPP (p<0.01) and mean CPP (p<0.01) with survival of coma (Mann-Whitney U test; NS = not significant at 5 per cent level). Open triangles represent two patients with posterior fossa haematomata who both made a cognitive recovery but were left with a spastic quadriparesis; open square represents patient in whom the ICP monitor was thought to have failed; filled triangles represent five patients who were surgically decompressed; filled circles represent all the other patients.

302

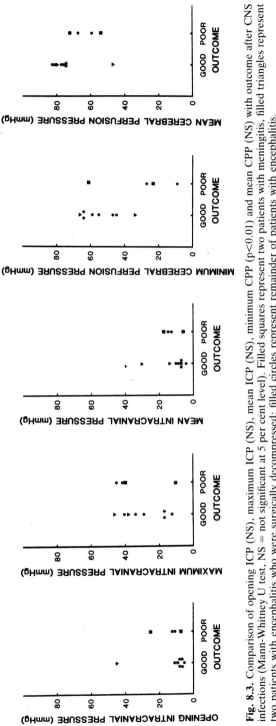

Fig. 8.3. Comparison of opening ICP (NS), maximum ICP (NS), mean ICP (NS), minimum CPP ($p<0.01$) and mean CPP (NS) with outcome after CNS infections (Mann-Whitney U test, NS = not significant at 5 per cent level). Filled squares represent two patients with meningitis, filled triangles represent two patients with encephalitis who were surgically decompressed; filled circles represent remainder of patients with encephalitis.

303

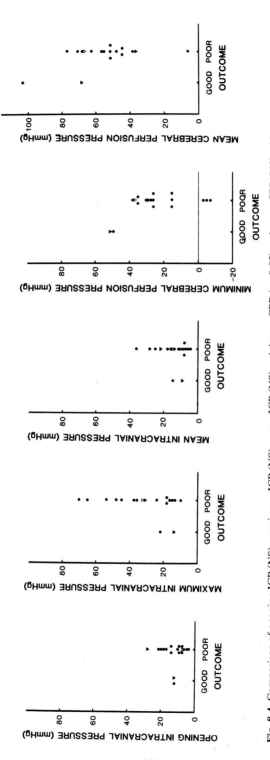

Fig. 8.4. Comparison of opening ICP (NS), maximum ICP (NS), mean ICP (NS), minimum CPP (NS) and mean CPP (p<0.05) with outcome after hypoxic-ischaemic encephalopathy (Mann-Whitney U test, NS = not significant). Open triangle represents patient with posterior fossa haematoma who made a cognitive recovery but was left with spastic quadriparesis; filled triangles represent two patients who were surgically decompressed; filled circles represent remainder of the patients.

Again, survival was more difficult to predict (nine false positives and two false negatives). Possible explanations for the false negative prediction of a good outcome may have included: (i) failure of the ICP monitor (considered in one patient in whom a subdural screw probably failed at high ICP and massive cerebral swelling was demonstrated at post-mortem examination—Miller *et al.* 1986), (ii) injury to the brainstem resulting from the original insult (considered in two patients with posterior fossa haematomata who made a cognitive recovery but were left with a spastic quadriparesis), and (iii) low CPP prior to insertion or after removal of the ICP monitor. The children whose mean CPP predicted that they would do badly but who did well were both surgically decompressed.

Pathophysiological changes with decreasing CPP. Poor outcome was seen in most children in whom mean CPP could not be maintained above 70mmHg, which is surprisingly high. All the children with good outcome spent short periods with CPP less than 70mmHg, but of the 12 who were not decompressed, CPP was above 60mmHg for at least 95 per cent and above 50mmHg for at least 97 per cent of the period over which they were monitored. The vasodilatory cascade hypothesis, put forward by Rosner and Becker (1984) to explain the occurrence of plateau waves, may be of relevance. At high MAP (or CPP), most of the resistance change occurring in response to a change in MAP (or CPP) takes place in the larger (>200μm) pial and intracerebral vessels, but at MAP (or CPP) values lower than 90mmHg, the smaller (<100μm) cerebral vessels also dilate, and at CPP less than 70mmHg, they are very dilated (Kontos *et al.* 1978), increasing the baseline CBV. The haemodynamics of the cerebral circulation may not be stable if CPP is beteen 40 and 70mmHg (Rosner 1987). A slow decline in CPP may be associated with further rapid autoregulatory vasodilatation (Kontos 1981), and as a small increase in CBV may be associated with a relatively large increase in ICP if baseline CBV is already high, a further sharp decrease in CPP occurs. These plateau waves are usually self-limiting because the vessels reach maximal dilatation and a compensatory Cushing response increases CBF and ICP initially; the increase in MAP causes vasoconstriction and then a fall in ICP. The Cushing response is variable and may fail after a series of pressure waves (Langfitt *et al.* 1965*b*), or if the systemic circulation is compromised because of poor cardiac function or fluid restriction (Rosner 1987).

As CPP decreases,below the lower limit of autoregulation reached between 40 and 60mmHg (Miller *et al.* 1972, Wagner and Traystman 1986), oxygen extraction increases (Kanno *et al.* 1988) and there is probably also a switch from aerobic to anaerobic metabolism, associated with lactate production and further vasodilatation (Zwetnow 1970). Adenosine, another potent vasodilator, may also be released at low CPP (Winn *et al.* 1980). Eventually, as CPP declines further, CO_2 reactivity is abolished (vasoparalysis) and as the vessels are maximally dilated, they cannot respond to an increase in metabolic demand with an increase in CBF. Ischaemia will occur if the capacity to increase oxygen extraction has been exceeded. The precise values for CPP at which these changes occur may vary in different circumstances, depending for example on whether there has been a recent previous plateau wave (Johnston *et al.* 1972) or seizure. At values of CPP below 30mmHg, the vessels collapse and there is severe and irreversible ischaemia.

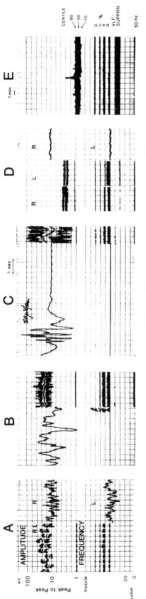

Fig. 8.5. Examples of cerebral function analysing monitor (CFAM) traces. Biparietal montage (P3-P4 on international 10–20 system) was used with paper speed 30cm/hour unless otherwise stated. A: normal or nearly normal (high-amplitude with all four frequencies present); compressed trace was alternating between right (F4-P4) and left (F3-P3) hemispheres every minute. EEG samples from right hemisphere (*upper*) and left hemisphere (*lower*). B: high-amplitude diffuse slowing. C: burst suppression. D. Low-amplitude trace. Compressed trace was alternating between right (F4-P4) and left (F3-P3) hemispheres every five minutes. EEG sample from right hemisphere (*upper trace*) and left hemisphere (*lower trace*). E: iso-electric trace.

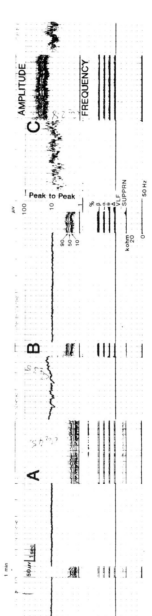

Fig. 8.6. CFAM trace from patient two hours after cardiac arrest. (Compressed trace, paper speed 6cm/hour.) A: PCO_2 of 34mmHg (4.5kPa), raw EEG was of low amplitude (mean amplitude of compressed trace 1.74 µV). B: when PCO_2 was decreased to 26mmHg (3.5kPa), amplitude increased slightly (mean amplitude of compressed trace 2.5µV). C: when PCO_2 was reduced to 21mmHg (2.8kPa), the EEG amplitude suddenly increased (mean amplitude of compressed trace 25.1µV). Patient was surgically decompressed on day 8 because of persistent intracranial hypertension at normocapnia and is now normal neurologically and intellectually.

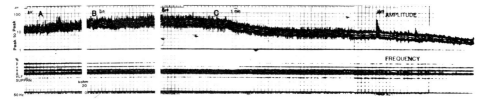

Fig. 8.7. CFAM trace from patient 20 hours after cardiac arrest lasting eight minutes (coming off bypass for a Fontan procedure). A: just after 11.00 compressed trace was of moderate amplitude (mean 13.2µV); and all frequencies were present. B: one hour later, amplitude had increased (mean approximately 25µV); there was increased percentage of delta and decreased percentage of faster frequencies, beta and alpha. C: from 13.00, amplitude of compressed trace progressively decreased (mean at 13.00 between 30 and 40µV and at 14.25, 2.5µV). During this period, MAP was maintained above 45mmHg but patient became anuric. ICP was not monitored, but it was postulated that the child's very large positive fluid balance may have contributed to cerebral oedema. There was no recovery of consciousness or of electrical activity and the patient fulfilled clinical criteria for brain death on two occasions the following day.

EEG

Tasker *et al.* (1988*b*) have suggested that serial eight-channel EEG recording might be useful in addition to ICP and CPP monitoring in non-traumatic coma as, in their series, prognosis was accurately predicted by EEG in the group with poor outcome despite a minimum CPP overlapping with the good outcome group. EEG appears to be useful in predicting outcome in children in coma due to cardiac arrest (Pampiglione and Harden 1968) or near-drowning (Kruus *et al.* 1979, Janati and Erba 1982). High-amplitude diffuse slowing is a pattern commonly seen in children in coma, and does not appear to be useful in discriminating outcome groups (Seshia *et al.* 1983).

Abnormal EEG patterns may be recognised on instruments designed for continuous cerebral function monitoring (Fig. 8.5). In a series of 89 children who had suffered a cardiac arrest, studied in three London centres between 1982 and 1985, 39 per cent recovered consciousness within one month, 27 per cent died a cardiac death whilst in coma, and the outcome in the remainder was either brain death or vegetative state. EEG was monitored in all using either a two- or three-channel tape system (Medilog, Oxford Medical) or a single- or dual-channel cerebral function analysing monitor (CFAM, Medaid Ltd). Eight-channel recordings were made whenever possible to verify the findings from the monitoring system. Four possible predictors of outcome—Glasgow coma score, brainstem score, EEG classified according to the system of Pampiglione and Harden (1968), and pH of the first gas—were used in a discriminant analysis. Recovery of consciousness was predicted with 89 per cent accuracy, and poor neurological outcome with 77 per cent accuracy. The main discriminants were the EEG grade and the pH of the first gas. This suggests that in unconscious children, it may not be possible to predict outcome early from clinical signs alone.

The main use of continuous EEG, however, is in following changes over long periods of time. After a cardiac arrest, the length of time taken for continuous EEG activity to return gives very useful prognostic information (Jorgensen and Malchow-Møller 1983) and the effects of various medical interventions on this

307

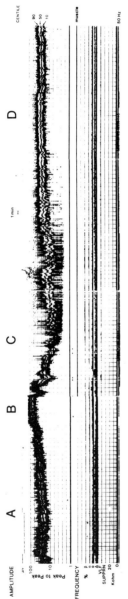

Fig. 8.8. CFAM trace from a child 48 hours after cardiac arrest lasting approximately 10 minutes (anaesthetic problem due to previously undiagnosed myopathy). MAP was maintained above 70mmHg but patient was becoming oliguric. A: high-amplitude diffuse slowing (mean amplitude between 20 and 35μV, minimum not below 7μV). B: amplitude of trace suddenly increased (mean approximately 90 μV); this was probably a subclinical seizure discharge. C: postictally, low-amplitude activity (mean 6 to 10μV, minimum approximately 2μV) persisted for nearly an hour. D: recovery of EEG to high-amplitude diffuse slowing was temporally associated with commencement of haemofiltration. No further seizures occurred; EEG amplitude remained high and child has recovered with residual language disorder.

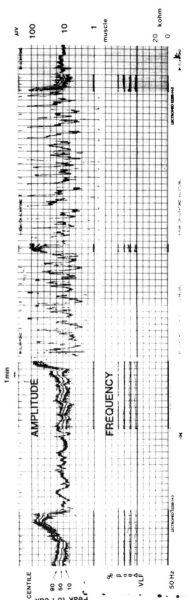

Fig. 8.9. CFAM trace from baby aged three months with Reye's syndrome, showing sudden increase in amplitude of compressed trace associated with rhythmical seizure discharge on the raw EEG playout.

308

recovery may be observed (Fig. 8.6). Deterioration of the EEG pattern may be followed, for example by loss of the faster frequencies, decrease in amplitude of the compressed trace, or a change to a pattern of graver prognostic significance (Prior and Maynard 1986). In our series of 89 children after cardiac arrest, 23 showed partial recovery of consciousness, recovery of brainstem function, and recovery of EEG pattern to diffuse slowing or better, and then deteriorated with poor eventual neurological outcome. This deterioration could be followed on the EEG (Fig. 8.7), and it may be possible to alter the course with immediate therapeutic interventions (Fig. 8.8); however, this is very difficult to prove. Seizures, which are often subclinical in the unconscious patient paralysed for ventilation, may also be seen as changes in the trace (Fig. 8.9) and treated (Tasker *et al.* 1989).

In the Guy's Hospital study there was more overlap between good and poor outcome groups when the minimum and mean CPP before EEG deterioration was examined (Fig. 8.10) and although there was a statistically significant difference for minimum and mean CPP between the two groups, discriminant analysis was less successful with seven false positives and five false negatives in predicting good outcome from minimum CPP prior to EEG deterioration and three false positives and three false negatives in predicting good outcome from mean CPP prior to EEG deterioration. This implies that low CPP was often seen after EEG deterioration had already occurred, which may limit the usefulness of this measurement in guiding management to attempt to prevent secondary deterioration. ICP was not always high and CPP was not always very low when EEG deteriorated (Fig. 8.10), suggesting that other factors may play an important role in secondary deterioration. Nevertheless, good outcome is likely if the initial EEG grade is diffuse slowing or better and mean CPP can be maintained above 70mmHg.

3. CEREBRAL BLOODFLOW AND METABOLISM

Prognosis of patients in non-traumatic coma. A single measurement of CBF does not appear to give useful prognostic information, either after cardiac arrest in adults (Brodersen and Jorgensen 1974, Beckstead *et al.* 1978) or in CNS infections (Paulson *et al.* 1974). Most authors have also found that single measurements of cerebral metabolism had no prognostic value unless they were less than one third of normal (Brodersen and Jorgensen 1974, Beckstead *et al.* 1978). Frewen *et al.* (1985a), in six children (four near-drowning), found cross-brain oxygen consumption and cerebral metabolic rate to be significantly different in surviving children compared with non-survivors, but the series was small, and cerebral metabolic rate in the non-surviving near-drowning victims was again very low indeed. Ducasse *et al.* (1984) suggested that a high arteriovenous oxygen difference may predict good outcome after cardiac arrest in adults. These findings will need confirmation in larger studies and their power to discriminate outcome will need to be compared with established methods, such as clinical examination and neurophysiology, which are on the whole less invasive and expensive.

Brain death. CBF measurements give clinically useful prognostic information when absent flow is demonstrated in brain death (Smith and Walker 1973). This may be demonstrated arteriographically (Rosenklint and Jorgensen 1974), using

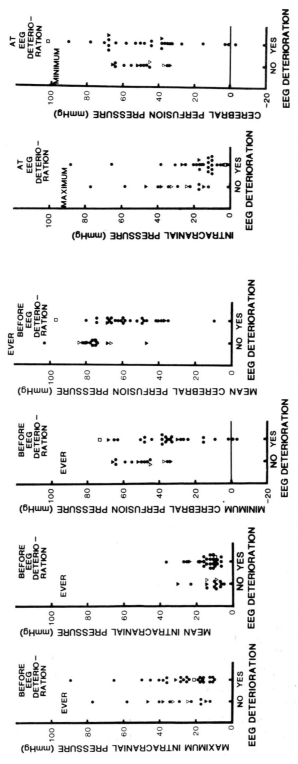

Fig. 8.10. Comparison of maximum ICP (NS), mean ICP (NS), minimum CPP (NS), mean CPP (p<0.01) before EEG deterioration (A) and of ICP (paradoxically significantly lower in those whose EEGs did deteriorate p<0.01) and CPP (NS) at EEG deterioration (B) in unconscious children whose EEGs did deteriorate with comparable values over the whole course of the child's illness in those whose EEGs did not deteriorate. (Statistical significance tested by Mann-Whitney U test, NS = not significant at 5 per cent level.) For discriminant analysis, see text. Open triangles represent two patients with posterior fossa haematomata who made a cognitive recovery but were left with a spastic quadriparesis; open square represents patient in whom the ICP monitor was thought to have failed; filled triangles represent five patients who were surgically decompressed; filled circles represent all other patients.

310

semi-quantitative CBF techniques such as isotope angiography (Goodman *et al.* 1969), xenon computed tomography (Ashwal *et al.* 1989), or with transcranial Doppler ultrasound. A characteristic Doppler sonogram is obtained from the MCA in brain death, with reverse flow throughout diastole (Fig. 8.11). The finding of such a signal for more than 30 minutes, with an MCA velocity of less than 10cm/sec and a direction of flow index (1-area of reverse flow/area of forward flow) of less than 0.8 was associated with clinical brainstem death and there were no false positives (Kirkham *et al.* 1987*a*). Other authors have reported similar findings (Bode *et al.* 1988, Hassler *et al.* 1988). The presence of forward flow throughout diastole does not preclude the diagnosis, however, and recovery has been seen when reverse flow throughout diastole has been seen over a short period of time (Kirkham *et al.* 1987*a*). Reverse flow throughout diastole may only be seen soon after brain death has occurred, and in many of these patients no signal could be obtained at all at a later stage. This is of no clinical use, as the same might be found with a technically unsatisfactory examination. Although the finding of reverse flow throughout diastole cannot be used as a confirmatory test, it may be helpful in guiding the timing of clinical examinations.

Cerebrovascular reserve. There has been considerable interest recently in the possibility of predicting patients at risk from cerebral ischaemia on haemodynamic grounds by assessing the reserve capacity of the cerebral circulation. In stroke patients, this may be done by measuring the ratio of CBV to CBF and the oxygen extraction ratio using PET (Gibbs *et al.* 1984), but this is not a practical approach in the unconscious patient. An alternative is to measure the reactivity of the cerebral circulation to carbon dioxide, using a CBF technique such as inhaled or intravenous ^{133}xenon, or using transcranial ultrasound, since changes in CBF produced by altering carbon dioxide appear to be followed by changes in MCA velocity.

The transcranial Doppler ultrasound technique has been used to measure the responses of the cerebral circulation to carbon dioxide in 57 normal patients (39 adults, 18 children) and in 26 patients in coma. The diagnoses in the abnormal patients are given in Table 8.IV (patients labelled *). All were in deep coma with a Glasgow coma score of less than 8, but had preserved brainstem function and diffuse slowing on the EEG, which we considered to be an intermediate grade (some had previously had a period when the EEG grade was of graver prognostic significance). MCA velocity was monitored during changes in arterial carbon dioxide tension produced by changing the ventilator settings. These changes were made on clinical grounds, in most cases, and the information was not allowed to influence the management of the patient: but in a few of the patients studied later in the series, CO_2 reactivity was studied prospectively and the study was aborted if the MCA velocity decreased with increasing PCO_2. In all, data werc obtaincd for 298 individual epochs in the abnormal patients (1 to 36 per patient). PCO_2 was measured using an infra-red end-tidal carbon dioxide analyser (Hewlett-Packard), but arterial PCO_2 was measured intermittently during the tests in all cases, and if the end-tidal measurements did not follow the arterial ones accurately, the former were discarded.

The curve describing the relationship between CBF and PCO_2 has been variously

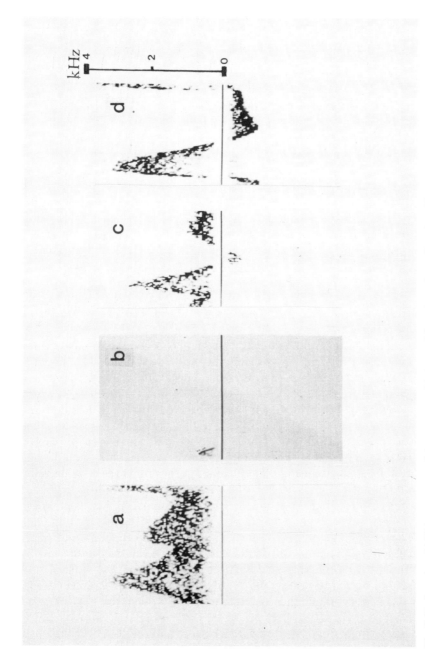

Fig. 8.11. Samples of MCA sonograms. (a) sonogram with forward flow throughout diastole, MCA velocity 55.2cm/sec, direction of flow index (DFI) 1.00, (b) sonogram with no flow in diastole, MCA velocity 2.4cm/sec, DFI 1.00, (c) sonogram with small amount of reverse flow in diastole, MCA velocity 24.8cm/sec, DFI 0.88, (d) sonogram with reverse flow throughout diastole, MCA velocity 2.3cm/sec, DFI 0.57. (From Kirkham *et al.* 1987, reproduced with the permission of the Editor of *Journal of Neurology, Neurosurgery and Psychiatry.*)

312

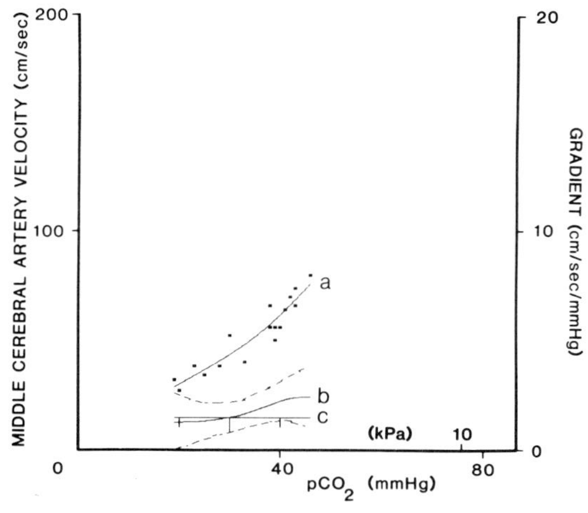

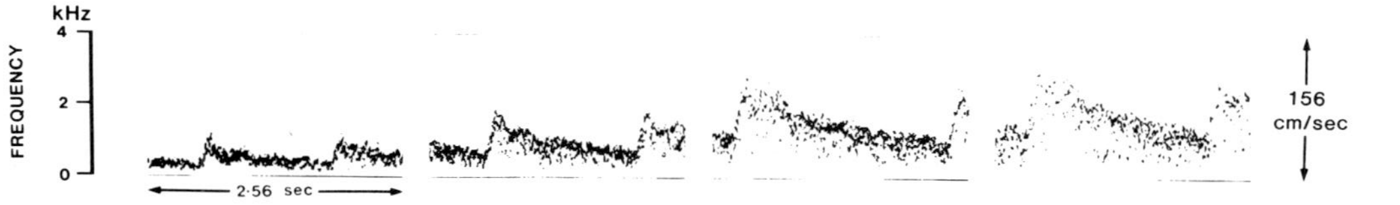

MAP	89	87	91	87	mmHg
pCO_2	20	38	42	46	mmHg
pCO_2	2.7	5.1	5.6	6.1	kPa
MCA $\bar{V}$	26	56	76	80	cm/sec

Fig. 8.12. Relationship between MCA velocity and arterial PCO_2 in normal adult. Four sonograms are shown; as PCO_2 increased, MAP remained nearly constant. MCA velocity has been plotted against PCO_2 and smoothed spline (line *a*) has been fitted through the points. Gradient (line *b*, with 95 per cent confidence limits shown as dotted lines) of this curve remained above zero over whole range of PCO_2 studied and at higher levels of PCO_2 tended to be greater than gradient at PCO_2 30mmHg (4.0kPa) (line c, gradient 1.22cm/sec/mmHg).

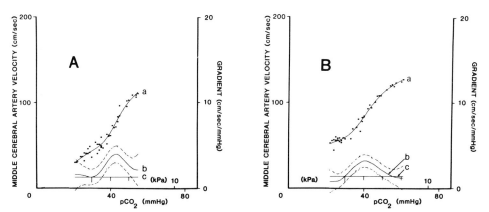

Fig. 8.13. Relationship between MCA velocity and end-tidal PCO_2 in normal adult (A) and normal child B. Smoothed spline (line *a*) has been fitted through points in each case. Gradient (line *b*, with 95 per cent confidence limits shown as dotted lines) remained above zero over whole range of PCO_2 in both. At top of the PCO_2 range, gradient started to decrease below gradient at PCO_2 30mmHg (4.0kPa) (line *c*, A: adult-gradient 1.79cm/sec/mmHg; B: child-gradient 1.62cm/sec/mmHg).

described as linear (Kummer 1984), sigmoid (Reivich 1964, Harper and Glass 1965) and exponential (Markwalder *et al.* 1984). In normal adults and children, we demonstrated a linear relationship between percentage change in maximum frequency envelope and arterial (four subjects, individually plotted) or end-tidal (15 adults and 18 children, whole population plotted together) PCO_2 (Kirkham *et al.* 1986), with gradients similar to those demonstrated by authors using CBF techniques to measure CO_2 reactivity and the same method of expressing their results (Harper and Glass 1965, Kummer 1984). We therefore felt justified in using changes in MCA velocity to measure changes in CBF due to changing PCO_2, but it became clear on plotting the relationship between MCA velocity and PCO_2 in a larger population of individual normal subjects and, more importantly in patients, that the relationship between MCA velocity and PCO_2 was curvilinear. Attempts at fitting polynomials and logistic curves met with varying degrees of success in the normal population, but failed totally in describing the relationship between MCA velocity and PCO_2 in the abnormal patients. These problems were overcome by using a smoothing spline curve fitting programme (Bathspline, Silverman 1985). In each case, a single smooth curve was obtained, and the gradient could then be calculated at any value of PCO_2. Figures 8.12, 8.13 and 8.14 show examples of the relationship between MCA velocity and arterial PCO_2 in a normal adult, the relationship between MCA velocity and end-tidal PCO_2 in a normal adult and a normal child, and the relationship between MCA velocity and PCO_2 in individuals in the abnormal population, plotted using the spline technique. Values for the normal range of absolute CO_2 reactivity at different values of PCO_2 at intervals of 5mmHg (0.66kPa) are given in Table 8.V (Fig. 8.23d).

When a straight line was plotted through the data for an individual abnormal epoch, a negative slope for carbon dioxide reactivity appeared to be associated with poor outcome (Kirkham *et al.* 1987*b*, 1989). The analysis has since been refined, with

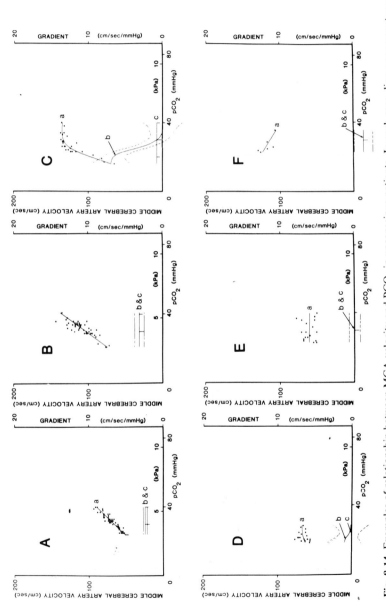

Fig. 8.14. Examples of relationship between MCA velocity and PCO_2 in unconscious patients. In each case, line a represents smoothed spline curve fitted through data points relating MCA velocity and PCO_2; line b (with 95 per cent confidence limits shown as dotted lines) represents gradient of line a at any point; and line c is gradient of line a at PCO_2 30mmHg (4.0kPa). Patient A: diagnosis encephalitis: relationship between MCA velocity and PCO_2 is straight line with gradient of 2.38cm/sec/mmHg. Blood pressure decreased by 5 per cent as PCO_2 increased from 24 to 40mmHg (3.2 to 5.3kPa). Patient B: diagnosis head injury; the relationship between MCA velocity and PCO_2 is straight line with gradient of 3.16cm/sec/mmHg, but blood pressure increased by 43 per cent as PCO_2 increased from 21 to 38mmHg (2.8 to 5.1kPa). Patient C: diagnosis encephalitis: initially MCA velocity increases with increasing PCO_2, but above PCO_2 of 35mmHg (4.7kPa) there is no further increase and gradient (b) of line a is zero. Gradient at PCO_2 30mmHg (4.0kPa) is 0.78cm/sec/mmHg. Patient D: diagnosis hypoxic-ischaemic encephalopathy: relationship between MCA velocity and PCO_2 is curve with gradient of 0.91cm/sec/mmHg at PCO_2 19mmHg (2.5kPa), decreasing to 0.3cm/sec/mmHg at PCO_2 24.5mmHg (3.3kPa) and tending to zero at values of PCO_2 above this. Patient E: diagnosis diabetes and ingestion of toluene: there is no relationship between MCA velocity and PCO_2, and gradient of straight line a is -0.04cm/sec/mmHg. Patient F: diagnosis head injury: relationship between MCA velocity and PCO_2 is straight line with negative slope of -1.41cm/sec/mmHg.

315

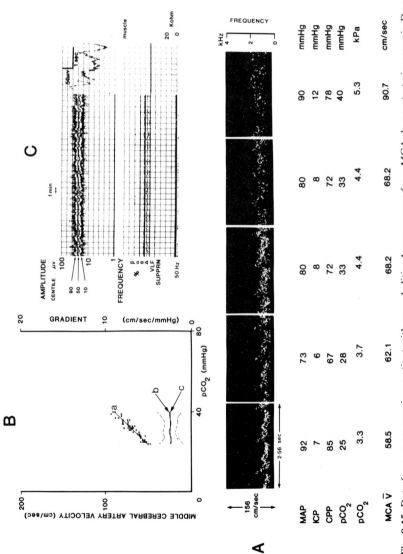

Fig. 8.15. Data from an unconscious patient with encephalitis. A: sonograms from MCA demonstrate increase in Doppler shift frequency with increasing PCO_2. B: Doppler shift frequency has been converted to velocity and plotted against PCO_2: relationship approximates to straight line (*a*) with gradient (*b*) of 2.38cm/sec/mmHg. EEG (CFAM trace C) showed high-amplitude diffuse slowing. Patient regained consciousness after three days in coma and made full recovery.

316

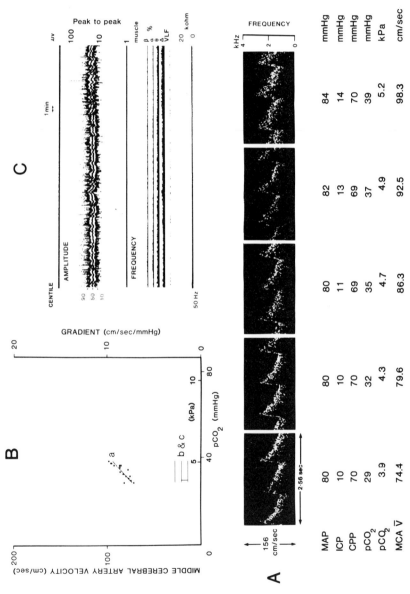

MAP	80	80	80	82	84	mmHg
ICP	10	10	11	13	14	mmHg
CPP	70	70	69	69	70	mmHg
pCO₂	29	32	35	37	39	mmHg
pCO₂	3.9	4.3	4.7	4.9	5.2	kPa
MCA V̄	74.4	79.6	86.3	92.5	98.3	cm/sec

Fig. 8.16. Data from unconscious patient who had suffered head injury. Day 1 A: sonograms (ordinate—Doppler shift frequency, abscissa—time) from the left MCA showing that Doppler shift frequency increased with increasing PCO₂. B: Doppler shift frequency has been converted to velocity and plotted against PCO₂; relationship was a straight line (*a*) with a gradient (*b*) of 2.08cm/sec/mmHg. Gradient (*c*) at PCO₂ 30mmHg (4.0kPa) is also shown. CFAM trace (C) was of normal amplitude and frequency plot showed all frequencies present.

317

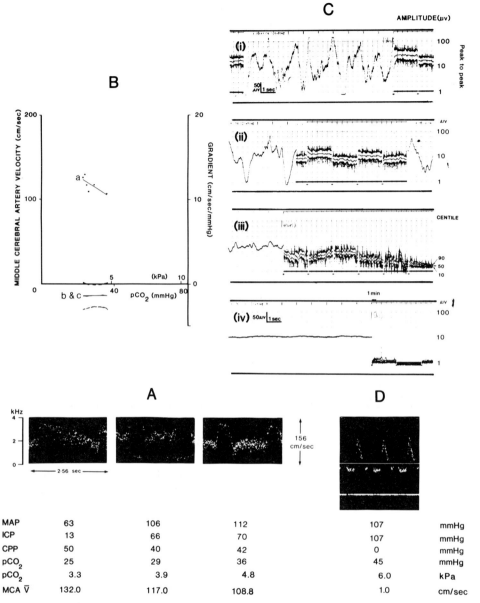

MAP	63	106	112	107	mmHg
ICP	13	66	70	107	mmHg
CPP	50	40	42	0	mmHg
pCO_2	25	29	36	45	mmHg
pCO_2	3.3	3.9	4.8	6.0	kPa
MCA $\bar{V}$	132.0	117.0	108.8	1.0	cm/sec

Fig. 8.17. Data from the same head-injured patient as Fig. 8.16. Day 4. A: sonograms (ordinate —Doppler shift frequency, abscissa—time) from the left MCA showing decreasing Doppler shift frequency with increasing PCO_2. B: Doppler shift frequency has been converted to velocity and plotted against PCO_2; relationship was a straight line (*a*) with a gradient (*b*) of −1.41cm/sec/mmHg. C: amplitude trace from CFAM on day 8. (i) At 10.40 amplitude was high (mean 27.5.μV) but it gradually decreased (ii) until at 14.40 it was 5.75 μV (iii) and just after 15.40 was less than 1μV (iv). D: sonogram obtained at 16.30 showing reverse flow throughout diastole (MCA velocity 1.4cm/sec, direction of flow index = 1—reverse flow/forward flow = 0.27). Patient fulfilled clinical criteria for brain death on two occasions and ventilation was discontinued on day 5.

318

TABLE 8.V

Relationship between middle cerebral artery velocity and PCO_2.
Normal range for gradient of spline curve (cm/sec/mmHg) at values of PCO_2 between 20 and 75mmHg
(2.7 and 10kPa)

PCO_2 mmHg	20	25	30	35	40	45	50	55	60	65	70	75
PCO_2 kPa	2.7	3.3	4.0	4.7	5.3	6.0	6.7	7.3	8.0	8.7	9.3	10.0
Minimum	0.70	0.39	0.54	0.74	0.92	0.20	−0.61	−0.25	−0.12	−0.99	0.20	0.17
Maximum	2.61	3.19	3.97	4.97	4.85	3.80	3.98	3.01	2.55	2.13	0.20	0.17
Mean	1.67	1.38	1.57	1.87	2.13	2.09	1.86	1.64	1.12	0.45	0.20	0.17
SD	0.64	0.65	0.71	0.91	1.01	0.87	0.90	0.94	1.08	1.28	0.20	0
Median	1.42	1.33	1.40	1.79	1.96	2.09	1.98	1.49	1.31	0.34	0.20	0.17
N	15	50	58	58	58	58	48	34	12	4	1	1
Tolerance limits (95% confidence)												
Lower limit		94	95	95	95	95	94	92				
Whole range		91	92	92	92	92	90	87				

TABLE 8.VI

Non-traumatic coma management of RICP

Maintenance of stable circulation with colloid and/or inotropes
Head positioned in midline and either flat or at 30°
Adequate paralysis and sedation
Aggressive management of seizures
Careful attention to fluid balance and plasma osmolarity
Ventilation to PCO_2 5.0kPa; hyperventilation for ICP spikes; careful weaning
Bolus doses of mannitol 0.25–1g/kg for ICP spikes
Maintenance of normothermia or mild hypothermia (35°C) (except in severe sepsis)
CSF drainage (via intraventricular catheter)
? Barbiturate coma
? Surgical decompression

a smoothed spline fitted to the points describing the relationship between MCA velocity and PCO₂ for each individual epoch.

In some patients, the EEG grade either remained the same or improved during the course of the child's illness, and this appeared to be associated with maintenance of a positive CO₂ reactivity slope (Fig. 8.15). In others, there was deterioration of the EEG, apparently in association with the finding of a flat or negative CO₂ response (Figs. 8.16, 8.17). Most of these patients went on to poor outcome (Figs. 8.17, 8.18), but two who were hyperventilated to very low PCO₂ eventually recovered (Fig. 8.19), as did two with negative CO₂ responses but preserved EEG who were surgically decompressed (Figs. 8.20, 8.21, 8.22). The latter two patients were also those with mean CPP which would have falsely predicted poor outcome using discriminant analysis (Fig. 8.1).

Most patients were hyperventilated, so the gradient at a PCO₂ of 30mmHg (4.0kPa) was chosen for comparisons between the good and poor outcome groups and the normals. There was no difference between good and poor outcome groups when the maximum CO₂ reactivity gradient at a PCO₂ of 30mmHg (4.0kPa) at any time during the patient's illness was compared with outcome, although both the good and poor outcome groups were significantly different from normal (Mann-

Whitney, both p<0.05, Fig. 8.23a). There was, however, a highly significant difference between good and poor outcome groups when the minimum CO_2 reactivity gradient at PCO_2 of 30mmHg (4.0kPa) obtained during the course of the child's illness were compared (p<0.01, Fig. 8.23b) and again both were significantly different from normal (p<0.01). Fig. 8.23c compares the CO_2 reactivity gradient at a PCO_2 of 30mmHg (4.0kPa), obtained before EEG deterioration, with the minimum CO_2 reactivity gradient at a PCO_2 of 30mmHg (4.0kPa) seen during the course of the child's illness in those whose EEGs did not deteriorate. There was a highly significant difference between these two groups (p<0.01).

Discriminant analysis has been used to attempt to predict outcome, using various combinations of three parameters (Fig. 8.24): (i) the gradient of the CO_2 reactivity curve at PCO_2 30mmHg (4.0kPa), (ii) whether or not the curve flattened off at the maximum PCO_2 achieved, and (iii) the maximum PCO_2 achieved or the PCO_2 at which the curve flattened off in those in which this occurred.

The curve with the maximum CO_2 reactivity slope at a PCO_2 30mmHg (4.0kPa) during the course of the child's illness was a poor discriminant of outcome, but the curve with the minimum CO_2 reactivity slope at a PCO_2 of 30mmHg (4.0kPa) during a child's illness was an excellent discriminant. For this curve, the model (i)*(ii)+(iii) demonstrated no false positives or negatives in the population studied retrospectively, whilst jack-knifing to predict the usefulness of the model in future studies suggested that 4 per cent false negatives and 4 per cent false positives would be expected (cut 0.1 to 0.9). Good discrimination was obtained, using the model (i)+(ii)*(iii) for the comparison of the curve prior to EEG deterioration in those whose EEGs did deteriorate, compared with the curve with the minimum slope at PCO_2 30mmHg (4.0kPa) in those in whom this did not happen. There was only one false positive for the retrospective population, and a 4 per cent false positive and false negative rate was expected when jack-knifing (cut 0.5) to predict the usefulness of the model in a prospective study.

These preliminary data suggest that poor outcome in coma may be predicted by analysis of the shape of the CO_2 reactivity curve, and in particular, its tendency to

Fig. 8.18 (*opposite*). Data from unconscious patient who had suffered hypoxic-ischaemic insult. B: MCA velocity has been plotted against PCO_2 from data collected at three separate times after cardiac arrest of approximately 10 minutes' duration. (i) 134 hours post-arrest, relationship between MCA velocity and PCO_2 was linear (*a*) with a gradient (*b*) of 5.15cm/sec/mmHg. (ii) 191 hours post-arrest, relationship was a curve with a lower gradient (*b*) (*e.g.* 0.62cm/sec/mmHg at PCO_2 25mmHg (3.3kPa) and decreasing still further at PCO_2 30mmHg (4.0kPa) (line *c*). (iii) 196 hours post-arrest, the relationship was a curve with a still lower gradient (*b*) (*e.g.* 0.34cm/sec/mmHg at PCO_2 25mmHg (3.3kPa) and tending towards zero at PCO_2 30mmHg (4.0kPa) (line *c*). Sonograms from which the data in (B) (iii) were taken are shown in (A). C: Samples of cerebral function monitor traces from same patient (i) 134 hours post-arrest—data collected simultaneously with Doppler data plotted in (B) (i); mean amplitude of cerebral function monitor trace was over 10μV. All four frequencies were present, although there was very scanty beta activity (ii) 191 hours post-arrest—data collected simultaneously with Doppler data plotted in (B) (ii)—mean amplitude remained above 10μV but minimum amplitude was lower. (iii) 197 hours post-arrest—one hour after collection of Doppler data plotted in (B) (iii); mean amplitude remained approximately 10μV but (iv) 200 hours post-arrest—four hours after collection of Doppler data plotted in (B) (iii)—mean amplitude had fallen to approximately 4μV and remained low during monitoring over next 12 hours. After this both CO_2 reactivity and amplitude of cerebral function monitor trace recovered to pre-existing values. At follow-up three years later, patient remained in a vegetative state.

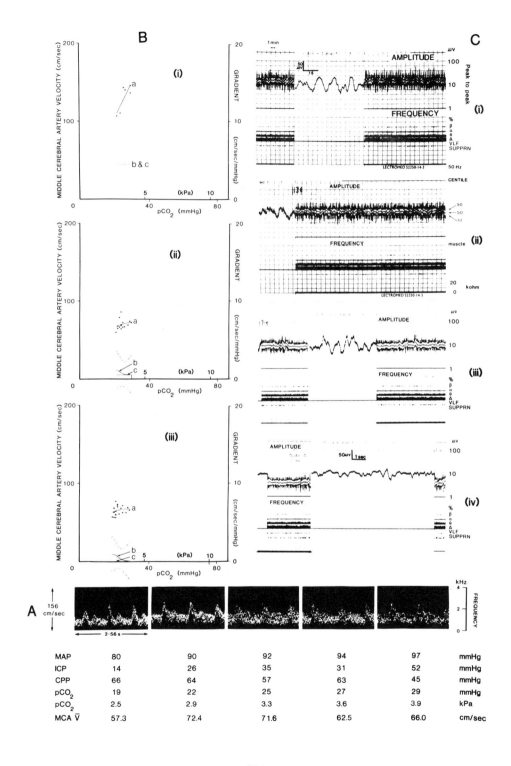

MAP	80	90	92	94	97	mmHg
ICP	14	26	35	31	52	mmHg
CPP	66	64	57	63	45	mmHg
pCO$_2$	19	22	25	27	29	mmHg
pCO$_2$	2.5	2.9	3.3	3.6	3.9	kPa
MCA V̄	57.3	72.4	71.6	62.5	66.0	cm/sec

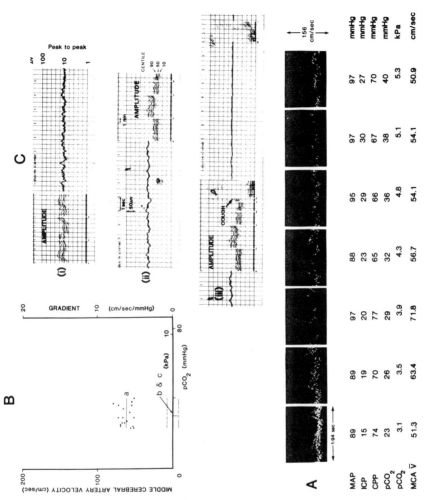

Fig. 8.19. Data from unconscious patient with diabetes who had ingested toluene. A: sonograms from left MCA on day 1. There was little change in Doppler shift frequency with increasing PCO₂. B: Doppler shift frequency was converted to velocity and plotted against PCO₂. Relationship was a straight line (*a*) with gradient (*b*) of −0.04cm/sec/mmHg. Gradient (*c*) at PCO_2 30mmHg (4.0kPa) is also shown. C: amplitude trace from cerebral function monitor trace later the same day. The machine presented compressed data from left and right hemispheres alternately every five minutes and played out 10 seconds of raw EEG data from right hemisphere every half hour. (i) Initially trace from both hemispheres was of moderate amplitude (mean just over 10μV) but six hours later (ii), amplitude had decreased a little and there was some asymmetry (mean amplitude on right 3.02μV and on left 8.32μV). 18 hours later (iii), after the patient had coughed, amplitude of CFAM trace decreased suddenly (mean 1.32μV). He was hyperventilated to very low PCO_2 (below 20mmHg); CFAM amplitude increased and patient recovered consciousness several days later and survived with no abnormal neurological signs (although he performed less well in school than previously and had a full-scale IQ of 80 at follow-up three years later).

322

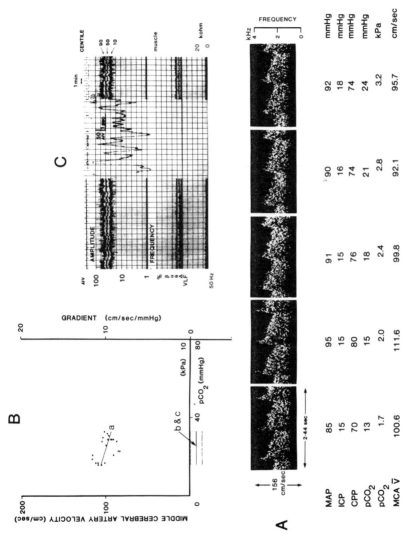

Fig. 8.20. Data from patient with encephalitis. A: sonograms from right MCA on day 1 of coma. There was no over-all increase of Doppler shift frequency when PCO₂ was increased from 13 to 24mmHg (1.7 to 3.2kPa). B: Doppler shift frequency has been converted to velocity and plotted against PCO₂: relationship was straight line (line *a*) with a gradient (line *b*) of −0.76cm/sec/mmHg. C: CFAM trace from same patient recorded simultaneously with Doppler data: trace was of high amplitude but with an excess of slower frequencies.

323

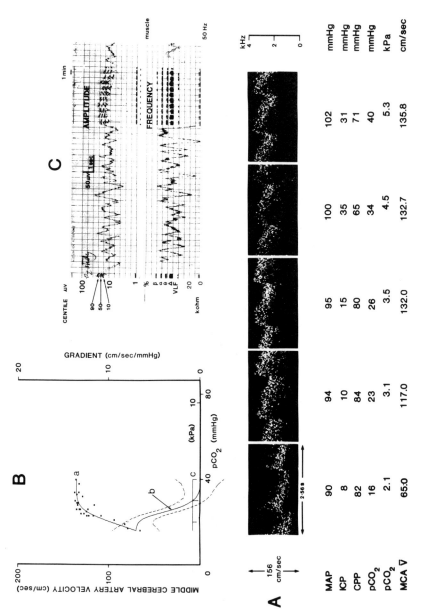

Fig. 8.21. Data from same patient with encephalitis as in Fig. 8.20. A: sonograms recorded on day 3: there was an initial increase in Doppler shift frequency (and therefore of time-averaged mean velocity) as PCO_2 increased from 17 to 30mmHg (2.3 to 4.0kPa) but no further increase over range of PCO_2 30 to 40mmHg (4.0 to 5.3kPa). B: Doppler shift frequency has been converted to velocity and plotted against PCO_2: relationship was curve (*a*) with gradient of 0.78cm/sec/mmHg at PCO_2 30mmHg (4.0kPa) (line *c*). The gradient (*b*, with 95 per cent confidence limits plotted as dotted lines of curve *a* was 6.93cm/sec/mmHg at PCO_2 17mmHg (2.3kPa), falling to zero at PCO_2 35mmHg (4.6kPa). C: CFAM trace recorded simultaneously with Doppler data: compressed trace alternated between right and left sides at one-minute intervals. Sample of EEG was played out (top–right, bottom–left): trace remained of high amplitude but with excess of slow frequencies. The patient was surgically decompressed 12 hours later because of continuing intracranial hypertension at normocapnia.

324

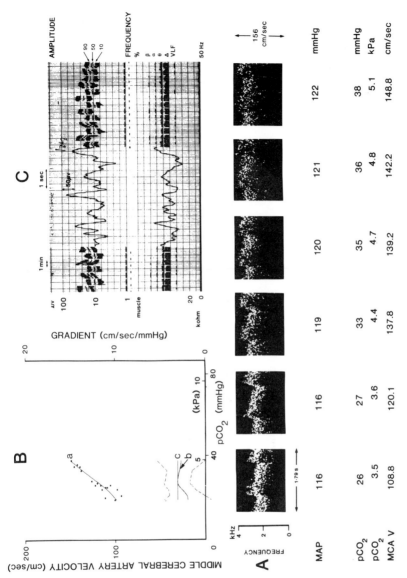

Fig. 8.22. Data from same patient with encephalitis as in Figs. 8.20. and 8.21 but obtained after surgical decompression. A: sonograms (ordinate—Doppler shift frequency, abscissa—time) on day 4, 10 hours after surgical decompression. Doppler shift frequency increased over range of PCO₂ 26 to 38mmHg (3.5 to 5.1kPa). B: Doppler shift frequency has been converted to velocity and plotted against PCO₂; relationship was curve (*a*) and gradient (*b*) has been plotted (with 95 per cent confidence limits as dotted lines). Gradient at PCO₂ 30mmHg (4.0kPa) was 3.12cm/sec/mmHg (line *c*). C: cerebral function monitor trace recorded simultaneously with Doppler data plotted in (B). Compressed trace alternated between the two hemispheres every minute. Sample of raw EEG was recorded (top–right, bottom–left): amplitude of trace remained high, with an excess of slower frequencies. Patient regained consciousness on day 7 and at follow-up three years later had no neurological deficit and had returned to a normal school.

325

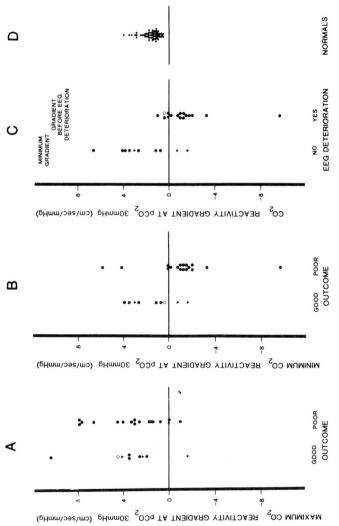

Fig. 8.23. A: relationship between maximum CO_2 reactivity at PCO_2 30mmHg (4.0kPa) during course of patients' illness and outcome. There was considerable overlap between good and poor outcome groups and no significant difference between them (Mann-Whitney). B: relationship between minimum CO_2 reactivity at PCO_2 30mmHg (4.0kPa) during course of patients' illness and outcome. There was a significant difference (Mann-Whitney) in values for minimum CO_2 reactivity at PCO_2 30mmHg (4.0kPa) between good and poor outcome groups. C: relationship between minimum CO_2 reactivity at PCO_2 30mmHg (4.0kPa) during the patients' illness in those whose EEGs did not deteriorate and between CO_2 reactivity gradient at PCO_2 30mmHg (4.0kPa) immediately before EEG deterioration in those patients in whom this occurred. There was a significant difference ($p<0.01$, Mann-Whitney) between these values in the two groups. D: normal range for CO_2 reactivity at PCO_2 30mmHg (4.0kPa): all patient groups differ significantly from normal but there was some overlap, even with minimum CO_2 reactivity in the poor outcome group (B) and with CO_2 reactivity immediately before EEG deterioration in those in whom this occurred (C). Closed triangles represent the patients who were surgically decompressed and open circle represents patient who was hyperventilated to very low PCO_2 levels (less than 20mmHg) after EEG had deteriorated and who made a good recovery (see Fig. 8.19).

326

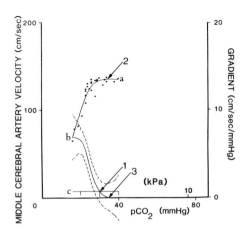

Fig. 8.24. Components of spline curve used in discriminant analysis. Curve *a* describes relationship between MCA velocity and PCO_2. Curve *b* is gradient of curve *a* (with 95 per cent confidence limits shown as dotted lines). Horizontal line *c* is gradient at PCO_2 30mmHg (4.0kPa) (for comparison with gradient at other values of PCO_2; 1: gradient at PCO_2 30mmHg (4.0kPa) of curve describing relationship between MCA velocity and PCO_2; 2: whether or not gradient of this curve reached zero as PCO_2 increased; 3: PCO_2 at which gradient of this curve reached zero if this occurred.

flatten off with increasing PCO_2 when maximal vasodilatation has been achieved. This might be used to test the reserve capacity of the cerebral circulation, and possibly to indicate the need for intervention when the reserve is exhausted. A prospective study is needed, and as it is time-consuming to process the data, a computer-aided system would be beneficial. There is an on-line system for monitoring MCA velocity in association with parameters such as MAP, ICP and end-tidal carbon dioxide (Ruben *et al.* 1989).

Management

It is worth making a distinction between the emergency resuscitation of the patient in non-traumatic coma (Table 8.II) and the management of the patient who remains unconscious for more than a few hours (Table 8.VI). Every paediatrician and casualty officer should be familiar with the priorities involved in the former, since if secondary ischaemic events can be avoided at this stage, coma may be quickly reversed and poor outcome prevented. There is much more controversy about long-term treatment, which is discussed below. Since the benefits and risks of various management strategies may need to be very carefully weighed up in the individual patient, and priorities may change during the course of a child's illness, treatment regimes may be very complex and should only be undertaken in ICUS where there is extensive experience of paediatric coma.

DIAGNOSIS AND MANAGEMENT OF THE UNDERLYING CAUSE

All patients in non-traumatic coma need a CT scan on admission to exclude surgically treatable aetiologies (*e.g.* intracerebral haemorrhage, hydrocephalus or tumour) and to look for evidence of cerebral oedema, although a normal CT scan does not exclude intracranial hypertension. The timing of other investigations (such as blood tests, EEG and MRI scan) will be governed by the clinical situation. An experienced physician should always be involved in these decisions and in those concerned with appropriate management of the underlying aetiology. If there is no obvious cause for coma, the child should receive acyclovir (750 to 1500mg/m²/day intravenously in three divided doses) to cover the possibility of HSV encephalitis.

It is dangerous to lumbar puncture an unconscious patient (Addy 1987) unless a CT scan has excluded a mass lesion and ICP is measured and can be managed (with a dose of 1g/kg 20 per cent mannitol and immediate ventilation) if the patient shows clinical signs of coning (Table 8.I) (McWilliam 1985). Broad spectrum antibiotics, either a modern cephalosporin such as ceftriaxone or ceftazidine (30 to 100mg/kg/day in two or three divided doses), or chloramphenicol (100mg/kg/day in four divided doses) and penicillin (300mg/kg/day in six divided doses), should be commenced after a septic screen but before CSF is obtained. In most cases, the organism causing meningitis can be identified clinically or from blood cultures or by countercurrent immunoelectrophoresis of CSF obtained at lumbar puncture when the patient is stable, and if necessary antibiotic regimes can be modified.

NURSING CARE

Patients should be nursed flat, as head elevation may reduce CPP (Rosner *et al.* 1986), and with the head in the midline so that the jugular venous drainage is not obstructed. Great care must be taken with endotracheal suction (Rudy *et al.* 1986). Adequate paralysis and sedation is essential. Transport to theatre or the radiology department must be very carefully supervised.

CIRCULATION AND FLUID BALANCE

It is most important that an adequate circulation is quickly restored, if necessary with volume expanders (plasma or blood) and vasopressor agents (*e.g.* dobutamine 10 to 20µg/kg/min), as shock is a commonly associated finding in the child presenting in non-traumatic coma (Lucking *et al.* 1986). Crystalloid fluids should be restricted to approximately 60 per cent of the age-appropriate requirements during the initial resuscitation, and hypo-osmolar fluids must be avoided. If the child remains unconscious for several days, arterial and central venous pressures and core and peripheral temperatures must be monitored, a careful fluid balance chart should be kept, the child should be weighed frequently using bedscales, and plasma electrolytes and osmolality must be measured at least twice daily.

Hyponatraemia can be associated with deterioration in conscious level due to cerebral oedema (Arieff 1985) and with poor outcome. Rapid correction may be associated with central pontine myelinolysis (Sterns *et al.* 1986) and hyponatraemia should therefore always be corrected slowly. There is controversy over whether low serum sodium in this situation is due to inappropriate ADH secretion (Kaplan and Feigin 1978) or to salt loss (Wijdicks *et al.* 1985); it is possible that the mechanism varies in different encephalopathies. There is evidence in some conditions, *e.g.* in subarachnoid haemorrhage (Wijdicks *et al.* 1985), that cerebral infarction is commoner in patients who are fluid-restricted, and it may be appropriate to give normal saline (Reeder and Harbaugh 1989). Few data are available to guide precise fluid management in other encephalopathies; there is however no doubt that severe dehydration must be avoided, and that patients should not be given large volumes of hypo-osmolar fluids, such as 10 per cent dextrose. Fluid prescriptions must be very regularly reviewed and revised according to the data from measurements of blood pressure, central venous pressure, core-peripheral temperature gap, plasma electrolytes and osmolality, body weight and fluid balance. Infusions of colloid may be required if central venous pressure is low or biochemical parameters indicate prerenal failure. If central venous pressure is normal or high, inotropes such as dobutamine (5 to 20µg/kg/min) and/or adrenaline (10µg/kg/min) and/or noradrenaline (100 to 1000ng/kg/min) may be required to maintain blood pressure. Low-dose dopamine (2µg/kg/min) can be useful in improving renal perfusion and preventing anuria. Therapy with other vasodilating drugs such as sodium nitroprusside is usually contraindicated, as these drugs also have an effect on the cerebral circulation, increasing ICP and altering the autoregulatory range (Marsh *et al.* 1979, Weiss *et al.* 1979). Prostacyclin is a vasodilator and has also been shown to improve tissue oxygenation (Bihari *et al.* 1986); in certain circumstances (*e.g.* meningococcal shock) this drug may be useful, but its precise role has yet to be defined. If there is a bleeding diathesis, infusions of platelets and/or fresh frozen plasma may be required. Careful attention must be paid to nutrition; there is no evidence that intracranial hypertension is worsened by parenteral feeding (Young *et al.* 1987). Acute renal failure may be a particular problem in hypoxic-ischaemic encephalopathy, when there is often acute tubular necrosis of the kidneys. Early peritoneal dialysis or haemofiltration enables fine control of fluid balance if renal failure becomes established.

CONTROL OF SEIZURES

Prolonged seizures appear to be associated with secondary deterioration, according to the Guy's Hospital study of hypoxic-ischaemic encephalopathy 1982–5 (Constantinou *et al.* 1989). During brief experimental seizures, CBF and cerebral metabolic rate usually increase and there is little evidence of ischaemia (Chapman 1985). The situation may be different after recurrent or prolonged seizures (Kreisman *et al.* 1983, Chapman 1985). In the unconscious patient, if there is already a degree of vasoparalysis, it is possible that the perfusion reserve is inadequate to meet the increased metabolic demand of a seizure and severe ischaemia might result. During seizures in coma in the Guy's study, MCA velocity increased in some in association with an increase in MAP (Fig. 8.25), but not in others (Fig. 8.26). Prognosis was very poor in the latter patients.

It may be difficult to know whether or not the unconscious patient is having fits, particularly if he is paralysed and sedated for ventilation. There may be a place for EEG monitoring in this situation (Tasker *et al.* 1989). Seizure control should be attempted with anticonvulsants such as phenobarbitone (loading dose of 20mg/kg then 5 to 10mg/kg/day) or phenytoin (loading infusion of 20mg/kg over 30 minutes then 5 to 10mg/kg/day); precise dosage must be guided by daily plasma levels. Bolus doses of diazepam (0.2 to 0.3mg/kg) or paraldehyde (0.3ml/kg in an equal volume of arachis oil) may be used to control individual seizures. Chlormethiazole by infusion (1ml/kg/hr) has a useful role, provided that the patient is not in renal failure, as a large volume of fluid must be given. Barbiturate coma (loading dose of 5 to 8mg/kg followed by an infusion of 2 to 10mg/kg/hr, guided by plasma levels) may be used in intractable status epilepticus (Tasker *et al.* 1989), but if this occurs

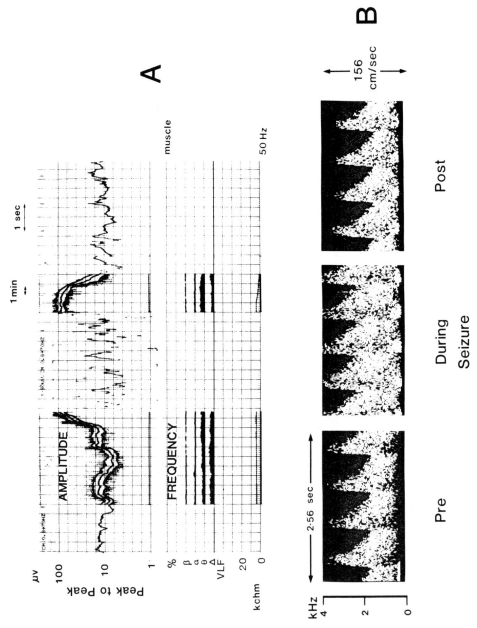

Fig. 8.25. Data from patient with Reye's syndrome. Day 3. A: cerebral function monitor trace. Mean amplitude of background activity was between 6 and 15 µV and all frequencies were present, although with very little beta activity (*a*). At *b*, mean amplitude increased to approximately 90µV and sample of raw EEG (*c*) showed spike and wave (*c*: 2Hz). At *d*, mean amplitude of compressed trace returned to mean amplitude just above 10µV. B: sonograms recorded from left MCA: before electrical discharge, MCA velocity was 102.2cm/sec and rose to 121.5cm/sec during discharge.

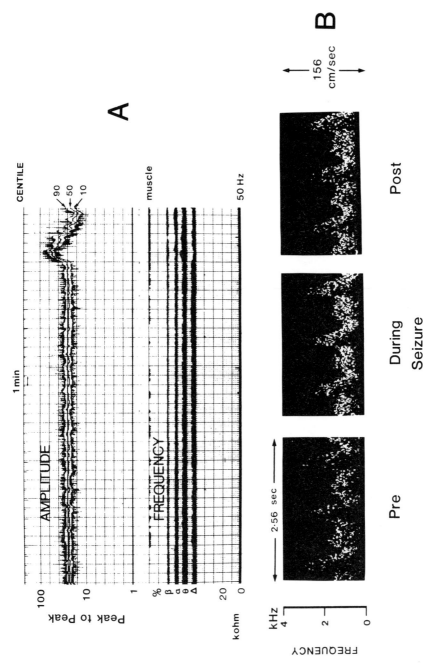

Fig. 8.26. Data from patient 30 hours after a cardiac arrest lasting 10 minutes. A: CFAM trace. At *a*, amplitude was high (mean approximately 40 μV) and all four frequencies were present, although there was little variation in either amplitude or frequency. At *d*, amplitude suddenly increased to a mean of between 50 and 60 μV. This was acompanied by a clinical myoclonic seizure (note increase in muscle band on the CFAM trace). B: sonograms from the right MCA: there was no increase in MCA velocity during clinical and electrical seizure.

331

as a consequence of hypoxic-ischaemic encephalopathy, the seizures may be impossible to control and the prognosis is very poor (Simon and Aminoff 1986).

STEROIDS

There is no evidence that steroids prevent cerebral oedema or improve outcome in terms of survival or of intellectual and motor function after cardiac arrest (Grafton and Longstreth 1988), in meningitis (de Lemos and Haggerty 1969, Belsey *et al.* 1969, Lebel *et al.* 1988) or in hepatic encephalopathy (Canalese *et al.* 1982). In meningitis, clinical (fever) and laboratory (CSF glucose, lactate and protein) parameters appeared to improve more rapidly in the steroid-treated group, and the incidence of deafness as a sequel was apparently reduced (Lebel *et al.* 1988), although there were methodological difficulties with these studies (Smith 1988) and these results need confirmation in a larger population (Kaplan 1989) as they may be partially explained by rapid CSF sterilisation by the cephalosporin, ceftriaxone (Schaad *et al.* 1990). In ischaemic encephalopathy there are concerns about the worsening of brain damage (Sapolsky and Pulsinelli 1985), which may be associated with hyperglycaemia, predisposing to cerebral lactic acidosis and infarction.

MANNITOL

It is probably reasonable to give a single dose of mannitol immediately after resuscitation from cardiac arrest or during the early phase following stroke, providing that blood pressure is adequate, to decrease the osmotic gradient between blood and brain during the reperfusion period and therefore perhaps to reduce cerebral oedema (Stephenson *et al.* 1988), for although the cerebral circulation may not necessarily be improved in severe ischaemia (Arai *et al.* 1986), there may well be an increase in CBF in moderately ischaemic regions (Meyer *et al.* 1987). Mannitol has been shown to decrease ICP in an experimental model of *Haemophilus influenzae* meningitis (Syrogiannopoulos *et al.* 1987), in line with clinical experience with osmotic agents in humans with meningitis (Williams *et al.* 1964), hepatic encephalopathy (Canalese *et al.* 1982) and head injury (Mendelow *et al.* 1985). There is no doubt that rapid administration (Roberts *et al.* 1987) of osmotic agents is beneficial in the short term in coma due to meningitis, encephalitis, status epilepticus and metabolic conditions and many previously unrousable children regain consciousness after a single dose of 0.5 to 1g/kg of mannitol. There is evidence that the main effect of mannitol is to reduce blood viscosity and induce cerebral vasoconstriction if autoregulation is intact (Muizelaar *et al.* 1984) rather than to reduce brain-water content. Prolonged use (more than 48 hours) may be associated with rebound intracranial hypertension, and it is better to give an occasional small (0.25g/kg) dose of mannitol in response to acutely raised ICP in this situation than to administer regular doses without guidance from an ICP monitor. Serum osmolality should not be allowed to rise above 300 milliosmoles, and mannitol should not be administered to children in established renal failure unless haemofiltration is in progress.

HYPERVENTILATION

ICP is thought to be decreased by hyperventilation because of the reduction of CBF and therefore of CBV, at least initially. One argument against the use of prolonged hyperventilation has been that in studies in unanaesthetised normal animals, the cerebral blood vessels are no longer constricted after approximately 20 hours (Muizelaar *et al*. 1988) and CBF and therefore CBV return to normal (Raichle *et al*. 1970, Albrecht *et al*. 1987). This phenomenon, however, has not been observed in anaesthetised animals (McDowell and Harper 1968), and although a similar effect on CBF and CBV was seen in dogs with an intracranial mass lesion, CSF pressure did not rise in parallel because CSF volume decreased, probably due to improved access to spinal reabsorption channels (Artru 1987). There are conflicting data about the effect of hyperventilation on ICP and CBF after global ischaemic insults in animals (Miller *et al*. 1980*b*) but CO_2 reactivity partially recovered at low PCO_2 in one study (Todd *et al*. 1985). This may be a marker for the recovery of the reserve capacity of the cerebral circulation, which may be important if other vasodilating events, such as seizures or waves of ICP, are expected. The effect of prolonged hyperventilation on cerebral haemodynamics in unconscious humans have not been studied.

There are worries that hyperventilation to a PCO_2 of less than 25mmHg (3.3kPa) may be associated with cerebral ischaemia, but although cerebral lactate is increased, the lactate-pyruvate ratio remains the same, which suggests that the increase in lactate is secondary to the stimulation of glycolysis (Albrecht *et al*. 1987). In addition, CMRO$_2$ either remains stable (Rosenberg 1988) or decreases in parallel with CBF during moderate hypocapnia (Albrecht *et al*. 1987) and is then maintained constant during severe hypocapnia, either because the oxygen extraction ratio is increased or because CBF no longer decreases (Rosenberg 1988). Haemodynamics are often altered in the unconscious patient, and if the CO_2 reactivity slope is negative, an increase in CBF may be obtained with a decrease in PCO_2. In one patient in our series, improvement in EEG was seen as soon as hyperventilation was commenced, two hours after cardiac arrest (Fig. 8.7).

There is therefore clear evidence that the reduction of CBF by hypocapnia is only temporary; however, the beneficial effects of hyperventilation noted by clinicians may be operating either by increasing CO_2 reactivity or by improving access to spinal channels of CSF absorption. There is an urgent need for clinical trials of hyperventilation in non-traumatic coma, as the available data suggest a short-term benefit only (Ede *et al*. 1986), and for further animal studies of prolonged hyperventilation in the presence of cerebral oedema or a mass lesion, but in the meantime the clinical use of hyperventilation in non-traumatic coma should be as follows:

1. If a patient is found acutely unconscious, s/he should be hyperventilated to a PCO_2 of 25 to 30mmHg (3.3 to 4.0kPa) as this achieves a rapid reduction of ICP. S/he should then be transferred to a paediatric ICU hyperventilated with very careful attention to airway management.

2. Patients who are paralysed and sedated for hyperventilation should always have ICP monitors inserted. This is paticularly important if the patient is to be weaned from the ventilator as CO_2 reactivity is increased by hyperventilation (Muizelaar *et al*. 1988), and ICP may increase greatly as PCO_2 is increased (Havill 1984). There may be a role for transcranial Doppler in monitoring the response of the cerebral circulation to weaning from the ventilator.

3. Patients with normal ICP should be weaned slowly from the ventilator.

4. It may be useful to be able to drain CSF from a ventricular catheter during weaning from the ventilator, as access to the spinal channels of CSF absorption may be suddenly cut off, causing a precipitous rise in ICP.

BARBITURATE COMA

At present, there is no indication for barbiturate coma in hypoxic ischaemic encephalopathy as a large controlled trial has shown that it is of no benefit (Brain Resuscitation Clinical Trial I Study Group 1986). It may occasionally be useful in the unconscious patient with intractable intracranial hypertension (Woodcock *et al.* 1982, Piatt and Schiff 1984) or status epilepticus (Lowenstein *et al.* 1988), provided that the systemic circulation can be maintained (Traeger *et al.* 1983). Patients must be very carefully selected (Eisenberg *et al.* 1988), and the cerebrovascular response to reduced CO_2 may be useful in this context (Nordstrom *et al.* 1988). The pharmacokinetics of thiopentone can make the clinical diagnosis of brainstem death impossible, as plasma levels may remain high for some time after an infusion has been discontinued (Harvey 1985).

HYPOTHERMIA

From animal data (Carlsson *et al.* 1976) and clinical experience in cardiac surgery, there is no doubt that hypothermia is protective if commenced before ischaemia occurs. It is less certain that hypothermia has a place in the resuscitation of the patient in non-traumatic coma. Cerebral metabolic rate increases directly with temperature and there is considerable experimental evidence for deranged metabolism if ischaemic brain is subjected to hyperthermia in addition (Hossmann 1988, Chopp *et al.* 1988). There is therefore a good case for the strict maintenance of normothermia or very mild (34 to 37°c) hypothermia. At lower temperatures, the potential benefits may be outweighed by side-effects, such as neutropenia and susceptibility to sepsis (Bohn *et al.* 1986), myocardial depression (Hildebrand *et al.* 1988) and haematological dysfunction. Some groups who originally advocated hypothermia as a treatment for the encephalopathies associated with Reye's syndrome and near-drowning (Conn *et al.* 1979) have since discontinued this modality (Bohn *et al.* 1986), but others still maintain that there is a place for hypothermia (Nussbaum and Maggi 1988). We have not found sepsis to be a problem in patients cooled to 35 or 36°c. One practical advantage of hypothermia over barbiturate coma for reducing cerebral metabolic rate is that the former is easily reversible for neurological examination. If a suitable maintenance temperature could be defined at which cerebral metabolism continued optimally but which was not associated with neutropenia, a prospective controlled trial, which has hitherto not been conducted, would be worthwhile.

CSF DRAINAGE

If an intraventricular catheter is inserted, CSF may be drained either in response to ICP peaks or continuously to maintain ICP below a certain level, predetermined by the height of the valve chamber. There is some evidence that oedema fluid may

334

disperse more quickly if CSF is allowed to drain in this way (Cao *et al*. 1984) There is a risk of infection, but continuous drainage of CSF may be an alternative to the side-effects and problems with rebound intracranial hypertension associated with prolonged drug therapy and hyperventilation.

SURGICAL DECOMPRESSION

Although surgical decompression has been successfully employed for the encephalopathies asociated with lead-poisoning (McLaurin and Nichols 1957), Reye's syndrome (Ausman *et al*. 1976) and encephalitis (Kirkham and Neville 1986), the results in traumatic coma have been disappointing (Venes and Collins 1975, Cooper *et al*. 1976), and there is animal evidence that cerebral oedema may be increased post-craniectomy (Cooper *et al*. 1979). It is possible that the patients in the previous series underwent surgery after irreversible secondary ischaemia had already occurred. Of the five cases decompressed at Guy's Hospital between 1982 and 1986, three with apparently compromised cerebral haemodynamics (mean CPP below 70mmHg at normocapnia and abnormal CO_2 reactivity) but preserved EEG activity are now normal intellectually and neurologically, whereas of the two patients decompressed after the minimum CPP had fallen below 40mmHg and the EEG amplitude had decreased, one is very severely disabled and one fulfilled clinical criteria for brainstem death. Craniectomy may also have a place in the management of the patient who has evidence of uncal herniation after stroke (Kondziolka and Fazl 1988). Surgical decompression may offer an alternative to prolonged medical management of intracranial hypertension in certain circumstances (Gower *et al*. 1988) and should be further explored.

OUTCOME

It is more difficult to show that treating RICP and maintaining CBF improves outcome. Despite early optimism, there is little evidence to show that the prognosis for the nearly drowned comatose child has been improved by brain resuscitation protocols. Similarly, the prognosis for most children with hypoxic ischaemic encephalopathy may be determined at the time of the original arrest. Early treatment of bacterial meningitis with adequate doses of antibiotics is more important than management of late cerebral oedema in this condition. It is important, however, to be aware of the potential for intracranial hypertension and poor cerebral perfusion in non-traumatic coma, as anticipation and early treatment may prevent secondary ischaemia and deterioration in those patients originally predicted to do well.

In summary, there are few data on which to base our clinical practice in managing the patient in non-traumatic coma. There is probably an intermediate group in deep coma, but with preserved brainstem reflexes and preserved EEG, in whom the prognosis may be improved with early recognition of haemodynamic compromise. In these patients, CPP must be maintained above 70mmHg and seizures should be controlled quickly. Further studies of pathophysiology and management are urgently required, as this is becoming an important problem in paediatrics.

ACKNOWLEDGEMENT: this work was supported by the British Heart Foundation, the Peek Trust, and the Handicapped Children's Aid Committee. I should like to thank my colleagues, Dr T. S. Padayachee, for helpful advice, Miss M. C. Kyme for excellent technical assistance, Miss M. Edwards for careful follow-up and Dr F. R. House for performing the statistical analysis.

REFERENCES

Aaslid, R., Markwalder, T. M., Nornes, H. (1982) 'Noninvasive transcranial Doppler ultrasound recording of flow velocity in basal cerebral arteries.' *Journal of Neurosurgery*, **57**, 769–774.
—— Lundar, T., Lindegaard, K. F., Nornes, H. (1986) 'Estimation of cerebral perfusion pressure from arterial blood pressure and transcranial Doppler recordings.' *In* Miller, J. D., Teasdale, G. M., Rowan, J.O., Galbraith, S. L., Mendelow, A. D. (Eds.) *Intracranial Pressure VI*. Berlin: Springer. pp. 226–229.
Adams, R. D., Kubic, C. S., Bonner, F. J. (1948) 'The clinical and pathological aspects of influenzal meningitis.' *Archives of Pediatrics*, **65**, 354–376, 408–441.
Addy, D. P. (1987) 'When not to do a lumbar puncture.' *Archives of Disease in Childhood*, **62**, 873–875.
Albrecht, R. F., Miletich, D. J., Ruttle, M. (1987) 'Cerebral effects of extended hyperventilation in unanaesthetized goats.' *Stroke*, **18**, 649–655.
Altman, D. I., Powers, W. J., Perlman, J. M., Herscovitch, P., Volpe, S. L., Volpe, J. J. (1988) 'Cerebral blood flow requirement for brain viability in newborn infants is lower than in adults.' *Annals of Neurology*, **24**, 218–226.
Ames, A. III, Wright, R. L., Kowada, M., Thurston, J. M., Majno, G. (1968) 'Cerebral ischaemia. 2: the no-reflow phenomenon.' *American Journal of Pathology*, **52**, 437–453.
Antoon, A.Y., Volpe, J. J., Crawford, J. D. (1972) 'Burn encephalopathy in children.' *Pediatrics*, **50**, 609–616.
Arai, T., Tsukahara, I., Nitta, K., Watanabe, T. (1986) 'Effects of mannitol on cerebral circulation after transient complete cerebral ischemia in dogs.' *Critical Care Medicine*, **14**, 634–637.
Arieff, A. I. (1985) 'Effects of water, electrolyte and acid-base disorders on the central nervous system.' *In* Arieff, A. I., De Fronzo, R. A. (Eds.) *Fluid, Electrolyte and Acid-Base Disorders*. New York: Churchill Livingstone. pp. 969–1040.
Artru, A. A. (1987) 'Reduction of cerebrospinal fluid pressure by hypocapnia: change in cerebral blood volume, cerebrospinal fluid volume, and brain tissue water and electrolytes.' *Journal of Cerebral Blood Flow and Metabolism*, **7**, 471–479.
Ashwal, S., Schneider, S., Thompson, J. (1989) 'Xenon computed tomography measuring cerebral blood flow in the determination of brain death in children.' *Annals of Neurology*, **25**, 539–546.
Astrup, J. (1982) 'Energy-requiring cell functions in the ischemic brain.' *Journal of Neurosurgery*, **56**, 482–497.
Ausman, J. I., Rogers, C., Sharp, H. L. (1976) 'Decompressive craniectomy for the encephalopathy of Reye's syndrome.' *Surgical Neurology*, **6**, 97–99.
Bale, J. F., Brasher, C., Siegler, R. L. (1980) 'CNS manifestions of the hemolytic-uremic syndrome.' *American Journal of Diseases of Children*, **134**, 869–872.
Barnett, G. H., Ropper, A. H., Romeo, J. (1988*a*) 'Intracranial pressure and outcome in adult encephalitis.' *Journal of Neurosurgery*, **68**, 585–588.
—— —— Johnson, K. A. (1988*b*) 'Physiological support and monitoring of critically ill patients during magnetic resonance imaging.' *Journal of Neurosurgery*, **68**, 246–250.
Barry, D. I., Lassen, N. A. (1984) 'Cerebral blood flow autoregulation in hypertension and effects of antihypertensive drugs.' *Journal of Hypertension*, **2**, 519–526.
Batjer, H. H., Devous, M. D., Meyer, Y. J., Purdy, P. D., Samson, D. S. (1988) 'Cerebrovascular hemodynamics in arteriovenous malformation complicated by normal perfusion pressure breakthrough.' *Neurosurgery*, **22**, 503–509.
Beckstead, J. E., Tweed, W. A., Lee, J. MacKeen, W. L. (1978) 'Cerebral blood flow and metabolism in man following cardiac arrest.' *Stroke*, **9**, 569–573.
Bell, T. S., Ellenberg, L., McComb, J. G. (1985) 'Neuropsychological outcome after severe pediatric near-drowning.' *Neurosurgery*, **17**, 604–608.
Belsey, M. A., Hoffpauir, C. W., Smith, M. H. D. (1969) 'Dexamethasone in the treatment of acute bacterial meningitis: the effect of study design on the interpretation of results.' *Pediatrics*, **44**, 503–513.

336

Bihari, D., Smithies, M., Gimson, A., Tinker, J. (1987) 'The effects of vasodilation with prostacyclin on oxygen delivery and uptake in critically ill patients.' *New England Journal of Medicine*, **317**, 397–403.

Bode, H., Sauer, M., Pringsheim, W. (1988) 'Diagnosis of brain death by transcranial Doppler sonography.' *Archives of Disease in Childhood*, **63**, 1474–1478.

—— Wais, U. (1988) 'Age dependence of flow velocities in basal cerebral arteries.' *Archives of Disease in Childhood*, **63**, 606–611.

Bohn, D. J., Biggar, W. D., Smith, C. R., Conn, A. W., Barker, A. (1986) 'Influence of hypothermia, barbiturate therapy, and intracranial monitoring on morbidity and mortality after near-drowning.' *Critical Care Medicine*, **14**, 529–534.

Boisvert, D. P. J., Pickard, J. D., Graham, D. I., Fitch, W. (1979) 'Delayed effects of subarachnoid haemorrhage on cerebral metabolism and the cerebrovascular response to hypercapnia in the primate.' *Journal of Neurology, Neurosurgery and Psychiatry*, **42**, 892–898.

Bos, A. P., Donckerwolcke, R. A., van Vught, A. J. (1985) 'The hemolytic-uremic syndrome; prognostic significance of neurological abnormalities.' *Helvetica Paediatrica Acta*, **40**, 381–389.

Bowton, D. L., Bertels, N. H., Prough, D. S., Stump, D. A. (1989) 'Cerebral blood flow is reduced in patients with sepsis syndrome.' *Critical Care Medicine*, **17**, 399–403.

Brain Resuscitation Clinical Trial 1 Study Group (1986) 'Randomized clinical study of thiopental loading in comatose survivors of cardiac arrest.' *New England Journal of Medicine*, **314**, 397–403.

Branston, N. M., Symon, L., Crockard, H. A., Pastzor, E. (1974) 'Relationship between the cortical evoked potential and local cerebral blood flow following acute middle cerebral artery occlusion in the baboon.' *Experimental Neurology*, **45**, 195–208.

Brazy, J. E. (1988) 'Effects of crying on cerebral blood volume and cytochrome aa3.' *Journal of Pediatrics*, **112**, 457–461.

—— Lewis, D. V. (1986) 'Changes in cerebral blood volume and cytochrome aa3 during hypertensive peaks in preterm infants.' *Journal of Pediatrics*, **108**, 983–987.

Brierley, J. B., Graham, D. I., Adams, J. H. (1971) 'Neocortical death after cardiac arrest.' *Lancet*, **2**, 560–565.

Brodersen, P., Jorgensen, E. O. (1974) 'Cerebral blood flow and oxygen uptake, and cerebrospinal fluid biochemistry in severe coma.' *Journal of Neurology, Neurosurgery and Psychiatry*, **37**, 384–391.

Bruce, D. A., Alavi, A., Bilaniuk, L., Dolinskas, C., Obrist, W., Uzzell, B. (1981) 'Diffuse cerebral swelling following head injuries in children: the syndrome of "malignant brain oedema". *Journal of Neurosurgery*, **54**, 170–178.

—— Schut, L., Sutton, L. N. (1983) 'Brain resuscitation in children: fact or fantasy?' *Concepts in Pediatric Neurosurgery*, **4**, 219–229.

Canalese, J., Gimson, A. E. S., Davis, C., Mellon, P. J., Davis, M., Williams, R. (1982) 'Controlled trial of dexamethasone and mannitol for the cerebral oedema of fulminant hepatic failure.' *Gut*, **23**, 625–629.

Cantu, R. C., Ames, A. III, Di Giacinto, G., Dixon, J. (1969) 'Hypotension: a major factor limiting recovery from cerebral ischaemia' *Journal of Surgical Research*, **9**, 525–529.

Cao, M., Lisheng, H., Shouzheng, S. (1984) 'Resolution of brain edema in severe brain injury at controlled high and low intracranial pressures.' *Journal of Neurosurgery*, **61**, 707–712.

Carlsson, C., Hagerdal, M., Siesjo, B. K. (1976) 'Protective effect of hypothermia in cerebral oxygen deficiency caused by arterial hypoxia.' *Anesthesiology*, **44**, 27–35.

Chandler, W. F., Kindt, G. W. (1976) 'Monitoring and control of intracranial pressure in non-traumatic encephalopathies.' *Surgical Neurology*, **5**, 311–314

Chapman, A. G. (1985) 'Cerebral energy metabolism and seizures.' *In* Pedley, P. A., Meldrum, B. F. (Eds.) *Recent Advances in Epilepsy*. London: Churchill Livingstone. pp. 19–63.

Cheung, J. Y., Bonventre, J. V., Malis, C. D., Leaf, A. (1986) 'Calcium and ischemic injury.' *New England Journal of Medicine*, **314**, 1670–1675.

Chodobski, A., Szmydynger-Chodobska, J., Skolasinska, K. (1986) 'Effect of ammonia intoxication on cerebral blood flow, its autoregulation and responsiveness to carbon dioxide and papaverine.' *Journal of Neurology, Neurosurgery and Psychiatry*, **49**, 302–309.

Chopp, M., Welch, K. M. A., Tidwell, C. D., Knight, R., Helpern, J. A. (1988) 'Effect of mild hyperthermia on recovery of metabolic function after global cerebral ischemia in cats.' *Stroke*, **19**, 1521–1525.

Chugani, H. T., Phelps, M. E., Mazziotta, J. C. (1987) 'Positron emission tomography study of human brain functional development.' *Annals of Neurology*, **22**, 487–497.

Clements, R. S., Blumenthal, S. A., Morrison, A. D., Winegrad, A. I. (1971) 'Increased cerebrospinal-fluid pressure during treatment of diabetic ketoacidosis.' *Lancet*, **2**, 671–675.

337

Cohan, S. L., Mun, S. K., Petite, J., Correia, J., Da Silva, A. T., Waldhorn, R. E. (1989) 'Cerebral blood flow in humans following resuscitation from cardiac arrest.' *Stroke*, **20**, 761–765.

Compton, J. S., Redmond, S., Symon, L. (1987) 'Cerebral blood velocity in subarachnoid haemorrhage: a transcranial Doppler study.' *Journal of Neurology, Neurosurgery and Psychiatry*, **50**, 1499–1503.

Conn, A. W., Edmonds, J. F., Barker, G. A. (1979) 'Cerebral resuscitation in near-drowning.' *Pediatric Clinics of North America*, **26**, 691–701.

—— Montes, J. E., Barker, G. A., Edmonds, J. F. (1980) 'Cerebral salvage in near-drowning following neurological classification by triage.' *Canadian Anaesthetists' Society Journal*, **27**, 201–209.

Constantinou, J. E. C., Gillis, J., Ouvrier, R. A., Rahilly, P. M. (1989) 'Hypoxic-ischaemic encephalopathy after near miss sudden infant death syndrome.' *Archives of Disease in Childhood*, **64**, 703–708.

Cooper, P. R., Rovit, R. L., Ransohoff, J. (1976) 'Hemicraniectomy in the treatment of acute subdural hematoma: a reappraisal.' *Surgical Neurology*, **5**, 25–28.

—— Hagler, H., Clark, W. K., Barnett, P. (1979) 'Enhancement of experimental cerebral edema after decompressive craniectomy: implications for the management of severe head injuries.' *Neurosurgery*, **4**, 296–300.

Crisp, D. E., Siegler, R. L., Bale, J. F., Thompson, J. A. (1981) 'Haemorrhagic cerebral infarction in the hemolytic-uremic syndrome.' *Journal of Pediatrics*, **99**, 273–276.

Crockard, H. A., Gadian, D. G., Frackowiak, R. S. J., Proctor, E., Allen, K., Williams, S. R., Ross Russell, R. W. (1987) 'Acute cerebral ischaemia: concurrent changes in cerebral blood flow, energy metabolites, pH, and lactate measured with hydrogen clearance and 31P and 1H nuclear magnetic resonance spectroscopy. II. Changes during ischaemia.' *Journal of Cerebral Blood Flow and Metabolism*, **7**, 394–402.

Day, N. E., Kerridge, D. F. (1967) 'A general maximum likelihood discriminant.' *Biometrics*, **23**, 313–323.

Dean, J. M., Kaufman, N. D. (1981) 'Prognostic indicators in pediatric near-drowning: the Glasgow coma scale.' *Critical Care Medicine*, **9**, 536–539.

—— McComb, J. G. (1981) 'Intracranial pressure monitoring in severe pediatric near-drowning.' *Neurosurgery*, **9**, 627–630.

de Lemos, R. A., Haggerty, R. J. (1969) 'Corticosteroids as an adjunct to treatment in bacterial meningitis: a controlled clinical trial.' *Pediatrics*, **44**, 30–34.

Dernbach, P. D., Little, J. R., Jones, S.C., Ebrahim, Z. Y. (1988) 'Altered cerebral autoregulation and CO_2 reactivity after aneurysmal subarachnoid hemorrhage.' *Neurosurgery*, **22**, 822–826.

Dodge, P. R., Swartz, M. N. (1965) 'Bacterial meningitis—a review of selected aspects. II. Special neurologic problems, postmeningitic complications and clinicopathological correlations.' *New England Journal of Medicine*, **272**, 1003–1009.

Ducasse, J. L., Marc-Vergnes, J. P., Cathala, B., Genestal, M., Lareng, L. (1984) 'Early cerebral prognosis of anoxic encephalopathy using brain energy metabolism.' *Critical Care Medicine*, **12**, 897–900.

Duck, S. C., Wyatt, D. T. (1988) 'Factors associated with brain herniation in the treatment of diabetic ketoacidosis.' *Journal of Pediatrics*, **113**, 10–14.

Ede, R. J., Gimson, A. E. S., Bihari, D., Williams, R. (1986) 'Controlled hyperventilation in the prevention of cerebral oedema in fulminant hepatic failure.' *Journal of Hepatology*, **2**, 43–51.

—— Williams, R. (1986) 'Occurrence and management of cerebral oedema in liver failure.' *In* Williams, R. (Ed.) *Liver Failure*. Edinburgh: Churchill Livingstone. pp. 26–46.

Eisenberg, H. M., Frankowski, R. F., Contant, C. F., Marshall, L. F., Walker, M. D. (1988) 'High-dose barbiturate control of elevated intracranial pressure in patients with severe head injury.' *Journal of Neurosurgery*, **69**, 15–23.

Emery, J. L., Campbell-Reid, D. A (1962) 'Cerebral oedema and spastic hemiplegia following minor burns in young children.' *British Journal of Surgery*, **50**, 53–56.

Enevoldsen, E. M., Cold, G., Jensen, F. T., Malmros, R. (1976) 'Dynamic changes in regional CBF, intraventricular pressure, CSF pH and lactate levels during the acute phase of head injury.' *Journal of Neurosurgery*, **44**, 191–214.

Eross, J., Silink, M., Dorman, D (1981) 'Cerebrospinal fluid lactic acidosis in bacterial meningitis.' *Archives of Disease in Childhood*, **56**, 692–698.

Fazekas, J. F., Ticktin, H. E., Ehrmantraut, W. R., Alman, R. W. (1956) 'Cerebral metabolism in hepatic insufficiency.' *American Journal of Medicine*, **21**, 843–849.

Feigin, R. D., Dodge, P. R. (1976) 'Bacterial meningitis: newer concepts of pathophysiology and neurologic sequelae.' *Pediatric Clinics of North America*, **23**, 541–556.

338

Fischer, E. G. (1973) 'Impaired perfusion following cerebrovascular stasis.' *Archives of Neurology*, **29**, 361–365.

Fitch, W., Ferguson, G. G., Sengupta, D., Garibi, J. (1975) 'Autoregulation of cerebral blood flow during controlled hypotension.' *In* Langfitt, T. W., McHenry, L. C. Jr., Reivich, M. Wollman, H. (Eds.) *Cerebral Blood Flow and Metabolism*. Berlin: Springer.

—— Mackenzie, E. T., Harper, A. M. (1976) 'Effects of decreasing arterial blood pressure on cerebral blood flow in the baboon.' *Circulation Research*, **37**, 550–557.

Frackowiak, R. S. J. (1986) 'PET scanning: can it help resolve management issues in cerebral ischemic disease?' *Stroke*, **17**, 803–807.

Franklin, B., Liu, J., Ginsberg-Fellner, F. (1982) 'Cerebral edema and ophthalmoplegia reversed by mannitol in a new case of insulin-dependent diabetes mellitus.' *Pediatrics*, **69**, 87–90.

Fraser, C. L., Arieff, A. I. (1985) 'Hepatic encephalopathy.' *New England Journal of Medicine*, **313**, 865–873.

Frates, R. C. (1981) 'Analysis of predictive factors in the assessment of warm-water near-drowning in children.' *American Journal of Diseases of Children*, **135**, 1006–1008.

Freeman, J., Ingvar, D. H. (1968) 'Elimination by hypoxia of cerebral blood flow autoregulation and EEG relationship.' *Experimental Brain Research*, **5**, 61–71.

Frewen, T. C., Sumabat, W. O., Del Maestro, R. F. (1985a) 'Cerebral blood flow, metabolic rate, and cross-brain oxygen consumption in brain injury.' *Journal of Pediatrics*, **107**, 510–513.

—— —— Han, V. K., Amacher, A. L., Del Maestro, R. F., Sibbald, W. J. (1985b) 'Cerebral resuscitation therapy in pediatric near-drowning.' *Journal of Pediatrics*, **106**, 615–617.

Fuhrmeister, U., Ruether, P., Dommasch, D., Gaab, M. (1980) 'Alterations of CSF hydrodynamics following meningitis and subarachnoid haemorrhage.' *In* Shulman, K., Marmarou, A., Miller, J. D., Becker, D. P., Hochwald, G. M., Brock, M. (Eds.) *Intracranial Pressure IV* . Berlin: Springer. pp. 241–243.

Gabor, A. J., Brooks, A. G., Scobey, R. P., Parsons, G. H. (1984) 'Intracranial pressure during prolonged seizures.' *Electroencephalography and Clinical Neurophysiology*, **57**, 497–506.

Gadian, D. G., Frackowiak, S. J., Crockard, H. A., Proctor, E. Allen, K., Williams, S. R., Ross Russell, R. W. (1987) 'Acute cerebral ischaemia: concurrent changes in cerebral blood flow, energy metabolites, pH, and lactate measured with hydrogen clearance and 31P and 1H nuclear magnetic resonance spectroscopy. I. Methodology.' *Journal of Cerebral Blood Flow and Metabolism*, **7**, 199–206.

Gibbs, J. M., Wise, R. J. S., Leenders, K. L., Jones, T. (1984) 'Evaluation of cerebral perfusion reserve in patients with carotid-artery occlusion.' *Lancet*, **1**, 182–186.

Gillard, J. H., Kirkham, F. J., Levin, S. D., Neville, B. G. R., Gosling, R. G. (1986) 'Anatomical validation of middle cerebral artery position as identified by transcranial pulsed Doppler ultrasound.' *Journal of Neurology, Neurosurgery and Psychiatry*, **49**, 1025–1029.

Giulioni, M., Ursino, M., Alvisi, C. (1988) 'Correlations among intracranial pulsatility, intracranial hemodynamics, and transcranial Doppler wave form: literature review and hypothesis for future studies.' *Neurosurgery*, **22**, 807–812.

Goitein, K. J., Fainmesser, P., Sohmer, H. (1983a) 'Cerebral perfusion pressure and auditory brain-stem responses in childhood CNS diseases.' *American Journal of Diseases of Children*, **137**, 777–781.

—— Amit, Y., Mussaffi, H. (1983b) 'Intracranial pressure in central nervous system infections and cerebral ischaemia of infancy.' *Archives of Disease in Childhood*, **58**, 184–186.

—— Tamir, I. (1983) Cerebral perfusion pressure in central nervous system infections of infancy and childhood.' *Journal of Pediatrics*, **103**, 40–43.

Goodman, J. M., Mishkin, F. S., Dyken, M. (1969) 'Determination of brain death by isotope angiography.' *Journal of the American Medical Association*, **209**, 1869–1872.

Gordon, N. S., Fois, A., Jacobi, G., Minns, R. A., Seshia, S. S. (1983) 'The management of the comatose child.' *Neuropediatrics*, **14**, 3–5.

Gower, D. J., Lee, K. S., McWhorter, J. M. (1988) 'Role of subtemporal decompression in severe closed head injury.' *Neurosurgery*, **23**, 417–422.

Grafton, S. T., Longstreth, W. T. Jr. (1988) 'Steroids after cardiac arrest: a retrospective study with concurrent, nonrandomized controls.' *Neurology*, **38**, 1315–1316.

Graham, D. I., Ford, I., Adams, J. H., Doyle, D., Teasdale, G. M., Lawrence, A. E., McLellan, D. R. (1989) 'Ischaemic brain damage is still common in fatal non-missile head injury.' *Journal of Neurology, Neurosurgery and Psychiatry*, **52**, 346–350.

Greenberg, J. H., Reivich, M., Noordergraaf, A. (1978) 'A model of cerebral blood flow control in hypercapnia.' *Annals of Biomedical Engineering*, **6**, 453–491.

339

Griswold, W. R., Viney, J., Mendoza, S. A., James, H. E. (1981) 'Intracranial pressure monitoring in severe hypertensive encephalopathy.' *Critical Care Medicine*, **9**, 573–576.

Grubb, R. L., Raichle, M. E., Phelps, M. E., Ratcheson, R. A. (1975) 'Effects of increased intracranial pressure in cerebral blood volume, blood flow, and oxygen utilization in monkeys.' *Journal of Neurosurgery*, **43**, 385–398.

Gutierrez, G., Andry, J. M. (1989) 'Nuclear magnetic resonance measurements–clinical applications.' *Critical Care Medicine*, **17**, 73–82.

Hanid, M. A., MacKenzie, R. L., Jenner, R. E., Chase, R. A., Mellon, P. J., Trewby, P. N., Janota, I., Davis, M., Silk, D. B. A., Williams, R. (1979) 'Intracranial pressure in pigs with surgically induced acute liver failure.' *Gastroenterology*, **76**, 123–131.

—— Davies, M., Mellon, P. J., Silk, D. B. A., Strunin, L. McCabe, J. J., Williams, R. (1980) 'Clinical monitoring of intracranial pressure in fulminant hepatic failure.' *Gut*, **21**, 866–869.

Harper, A. M. (1965) 'The inter-relationship between $PaCO_2$ and blood pressure in the regulation of blood flow through the cerebral cortex.' *Acta Neurologica Scandinavica*, **14** (Suppl.), 94–103.

—— Glass, H. I. (1965) 'Effect of alterations in the arterial carbon dioxide tension on the blood flow through the cerebral cortex at normal and low arterial blood pressures.' *Journal of Neurology, Neurosurgery and Psychiatry*, **28**, 449–452.

—— Deshmukh, V. D., Sengupta, D., Rowan, J. O., Jennett, W. B. (1972) 'The effect of experimental spasm on the CO_2 response of cerebral bloodflow in primates.' *Neuroradiology*, **3**, 134–136.

Harris, G. D., Fiordalisi, I., Finberg, L. (1988) Safe management of diabetic ketoacidemia.' *Journal of Pediatrics*, **113**, 65–68.

Harvey, S. C. (1985) 'Drugs acting on the CNS. Hypnotics and sedatives.' *In* Gilman, A. G., Goodman, L. S., Rall, T. W., Murad, F. (Eds.) *The Pharmacological Basis of Therapeutics. 7th Edn.* London: Macmillan.

Hashi, K., Meyer, J. S., Shinmaru, S., Welch, K. M. A., Teraura, T. (1972) 'Changes in cerebral vasomotor reactivity to CO_2 and autoregulation following experimental subarachnoid haemorrhage.' *Journal of the Neurological Sciences*, **17**, 15–22.

Hassler, W., Steinmetz, H., Gawlowski, J. (1988) 'Transcranial Doppler ultrasonography in raised intracranial pressure and in intracranial circulatory arrest.' *Journal of Neurosurgery*, **68**, 745–751.

Havill, J. H. (1984) 'Prolonged hyperventilation and intracranial pressure.' *Critical Care Medicine*, **12**, 72–74.

Herold, S., Brown, M. M., Frackowiak, R. S. J., Mansfield, A. O., Thomas, D. J., Marshall, J. (1988) 'Assessment of cerebral haemodynamic reserve: correlation between PET parameters and CO_2 reactivity measured by the intravenous [133]xenon technique.' *Journal of Neurology, Neurosurgery and Psychiatry*, **51**, 1045–1050.

Herson, V. C., Todd, J. K. (1977) 'Prediction of morbidity in *Hemophilus influenzae* meningitis.' *Pediatrics*, **59**, 35–39.

Hildebrand, C. A., Hartmann, A. G., Arcinue, E. L., Gomez, R. J., Bing, R. J. (1988) 'Cardiac performance in pediatric near-drowning.' *Critical Care Medicine*, **16**, 331–335.

Horwitz, S. J., Boxerbaum, B., O'Bell, J. (1980) 'Cerebral herniation in bacterial meningitis in childhood.' *Annals of Neurology*, **7**, 524–528.

Hossmann, K. A. (1988) 'Resuscitation potentials after prolonged global cerebral ischaemia in cats.' *Critical Care Medicine*, **16**, 964–971.

Janati, A., Erba, G. (1982) 'Electroencephalographic correlates of near-drowning encephalopathy in children.' *Electroencephalography and Clinical Neurophysiology*, **53**, 182–191.

Javaheri, S., Clendening, A., Papadakis, N., Brody, J. S. (1984) 'pH changes on the surface of brain and in cisternal fluid in dogs in cardiac arrest.' *Stroke*, **15**, 553–557.

Jennett, B., Plum, F. (1972) 'Persistent vegetative state after brain damage: a syndrome in search of a name.' *Lancet*, **1**, 734–737.

Johansson, B. B., Fredriksson, K. (1985) 'Cerebral arteries in hypertension: structural and hemodynamic aspects.' *Journal of Cardiovascular Pharmacology*, **7**, S90–S93.

Johnston, I. H., Rowan, J. O., Harper, A. M., Jennett, W. B. (1972) 'Raised intracranial pressure and cerebral blood flow. 1. Cisterna magna infusion in primates.' *Journal of Neurology, Neurosurgery and Psychiatry*, **35**, 285–296.

Jones, T. H., Morawetz, R. B., Crowell, R. M., Marcoux, F. W., FitzGibbon, S. J., DeGirolami, U., Ojemann, U. (1981) 'Thresholds of focal ischemia in awake monkeys.' *Journal of Neurosurgery*, **54**, 773–782.

Jorgensen, E. O., Malchow-Møller, A. (1981) 'Natural history of global and critical brain ischaemia. Part I: EEG and neurological signs during the first year after cardiopulmonary resuscitation in patients subsequently regaining consciousness.' *Resuscitation*, **9**, 133–153.

Kanno, I., Uemura, K., Higano, S., Muramaki, M., Iida, H., Muira, S., Shishido, F., Inugami, A., Sayama, I. (1988) 'Oxygen extraction fraction of maximally vasodilated tissue in the ischemic brain estimated from the regional CO_2 responsiveness measured by positron emission tomography.' *Journal of Cerebral Blood Flow and Metabolism*, **8**, 227–235.

Kaplan, S. L. (1989) 'Dexamethasone for children with bacterial meningitis: should it be routine therapy?' *American Journal of Diseases in Children*, **143**, 290–291.

Kay, S., Rao, S. S., Lord, D., Greenhough, S. (1986) 'Intracranial pressure monitoring as an aid to resuscitation in the burnt and asphyxiated child: three case reports.' *Burns*, **12**, 212–213.

—— Feigin, R. D. (1978) 'The syndrome of inappropriate secretion of antidiuretic hormone in children with bacterial meningitis.' *Journal of Paediatrics*, **92**, 758–761.

Kennard, C., Swash, M. (1981) 'Acute viral encephalitis: its diagnosis and outcome.' *Brain*, **104**, 129–148.

Kennedy, C. R., Duffy, S. W., Smith, R., Robinson, R. O. (1987) 'Clinical predictors of outcome in encephalitis.' *Archives of Disease in Childhood*, **62**, 1156–1162.

Kennedy, C., Sokoloff, L. (1957) 'An adaptation of the nitrous oxide method to the study of the cerebral circulation in children; normal values for cerebral blood flow and cerebral metabolic rate in childhood.' *Journal of Clinical Investigation*, **36**, 1130–1137.

Kirkham, F. J., Neville, B. G. R. (1986) 'Successful management of severe intracranial hypertension by surgical decompression.' *Developmental Medicine and Child Neurology*, **28**, 506–509.

—— Padayachee, T. S., Parsons, S., Seargeant, L. S., House, F. R., Gosling, R. G. (1986) 'Transcranial measurement of blood velocities in the basal cerebral arteries using pulsed Doppler ultrasound: velocity as an index of flow.' *Ultrasound in Medicine and Biology*, **12**, 15–21.

—— Levin, S. D., Padayachee, T. S., Kyme, M. C., Neville, B. G. R., Gosling, R. G. (1987a) 'Transcranial pulsed Doppler ultrasound findings in brainstem death.' *Journal of Neurology, Neurosurgery and Psychiatry*, **50**, 1504–1513.

—— Kyme, M. C., Levin, S. D., Neville, B. G. R., Gosling, R. G. (1987b) 'Clinical importance of vasoparalysis demonstrated using transcranial ultrasound.' *Journal of Cerebral Blood Flow and Metabolism*, **7** (Suppl.) S655.

—— —— —— Padayachee, T. S., House, F. R., Neville, B. G. R., Gosling, R. G. (1989) 'Monitoring of changes in blood velocity in the unconscious child.' *In* Eden, A., Aaslid, R., Fieschi, C., Zanetti, E. (Eds.) *Advances in Transcranial Pulsed Doppler Ultrasound*. Berlin: Springer.

Kirsch, J. R., Traystman, R. J., Rogers, M. C. (1985) 'Cerebral blood flow measurement techniques in infants and children.' *Pediatrics*, **75**, 887–895.

Klingelhofer, J., Conrad, B., Benecke, R., Sander, D., Markakis, E. (1988) 'Evaluation of intracranial pressure from transcranial Doppler studies in cerebral disease.' *Journal of Neurology*, **235**, 159–162.

Koch, K. A., Jackson, D. L., Schmiedl, M., Rosenblatt, J. I. (1984) 'Total cerebral ischemia: effect of alterations in arterial PCO_2 on cerebral microcirculation.' *Journal of Cerebral Blood Flow and Metabolism*, **4**, 343–349.

Koehler, R. C., Traystman, R. J. (1982) 'Bicarbonate ion modulation of cerebral blood flow during hypoxia and hypercapnia.' *American Journal of Physiology*, **243**, H33–H40.

Kogure, K., Scheinberg, P., Reinmuth, O. M., Fujishima, M., Busto, R. (1970) 'Regional cerebral blood flow in dogs.' *Archives of Neurology*, **22**, 528–540.

Kondziolka, D., Fazl, M. (1988) 'Functional recovery after decompressive craniectomy for cerebral infarction.' *Neurosurgery*, **23**, 143–147.

Kontos, H. A. (1981) 'Regulation of the cerebral circulation.' *Annual Review of Physiology*, **43**, 397–407.

—— Wei, E. P., Navari, R. M., Levasseur, J. E., Rosenblum, W. I., Patterson, J. L. Jr. (1978) 'Responses of cerebral arteries and arterioles to acute hypotension and hypertension'. *American Journal of Physiology*, **234**, H371–H383.

Krane, E. J., Rockoff, M. A., Wallman, J. K., Wolsdorf, J. I. (1985) 'Subclinical brain swelling in children during treatment of diabetic ketoacidosis.' *New England Journal of Medicine*, **312**, 1147–1151.

Kreisman, N. R., Rosenthal, M., LaManna, J. C., Sick, T. J. (1983) 'Cerebral oxygenation during recurrent seizures.' *In* Delgado-Escueta, A. V., Wasterlain, C. G., Treiman, D. M., Porter, R. J. (Eds.) *Advances in Neurology*. New York: Raven. pp. 231–239.

Kruus, S., Bergstrom, L., Suutarinen, T., Hyvonen, R. (1979) 'The prognosis of near-drowned children.' *Acta Paediatrica Scandinavica*, **68**, 315–322.

Kuhl, D. E., Alavi, A., Hoffman, E. J., Phelps, M. E., Zimmerman, R. A., Obrist, W. D., Bruce, D. A., Greenberg, J. H., Uzzell, B. (1980) 'Local cerebral blood volume in head-injured patients.'

Journal of Neurosurgery, **52**, 309–320.

Kummer, R. V. (1984) 'Local vascular response to change in carbon dioxide tension. Long term observation in the cat's brain by means of the hydrogen clearance technique.' *Stroke*, **15**, 108–114.

Langfitt, T. W., Kassell, N. F., Weinstein, J. D. (1965a) 'Cerebral blood flow with intracranial hypertension.' *Neurology*, **15**, 761–773.

—— Weinstein, J. D., Kassell, N. F. (1965b) 'Cerebral vasomotor paralysis produced by intracranial hypertension.' *Neurology*, **15**, 622–641.

—— Kassell, N. F. (1968) 'Cerebral vasodilatation produced by brain-stem stimulation: neurogenic control vs. autoregulation.' *American Journal of Physiology*, **215**, 90–97.

—— Kumar, V. S., James, H. E., Miller, J. D. (1971) 'Continuous recording of intracranial pressure in patients with hypoxic brain damage.' *In* Brierley, J. B., Meldrum, B. S. (Eds.) *Brain Hypoxia*. London: Spastics International Medical Publications. pp. 118–135.

—— Obrist, W. D., Alavi, A., Grossman, R. I., Zimmerman, R., Jaggi, J., Uzzell, B., Reivich, M., Patton, D. R. (1986) 'Computerized tomography, magnetic resonance imaging, and positron emission tomography in the study of brain trauma.' *Journal of Neurosurgery*, **64**, 760–767.

Lassen, N. A. (1959) 'Cerebral blood flow and oxygen consumption in man.' *Physiological Reviews*, **39**, 183–238.

—— (1966) 'The luxury perfusion syndrome and its possible relation to acute metabolic acidosis localised within the brain.' *Lancet*, **2**, 1113–1115.

Lebel, M. H., Freij, B. J., Syrogiannopoulos, G. A., Chrane, D. F., Hoyt, M. J., Stewart, S. M., Kennard, B. D., Olsen, K. D., McCracken, G. H. Jr. (1988) 'Dexamethasone therapy for bacterial meningitis.' *New England Journal of Medicine*, **319**, 964–971.

—— Hoyt, J., Waagner, D. C., Rollins, N. K., Finitzo, T., McCracken, G. H. Jr. (1989) 'Magnetic resonance imaging and dexamethasone therapy for bacterial meningitis.' *American Journal of Diseases of Children*, **143**, 301–306.

Levy, D. E., Bates, D., Caronna, J. J., Cartlidge, N. E. F., Knill-Jones, R. P., Lapinski, R. H., Singer, B. H., Shaw, D. A., Plum, F. (1981) 'Prognosis in nontraumatic coma.' *Annals of Internal Medicine*, **94**, 293–301.

—— Sidtis, J. J., Rottenberg, D. A., Jarden, J. O., Strother, S. C., Dhawan, V., Ginos, J. Z. Tramo, M. J., Evans, A. C., Plum, F. (1987) 'Differences in cerebral blood flow and glucose utilization in vegetative versus locked-in patients.' *Annals of Neurology*, **22**, 673–682.

Lewelt, W., Jenkins, L. W., Miller, J. D. (1982) 'Effects of experimental fluid-percussion injury of the brain on cerebrovascular reactivity to hypoxia and to hypercapnia.' *Journal of Neurosurgery*, **56**, 332–338.

Lindegaard, K. F., Lundar, T., Wiberg, J., Sjoberg, D., Aaslid, R., Nornes, H. (1987) 'Variations in middle cerebral artery blood flow investigated with noninvasive transcranial blood velocity measurements.' *Stroke*, **18**, 1025–1030.

Livingston, J. H., Brown, J. K. (1986) 'Intracerebral haemorrhage after the neonatal period.' *Archives of Disease in Childhood*, **61**, 538–544.

Lowenstein, D. H., Aminoff, M. J., Simon, R. P. (1988) 'Barbiturate anesthesia in the treatment of status epilepticus: clinical experience with 14 patients.' *Neurology*, **38**, 395–400.

Lucking, S. E., Pollack, M. M., Fields, A. I. (1986) 'Shock following generalized hypoxic-ischaemic injury in previously healthy infants and children.' *Journal of Pediatrics*, **108**, 359–364.

Markwalder, T. M. Grolimund, P., Seiler, R. W., Roth, F., Aaslid, R. (1984) 'Dependency of blood flow velocity in the middle cerebral artery on end-tidal carbon dioxide partial pressure–A transcranial ultrasound Doppler study.' *Journal of Cerebral Blood Flow and Metabolism*, **4**, 368–372.

Marsh, M. L., Shapiro, H. M., Smith, R. W., Marshall, L. F. (1979) 'Changes in neurologic status and intracranial pressure associated with sodium nitroprusside administration.' *Anesthesiology*, **51**, 336–338.

Maynard, D. E., Jenkinson, J. L. (1984) 'The cerebral function analysing monitor.' *Anaesthesia*, **39**, 678–690.

McDowell, D. G., Harper, A. M. (1968) 'CBF and CSF pH in the monkey during prolonged hypocapnia.' *Scandinavian Journal of Clinical and Laboratory Investigation*, (Suppl. 102) 8E.

McKee, A. C., Winkelman, M. D., Banker, B. Q. (1988) 'Central pontine myelinolysis in severely burned patients: relationship to serum hyperosmolality.' *Neurology*, **38**, 1211–1217.

McLaurin, R. L., Nichols, J. B. Jr. (1957) 'Extensive cranial decompression in the treatment of severe lead encephalopathy.' *Pediatrics*, **39**, 653–667.

McWilliam, R. (1985) 'Timing of lumbar puncture in severe childhood meningitis.' *British Medical Journal*, **291**, 1124.

342

—— Stephenson, J. B. P. (1984) 'Rapid bedside technique for intracranial pressure monitoring.' *Lancet*, **2**, 73–75.

Mendelow, A. D., Teasdale, G. M., Russell, T., Flood, J., Patterson, J., Murray, G. D. (1985) 'Effect of mannitol on cerebral blood flow and cerebral perfusion pressure in human head injury.' *Journal of Neurosurgery*, **63**, 43–48.

Messeter, K., Nordstrom, C. H., Sundbarg, G., Algotsson, L., Ryding, E. (1986) 'Cerebral hemodynamics in patients with acute severe head trauma.' *Journal of Neurosurgery*, **64**, 231–237.

Meyer, F. B., Anderson, R. E., Sundt, T. M. Jr., Yaksh, T. L. (1987) 'Treatment of experimental focal cerebral ischemia with mannitol.' *Journal of Neurosurgery*, **66**, 109–115.

Miller, C. L., Lampard, D. G., Alexander, K., Brown, W. A. (1980a) 'Local cerebral blood flow following transient cerebral ischemia. I: onset of impaired reperfusion within the first hour following global ischemia.' *Stroke*, **11**, 534–541.

—— Alexander, K., Lampard, D. G., Brown, W. A. Griffiths, R. (1980b) 'Local cerebral blood flow following transient cerebral ischemia. II: effect of arterial pCO_2 on reperfusion following global ischemia.' *Stroke*, **11**, 542–552.

Miller, J. D., Stanek, A., Langfitt, T. W. (1972) 'Concepts of cerebral perfusion pressure and vascular compression during intracranial hypertension.' *Progress in Brain Research*, **35**, 411–432.

—— Bobo, H., Kapp, J. P. (1986) 'Inaccurate pressure readings from subarachnoid bolts.' *Neurosurgery*, **19**, 253–255.

Minns, R. A., Brown, J. K. (1978) 'Intracranial pressure changes associated with childhood seizures.' *Developmental Medicine and Child Neurology*, **20**, 561–569.

—— Engleman, H. M., Stirling, H. (1989) 'Cerebrospinal fluid pressure in pyogenic meningitis.' *Archives of Disease in Childhood*, **64**, 814–820.

Mohnot, D., Snead, O. C. III, Benton, J. W. (1982) 'Burn encephalopathy in children.' *Annals of Neurology*, **12**, 42–47.

Montes, J. E., Conn, A. W. (1980) 'Near-drowning: an unusual case.' *Canadian Anaesthetists' Society Journal*, **27**, 172–174.

Moossy, J., Safar, P., Adler, S., Arfors, K. E., Baethmann, A., Basford, R. E., Bontempo, F., Cerchiari, E., Chandra, N., Garcia, J. H., Hossmann, K. A., Jennings, R. B., Kang, Y., Negovsky, V. A., Nemoto, E. M., Obrist, W., Pettegrew, J. W., Pinsky, M. R., Severinghaus, J. W., Siesjo, B. K., Weil, M. H., White, B. C. Wolf, G. L., Wolfson, S. (1988) 'Pathophysiologic limits to the reversibility of clinical death.' *Critical Care Medicine*, **16**, 1022–1033.

Muizelaar, J. P., Lutz, H. A. III, Becker, D. P. (1984) 'Effect of mannitol on ICP and CBF and correlation with pressure autoregulation in severely head-injured patients.' *Journal of Neurosurgery*, **61**, 700–706.

—— Van der Poel, H. G., Li, Z., Kontos, H. A., Levasseur, J. E. (1988) 'Pial arteriolar vessel diameter, and CO_2 reactivity during prolonged hyperventilation in the rabbit.' *Journal of Neurosurgery*, **69**, 923–927.

—— Marmarou, A., DeSalles, A. A. F., Ward, J. D., Zimmerman, R. S., Li, Z., Choi, S. C., Young, H. F. (1989a) 'Cerebral blood flow and metabolism in severely head-injured children. Part 1: relationship with GCS score, outcome, ICP, and PVI.' *Journal of Neurosurgery*, **71**, 63–71.

—— Ward, J. D., Marmarou, A., Newlon, P. G., Wachi, A. (1989b) 'Cerebral blood flow and metabolism in severely head-injured children. Part 2: autoregulation.' *Journal of Neurosurgery*, **71**, 72–76.

Mullan, S., Hanlon, K., Brown, F. (1978) 'Management of 136 consecutive supratentorial berry aneurysms.' *Journal of Neurosurgery*, **49**, 794–804.

Mullie, A., Verstringe, P., Buylaert, W., Houbrechts, H., Michem, N., Delooz, H., Verbruggen, H., Van Den Broeck, L., Corne, L., Lauwaert, D., De Cock, R., Weeghmans, M., Mennes, J., Bossaert, L., Quets, A., Lewi, P. (1988) 'Predictive value of Glasgow coma score for awakening after out-of-hospital cardiac arrest.' *Lancet*, **1**, 137–140.

Myers, R. E. (1979) 'A unitary theory of causation of anoxic and hypoxic brain pathology.' *Advances in Neurology*, **26**, 195–213.

Nemoto, E. M. (1978) 'Pathogenesis of cerebral ischemia-anoxia.' *Critical Care Medicine*, **6**, 203–214.

Nordstrom, C. H., Messeter, K., Sundbarg, G., Schalen, W., Werner, M., Ryding, E. (1988) 'Cerebral blood flow, vasoreactivity, and oxygen consumption during barbiturate therapy in severe traumatic brain lesions.' *Journal of Neurosurgery*, **68**, 424–431.

Nugent, S. K., Bausher, J. A., Moxon, E. R., Rogers, M. C. (1979) 'Raised intracranial pressure. Its management in *Neisseria meningitidis* meningoencephalitis.' *American Journal of Diseases of Children*, **133**, 260–262.

—— Rogers, M. C (1980) 'Resuscitation and intensive care monitoring following immersion hypothermia.' *Journal of Trauma*, **20**, 814–815.

Nussbaum, E. (1985) 'Prognostic variables in nearly drowned, comatose children.' *American Journal of Diseases of Children*, **139**, 1058–1059.

—— Galant, S. P. (1983) 'Intracranial pressure monitoring as a guide to prognosis in the nearly drowned, severely comatose child.' *Journal of Pediatrics*, **102**, 215–218.

—— Maggi, J. C. (1988) 'Pentobarbital therapy does not improve neurologic outcome in nearly drowned, flaccid-comatose children.' *Pediatrics*, **81**, 630–634.

Oakes, D. D., Sherck, J. P., Maloney, J. R., Charters, A. C. (1982) 'Prognosis and management of victims of near-drowning.' *Journal of Trauma*, **22**, 544–549.

Obrist, W. D., Gennarelli, T. A., Segawa, H., Dolinskas, C. A., Langfitt, T. W. (1979) 'Relation of cerebral blood flow to neurological status and outcome in head-injured patients.' *Journal of Neurosurgery*, **51**, 292–300.

—— Langfitt, T. W., Jaggi, J. L., Cruz, J., Gennarelli, T. A. (1984) 'Cerebral blood flow and metabolism in comatose patients with acute head injury.' *Journal of Neurosurgery*, **61**, 241–253.

Ogata, N., Yonekawa, Y.,Taki, W., Kannagi, R., Murachi, T., Hamakubo, T., Kikuchi, H. (1989) 'Degradation of neurofilament protein in cerebral ischemia.' *Journal of Neurosurgery*, **70**, 103–107.

Orlowski, J. P. (1987) 'Drowning, near-drowning, and ice-water submersions.' *Pediatric Clinics of North America*, **34**, 75–92.

Ostrup, R. C., Luerssen, T. G., Marshall, L. F., Zornow, M. H. (1987) 'Continuous monitoring of intracranial pressure with a miniaturized fiberoptic device.' *Journal of Neurosurgery*, **67**, 206–209.

Padayachee, T. S., Kirkham, F. J., Lewis, R. R., Gillard, J. H., Hutchinson, M. C. E., Gosling, R. G. (1986) 'Transcranial measurement of blood velocities in the basal cerebral arteries using pulsed Doppler ultrasound: a method of assessing the circle of Willis.' *Ultrasound in Medicine and Biology*, **12**, 5–14.

Pampiglione, G., Harden, A. (1968) 'Resuscitation after cardiocirculatory arrest. Prognostic evaluation of early electroencephalographic findings.' *Lancet*, **1**, 1261–1264.

Paulson, O. B., Broderson, P., Hansen, E. L., Kristensen, H. S. (1974) 'Regional cerebral blood flow, cerebral metabolic rate of oxygen, and cerebrospinal fluid acid-base variables in patients with acute meningitis and with acute encephalitis.' *Acta Medica Scandinavica*, **196**, 191–198.

Pavlakis, S. G., McCormick, K. L., Bromberg, K., Peter, G. (1980) 'Cerebrospinal fluid anion gap in meningitis.' *Journal of Pediatrics*, **96**, 874–876.

Pearn, J. (1985) 'The management of near-drowning.' *British Medical Journal*, **291**, 1447–1452.

Pesso, J. L., Floret, D., Cochat, P., Dumont, C. (1988) 'Meningite suppurée à pneumocoque chez le nourrisson et l'enfant: complications et facteurs pronostiques.' *Pédiatrie*, **43**, 263–267.

Peterson, B. (1977) 'Morbidity of childhood near-drowning.' *Pediatrics*, **59**, 364–370.

Piatt, J. H. Jr., Schiff, S. J. (1984) 'High dose barbiturate therapy in neurosurgery and intensive care.' *Neurosurgery*, **15**, 427–444.

Plum, F. (1983) 'What causes infarction in ischemic brain?' *Neurology*, **33**, 222–233.

—— Posner, J. B. (1980) *The Diagnosis of Stupor and Coma*. Philadelphia: F. A. Davis.

Posner, J. B., Plum, F. (1960) 'The toxic effects of carbon dioxide and acetazolamide in hepatic encephalopathy.' *Journal of Clinical Investigation*, **39**, 1246–1258.

Powers, W. J., Grubb, R. L. Jr., Darriet, D., Raichle, M. E. (1985) 'Cerebral blood flow and cerebral metabolic rate of oxygen requirements for cerebral function and viability in humans.' *Journal of Cerebral Blood Flow and Metabolism*, **5**, 600–608.

—— Raichle, M. E. (1985) 'Positron emission tomography and its application to the study of cerebrovascular disease in man.' *Stroke*, **16**, 361–376.

Prior, P. F., Maynard, D. E. (1986) *Monitoring Cerebral Function*. Amsterdam: Elsevier.

Raichle, M. E. (1983) 'The pathophysiology of brain ischemia.' *Annals of Neurology*, **13**, 2–10.

—— Posner, J. B., Plum, F. (1970) 'Cerebral blood flow during and after hyperventilation.' *Archives of Neurology*, **23**, 394–403.

Rebaud, P., Berthier, J. C., Hartemann, E. Floret, D. (1988) 'Intracranial pressure in childhood central nervous system infections.' *Intensive Care Medicine*, **14**, 522–525.

Reddy, S. V. R., Yaksh, T. L., Anderson, R. E., Sundt, T. M. Jr. (1986) 'Effect in cat of locus coeruleus lesions on the response of cerebral blood flow and cardiac output to altered $PaCO_2$.' *Brain Research*, **365**, 278–288.

Reeder, R. F., Harbaugh, R. E. (1989) 'Administration of intravenous urea and normal saline for the treatment of hyponatremia in neurosurgical patients.' *Journal of Neurosurgery*, **70**, 201–206.

Rehncrona, S., Rosen, I., Siesjo, B. K. (1980) 'Excessive cellular acidosis: an important mechanism of neuronal damage in the brain?' *Acta Physiologica Scandinavica*, **110**, 435–437.

Reinmuth, O. M., Vaagenes, P., Abramson, N. S., Andrejev, G., Bar-Joseph, G., Cerchiari, E.,

344

Chandra, N., Diven, W. F., Edgren, E., Gisvold, S. E., Latchaw, R. E., Novak, R., Obrist, W. D., Safar, P., Sclabassi, R. J., Shoemaker, W. C., White, R. (1988) 'Predicting outcome after resuscitation from clinical death.' *Critical Care Medicine*, **16**, 1043–1052.

Reivich, M. (1964) 'Arterial PCO_2 and cerebral hemodynamics.' *American Journal of Physiology*, **206**, 25–35.

Ringelstein, E. B. (1988) 'Transcranial Doppler ultrasonography and hyperostosis of the skull.' *Stroke*, **19**, 1445.

Roberts, P. A., Pollay, M., Engles, C., Pendelton, B., Reynolds, E., Stevens, F. A (1987) 'Effect on intracranial pressure of furosemide combined with varying doses and administration rates of mannitol.' *Journal of Neurosurgery*, **66**, 440–446.

Robertson, C. S., Grossman, R. G., Goodman, J. C., Narayan, R. K. (1987) 'The predictive value of cerebral anaerobic metabolism with cerebral infarction after head injury.' *Journal of Neurosurgery*, **67**, 361–368.

—— Narayan, R. K., Gokaslan, Z. L., Pahwa, R., Grossman, R. G., Caram P. Jr., Allen, E. (1989) 'Cerebral arteriovenous oxygen difference as an estimate of cerebral blood flow in comatose patients.' *Journal of Neurosurgery*, **70**, 222–230.

Rolfsen, M. L., Davis, W. R. (1989) 'Cerebral function and preservation during cardiac arrest.' *Critical Care Medicine*, **17**, 283–292.

Rooney, J. C., Anderson, R. McD., Hopkins, I. J. (1971) 'Clinical and pathological aspects of central nervous system involvement in the haemolytic uraemic syndrome.' *Australian Paediatric Journal*, **7**, 28–33.

Ropper, A. H., King, R. B. (1984) 'Intracranial pressure monitoring in comatose patients with cerebral hemorrhage.' *Archives of Neurology*, **41**, 725–728.

—— Shafran, B. (1984) 'Brain edema after stroke.' *Archives of Neurology*, **41**, 26–29.

—— King, R. B. (1985) 'Intracranial pressure monitoring in patients with cerebral hemorrhage.' *Archives of Neurology*, **42**, 1134–1135.

Rosenberg, A. A. (1988) 'Response of the cerebral circulation to profound hypocarbia in neonatal lambs.' *Stroke*, **19**, 1365–1370.

Rosenklint, A., Jorgensen, P. B. (1974) 'Evaluation of angiographic methods in the diagnosis of brain death. Correlation with local and systemic arterial pressure and intracranial pressure.' *Neuroradiology*, **7**, 215–219.

Rosner, M. J. (1987) 'Cerebral perfusion pressure: link between intracranial pressure and systemic circulation.' *In* Wood, J. H. (Ed.) *Cerebral Blood Flow*. New York: McGraw-Hill. pp. 425–448.

—— Becker, D. P. (1984) 'Origin and evolution of plateau waves.' *Journal of Neurosurgery*, **60**, 312–324.

—— Coley, I. B. (1986) 'Cerebral perfusion pressure, intracranial pressure, and head elevation.' *Journal of Neurosurgery*, **65**, 636–641.

Rothman, S. M., Olney, J. W. (1986) 'Glutamate and the pathophysiology of hypoxic-ischemic brain damage.' *Annals of Neurology*, **19**, 105–111.

Ruben, D., Doubell, S., Kirkham, F. J., Kontis, S., Clark, A. D., Gosling, R. G. (1989) 'On-line Doppler blood velocity analysis in a data-logging computer system for cerebral management in paediatric ITU.' *In* Eden, A., Aaslid, R., Fieschi, C., Zanetti, E. (Eds.) *Advances in Transcranial Pulsed Doppler Ultrasound*. Berlin: Springer.

Rudy, E. B., Baun, M., Stone, K., Turner, B. (1986) 'The relationship between endotracheal suctioning and changes in intracranial pressure: a review of the literature.' *Heart and Lung*, **15**, 488–494.

Safar, P. (1986) 'Cerebral resuscitation after cardiac arrest: a review.' *Circulation*, **74**, 138–153.

Sandyk, R., Brennan, M. J. W. (1983) 'Fulminating encephalopathy associated with *Shigella flexneri* infection.' *Archives of Disease in Childhood*, **58**, 70–71.

Sapolsky, R. M., Pulsinelli, W. A. (1985) 'Glucocorticoids potentiate ischemic injury to neurons: therapeutic implications.' *Science*, **299**, 1397–1400.

Sarnaik, A. P., Preston, G., Lieh-Lai, M., Eisenbrey, A. B. (1985) 'Intracranial pressure and cerebral perfusion pressure in near-drowning.' *Critical Care Medicine*, **13**, 224–227.

Saunders, M. L., Miller, J. D., Stablein, D., Allen, G. (1979) 'The effects of graded experimental trauma on cerebral blood flow and responsiveness to CO_2.' *Journal of Neurosurgery*, **51**, 18–26.

Schaad, U. B., Suter, S., Gianella-Borradori, A., Pfenninger, J., Auckenthaler, R., Bernath, O., Cheseaux, J. J., Wedgwood, J. (1990) 'A comparison of ceftriaxone and cefuroxime for the treatment of bacterial meningitis in children.' *New England Journal of Medicine*, **322**, 141–147.

Schmidt-Kastner, R., Ophoff, B. G., Hossmann, K. A. (1986) 'Delayed recovery of CO_2 reactivity after one hour's complete ischaemia of cat brain.' *Journal of Neurology*, **233**, 367–369.

—— Hossman, K. A., Ophoff, B. G. (1987) 'Pial artery pressure after one hour of global ischemia.'

345

Journal of Cerebral Blood Flow and Metabolism, **7**, 109–117.

Seiler, R. W., Grolimund, P., Aaslid, R., Huber, P., Nornes, H. (1986) 'Cerebral vasospasm evaluated by transcranial ultrasound correlated with clinical grade and CT-visualized subarachnoid hemorrhage.' *Journal of Neurosurgery*, **64**, 594–600.

Seki, H., Yoshimoto, T., Ogawa, A., Suzuki, J. (1984) 'The CO_2 response in focal cerebral ischemia–sequential changes following recirculation'. *Stroke*, **15**, 699–704.

Senter, H. J.,Wolf, A., Wagner, F. C. (1981) 'Intracranial pressure in nontraumatic ischemic and hypoxic cerebral insults.' *Journal of Neurosurgery*, **54**, 489–493.

Seshia, S. S., Chow, P. N., Sankaran, K. (1979) 'Coma following cardiorespiratory arrest in childhood.' *Developmental Medicine and Child Neurology*, **21**, 143–153.

—— Johnston, B., Kasian, G. (1983) 'Non-traumatic coma in childhood: clinical variables in prediction of outcome.' *Developmental Medicine and Child Neurology*, **25**, 493–501.

Settergren, G., Lindblad, B. S., Persson, B. (1980) 'Cerebral blood flow and exchange of oxygen, glucose, ketone bodies, lactate, pyruvate and amino acids in anesthetized children.' *Acta Paediatrica Scandinavica*, **69**, 457–465.

Severinghaus, J. W., Lassen, N. (1967) 'Step hypocapnia to separate arterial from tissue PCO_2 in the regulation of cerebral blood flow.' *Circulation Research*, **20**, 272–282.

Shalit, M. N., Reinmuth, O. M., Shimojyo, S., Sheinberg, P. (1967) 'Carbon dioxide and cerebral circulatory control.' *Archives of Neurology*, **17**, 342–353.

Shapiro, W., Eisenberg, S. (1969) 'Pathophysiology of St. Louis encephalitis: III. Cerebral blood flow and metabolism.' *Annals of Internal Medicine*, **71**, 691–702.

Siesjo, B. K. (1984) 'Cerebral circulation and metabolism.' *Journal of Neurosurgery*, **60**, 883–908.

—— (1988) 'Mechanisms of ischemic brain damage.' *Critical Care Medicine*, **16**, 954–963.

Silverman, B. W. (1985) 'Some aspects of the spline smoothing approach to non-parametric regression curve fitting.' *Journal of the Royal Statistical Society*, **47**, 1–52.

Simon, R. P., Aminoff, M. J. (1986) 'Electrographic status epilepticus in fatal anoxic coma.' *Annals of Neurology*, **20**, 351–355.

Simpson, D., Reilly, P. (1982) 'Paediatric coma scale.' *Lancet*, **2**, 450.

Skinhoj, E., Paulson, O. B. (1969) 'Carbon dioxide and cerebral circulatory control.' *Archives of Neurology*, **20**, 249–252.

Smith, A. J. K., Walker, A. E. (1973) 'Cerebral blood flow and brain metabolism as indicators of cerebral death: a review.' *Johns Hopkins Medical Journal*, **133**, 107–119.

Smith, A. L. (1988) 'Neurologic sequelae of meningitis.' *New England Journal of Medicine*, **319**, 1012–1013.

Snyder, J. V., Nemoto, E. M., Carroll, R. G., Safar, P. (1975) 'Global ischemia in dogs: intracranial pressures, brain blood flow and metabolism.' *Stroke*, **6**, 21–27.

Stanley, N. N., Salisbury, B. G., McHenry, L. C., Cherniack, N. S. (1975) 'Effect of liver failure on the response of ventilation and cerebral circulation to carbon dioxide in man and the goat.' *Clinical Science and Molecular Medicine*, **49**, 157–169.

Steele, B. T., Murphy, N., Chuang, S. H., McGreal, D., Arbus, G. S. (1983) 'Recovery from prolonged coma in hemolytic uremic syndrome.' *Journal of Pediatrics*, **102**, 402–405.

Steinberg, A., Ish-Horowitcz, M., El-Peleg, O., Mor, J., Branski, D. (1986) 'Stroke in a patient with hemolytic-uremic syndrome with a good outcome.' *Brain and Development*, **8**, 70–72.

Stephenson, H. E., Safar, P., Arfors, K. E., Baethmann, A., Basford, R. E., Bontempo, F., Dindzans, V., Hossmann, K. A., Jennings, R. B., Knickerbocker, G., Kochanek, P. M., Pinsky, M. R., Rosborough, J. P., Severinghaus, J. W. Siesjo, B. K., White, B. C., White, R. (1988) 'Treatment potentials for reversing clinical death.' *Critical Care Medicine*, **16**, 1034–1042.

Sterns, R. H., Riggs, J. E., Schochet, S. S. (1986) 'Osmotic demyelination syndrome following correction of hyponatraemia.' *New England Journal of Medicine*, **314**, 1535–1542.

Stovring, J., Snyder, R. D. (1980) 'Computed tomography in childhood bacterial meningitis.' *Journal of Pediatrics*, **96**, 820–823.

Strandgaard, S., MacKenzie, E. T., Sengupta, D., Rowan, J. O., Lassen, N. A., Harper, A. M. (1974) 'Upper limit of autoregulation of cerebral blood flow in the baboon.' *Circulation Research*, **34**, 435–440.

—— Jones, J. V., MacKenzie, E. T., Harper, A. M. (1975) 'Upper limit of cerebral blood flow autoregulation in experimental renovascular hypertension in the baboon.' *Circulation Research*, **37**, 164–167.

—— Paulson, O. B. (1984) 'Cerebral autoregulation.' *Stroke*, **15**, 413–416.

Syrogiannopoulos, G. A., Olsen, K. D., McCracken, G. H. Jr. (1987) 'Mannitol treatment in experimental *Haemophilus influenzae* type b meningitis.' *Pediatric Research*, **22**, 118–122.

346

Talwar, D., Torres, F. (1988) 'Continuous electrophysiologic monitoring of cerebral function in the pediatric intensive care unit.' *Pediatric Neurology*, **4**, 137–147.

Tasker, R. C., Matthew, D. J., Helms, P., Dinwiddie, R., Boyd, S. (1988a) 'Monitoring in non-traumatic coma. Part I: invasive intracranial measurements.' *Archives of Disease in Childhood*, **63**, 888–894.

—— Boyd, S., Harden, A., Matthew, D. J. (1988b) 'Monitoring in non-traumatic coma. Part II: electroencephalography.' *Archives of Disease in Childhood*, **63**, 895–899.

—— —— —— (1989) 'EEG monitoring of prolonged thiopentone adminstration for intractable seizures and status epilepticus in infants and young children.' *Neuropediatrics*, **20**, 147–153.

Todd, M. M., Tommasino, C., Shapiro, H. M. (1985) 'Cerebrovascular effects of prolonged hypocarbia and hypercarbia after experimental global ischemia in cats.' *Critical Care Medicine*, **13**, 720–723.

Torphy, D. E., Minter, M. G., Thompson, B. M (1984) 'Cardiorespiratory arrest and resuscitation of children.' *American Journal of Diseases of Children*, **138**, 1099–1102.

Trevathan, E., Dooling, E. C. (1987) 'Large thrombotic strokes in hemolytic-uremic syndrome.' *Journal of Pediatrics*, **111**, 863–866.

Trewby, P. N., Hanid, M. A., Mackenzie, R. L., Mellon, P. J., Williams, R. (1978) 'Effects of cerebral oedema and arterial hypotension on cerebral blood flow in an animal model of hepatic failure.' *Gut*, **19**, 999–1005.

Turner, G. R., Levin, D. L. (1985) 'Improvement of neurologic status after pediatric near-drowning accidents.' *Critical Care Medicine*, **13**, 1080.

Upadhyaya, K., Barwick, K., Fishaut, M., Kashgarian, M., Siegel, N. J. (1980) 'The importance of nonrenal involvement in hemolytic-uremic syndrome.' *Pediatrics*, **65**, 115–120.

Van Der Meulen, J. A., Klip, A., Grinstein, S. (1987) 'Possible mechanisms for cerebral oedema in diabetic ketoacidosis.' *Lancet*, **2**, 306–308.

Venes, J. L., Collins, W. F. (1975) 'Bifrontal decompressive craniectomy in the management of head trauma.' *Journal of Neurosurgery*, **42**, 429–433.

Voldby, B., Enevoldsen, E. M., Jensen, F. T. (1985) 'Cerebrovascular reactivity in patients with ruptured intracranial aneurysms.' *Journal of Neurosurgery*, **62**, 59–67.

Wagner, E. M., Traystman, J. (1986) 'Hydrostatic determinants of cerebral perfusion.' *Critical Care Medicine*, **14**, 484–490.

Ware, A. J., D'Agostino, A. N., Combes, B. (1971) 'Cerebral edema: a major complication of massive hepatic necrosis.' *Gastroenterology*, **61**, 877–884.

Warrell, D. A., White, N. J., Veall, N., Looareesuwan, S., Chanthavanich, P., Phillips, R. E., Karbwang, J., Pongpaew, P. (1988) 'Cerebral anaerobic glycolysis and reduced cerebral oxygen transport in human cerebral malaria.' *Lancet*, **2**, 534–538.

Weiss, M. H., Spence, J., Apuzzo, M. L. J., Heiden, J. S., McComb, J. G., Kueze, T. (1979) 'Influence of nitroprusside on cerebral pressure autoregulation.' *Neurosurgery*, **4**, 56–59.

White, N. J., Warrell, D. A., Looareesuwan, S., Chanthavanich, P., Phillips, R. E., Pongpaew, P. (1985) 'Pathophysiological and prognostic significance of cerebrospinal-fluid lactate in cerebral malaria.' *Lancet*, **1**, 776–778.

Whitley, R. J., Alford, C. A., Hirsch, M. S., Schooley, R. T., Luby, J. P., Aoki, F. Y., Hanley, D., Nahmias, A. J., Soong, S.-J. (1986) 'Vidarabine versus acyclovir therapy in herpes simplex encephalitis.' *New England Journal of Medicine*, **314**, 144–149.

Wijdicks, E. F. M., Vermeulen, M., Hijdra, A., Van Gijn, J. (1985) 'Hyponatraemia and cerebral infarction in patients with ruptured cerebral aneurysms; is fluid restriction harmful?' *Annals of Neurology*, **17**, 137–140.

Wilkins, R. H. (1980) *Cerebral Artery Spasm*. Baltimore: Williams and Wilkins.

Williams, C. P. S., Swanson, A. G., Chapman, J. T. (1964) 'Brain swelling with acute purulent meningitis: report of treatment with hypertonic intravenous urea.' *Pediatrics*, **34**, 220–227.

Winney, R. J., Kean, D. M., Best, J. J., Smith, M. A. (1986) 'Changes in brain water with haemodialysis.' *Lancet*, **2**, 1107–1108.

Winn, H. R., Welsh, J. E., Rubio, R., Berne, R. M. (1980) 'Brain adenosine production in rat during sustained alteration in systemic blood pressure.' *American Journal of Physiology*, **239**, H636–H641.

Woodcock, J., Ropper, A. H., Kennedy, S. K. (1982) 'High dose barbiturates in non-traumatic brain swelling: ICP reduction and effect on outcome.' *Stroke*, **13**, 785–787.

Wyatt, J. S., Cope, M., Delpy, D. T., Wray, S., Reynolds, E. O. R. (1986) 'Quantification of cerebral oxygenation and haemodynamics in sick newborn infants by near infrared spectrophotometry.' *Lancet*, **2**, 1063–1066.

Yao, H., Sadoshima, S., Fujii, K., Kasuda, K., Ishitsuka, T., Tamaki, K., Fujishima, M. (1987)

'Cerebrospinal fluid lactate in patients with hepatic encephalopathy.' *European Neurology*, **27**, 182–187.

—— —— Nishimura, Y., Fujii, K., Oshima, M., Ishitsuka, T., Fujishima, M. (1989) 'Cerebrospinal fluid lactate in patients with diabetes mellitus and hypoglycaemic coma.' *Journal of Neurology, Neurosurgery and Psychiatry*, **52**, 372–375.

Young, B., Ott, L., Haack, D., Turyman, D., Combs, D., Oexman, J. B., Tibbs, P., Dempsey, R. (1987) 'Effect of total parenteral nutrition upon intracranial pressure in severe head injury.' *Journal of Neurosurgery*, **67**, 76–80.

Young, E., Bradley, R. F. (1967) 'Cerebral edema with irreversible coma in severe diabetic ketoacidosis.' *New England Journal of Medicine*, **276**, 665–669.

Young, R. S. K., Zalneraitis, E. L., Dooling, E. C. (1980) 'Neurological outcome in cold water drowning.' *Journal of the American Medical Association*, **244**, 1233–1235.

Zwetnow, N. N. (1970) 'Effects of increased cerebrospinal fluid pressure on the blood flow and on the energy metabolism of the brain. An experimental study.' *Acta Physiologica Scandinavica* (Suppl. 339) 1–31.

9
A SURVEY OF THE TREATMENT OF INFANTILE HYDROCEPHALUS

Concezio Di Rocco

In the late 1950s, the treatment of hydrocephalus entered a new era with a revolutionary technique for shunting CSF into the right cardiac auricle. The shunting system had a valve assembly to ensure one-way CSF flow, preventing blood reflux and keeping ICP relatively constant (Pudenz *et al.* 1957). Although nowadays CSF is more often shunted into the peritoneal cavity, and Pudenz's operation is rarely performed, its introduction remains a landmark—not just because of the resultant increase in the life-expectancy of hydrocephalic patients, but also because of the way it changed the adverse attitude towards the surgical therapy of the condition. It has also led to a whole new series of problems related to the prevention, identification and treatment of the numerous CSF-shunting complications.

Current options in the treatment of hydrocephalus
Medical treatment
Since the first descriptions by Hippocrates, the therapeutic suggestions for the care of those suffering from hydrocephalus have combined both medical and surgical proposals (Di Rocco 1987). Non-surgical methods include the administration of drugs, such as those which reduce CSF formation, induce diuresis or counteract a blockage of the CSF pathways (in cases of hydrocephalus resulting from intracranial haemorrhage or infections), as well as physical measures which tend to favour CSF absorption, such as the tight bandaging of the head.

PHARMACOLOGICAL METHODS
The attempts to reduce CSF formation are essentially based on two drugs: acetazolamide and isosorbide. Other chemical agents have been tried, to very little effect.

Acetazolamide (Diamox) is an inhibitor of carbonic anhydrase, an enzyme present in the glial cells of the brain and the choroidal epithelium, which was first synthesised by Rubin and Clapp in 1950 (Birzis *et al.* 1958, Rapoport 1976). A series of laboratory experiments carried out in the 1950s and early 1960s demonstrated that when the agent was administered in large doses, it could decrease CSF pressure by reducing its production, without interfering with CSF circulation and absorption (Kister 1956, Tschirgi *et al.* 1957, Pollay and Davson 1963). Though a secondary vasoconstriction of the choroidal arteries could not be ruled out (Macri *et al.* 1956), the reduction in CSF production was regarded as mainly due to a specific inhibition of the enzyme carbonic anhydrase at the level of the choroid plexus. Following the demonstration by Rubin *et al.* (1966) of a 6 to 50 per cent reduction in the CSF production in man after the intravenous administration of 300 to 500mg of the drug, several clinical trials were carried out to control neonatal and childhood hydrocephalus. The results proved to be very unreliable, varying from success in infants with slowly progressive hydrocephalus (Huttenlocher 1965, Nalin and Gatti 1977, Donat 1980) to obvious failures (Mealy and Barker 1968, Schain 1969). In several cases, ventricular dilatation persisted throughout the entire period of administration of the drug and continued to increase again after discontinuation of the therapy (Donat 1980). The drug also has serious side-effects such as an immediate increase in ICP following the administration of the agent, presumably due to the inhibition of carbonic anhydrase within the red blood cells, with secondary interference on respiratory function leading to hypercapnia (responsible in turn for cerebral vasodilatation), vomiting, anorexia, dehydration, metabolic acidosis, growth failure, paraesthesiae, and calcium-phosphate lithiasis.

The clinical introduction of *isosorbide*, a sugar derivative dihydric alcohol derived from sorbital), was accompanied by considerable interest because of the proven effectiveness of the drug in lowering CSF pressure both in laboratory animals (Shinaberger *et al.* 1965, Wise *et al.* 1966) and humans (Troncale *et al.* 1966, Wise *et al.* 1977). Preliminary clinical trials, mostly performed in myelodysplasic subjects or in advanced cases of hydrocephalus, seemed encouraging. In fact, multiple doses of oral isosorbide appeared to have a cumulative effect, by inducing a prolonged reduction in CSF pressure, which persisted until about 18 hours after discontinuation of the therapy. No rebound responses were observed. With the progress in experience, however, the abnormal growth of the head was seen to recur consistently when the drug was withdrawn, and the final outcome of the hydrocephalus appeared to be substantially unaffected by the administration of the agent (Shurtleff *et al.* 1973, Lorber *et al.* 1983). Furthermore, toxicity was observed in about a third of cases, clinically manifested by irritability and decreased tissue turgor. In such cases, laboratory examinations demonstrated an increase in serum sodium. In infants, vomiting, weight loss and loose stools could be so serious as to suggest that the CSF pressure reduction could depend on total body dehydration rather than on preferential dehydrating effect on the brain.

Later a cardiac glycoside, *digoxin*, was proposed to decrease the rate of CSF formation in hydrocephalic patients (Neblett *et al.* 1972). The agent has a specific activity for, and binds to, the magnesium-dependent, ouabain-sensitive, sodium-potassium-activated enzyme ATPase, which is found in the choroid plexus of mammals and is necessary for the active production of CSF (Yates *et al.* 1964, Oppelt and Palmer 1966). In experimental animals, small amounts of digoxin stimulated the formation of CSF, while large amounts had an inhibitory effect (Oppelt and Palmer 1966, Wright 1972). Even though clinical trials carried out on very small populations of infants with moderate ventricular dilatation confirmed the possibility of reducing the CSF production with the drug (Allonen *et al.* 1977), the results were even more deceptive than those obtained with acetazolamide and isosorbide. In fact, the action of the digoxin was characterised by a slow onset and an extremely brief duration; furthermore the doses required to reduce the production of CSF were so high as to reach a toxic effect (Bass *et al.* 1979).

In spite of the lack of any experimental evidence on their actual role in preventing arachnoiditis, *corticosteroids* have been widely used in cases of post-inflammatory or post-haemorrhagic hydrocephalus (Sehgal *et al.* 1962, Kulick 1965, Rasi 1971, Wilkinson *et al.* 1974, Kaufman and Carmel 1978, Julow 1979). Intrathecal hydrocortisone or systemic steroids have also been associated with other drugs, such as *hyaluronidase* or *urokinase*, with the aim of counteracting a blockage in the CSF pathways (Schwatzman 1949, Lapin 1950, Fostad *et al.* 1978, Gourie-Dev and Satish 1980). Hyaluronidase hydrolyses the glucosaminidic bonds of hyaluronic acid of the ground substance; it is therefore thought to favour the absorption of exudate and to prevent the formation of adhesions in post-infective hydrocephalus. The good results claimed with the use of this substance have been mostly obtained in cases of hydrocephalus resulting from tuberculous leptomen-ingitis (Gourie-Dev and Satish 1980). The therapeutic proposal of urokinase was based on clinical and laboratory observations made in the late 1970s. At that time the clinical introduction of antifibrinolytic agents, to prevent the lysis of the clot around a ruptured intracranial aneurysm, was noted to be followed by an increased incidence of post-haemorrhagic hydrocephalus, due to enhanced subarachnoid fibrosis (Fostad *et al.* 1978, Park 1979).

Julow (1979) injected blood into the cisterna magna of dogs, and found that subarachnoid fibrosis could be prevented or at least reduced by an intrathecal injection of urokinase. The interference of urokinase with the pathomechanism of subarachnoid fibrosis is similar to that of other plasminogen activators, such as streptokinase; nevertheless, urokinase has the advantage of being a human protein with no antigenic effect. However, the experience with urokinase (or strepto-kinase) in the treatment of hydrocephalus is too limited to allow any definitive conclusion (Furukawa 1968, Ringelova 1976).

PHYSICAL METHODS

Heliotherapy was one of the first physical treatment methods for hydrocephalus. In 1564 Riverius (cited by Torack 1982) suggested the application of a compressive wrapping round the head to control the abnormal growth of the skull. A meticulous description of the technique was provided by Barnard (1838). In recent years, head-wrapping has again been proposed (Epstein *et al.* 1973) on the assumption that the artificial resistance to the enlargement of the skull could stimulate the development of alternative mechanisms for CSF absorption, in relation to the secondary increase in CSF pressure. The theoretical basis for the proposal was furnished by experimental observations on hydrocephalic cats, in which the partial removal of the skull was followed by an impressive increase in ventricular volume (Hochwald *et al.* 1972).

The clinical results have been controversial. Epstein *et al.* (1973) reported an arrest of the abnormal head-growth with the ventricular size remaining essentially unchanged in five infants selected according to three criteria: progressive hydrocephalus with normal or slightly increased intraventricular pressure; mild to moderate ventriculomegaly; good general clinical condition. However Meyer *et al.*

TABLE 9.I

The treatment of hydrocephalus

Physiological procedures
    Operations on the choroid plexus
        Open surgical extirpation of the choroid plexus
        Endoscopic cauterisation of the choroid plexus
        Radioactive destruction of the choroid plexus
    Third ventriculostomy
        Open surgical third ventriculostomy
        Percutaneous third ventriculostomy
            Endoscopic guidance
            Radiological guidance
    Direct surgical attack on obstructions to CSF flow
    Transcerebral fistula
    Biological methods of draining CSF
        Lumbo-omental pedicle graft
        The pericranium flap operation

(1973) described a deterioration of the neurological state in two infants following head-wrapping attempts. It is worth noting that most of the claimed success has been obtained in subjects with hydrocephalus associated with myelodysplasia (Epstein *et al.* 1973, 1974*b*; Porter 1975), that is a particular type of hydrocephalus characterised by a slow and intermittent clinical course. In myelodysplasic patients the hydrocephalus is often accompanied by a dilatation of the central spinal canal, which is thought to serve as an extra space to compensate for the CSF accumulation. Therefore particular attention should be given to the suggestion by Boltshauser and Cavanagh (1976) that head-wrapping in infants with myelodysplasia could favour the formation of hydromyelia, thus slowing down the progression of the hydrocephalus at the expense of additional spinal damage.

Surgical treatment
The numerous attempts to treat hydrocephalus by means of surgical procedures are traditionally divided into two main groups: the so-called 'physiological' operations, and those which use mechanical valves and tubes. The main aim of the first type of operation is to reduce CSF formation or to restore CSF circulation to within the natural pathways; the second type is devoted to by-passing an eventual block in CSF circulation, or to favouring CSF absorption by diverting CSF into other body cavities.

PHYSIOLOGICAL OPERATIONS (Table 9.I)
The 'physiological' treatment of hydrocephalus may be regarded as beginning with Dandy, who devised an impressive variety of surgical procedures: he performed the surgical extirpation of the choroid plexus from both lateral cerebral ventricles (Dandy 1918), he cannulated the aqueduct (Dandy 1920) and opened the floor of the third ventricle (Dandy 1922). Two main theories divided scientists at the beginning of the century (Di Rocco 1987): according to some, CSF resulted from a process of simple filtration through an animal membrane, like other body fluids; according to others, CSF was produced by the choroid plexus through an active process of cellular secretion.

Dandy and Blackfan (1914) integrated the two theories by suggesting that the choroid plexus generated CSF by filtration *and* secretion. They also stressed the necessity of communication between the ventricular system (which they considered to be the site of CSF production) and the peripheral subarachnoid spaces (identified as the site of CSF absorption).

All three types of operation introduced by Dandy—choroid plexectomy, third ventriculostomy and cannulation of the fourth ventricle—were based on the concept of the choroid plexus as the only source of CSF. They are still occasionally performed today.

Choroid plexectomy (Dandy 1918, 1932; Sachs 1942; Davidoff 1948) was followed by equivocal results. The failures, however, did not discourage the development of new techniques aimed at eliminating the 'source' of CSF, such as the endoscopic removal (Feld 1957) or the endoscopic cauterisation (Putnam 1934) of the choroid plexus. Nor did failures impede the proposal of alternative methods such as the radioactive destruction of the choroid plexus, which was propounded on the basis of the experimental evidence of the accumulation of radioactive colloidal gold in the choroidal cells when instilled directly into the cerebral ventricles (McClure 1955, Rish and Meacham 1967, Weiss *et al.* 1972).

The unreliability of choroidal plexectomy prompted some authors to criticise the 'physiological' basis of the operation. For example, the possible role of a fistula (ventriculostomy), created by operating on the choroid plexus and allowing CSF to escape from the lateral ventricle into the subarachnoid spaces of the cerebral convexity, was proposed as an alternative explanation for interpreting the success of plexectomy (Hyndman 1946). When Hassin *et al.* (1937) repeated Dandy and Blackfan's experiments, they got completely different results, leading them to postulate an extra-choroidal source of the CSF. This extra-choroidal source was unequivocally demonstrated 30 years later, when several different groups of investigators (Pollay and Curl 1967, Sato and Bering 1967, Sonnenberg *et al.* 1967) demonstrated that most of the CSF is formed at the level of the ependyma, thus explaining the limited value of plexectomy in curing hydrocephalus (Milhorat 1969, 1974).

Scarff (1970) compared the outcomes of 39 personal cases treated with plexectomy, and 42 subjects described by Feld (1957) and Putnam (1934), with the results of operations which used a CSF-shunting valve system. Though the short postoperative course recorded in the patients whose clinical histories had been collected from the literature precluded a reliable comparison, Scarff stressed the decreased number of surgical deaths (5 per cent mortality rate) among his recent operations (after World War II) and the high percentage (50 to 80 per cent) of 'arrest' of hydrocephalus.

However, it should be pointed out that among the successful results (16 cases) claimed by the author, only one in four presented a satisfactory mental development later. This finding, together with a mortality rate which is unacceptable today, is sufficient to rule out the validity of choroid plexectomy as an elective procedure in the treatment of hydrocephalus. Indeed, the operation is now confined to those cases of post-infective loculated hydrocephalus which are unsuitable for CSF shunting, and which may benefit even from a limited reduction in CSF formation.

Third ventriculostomy—the opening of the anterior third ventricle—is still performed. Its aim is to create a fistula between the ventricular system and the basal cisterns in cases of internal obstructive hydrocephalus.

The procedure, as devised by Dandy (1922), allowed the fenestration of the floor and the lateral wall of the third ventricle, just behind the pituitary stalk, through a craniotomy and a subfrontal approach, with the deliberate resection of one optic nerve. A substantial advance in the technique, with the elimination of the unacceptable sacrifice of the optic nerve, was due to Stookey and Scarff (1936), who introduced the puncture of the lamina terminalis and the floor of the third ventricle. Nowadays, the direct approach to the lamina terminalis and basal membrane of the floor of the third ventricle through a craniotomy is still used, but with the aid of the operating microscope (Avman and Kampolat 1979, Kuwabara *et al.* 1982). Its main advantage is that the opening of the third ventricle is carried out under direct vision, with a decreased risk of damaging the hypothalamus and the possibility of performing an additional opening in the arachnoid of the chiasmatic cistern and Liliequist's membrane, which may favour the circulation of the CSF. Furthermore, the better control of local bleeding may reduce the possibility of a secondary obliteration of the surgically created fistula.

Third ventriculostomy is currently performed with the percutaneous approach, either with endoscopic or radiological guidance. The endoscopic third ventriculostomy, first performed by Mixter (1923), has been significantly improved over the last few years with better lighting systems and the development of flexible endoscopes (Guiot *et al.* 1968, Vries 1978). Radiological guidance for the percutaneous opening of the third ventricle, first used by McNickle (1947), has gained great favour with neurosurgeons because of its high rate of immediate success (75 to 95 per cent) and low mortality rate (4 per cent) (Guiot 1968, Pierre-Kahn *et al.* 1975, Poblete and Zamboni 1975, Sayers and Kosnik 1976, Hoffman *et al.* 1980). The aetiology of the hydrocephalus correlates with outcomes of the operation, as the worst results are obtained in children with hydrocephalus following intracranial haemorrhages or infections, and in cases of hydrocephalus apparent at birth (Pierre-Kahn *et al.* 1975). The best candidates for a potentially successful outcome are those subjects presenting with an obstructive hydrocephalus (with the obstruction at the level of the aqueduct or the outlets of the fourth ventricle, without any neoplastic mass within the third ventricle) and those with a grossly dilated third ventricle (with its floor bulging into the interpeduncular cistern) (Hoffman *et al.* 1980, Frerebeau *et al.* 1982). The absence of a previously inserted CSF shunt device further contributes to the surgical success.

Percutaneous third ventriculostomy has undoubted advantages when compared to other methods of treating hydrocephalus (Di Rocco 1987). Besides the low operative mortality, the low incidence of infective complications, and the low rate of surgical revision procedures, the operation does not require the insertion of foreign material within the body, and does not have severe complications such as excessive CSF drainage and secondary craniosynostosis.

TABLE 9.II

The treatment of hydrocephalus

CSF shunting procedures with mechanical valves and tubes
    Intrathecal CSF shunts
        Ventriculocisternostomy
        Cannulation of the aqueduct (interventriculostomy)
        Ventriculo-subdural CSF shunt
        CSF shunting to the epidural space
        CSF shunting from the cerebral ventricles or cisterns
            to the intracranial venous sinuses
        Other intracranial CSF shunts
    Extrathecal CSF shunting
        CSF shunting outside the organism
            CSF shunt to ureter
            CSF shunt to the urinary bladder
        CSF shunting to the bloodstream
            CSF shunt to the scalp and neck veins
            CSF shunt to the thoracic duct
            CSF shunt to the jugular vein, superior vena
                cava and cardiac atrium
        CSF shunting to body cavities and structures
          other than blood circulation
            CSF shunt to the subaponeurotic layers of the
                scalp and skin
            CSF shunt to the salivary duct
            CSF shunt into the gastric cavity
            CSF shunt to the gall bladder
            CSF shunt to the ileum
            CSF shunt to the pleural cavity
            CSF shunt to the peritoneal cavity
                Ventriculo-peritoneal CSF shunt
                Lumbo-peritoneal CSF shunt

Its disadvantages are a precocious obliteration of the artificial communication between the third ventricle and the interpeduncular cistern (demonstrated in about one sixth of subjects) (Pierre-Kahn *et al.* 1975). The effect on the ventriculomegaly is very slight. Actually, abnormal head-growth may persist even in children who appear to have benefited from the procedure. The finding suggests that the peripheral subarachnoid spaces are unable to absorb the shunted CSF in a large percentage of patients. While the incidence of secondary obstruction of the stoma may be decreased by reducing the local bleeding with the use of relatively atraumatic tools (Cl. Bertrand's leukotome, Fogarty's balloon) to perforate the lamina terminalis and the floor of the third ventricle, the preoperative determination of the patency of the peripheral subarachnoid spaces has still not been fully solved (Patterson and Bergland 1968). The validity of preoperative isotope cisternography, as proposed by Akerman *et al.* (1972) has not been confirmed by other authors (Pierre-Kahn *et al.* 1975, Des Plantes and Crezee 1978). The subarachnoid spinal-infusion test may be unreliable in aqueductal stenosis when testing CSF absorption within the peripheral subarachnoid spaces, which are functionally inactive because of the compression exerted by the expanded cerebral hemispheres.

Other 'physiological' methods for treating hydrocephalus (Table 9.I) such as the *direct surgical attack on obstructions in the* CSF flow, the creation of a *transcerebral fistula*, and the *biological methods of draining the* CSF, are of historical interest only.

CSF DIVERSION OPERATIONS USING MECHANICAL VALVES AND TUBES (Table 9.II)

The introduction of silicone rubber tubing for CSF-shunting operations (Pudenz *et al.* 1957) marked a great improvement in the possibility of treating hydrocephalus using artificial systems for CSF drainage. The new material seemed almost to annihilate the inflammatory responses of the host, thus dramatically reducing the incidence of complications due to the interreaction of the patient's tissues with the inserted CSF shunting device. The availability of silastic tubes and valves stimulated the application of procedures aimed at draining CSF from the intracranial or intraspinal spaces to other body cavities, suitable for absorbing the excess fluid (extrathecal CSF shunts) (Table 9.II). It also contributed to reviving techniques for by-passing anatomical obstacles in the CSF circulation within the skull (intrathecal CSF shunts) (Table 9.II).

1. INTRATHECAL CSF SHUNTS

Among the variety of techniques for by-passing such an obstacle, or for diverting CSF from the ventricular system to the cisterns, the subdural or epidural spaces, the intracranial venous sinuses, and the osseous structures of the skull and the spine by means of artificial systems, only cannulation of the aqueduct (interventriculostomy) and third ventriculostomy maintain their place in the management of hydrocephalus (Di Rocco 1987).

Cannulation of the aqueduct was first performed by Dandy (1920), who dilated a strictured aqueduct by using a rubber catheter which was left in place for a few weeks in an attempt to prevent the channel from narrowing again.

A variant of the operation was introduced by Leksell (1949), who used a rubber catheter covered by a spiral of tantalium. This latter part of the device could remain permanently *in situ* within the aqueduct to maintain dilatation, while the rubber catheter could be withdrawn to reduce the risk of inflammatory reactions.

Subsequent experience proved that interventriculostomy was relatively safe and effective as far as the function of the catheter within the aqueduct was concerned (Elvidge 1966), while most of the failures could be attributed to a congenital or acquired incompetence of the subarachnoid spaces of the cerebral convexity (Crosby *et al.* 1973). As with the third ventriculostomy, insertion of an extrathecal CSF shunt device before the cannulation of the aqueduct was suggested in order to ease CSF absorption within the peripheral subarachnoid spaces (Crosby *et al.* 1973). Further suggestions were aimed at decreasing the surgical death rate, such as the gently progressive dilatation of the aqueduct, to be achieved by inserting progressively larger catheters one after the other, and preventing the upward or downward spontaneous migration of the tube left within the aqueduct by using special catheters with rostral and/or caudal cuffs (Crosby *et al.* 1973, Lapras *et al.* 1975).

Cannulation of the aqueduct is still used almost exclusively in subjects already harbouring a CSF extrathecal drainage system, in cases where it is necessary to transform an obstructive hydrocephalus into a communicating one. This may be necessary in patients with transient episodes of shunt malfunction apparently due to an excessive reduction in volume of the lateral cerebral ventricle (slit ventricle syndrome) (Lapras *et al.* 1975), or in children with post-inflammatory hydrocephalus, when scarring adhesions (membranes) isolate the fourth ventricle by occluding the aqueduct and its exit foramina as well (entrapped fourth ventricle).

Besides the insertion of the catheter into the aqueduct under direct vision through the direct suboccipital approach, current methods for carrying out interventriculostomy use percutaneous techniques from above (from the lateral through the third ventricle) (Cuatico and Richardson 1979, Bret 1981), as well as stereotactic techniques (Backlund *et al.* 1981).

Among the various procedures of *ventriculocisternostomy* which have been developed in the course of the years (Di Rocco 1987) (Table 9.II), that proposed by Torkildsen (1939) for the management of obstructive hydrocephalus due to a mass within the third ventricle, or at the level of the aqueduct, has been by far the most widely used. The operation, which allows CSF shunting from one lateral ventricle into the cisterna magna by means of a tube, is still performed as originally described by the author. Only two variants of the operation have been introduced. The first, by Swanson and Perrett (1950), used two ventricular catheters connected by a Y junction to the distal limb of the shunt system, in subjects where the CSF circulation was obstructed by a mass occluding both foramina of Monro. The second modification, by Matson (1969), was designed to help the surgical procedure in infants by avoiding the opening of the dura mater of the posterior cranial fossa with its abundant venous lakes and sinuses, and inserting the distal end of the tube into the antero-lateral cervical gutter through a c_1-c_3 hemilaminectomy.

Torkildsen's procedure has some obvious advantages, such as low cost, the reduced rate of late complications, and the absence of malfunction due either to CSF overdrainage or to dislocation of the shunt device secondary to the physical growth of the child. However, its technical simplicity has not led to its being widely used except in patients with inoperable endocranial neoplasms. Matson (1969) was convinced that a child's peripheral subarachnoid spaces could not accommodate the diverted CSF, and this might help to explain the reduced clinical application of the procedure in the paediatric population. Neurosurgeons have also been reluctant to use Torkildsen's ventriculostomy in children with congenital aqueductal stenosis, because of the difficulty of pre-operatively evaluating the 'competence' of the peripheral subarachnoid spaces, the same disadvantage experienced with other types of internal shunts already mentioned.

2. EXTRATHECAL CSF SHUNTS

Most of the old procedures for diverting CSF from the cerebral ventricles and subarachnoid spaces are currently only of historical interest (Di Rocco 1987). Heile's procedure (1925) involved shunting CSF outside the body, thus eliminating it once and for all; this technique was modified by Matson (1951, 1953), who diverted

CSF from the arachnoid lumbar space or the cerebral ventricles into the ureter, and by West (1980), who diverted it from the cerebral ventricles to the urinary bladder) (Table 9.II).

Other CSF-diversion procedures were designed to shunt the fluid into the bloodstream, either directly (CSF shunt to the scalp and neck veins, to the jugular vein, the superior vena cava and cardiac atrium) or by way of the thoracic duct (CSF ventriculo-lymphatic shunt) (Table 9.II). Of these procedures, only the CSF *shunting into the right cardiac auricle (ventriculo-atrial shunt)* (Pudenz *et al.* 1957) maintains its place in the current management of hydrocephalus.

The first successful diversion of CSF from one lateral cerebral ventricle into the internal jugular vein, performed by Nulsen and Spitz (1952), had already met some of the criteria on which the success of the ventriculo-atrial CSF shunting is based. The authors used a CSF shunt device with a valve to ensure one-way CSF flow, thus preventing a blood reflux within the shunt, and maintaining the CSF pressure within predetermined ranges; the location of the distal tip of the shunt apparatus had been chosen in order to minimise its secondary blockage by blood clots. However, this latter complication appeared to be effectively prevented only when the cardiac tip of the CSF shunt apparatus was located within the free circulation of the blood of large vessels such as the superior vena cava, or within the cardiac atrium.

The accurate placement of the distal end of the shunt apparatus is of paramount importance in this type of operation for maintaining the system patent, thus explaining the continuous research of reliable methods of control. Pudenz had suggested the use of chest x-ray examinations, some authors have introduced neurophysiological techniques (Robertson *et al.* 1961), and others have advocated the direct transthoracic intra-auricular introduction of the cardiac end of the shunt system (Weineman and Paul 1967). Nevertheless, the accumulated experience indicates that, in spite of a proper preoperative placement of the cardiac catheter, the ventriculo-atrial shunt is exposed to the inevitable complication of the venous catheter blockage in the growing infant, when the catheter secondarily 'migrates' into the jugular vein. The cardiac catheter obstruction usually begins when the chest x-ray examination demonstrates the tip of the catheter to be at the level of the fourth thoracic vertebra, and becomes very frequent when the tip is at the level of the third thoracic vertebra (Becker *et al.* 1968). Attempts to prevent or delay this type of complication, by placing the tip of the cardiac catheter in a lower position at the operation, have resulted in a high incidence of bacteraemia, probably related to the damage to the tricuspid valve or to enmeshing of the catheter in infected vegetation and thrombi (Becker *et al.* 1968).

To obviate the precocious blockage of the ventriculo-atrial shunt secondary to the patient's physical growth, the prophylactic lengthening of the shunt system has been advocated, on the grounds that the operative risk is minimal compared with revision procedures carried out for removing venous obstruction (Becker *et al.* 1968, Tsingoglou and Forrest 1968).

Modifications to the shunt system, which allow it to elongate during the growth of the child (the so-called telescopic ventriculo-atrial shunt) (Wise 1974), and surgical techniques for lengthening the shunt, by pushing its tip down to a lower level by means of a specific device, have also been introduced (Hooper 1969, Yamada and Tajima 1974).

The ventriculo-atrial CSF shunt is still performed as originally described by Pudenz *et al*. 1957); but following the technique for cannulating the subclavian vein for continuous monitoring of the central venous pressure (Borja and Hinshaw 1970), simplified methods of performing the operation have been developed, such as the percutaneous placement of the cardiac catheter into the subclavian, internal or external jugular veins (Ashker and Fox 1981, Epstein *et al*. 1981, Tomita 1984).

The multitude of unsuccessful CSF-shunting techniques demonstrates how difficult the problem has been for neurosurgeons (Di Rocco 1987). Virtually no body cavities or structures have been spared (Table 9.II), but out of these numerous procedures, only a few (CSF shunts to the peritoneal cavity, and to a lesser extent, those to the pleural cavity) survive today. Some procedures, such as the CSF shunt to the subaponeurotic layers of the scalp and skin, have occasionally been revived, but have very little clinical application.

The history of CSF *peritoneal shunts* coincides with the availability of silicone catheters (Ames 1967). However, their pioneer applications can be traced back as far as the end of the 19th century, when Ferguson (1898) first made a lumbo-peritoneal CSF shunt, by removing the arch of the fifth lumbar vertebra and drilling a small hole to pass a loop of silver wire through it from the subarachnoid space into the peritoneal cavity. In 1908 Kausch carried out the first ventriculo-peritoneal CSF shunt by means of a rubber tube, which resulted in the patient dying because of an excessive fluid drainage. Cushing (1908) used a laparotomy to introduce the catheter into the peritoneal cavity. Though his results unequivocally demonstrated the effectiveness of the operation, he commented negatively on this type of operation. In fact, he believed that the few cases of intussusception he had recorded were due to the presence of some substances in the CSF which could stimulate an abnormal peristalsis.

This negative attitude deeply influenced neurosurgeons, to the extent that the diversion of CSF into the peritoneal cavity was practically discarded for more than 30 years. However a series of new attempts was carried out with the introduction of new procedures, such as CSF shunting into the fallopian tube (Harsch 1954) or the omental bursa (Picaza 1956), as well as the development of measures (resection of the omentum, utilisation of different tubing material, special coverings for the tip of the peritoneal end of the shunt device) to improve the efficiency of the operation by decreasing an excessively high rate of secondary obstruction (Di Rocco 1987).

In 1967, Ames reported on the first large series of *ventriculo-peritoneal shunts* using silicone tubes. The author pointed out the very low mortality rate, the absence of 'rejection' of the shunt by the peritoneum, and the lack of inflammatory reactions of the omentum leading to the obstruction of the peritoneal tip. In the same year, Raimondi and Matsumoto (1967) introduced a simplified technique for performing the operation, using the percutaneous puncture of the abdominal wall for inserting the distal end of the CSF shunt apparatus into the peritoneal cavity. In the seventies, the *ventriculo-peritoneal* CSF shunt and its variant the *lumbo-peritoneal shunt*, performed by means of a hemilaminectomy (Eisenberg *et al*. 1971) or by using a percutaneous technique (Murtagh and Lechman 1967, Selman *et al.* 1980) became the preferred type of CSF shunt in nearly all centres, owing to the simplicity of the technique, and to the lower incidence of serious complications than that recorded with venous shunts.

Results

The variety of factors which may influence the prognosis of infantile hydrocephalus prevents one from evaluating the relationship between outcomes and modalities of treatment adopted. Some of these factors are very significant, such as the aetiology of the hydrocephalus, the age and general condition of the patient at the time of treatment, the quality of supervision of the shunt function, the occurrence of complications, and the socio-economic environment of the child.

Before the introduction of the CT scan and MRI techniques, the most obvious limit in determining outcomes was inadequate diagnosis, which affected the choice of the most appropriate therapeutic modality and hindered the early detection and proper treatment of complications.

The appraisal of a series of 6005 cases of non-tumoural infantile hydrocephalus, collected from reports published between 1960 and 1978 and concerning children given ventriculo-atrial and ventriculo-peritoneal shunts, demonstrates that long-term survivals range from 53 to 88 per cent (Di Rocco 1987). The most recent figures agree on a percentage of 15 to 20 per cent of children doomed to perish at some time from causes directly or indirectly related either to the progression of the original disease or its treatment. However, the most interesting finding is that most of the deaths are recorded in the first two years following surgical treatment, thus suggesting the important role of both the aetiology of the hydrocephalus and the condition of the patient at the time of the first operation.

In a series of 496 children with non-tumoural hydrocephalus operated on by Hemmer (1979), the over-all mortality rate was 16 per cent. However, 49 per cent of the deaths occurred in newborns, 34 per cent in infants, and only 17 per cent in children. Mortality not associated with the CSF shunt was 43 per cent.

Myelodysplasic subjects, who are usually operated on within the first hours of life, show a higher incidence of surgically related deaths (29 to 47 per cent) (Weissenfels and Hemmer 1981, Amacher and Wellington 1984). These deaths are due to a symptomatic Chiari type II malformation or, more commonly, to infective complications directly depending on the associated spinal defect and favoured by the relatively insufficient immunological response of the newborn infant. Similar considerations could be made for other types of hydrocephalus, when treated surgically during the first week of life, and for hydrocephalus secondary to leptomeningitis (Di Rocco 1987).

The choice of the CSF shunt procedure may influence the mortality rate, as demonstrated by a series of reports clearly indicating a higher death rate associated with ventriculo-atrial CSF shunts (Ignelzi and Kirsch 1975, Caldarelli *et al.* 1979, Keucher and Mealy 1979, Mazza *et al.* 1980, Amacher and Wellington 1984) than with ventriculo-peritoneal CSF shunts. Most deaths associated with ventriculo-atrial CSF shunts result from lethal complications such as formation of thrombi or emboli, perforation of the cardiac atrial or ventricular wall, detachment and migration of a segment of the shunt device within the heart and/or the pulmonary artery, and acute and chronic septicaemia.

On the other hand, the number of surgical procedures does not significantly affect the mortality rate (Occhipinti *et al.* 1981). Indeed, most deaths are recorded after the first or second operation, further stressing the importance of the aetiological factor (Di Rocco 1987).

Follow-up studies on a large series of operated hydrocephalic subjects show that survivors have a lower mean IQ, with a greater variability, than normal subjects. These series, however, especially the most recent ones, include several severely retarded patients, who, in the past, were destined to die because of the relative inadequacy of surgical treatment. The great variability in IQ scores can be seen in the report by Tromp *et al.* (1979), who noticed a mean IQ of 80.6 in 194 unselected hydrocephalic children, with a standard deviation of 29.9, *i.e.* twice the normal value; this variability may be explained by again considering the number of factors which may influence the long-term prognosis. The aetiology of hydrocephalus plays an important role in the mental development of survivors. The highest IQS are recorded in children with hydrocephalus secondary to myelomeningocele (Raimondi and Soare 1974, Shurtleff *et al.* 1975, Weissenfels and Hemmer 1981), and the lowest in subjects with post-infective and post-traumatic hydrocephalus, or with hydrocephalus associated with severe cerebral malformations (Tromp *et al.* 1979, McLone and Raimondi 1983, Amacher and Wellington 1984).

Tromp *et al.* (1979) found a significant correlation between children's IQ scores and the educational and professional level of parents. Raimondi and Soare (1974) demonstrated that the IQs of operated hydrocephalic children did not differ significantly from those of their siblings.

The time of the operation also influences the development of intellectual capacity. All the authors agree on the existence of a 'crucial period' after which the surgical therapy may be insufficient to prevent intellectual impairment. Unfortunately, the limits of such a period have not been clearly established, even though some indications have been supplied. Lorber (1968), for example, stated that the operation should be performed within the 'first few months of life'. Nulsen and Rekate (1982) reported their best outcomes in children shunted prior to five months of age and established 18 months as the upper age-limit, after which they no longer observed a re-expansion of the cerebral mantle.

On the other hand, cumulated experience has demonstrated that intellectual performances are not significantly affected by the severity of hydrocephalus (which is based on the thickness of the cortical mantle at the time of the operation) or by the number of surgical revisions.

Surveillance of CSF shunt function
The development of echoencephalography, CT and MRI has resulted not only in a better surgical indication but also in an improved capacity for assessing the function of the inserted CSF shunt device, thus contributing to better surgical results.

Traditionally, the evaluation of the function of CSF shunts is based on the combination of clinical observations and on laboratory investigations. Besides the obvious signs of increased intracranial pressure, which can correspond to a malfunctioning shunt, some information about the functioning of the shunt apparatus can be provided by observing the characteristics of the *head-growth curve* following the implantation of the CSF shunt device. There are three main patterns suggesting efficient CSF drainage: head growth is temporarily arrested, resuming again at a normal rate when the child's body has caught up to the size of the head; the head volume becomes actually smaller after surgical treatment, with a delayed resumption of normal growth when the body has caught up; and finally, the rate of head growth decreases but remains such as to constantly maintain the head circumference at a percentile above the normal values (Schick and Matson 1961).

Even though evaluation of head growth is an important parameter in the follow-up observation of operated-on hydrocephalic children, its value is limited by its exclusive application to children with still expansible skulls. Furthermore, the time required to assess with certainty an abnormal head growth may be too long, thus possibly exposing the brain to a chronically elevated CSF pressure.

In infants the anterior fontanelle offers a natural window for evaluating the size of the cerebral ventricle by ultrasound. Modern *echoencephalography* machines provide accurate 2D images of the brain with no discomfort for the patient, no exposure to ionising radiation, and no need for sedation. The only disadvantage is the short period during which the examination can be used.

The direct *radiological examination* of the skull may furnish reliable findings, by demonstrating obvious calvarial changes and a certain degree of remodelling of the base of the skull after the operation. Typical calvarial changes are the thickening of the vault (inner table), the attenuation of digital and vascular markings, the fusion of cranial sutures and the eventual asymmetry of the skull, due to the hemicranium harbouring the CSF shunt being smaller than the contralateral one. The most prominent changes of the base of the skull consist of thickening of the sphenoid plane, wings and posterior clinoids, the reduction in size of the *aditus ad sellam*, the reduction in diameter of the basal foramina, and the increase in volume of the paranasal sinuses.

The direct radiological examination of the skull may also demonstrate secondary craniosynostosis due to excessive CSF drainage, while an x-ray evaluation of the shunt assembly may reveal complications such as displacement, kinking and disconnection when the CSF shunt device is made of radiopaque material or provided with radiopaque markers or wire springs. It can also find the 'fixed' position of the tip of the peritoneal catheter at serial examinations. The lack of mobility of the catheter is thought to result from inflammatory adhesions of the shunt to a wall of a viscus, which may eventually lead to a decubitus perforation.

The advent of the CT scan and MRI techniques has made any invasive technique obsolete, and practically replaced all previous radiological procedures (Naidich *et al.* 1982). They both demonstrate the reduction in ventricular volume following the insertion of the CSF shunt apparatus, as well as any eventual changes in the subarachnoid spaces, the exact position of the intracranial catheter, and the integrity of the CSF shunt assembly. The CT scan may also document the modifications of the skull bones induced by the decrease in CSF pressure brought about by the operation.

Unfortunately both CT scan and MRI are relatively expensive and require the deep sedation of the very young patients.

Invasive methods of radiological evaluation of the shunt functions are usually aimed at demonstrating the free movement of a contrast medium, injected into the CSF shunt assembly or into the subarachnoid spaces. The injection of contrast medium into the shunt device (valvulography) (Amador *et al.* 1969) is a relatively safe manoeuvre when the injection is performed through an unidirectional reservoir which prevents the reflux of the agent within the ventricular system. The visualisation of the CSF stream using isotopic substances, such as RHISA or ^{99m}Tc-pertechnetate (Migliore *et al.* 1962, Amador *et al.* 1969, Frick *et al.* 1974, Harbert and McCullough 1984), is very reliable but requires sophisticated equipment. However, with invasive radiological methods there is a risk of iatrogenic contamination of the valve assembly, besides the obvious discomfort for the patient when the examination is performed by means of the percutaneous puncture of the reservoir or by the ventricular or lumbar tap.

Non-invasive methods of CSF-flow determination are based on gross and relatively unreliable manoeuvres, such as the pumping of a flushing device inserted along the shunt tubing (Osaka *et al.* 1977), or on sophisticated techniques such as the study of the transfer of the thermic gradient due to the movement of CSF (Go *et al.* 1968, Caldarelli *et al.* 1981), or the ultrasonic determination of the presence of a fluid stream within the shunt apparatus (Flitter *et al.* 1975).

More reliable, but weighted again by the risk of bacterial contamination, is the *study of the* CSF *dynamics* through the assessment of CSF absorption (infusion test) (Caldarelli *et al.* 1979*a*), or the direct evaluation of the intracranial pressure behaviour (by means of short- and long-term recordings of ICP using the puncture of subcutaneous reservoirs) (Daniels *et al.* 1981, Longatti *et al.* 1982).

Finally, indirect information on the function of the CSF shunt may be obtained through *electrophysiological* or *metabolic studies*. While the latter are of little practical importance because of technical difficulties, the former have been used in clinical practice (Rossini *et al.* 1978, Ehle *et al.* 1979). This kind of examination is aimed at evaluating the normalisation of physiological parameters, brought about by the shunt procedure, such as the latencies of visual and auditory-evoked potentials or the blink reflex. In cases of ventricular dilatation the normal pathways for the above-mentioned reflexes are elongated in relation to the distortion of paraventricular anatomical structures.

Complications of CSF shunting
Complications common to all types of shunts
The most common complication is *mechanical malfunction*, resulting either from obstruction or from disconnection of the different components of the shunt assembly.

Obstruction is common at the level of the ventricular catheter, resulting from improper placement, secondary malpositioning due to ventricular coarctation, and choroidal and ependymal reaction. Prophylaxis includes accurate placement of the ventricular catheter, use of special ventricular catheters and, when necessary, the choice of surgical procedures which prevent the excessive collapse of the cerebral ventricles.

Obstruction of the distal end of the shunt system also occurs; its incidence and significance vary according to the environment from where the CSF is drained. The patency of the venous catheter appears directly related to the calibre of the vein where its tip is located and to the magnitude of bloodflow around it. Early occlusion of the distal end of ventriculo-peritoneal shunts often corresponds to overt or occult shunt infections leading to the fibrous encapsulation of the tip of the shunt.

The physiological growth of the child results in the dislocation of the distal end of the shunt apparatus. In children with ventriculo-atrial shunts this event is regarded as the commonest cause of obstruction, while in subjects with ventriculo-peritoneal shunts the CSF may continue to flow within the 'tube' formed by the connective tissue reaction around the shunt catheter, thus eventually masking the malfunction of the CSF shunt device for a variable period of time.

The disconnection of the various components of the CSF shunt assembly may be due to technical errors during implantation, as well as to the poor quality of the material or its improper management, e.g. continuous and excessive manoeuvres of pumping on the flushing device (Haase 1976). In very active young children, the traction forces exerted during physical activity at the weak points of the CSF shunt assembly (ligatures of the different plastic components which may favour tearing of the catheters, interfaces between the silicone and metallic components of the apparatus) may result in the disruption of the CSF shunt device, generally revealed by signs of increased ICP or local swelling of the tissue overlying the shunt tube, because of the subcutaneous accumulation of fluid. Though there is no evidence of any harm related to the presence of a detached catheter remaining in place within the ventricular or the peritoneal cavity (with the exception of infected tubes), the detachment of the distal component of the venous shunt may be the cause of very serious complications. This explains the increasing adoption of one-piece CSF shunts, which has considerably reduced the incidence of disconnection in the last years (Raimondi *et al.* 1977).

Overdrainage of CSF, either acute or chronic, is one of the most serious complications of the surgical treatment of hydrocephalus. In its acute form, overdrainage is revealed by dramatic clinical symptoms such as deterioration in the level of consciousness, respiratory and cardiac arrest, and tachycardia. The symptoms are regarded as being due to brainstem and hypothalamic involvement, when these structures are shifted or distorted because of the rapid decompression of the lateral cerebral ventricles (ventriculo-atrial or ventriculo-peritoneal CSF shunts) or the abrupt decrease in pressure in the spinal compartment (lumbo-peritoneal CSF shunt). The reversibility of the clinical manifestations with manoeuvres which counteract CSF hypotension, such as the injection of saline solution, the closure of the drainage, and putting the patient's head down, clearly indicates the excessively rapid removal of relatively large amounts of CSF as the pathogenic mechanism accounting for this type of complication. Also related to an excessive and rapid subtraction of CSF is the formation of epidural or subdural haematomas. The former, which are particularly life-threatening, characteristically occur in the first few hours after the operation and prefer the fronto-parietal location, probably because of a peculiar loose adherence of the dura to the internal table of the calvarium in these regions. The latter are commonly recorded after decompression of large cerebral ventricles under tension, when the centripetal movement of the cerebral hemispheres causes the stretching and tearing of the bridging veins in the subdural space. The clinical manifestations are generally less dramatic and the lapse of time from the insertion of the shunt is usually greater than in cases of an epidural haematoma.

The commonest prophylactic measures are the careful evacuation of the dilated ventricles, refilling them with saline solution, and the use (when possible) of high-pressure opening valve systems. Therapeutic measures consist of removing the clot, temporarily closing the drainage and eventually inserting a subdural shunting device.

The chronic form of CSF overdrainage has different types of complications. Low ICP is usually a transient phenomenon, with repeated episodes of headache, nausea and vomiting, eventually induced by the patient changing from lying to standing. These episodes are experienced by some children after the shunting operation. The clinical manifestations, which usually fade away progressively, are thought to express a relatively slow adaptation to the new levels of ICP determined by the presence of the CSF shunt system.

The low-pressure syndrome in infants may be associated with an obvious reduction in skull size, with sunken fontanelles and the overriding of cranial bones. With persistently low ICP values, the condition may evolve towards a true microcrania. In older children, however, excessive reduction in the size of the skull, with its eventual disproportion to the contained structures, may result from a remodelling of the calvarium through reabsorption by osteoclasts and new bone formation osteoblasts. Besides the obvious reduction of the neurocranium, radiologically this complication is revealed by the apposition of laminated layers of new bone along the inner table of the skull. Additional findings are the appearance of dense parasutural bone, the reduction of convolutional and endocranial vascular landmarks, and a widening of the diploic space. A particular type of microcrania, limited to the posterior fossa, has also been described in children with valveless lumbo-peritoneal shunts (Hoffman and Tucker 1976).

The therapy for craniosynostosis secondary to excessive CSF drainage may require the craniectomy of the sutural lines or more complex procedures of cranioplasty, apt to increase the volume of the skull.

A particular clinical syndrome referred to as chronic CSF hyperdrainage is the *slit-ventricle syndrome*, defined as the intermittent appearance of headache, vomiting and lethargy in shunted hydrocephalic subjects. The symptomatology is associated with the CT scan evidence of barely recognisable lateral cerebral ventricles, which may also be found in a large proportion of shunted asymptomatic patients. The marked reduction in volume of the cerebral ventricles, brought about by the insertion of the CSF shunt device, may represent the first pathogenic event, leading to the transient obstruction of the indwelling ventricular catheter by the ventricular wall. This would occur especially when the cerebral parenchyma becomes enlarged because of a transitory increase in CBF or during phases of cerebral oedema, like those which take place in pseudotumor cerebri. Alternative hypotheses point to the reduction of the area of the ventricular walls following the shunt insertion, which would cut off the compensatory mechanism for CSF absorption related to the transependymal transfer of CSF from the ventricular system, as well as to changes in the elasticity of the ventricular walls (decreased ventricular compliance), resulting in their abnormal rigidity and exposing the patient to sudden increases in intraventricular pressure.

The two main therapeutic approaches are to try to increase the brain compliance and the ventricular volume by means of a subtemporal decompressive craniectomy (Epstein *et al.* 1974*a*), or to decrease the CSF drainage by using a higher-pressure valve (Salmon 1978) or by adding an antisiphon device to the shunt system (Gruber *et al.* 1984).

Chronic subdural hygromas and haematomas are often found in asymptomatic shunted hydrocephalic subjects, especially in cases where the ventricular dilatation has persisted for a long time prior to surgery, and when the operation has been performed after the fusion of the cranial sutures. The asymptomatic subdural fluid collections are commonly extended over two cerebral hemispheres; they are regarded as being an expression of a limited re-expansion of the cerebral hemispheres. Their treatment is controversial, except when they are associated with signs of increased ICP or epileptic seizures; in these cases, the simple drainage from the subdural space, either with an external (temporary) or internal (permanent) shunt, may suffice to determine the disappearance of the lesion. It is seldom necessary to close the ventricular CSF shunt device temporarily, or to substitute it with another one provided with a higher-pressure opening valve system. Chronic subdural haematomas in children are often more symptomatic than the subdural hygromas, and are revealed by the appearance of epileptic seizures, psychomotor deterioration and signs of intracranial hypertension. The surgical treatment consists of evacuating the blood collection through burr holes or, more frequently, through a craniotomy with removal of the fibrous membranes which surround the haematoma. The persistence of these membranes may cause the recurrence of the lesions impeding the normal development of the brain, and in some cases even favour the deposition of calcium, thus inducing a 'shell' formation encasing the underlying cerebral hemisphere.

Infection is the second most frequent complication of CSF shunts but probably the most important as far as survival and neurological outcomes are concerned. Though recent years have seen a decrease in its incidence, this type of complication still affects as many as 10 to 20 per cent of the cases (see Chapter 12).

Isolated ventricles, i.e. the exclusion of some portions of the ventricular system, can be seen on CT scan MR examinations. This complication results from the development of post-inflammatory membranes and/or from the distortion of cerebral structures, which create a block in CSF circulation, preventing CSF from reaching the chamber where the ventricular catheter is located. The clinical manifestations include signs of increased intracranial pressure and/or focal neurological deficits, related to the local mass effect of the 'cyst'.

Septations of the lateral ventricle often determine a block within the ventricular body, just posterior to the foramen of Monro, thus separating the frontal horn from a blind posterior compartment. More frequently, however, the ventricular system appears multiloculated, making effective drainage of all cavities very difficult.

The isolation of the entire lateral cerebral ventricle may depend on the inflammatory occlusion of one foramen of Monro, but more often it results from a functional block of the interventricular communication due to an excessive coarctation of the shunted contralateral ventricle, with a distortion of the midline structures.

The *entrapment of the fourth ventricle* may be caused by a functional obstruction of the aqueduct, due to kinking of the mesencephalon caused by an excessive drainage of the lateral cerebral ventricles, in association with a congenital or inflammatory obstruction of the foramina of Magendie and Luschka (Oi *et al.* 1986). Such entrapment and cystic dilatation, however, has more frequently been described under several denominations (double compartment hydrocephalus, isolated fourth ventricle, cystic fourth ventricle, trapped fourth ventricle) in a series of conditions apt to determine the inflammatory obstruction of the aqueduct.

The clinical manifestations may be subtle, but can abruptly worsen into life-threatening conditions because of the compression exerted on the brainstem structures. The treatment consists of canalising the aqueduct, shunting the fourth ventricle or correcting the overdrainage of the lateral cerebral ventricles.

Complications unique to vascular shunts
Shunt nephritis, pulmonary thrombo-embolism, thrombosis, and cardiac tamponade are the main complications characteristic of vascular shunts. Two further complications—septicaemia and the misplacement of the distal end of the shunt secondary to the physiological growth of the child—assume a particular importance with this type of shunt: the former because it represents the most frequent cause of death, and the latter because of its inevitability.

Shunt nephritis was first identified by Black *et al.* (1965), who pointed out the relationship between nephritis and the colonisation of the shunt by *Staphylococcus albus* in two patients with ventriculo-atrial shunts. The clinical manifestations, which may occur days or years after the operation, include signs of septicaemia, spiking fever, anaemia, hepato-splenomegaly, and in some cases oedema due to the nephrotic syndrome. Proteinuria, systemic hypertension and azotaemia are the characteristic laboratory findings when the syndrome is fully established. Blood cultures are usually positive for coagulase-negative staphylococci, but are more rarely so for other bacteria such as *Staphylococcus aureus, Pseudomonas aeruginosa, Propionibacterium acnes*, and others. Infants and children are more frequently affected, though the syndrome has been reported even in adolescents and adults. The pathogenesis of this complication has been identified as an immunological process, depending on the formation of antigen antibody complexes (from bacteria of low virulence) in antibody excess, and resulting in the secondary activation of the complement system and deposits in the glomerular capillary wall. The microscopic examination of the kidney demonstrates mesangial cell proliferation, a widening of the mesangial matrix and a thickening of the glomerular basement membrane. Removal of the shunt, together with an appropriate antibiotic treatment, are the principal therapies to adopt, with the eventual association of immunosuppressive drugs and steroids. In a few patients, however, impairment of renal function at the time of the diagnosis may be so critical that even shunt removal may not prevent death. In other patients, conversion of the ventriculo-atrial shunt to a ventriculo-peritoneal shunt may not be sufficient to stop complement activation.

Pulmonary thrombo-embolism with possible heart failure was first described by Anderson (1959). Though pulmonary embolisation is found in more than half the shunted patients, few exhibit complications and even fewer develop an obvious pulmonary hypertension. Pulmonary hypertension is clinically revealed by an accentuated second heart sound, with the disappearance of the normal splitting; murmurs and insufficiency of the pulmonary or tricuspid valve characterise the most severe cases. Periodic chest x-rays and electrocardiograms may help the early identification of the condition. Infection, together with the mechanical effect of the indwelling shunt, are major causes of ulceration of the atrial wall, in turn responsible for thrombus formation within the cardiac atrium.

The progressive pulmonary-vascular occlusive disease due to embolisation, originating in the right atrium in patients with ventriculo-atrial shunt, may be arrested only by the immediate removal of the shunt.

Prophylactic measures include the avoidance of risk factors (history of bacterial endocarditis, cardiac-valvular anomalies, cyanotic heart disease) and the administration of salicylates to reduce platelet aggregation and adhesion.

Thrombosis is a very frequent complication of ventriculo-atrial shunts; autopsy observations have demonstrated the presence of fibrinous material and clots surrounding the tip of the catheter within the heart, sometimes extending into the auricle, in 60 to 100 per cent of subjects. The main risk of this complication, besides the possible obstruction of the catheter, is the formation of emboli, aggravated by the movement of the tip of the atrial shunt.

Cardiac tamponade, secondary to the perforation of the atrial wall, was first reported by Anderson (1959). The pathogenetic mechanism has been established in a gradual erosion of the cardiac wall, when the shunt tip is located in a position which reduces its movement or when a clot inside it results in major stiffness. Only rarely does the complication immediately follow the operation—perhaps because of forceful introduction of the catheter with stylet. The condition may be treated successfully by pericardial aspiration, after an early radiological demonstration of an enlarged heart shadow (Tsingoglou and Eckstein 1971).

The *misplacement* of the cardiac tube, when its tip migrates from the atrium into the superior vena cava because of the growth of the child, is the principal cause of failure of the vascular shunts. As the complication has to be regarded as a 'physiological' event, the elective lengthening of the shunt has been proposed as a routine policy. But misplacement may also result from a technical error during surgery, if the catheter progresses into the subclavian vein rather than into the cardiac atrium after its insertion into the jugular vein, or if it is placed within the cardiac ventricle, a condition which may lead to permanent cardiac arrhythmia and pulmonary valve infection. Misplacement may be caused by the detachment of the distal catheter; the detached segment of the shunt assembly may remain within the right chambers of the heart (and eventually be removed by thoracotomy or percutaneously) or migrate into the pulmonary artery, thus becoming a life-threatening complication.

Septicaemia from valve colonisation occurs in about a sixth of patients operated on through a ventriculo-atrial CSF shunt (Luthardt 1970). Two main clinical courses, acute and chronic, have been described in relation to the causative organism, the extent of the anatomical structures involved and the inflammatory response of the subject. In general, septicaemia due to *Staphylococcus epidermidis*, the bacterium most frequently involved in shunt colonisation, is chronic and indolent, and often clinically manifested only by fever, while that due to *Staphylococcus aureus* is usually acute or fulminating. Bacteraemia is a frequent finding, in contrast to colonised ventriculo-peritoneal shunts. The treatment of acute septicaemia requires the immediate removal of the CSF shunt valve system, while in cases of chronic septicaemia different modalities of treatment have been suggested, either with removal of the shunt (shunt removal with immediate or delayed replacement in the same or different site plus antibiotic therapy) or without (systemic antibiotic therapy plus eventual intrathecal or intra-shunt antibiotic therapy).

Complications unique to peritoneal shunts
Obstruction of the peritoneal catheter is by far the most frequent complication of ventriculo-peritoneal shunts. Sometimes the complication arises when the tip of the shunt is displaced from the peritoneal cavity into the tissues of the abdominal wall because of the physiological growth of the child; but more often, obstruction depends on the presence of foreign material in the lumen of the catheter, from fibrous encapsulation or kinking, due to incorrect surgical placement. A variety of substances may be found embedded in the yellowish-white material obstructing the peritoneal catheter at the level of the set valve; *e.g.* hair (from the patient or operating-room personnel), cotton fibres (from cottonoids and sponges), talc granules (from surgical gloves), and mesothelial cells (from the peritoneal cavity).

Visceral perforation was first described by Wilson and Bertan (1966) in two children whose peritoneal catheters had extruded through the anus. The gastrointestinal tract, the vagina and the bladder (especially in children with myelomeningocele) may be involved either during the shunt insertion (direct perforation of the viscus) or at different times after the operation (decubitus ulceration).

Clinical manifestations vary from signs of chronic shunt malfunction to the evidence of superimposed infective complications, such as leptomeningitis or peritonitis: though in most cases of bowel perforation peritonitis is absent, in

369

contrast with its frequent occurrence in cases of perforation of the bladder. Indeed, in most cases of bowel perforation, the perforating catheter is encased within an inflammatory reaction which is thought to act as an anatomical defence preventing material from the visceral lumen from penetrating into the peritoneal cavity. The complication may be aggravated by adhesion of the catheter to the viscus wall, especially when due to local inflammatory processes.

In most patients, removal of the perforating catheter associated with antibiotic administration is a simple and quite effective treatment; however a significant mortality has been recorded with more difficult procedures, such as the removal of the catheter through a laparotomy.

Inguinal hernia and/or hydrocele, which occur in about 1.2 per cent of the normal paediatric population, are recorded in 4 to 17 per cent of children operated on for a CSF ventriculo-peritoneal shunt (Di Rocco *et al.* 1982). The complication may occur on the day of the operation or several months after the shunt insertion, with a mean of three months (Di Rocco *et al.* 1982). Infants and young children are more frequently affected, because of the high incidence of a patent processus vaginalis in this age-group. It may also be caused by insufficient CSF absorption within the peritoneal cavity. Surgical repair of the hernia with bilateral exploration is the treatment of choice.

Pseudocyst formation, *i.e.* the formation of encapsulated CSF containing intra-abdominal lesions, occurs in about 1 per cent of patients with peritoneal shunts. It is clinically revealed by the failure of the shunt, by signs of intestinal obstruction, or by dysfunction of other intra-abdominal organs, as well as by inspection or palpable evidence of an intra-abdominal mass. The laboratory diagnosis is based on non-invasive methods such as cyst aspiration under echographic control, which allows the culture and cyto-chemical examination of the contained fluid.

A history of previous shunt infection is frequently found; in its absence, pseudocysts are thought to originate from inflammatory reactions to the shunt catheter or to some component of the CSF, especially proteins. Various therapeutic measures have been adopted: direct excision of the cyst wall through laparotomy with displacement and reposition of the shunt into a different site of the peritoneal cavity (or its conversion to another type of shunt), the aspiration of the cyst through the shunt catheter itself, and the puncture and evacuation of the cyst through a needle.

Ascites is a rare complication, often associated with an increased protein content in the abdominal fluid, especially in cases of hydrocephalus due to CSF neoplasms and infections. However, in less than a quarter of cases, ascites occurs in subjects with normal or even low ascitic-fluid protein content. The best method of treatment is to convert the ventriculo-peritoneal to a ventriculo-atrial CSF shunt, a manoeuvre which results in the spontaneous resolution of the ascites in practically all subjects.

Conclusion
In the past the main difficulty for the neurosurgeon faced with hydrocephalus was to achieve a correct diagnosis. Thus most of the therapeutic modalities adopted

were directed towards treating hydrocephalus as a single disorder rather than as different specific entities, each with a different pathogenesis.

The development of concepts such as the 'communicating' or 'obstructive' nature of hydrocephalus, which led to greater understanding of the CSF's physiology, was paralleled by the discovery of more adequate ways of treatment. The introduction of modern diagnostic tools for neuro-imaging has led to improved diagnosis of hydrocephalus, and to more appropriate modalities of controlling the results of medical and surgical treatment.

Medical treatment has practically been abandoned, due to inconsistent results and the adverse effects of pharmacological and physical agents. Drugs to reduce CSF secretion are used only temporarily, to control the progression of the ventricular dilatation when CSF alterations (infection, presence of blood, high protein content) or poor general condition do not allow a surgical procedure to be performed.

Surgical treatment of hydrocephalus has become very reliable and safe, with the introduction of new materials well tolerated by the organism, together with the availability of more competent valve systems. In the majority of hydrocephalic children it is currently possible to obtain the reduction of macrocrania, with a concomitant decrease in volume of the cerebral ventricles and the re-expansion of the cerebral parenchyma, accompanied by a satisfactory psychomotor development. Numerous minor and major complications may necessitate several operative procedures in the same subject: however, some of these complications may be minimised by careful and appropriate surgery, the correct choice of CSF shunt system, and attentive postoperative surveillance.

REFERENCES

Akerman, M., de Tovar, G., Guiot, G. (1972) 'Radio-isotope cisternography and ventriculography in non communicating hydrocephalus.' *In* Harbert, J. C. *Cisternography and Hydrocephalus: A Symposium.* Springfield, Ill: C. Thomas. p. 483.

Allonen, H., Andersson, K. E., Iisalo, E., Kanto, J., Strömblad, L. G., Wettrell, G. (1977) 'Passage of digoxin into cerebrospinal fluid in man.' *Acta Pharmacologica et Toxicologica*, **41**, 193–202.

Amacher, A. L., Wellington, J. (1984) 'Infantile hydrocephalus: long-term results of surgical therapy.' *Child's Brain*, **11**, 217–229.

Amador, L. V., Jara, O., Porras, C. L. (1969) 'Valvulography: a test for patency of Holter valve shunts.' *American Journal of Diseases of Children*, **117**, 190–193.

Ames, R. H. (1967) 'Ventriculo-peritoneal shunts in the management of hydrocephalus.' *Journal of Neurosurgery*, **27**, 525–529.

Anderson, F. M. (1959) 'Ventriculo-auriculostomy in treatment of hydrocephalus.' *Journal of Neurosurgery*, **16**, 551–557.

Ashker, K., Fox, J. L. (1981) 'Percutaneous technique for insertion of an atrial catheter for CSF shunting: technical note.' *Journal of Neurosurgery*, **55**, 488–490.

Avman, N., Kanpolat, Y. (1979) 'Third ventriculostomy by microtechnique.' *Acta Neurochirurgica*, Suppl. 28, 588–595.

Backlund, F. O., Grepe, A., Lunsford, D. (1981) 'Stereotaxic reconstruction of the aqueduct of Sylvius.' *Journal of Neurosurgery*, **55**, 800–810.

Barnard, J. F. (1838) 'Strapping the head in chronic hydrocephalus.' *Lancet*, **2**, 685.

Bass, N. H., Fällström, S. P., Lundborg, P. (1979) 'Digoxin-induced arrest of cerebrospinal fluid circulation in the infant rat: implications for medical treatment of hydrocephalus during early postnatal life.' *Pediatric Research*, **13**, 26–30.

Becker, D. P., Nulsen, F. E. (1968) 'Control of hydrocephalus by valve-regulated venous shunt:

avoidance of complications in prolonged shunt maintenance.' *Journal of Neurosurgery*, **28**, 215–226.

Birzis, L., Carter, C. H., Maren, T. H. (1958) 'Effect of acetazolamide on CSF pressure and electrolytes in hydrocephalus.' *Neurology*, **8**, 522–528.

Black, J. A., Challacombe, D. N., Ockenden, B. G. (1965) 'Nephrotic syndrome associated with bacteremia after shunt operation for hydrocephalus.' *Lancet*, **2**, 921–924.

Boltshauser, E., Cavanagh, N. (1976) 'Hydrocephalus treated by compressive head wrapping.' *Archives of Disease in Childhood*, **51**, 399.

Borja, A. R., Hinshaw, J. R. (1970) 'A safe way to perform infraclavicular subclavian vein catheterization.' *Surgery, Gynecology and Obstetrics*, **130**, 673–673.

Bret, J. (1981) 'Recanalization of the Sylvian aqueduct.' *European Journal of Radiology*, **1**, 67–70.

Caldarelli, M., Di Rocco, C., Rossi, G. F. (1979a) 'Lumbar subarachnoid infusion test in pediatric neurosurgery.' *Developmental Medicine and Child Neurology*, **21**, 71–82.

—— —— Iannelli, A., Velardi, F. (1979b) 'Follow-up comparison of ventriculo-atrial and ventriculo-peritoneal shunts in the treatment of hydrocephalus in children.' *Acta Medica Roma*, **17**, 42.

—— —— Cellini, N., De Santis, M. (1981) 'A technique for evaluation of CSF shunt patency using telethermography.' *Neuropediatrics*, **12**, 303–307.

Crosby, R. M. N., Henderson, C. M., Paul, R. L. (1973) 'Catheterization of the cerebral aqueduct for obstructive hydrocephalus in infants.' *Journal of Neurosurgery*, **38**, 596–601.

Cuatico, W., Richardson, N. K. (1979) 'Transcutaneous therapeutic canalization of aqueductal stenosis in a hydrocephalic: case report and technical note.' *Acta Neurochirurgica*, **47**, 181–186.

Cushing, H. (1908) 'Surgery of the head.' *In* Keen, W. W. (Ed.) *Surgery, its Principles and Practice*. Philadelphia: W. B. Saunders. pp. 17–276.

Dandy, W. E. (1918) 'Extirpation of the choroid plexus of the lateral ventricles in communicating hydrocephalus.' *Annals of Surgery*, **68**, 569–579.

—— (1920) 'The diagnosis and treatment of hydrocephalus resulting from strictures of the aqueduct of Sylvius.' *Surgery, Gynecology and Obstetrics*, **31**, 340–358.

—— (1922) 'An operative procedure for hydrocephalus.' *Johns Hopkins Hospital Bulletin*, **33**, 189.

—— Blackfan, K. D. (1914) 'Internal hydrocephalus: an experimental, clinical and pathological study.' *American Journal of Diseases of Children*, **8**, 406–482.

—— (1932) 'The brain.' *In* Lewis, D. (Ed.) *Practice of Surgery*. Hagerstown: W. F. Prior. p. 247.

Daniels, H. V., Pothmann, R., Kauther, K., Lim, D. P. (1981) 'The applanation tonometry of the fontanelle: a new non-invasive instrument for the management of hydrocephalus in infancy. *Zeitschrift für Kinderchirurgle*, **34**, 144–146.

Davidoff, L. M. (1948) 'Hydrocephalus and hydrocephalus with meningocele: their treatment by choroid plexectomy.' *Surgical Clinics of North America*, **28**, 416–431.

Des Plantes, B. G. Z., Crezee, P. (1978) 'Transfrontal perforation of the lamina terminalis.' *Neuroradiology*, **16**, 51–53.

Di Rocco, C. (1987) *The Treatment of Infantile Hydrocephalus*. Boca Raton, Florida: CRC Press. pp. 1–16.

—— Iannelli, A., Puca, A., Calisti, A. (1982) 'Idrocele ed ernia inguinale dopo derivazione ventricolo peritoneale in età pediatrica.' *Pediatria del Medico Chirurgica*, **4**, 661.

Donat, J. F. (1980) 'Acetazolamide-induced improvement in hydrocephalus.' *Archives of Neurology*, **37**, 376.

Ehrle, A., Sklar, F. (1979) 'Visual evoked potentials in infants with hydrocephalus.' *Neurology*, **29**, 1541–1543.

Eisenberg, H. M., Davidson, R. I., Shillito, J. R. (1971) 'Lumboperitoneal shunts. Review of 34 cases.' *Journal of Neurosurgery*, **35**, 427–431.

Elvidge, A. R. (1966) 'Treatment of obstructive lesions of the aqueduct of Sylvius and the fourth ventricle by interventriculostomy.' *Journal of Neurosurgery*, **24**, 11–23.

Epstein, F., Hochwald, G. M., Ransohoff, J. (1973) 'Neonatal hydrocephalus treated by compressive head wrapping.' *Lancet*, **1**, 634–636.

—— Fleischer, A. S., Hochwald, G. M., Ransohoff, J. (1974a) 'Subtemporal craniectomy for recurrent shunt obstruction secondary to small ventricles.' *Journal of Neurosurgery*, **41**, 29–31.

—— Wald, A., Hochwald, G. (1974b) 'Intracranial pressure during compressive head wrapping in treatment of neonatal hydrocephalus.' *Pediatrics*, **54**, 786–790.

Epstein, N., Epstein, F., Trehan, N. (1981) 'Percutaneous placement of the atrial end of a vascular shunt utilising the Swan-Ganz introduzer.' *Neurosurgery*, **9**, 564–565.

Feld, M. (1957) 'La coagulation des plexus choroïdes par ventriculoscopie directe dans l'hydrocéphalie nonobstructive du nourisson.' *Neurochirurgie*, **3**, 70–79.

372

Ferguson, A. H. (1898) 'Intraperitoneal diversion of the cerebrospinal fluid in cases of hydrocephalus (review).' *New York Medical Journal*, **67**, 902.

Flitter, M. A., Buchheit, W. A., Murtagh, F., Lapayowker, M. S. (1975) 'Ultrasound determination of cerebrospinal fluid shunt patency. Technical note.' *Journal of Neurosurgery*, **42**, 728–730.

Fodstad, H., Liliequist, B., Schannong, M., Thulin, C. A. (1978) 'Tranexamic acid in the preoperative management of ruptured intracranial aneurysm.' *Surgical Neurology*, **10**, 9–15.

Frerebeau, Ph., Guillen, M., Privat, J. M., Benezech, J. (1982) 'Ventriculostomie percutanée non stéréotaxique par sonde à ballonet gonflable.' *Neurochirurgie*, **28**, 331–334.

Frick, M., Rösler, H., Kinser, J. (1974) 'Functional evaluation of ventriculo-atrial and ventriculo-peritoneal shunts with ^{99m}Tc-pertechnetate.' *Neuroradiology*, **7**, 145–152.

Furukawa, N. (1968) 'Experience with intrathecal administration of urokinase.' *Medical Postgraduates (Osaka)* **6**, 204.

Go, K. G., Lakke, J. P. W., Beks, J. W. F. (1968) 'A harmless method for the assessment of the patency of ventriculo-atrial shunt in hydrocephalus.' *Developmental Medicine and Child Neurology*, Suppl. 16, 100–106.

Gourie-Dev, M., Satish, P. (1980) 'Hyaluronidase as an adjuvant in the treatment of cranial arachnoiditis (hydrocephalus and optochiasmatic arachnoiditis) complicating tuberculous meningitis.' *Acta Neurologica Scandinavica*, **62**, 368–381.

Griffith, H. B. (1975) 'Technique of fontanelle and persutural ventriculoscopy and endoscopic ventricular surgery in infants.' *Child's Brain*, **1**, 359–363.

Gruber, R., Jenny, P., Herzog, B. (1984) 'Experiences with the antisiphon device (ASD) in shunt therapy of pediatric hydrocephalus.' *Journal of Neurosurgery*, **61**, 156–162.

Guiot, G. (1968) 'Techinique simplifiée de ventriculo-cisternostomie pour hydrocéphalie obstructive.' *Revue Neurologique*, **118**, 391–392.

—— Derome, P., Hertzog, E., Bambberg, C., Akerman, M. (1968) 'Ventriculo-cisternostomie sous contrôle radioscopique pour hydrocéphalie obstructive.' *Presse Médicale*, **76**, 1923–1926.

Haase, J. (1976) 'Damage to a Hakim valve. Case report.' *Journal of Neurosurgery*, **44**, 522.

Harbert, J. C., McCullough, D. C. (1984) 'Radionuclide tests of cerebral fluid shunt patency.' *Journal of Nuclear Medicine*, **25**, 112–114.

Harsch, G. R. III (1954) 'Peritoneal shunt for hydrocephalus utilizing the fimbria of the fallopian tube for entrance to the peritoneal cavity.' *Journal of Neurosurgery*, **11**, 284–294.

Hassin, G. B., Oldberg, E., Tinsley, M. (1937) 'Changes in the brain in plexectomized dogs with comments on the cerebrospinal fluid.' *Archives of Neurology and Psychiatry*, **38**, 1224–1239.

Heile, B. (1925) 'Über neue operative Wege zur Druckenblasting bei angeborenem Hydrocephalus (Ureter–Duraanastomose).' *Zentralblatt für Chirurgie*, **52**, 2229.

Hemmer, R. (1970) 'Postoperative causes of death in hydrocephalic children. Analysis and conclusions about therapy.' *In* Richman, P. P., Hecker, W. C., Prévot, J. (Eds.) *Causes of Postoperative Death in Children*. Baltimore: Urban & Schwarzenberg. p. 95.

Hochwald, G. M., Epstein, F., Malhan, C., Ransohoff, J. (1972) 'The role of the skull and dura in experimental feline hydrocephalus.' *Developmental Medicine and Child Neurology*, **14**, Suppl. 27, 65–69.

Hoffman, H. J., Tucker, W. J. (1976) 'Cephalocranial disproportion.' *Child's Brain*, **2**, 167–176.

—— Harwood-Nash, D., Gilday, D. L. (1980) 'Percutaneous third ventriculostomy in the management of non communicating hydrocephalus.' *Neurosurgery*, **7**, 313–321.

Hooper, R. (1969) 'A lengthening procedure for ventriculo-atrial shunts. Technical note.' *Journal of Neurosurgery*, **30**, 93–95

Huttenlocher, P. R. (1965) 'Treatment of hydrocephalus with acetazolamide.' *Journal of Pediatrics*, **66**, 1023–1030.

Hyndman, O. R. (1946) 'Hydrocephalus: a contribution related to treatment.' *Journal of Neurosurgery*, **4**, 426–443.

Ignelzi, R. J., Kirsch, W. M. (1975) 'Follow-up analysis of ventriculoperitoneal and ventriculoatrial shunts for hydrocephalus.' *Journal of Neurosurgery*, **42**, 679–682.

Jackson, I. J., Snodgrass, S. R. (1955) 'Peritoneal shunts in the treatment of hydrocephalus and increased intracranial pressure: a 4-year survey of 62 patients.' *Journal of Neurosurgery*, **12**, 216–222.

Julow, J. (1979a) 'The influence of dexamethasone on subarachnoid fibrosis after subarachnoid hemorrhage.' *Acta Neurochirurgica*, **51**, 43–52.

—— (1979b) 'Prevention of subarachnoid fibrosis after subarachnoid haemorrhage with urokinase. Scanning electron microscopic study in the dog.' *Acta Neurochirurgica*, **51**, 51–63.

Kaufman, H. H., Carmel, P. W. (1978) 'Aseptic meningitis and hydrocephalus after posterior fossa surgery.' *Acta Neurochirurgica*, **44**, 179–196.

Kausch, W. (1908) 'Die Behandlung des Hydrocephalus der kleinen Kinder.' *Archiv für Klinische Chirurgie*, **87**, 709–796.

Keucher, T. R., Mealey, J. (1979) 'Long-term results after ventriculoatrial and ventriculoperitoneal shunting for infantile hydrocephalus.' *Journal of Neurosurgery*, **50**, 179–186.

Kister, S. J. (1956) 'Carbonic anhydrase inhibition. VI: The effect of acetazolamide on cerebrospinal fluid flow.' *Journal of Pharmacology and Experimental Therapeutics*, **117**, 402–405.

Kulick, S. A. (1965) 'The clinical use of intrathecal methylprednisolone-acetate following lumbar puncture.' *Journal of the Mount Sinai Hospital*, **32**, 75–78.

Kuwabara, T., Fujitsu, K., Pak, S., Masuda, H., Kuwana, N. (1982) 'Microsurgical third ventriculostomy in the treatment of obstructive hydrocephalus.' *Shoni Suitosho no Byotai Oyobi Chiryo*, **77**.

Lapin, J. H. (1950) 'Successful medical treatment of obstructive hydrocephalus in tuberculous meningitis.' *New York State Journal of Medicine*, **50**, 1615–1616.

Lapras, C., Poirier, N., Deruty, R., Bret, P., Joyeux, O. (1975) 'Le cathétérisme de l'aqueduc de Sylvius. Sa place actuelle dans le traitement chirurgical des sténoses de l'aqueduc de Sylvius, des tumeurs de la F.C.P. et de la syringomyélie.' *Neurochirurgie*, **21**, 101–109.

Lecksell, L. (1949) 'A surgical procedure for atresia of the aqueduct of Sylvius.' *Acta Psychiatrica et Neurologica Scandinavica*, **24**, 559–568.

Longatti, P. L., Scanarini, M., Gerosa, M., Ori, C., Carteri, A. (1982) 'ICP monitoring and function of CSF shunts.' *In* Paraicz, E. (Ed.) *Intracranial Pressure in Infancy and Childhood. Monographs in Pediatrics, vol. 15.* Basel: Karger. p. 144.

Lorber, J. (1968) 'The results of early treatment of extreme hydrocephalus.' *Developmental Medicine and Child Neurology*, Suppl. 16, 21–29.

—— Salfield, S., Lonton, T. (1983) 'Isosorbide in the management of infantile hydrocephalus.' *Developmental Medicine and Child Neurology*, **25**, 502–511.

Luthardt, T. (1970) 'Bacterial infections in ventriculo-atrial shunt systems.' *Developmental Medicine and Child Neurology*, Suppl. 22, 105–109.

Macri, F. J., Politoff, A., Rubin, R. C. (1966) 'Preferential vasoconstrictor properties of acetazolamide on the arteries of the choroid plexus.' *International Journal of Neuropharmacology*, **5**, 109–115.

Matson, D. D. (1951) 'Ventriculo-ureterostomy.' *Journal of Neurosurgery*, **8**, 398–404.

—— (1953) 'Hydrocephalus treated by arachnoid-ureterostomy: report of fifty cases.' *Pediatrics*, **12**, 326–334.

—— (1969) *Neurosurgery of Infancy and Childhood, 2nd edn.* Springfield, Ill: C. Thomas. p. 233.

Mazza, C., Pasqualin, A., Da Pian, R. (1980) 'Results of treatment with ventriculo-peritoneal shunt in infantile non-tumor hydrocephalus.' *Child's Brain*, **7**, 1–14.

McClure, C. C. Jr., Carothers, E. C., Hahn, P. F. (1955) 'Distribution and pathology resulting from the intracerebral and intraventricular injection of radioactive gold and silver coated radiogold colloids.' *American Journal of Roentgenology*, **73**, 81–87.

McLone, D. G., Raimondi, A. J. (1983) 'Infezioni del Sistema Nervoso Centrale e loro ruolo come fattore limitante lo sviluppo intellettivo nel bambino con mielomeningocele.' *In* Di Rocco, C., Caldarelli, M. (Eds.) *Mielomeningocele.* Rome: Casa del Libro. p. 245.

McNickle, H. F. (1947) 'The surgical treatment of hydrocephalus: a simple method of performing third ventriculostomy.' *British Journal of Surgery*, **34**, 302–307.

Mealy, J., Barker, D. T. (1968) 'Failure of oral acetazolamide to avert hydrocephalus in infants with myelomeningocele.' *Journal of Pediatrics*, **72**, 257–259.

Meyer, H., Price, B. E., Reubel, C. D. (1973) 'Complications arising from head wrapping for the treatment of hydrocephalus.' *Pediatrics*, **52**, 867–868.

Migliore, A., Paoletti, P., Villani, R. (1962) 'Radioisotopic method for evaluating the patency of the Spitz-Holter valve.' *Journal of Neurosurgery*, **19**, 605.

Milhorat, T. H. (1969) 'The choroid plexus and cerebrospinal fluid production.' *Science*, **166**, 1514–1516.

—— (1974) 'Failure of choroid plexectomy as treatment for hydrocephalus.' *Surgery, Gynecology and Obstetrics*, **139**, 505–508.

Mixter, W. J. (1923) 'Ventriculoscopy and puncture of the floor of the third ventricle. Preliminary report of a case.' *Boston Medical and Surgical Journal*, **188**, 277–278.

Murtagh, F., Lechman, R. (1967) 'Peritoneal shunts in the management of hydrocephalus.' *Journal of the American Medical Association*, **202**, 1010–1014.

Naidich, T. P., Schott, L. H., Baron, R. L. (1982) 'Computed tomography in evaluation of hydrocephalus.' *Radiologic Clinics of North America*, **20**, 143–167.

Nalin, A., Gatti, G. (1977) 'Effects of treatment with acetazolamide (Diamox) in cases of non tumorous hydrocephalus early diagnosed and controlled by encephalography.' *Acta Universitae Carolinae Medica*, **75**, 170.

Neblett, C. R., McNeel, D. P., Waltz, T. A. Jr., Harrison, G. M. (1972) 'Effect of cardiac glycosides on human cerebrospinal fluid production.' *Lancet*, **2**, 1008–1009.

Nulsen, F. E., Spitz, E. B. (1952) 'Treatment of hydrocephalus by direct shunt from ventricle to jugular vein.' *Surgical Forum of the American College of Surgeons*, **2**, 399–403.

—— Rekate, H. L. (1982) 'Results of treatment for hydrocephalus as a guide to future management.' *In Pediatric Neurosurgery*. New York: Grune & Stratton. p. 229.

Occhipinti, E., Fontana, M., Riccio, A., Giuffre, R., Palam, L., Giudetti, B., Luccavelli, G., Moise, A., Migliavacca, F., Gaini, S., Tomei, G., Villani, R., Pagni, C. A., Longatti, L., Carteri, I., Licata, C., Cognoni, G., Benvenuti, L., Briani, S. (1981) 'Long-term follow-up of 108 patients operated on for infantile non tumoural hydrocephalus: a cooperative study by 6 Italian neurosurgical centres.' *Zeitschrift für Kinderchirurgie*, **34**, 104–107.

Oi, S., Matsumoto, S. (1986) 'Isolated fourth ventricle.' *Journal of Pediatric Neurosciences*, **2**, 125.

Oppelt, W. W., Palmer, R. F. (1966) 'Stimulation of cerebrospinal fluid production by low doses of intraventricular ouabain.' *Journal of Pharmacology and Experimental Therapeutics*, **154**, 581–589.

Osaka, K., Yamasaki, S., Hirayama, A., Sato, N., Ohi, Y., Matsumoto, S. (1977) 'Correlation of the response of the flushing device to compression with the clinical picture in the evaluation of the functional status of the shunting system.' *Child's Brain*, **3**, 25–30.

Park, B. E. (1979) 'Spontaneous subarachnoid hemorrhage complicated by communicating hydrocephalus: epsilon aminocaproic acid as a possible predisposing factor.' *Surgical Neurology*, **11**, 73–80.

Patterson, R. H. Jr., Bergland, R. M. (1968) 'The selection of patients for third ventriculostomy based on experience with 33 operations.' *Journal of Neurosurgery*, **29**, 252–254.

Picaza, J. A. (1956) 'The posterior-peritoneal shunt technique for the treatment of internal hydrocephalus in infants.' *Journal of Neurosurgery*, **13**, 289–293.

Pierre-Kahn, A., Renier, D., Bombois, B., Askienazy, S., Moreau, R., Hirsch, J. F. (1965) 'Place de la ventriculo-cisternostomie dans le traitement des hydrocéphalies non communicantes.' *Neurochirurgie*, **21**, 557–569.

Poblete, M., Zamboni, R. (1975) 'Stereotaxic third ventriculostomy.' *Confinia Neurologia*, **37**, 150–155.

Pollay, M., Davson, H. (1963) 'The passage of certain substances out of the cerebrospinal fluid.' *Brain*, **86**, 137–150.

—— Curl, F. (1967) 'Secretion of cerebrospinal fluid by ventricular ependyma of the rabbit.' *American Journal of Physiology*, **213**, 1031–1038.

Porter, F. N. (1975) 'Hydrocephalus treated by compressive head wrapping.' *Archives of Disease in Childhood*, **50**, 816–818.

Pudenz, R. H., Russell, F. E., Hurd, A. H., Shelden, C. H. (1957) 'Ventriculo-auriculostomy: a technique for shunting cerebrospinal fluid into the right auricle: preliminary report.' *Journal of Neurosurgery*, **14**, 171–179.

Putnam, T. J. (1934) 'Treatment of hydrocephalus by endoscopic coagulation of the choroid plexus: description of a new instrument and preliminary report of results. *New England Journal of Medicine*, **210**, 1373–1376.

Raimondi, A. J., Matsumoto, S. (1967) 'A simplified technique for performing the ventriculo-peritoneal shunt: technical note.' *Journal of Neurosurgery*, **26**, 357–360.

—— Soare, P. (1974) 'Intellectual development in shunted hydrocephalic children.' *American Journal of Diseases of Children*, **127**, 664–671.

—— Robinson, J. S., Kuwamura, K. (1977) 'Complications of ventriculo-peritoneal shunting and a critical comparison of the three-piece and one-piece systems.' *Child's Brain*, **3**, 321–342.

Rapoport, S. I. (1976) *Blood-brain Barrier in Physiology and Medicine*. New York: Raven Press. p. 316.

Rasi, F. (1971) 'Un caso di idrocefalia trattato con cortisonici.' *Minerva Pediatria*, **23**, 1367–1368.

Ringelova, J. (1976) 'Streptokinase in therapy of purulent meningitis of newborn and sucklings.' *Československá Pediatrie*, **31**, 163–166.

Rish, B. L., Meacham, W. F. (1967) 'Experimental study of intraventricular instillation of radioactive gold.' *Journal of Neurosurgery*, **27**, 15–20.

Robertson, J. T., Schick, R. W., Morgan, F., Matson, D. D. (1961) 'Accurate placement of ventriculoatrial shunt for hydrocephalus under electrocardiographic control.' *Journal of Neurosurgery*, **18**, 255–257.

Rossini, P., Gambi, D., Di Rocco, C., Sollazzo, D. (1978) 'Studio dei potenziali evocati visivi in bambini con idrocefalo.' *Rivista Neurologica*, **48**, 594–598.

Rubin, R. C., Henderson, E. S., Ommaya, A. K., Walker, M. D., Rall, D. P. (1966) 'The production of cerebrospinal fluid in man and its modification by acetazolamide.' *Journal of Neurosurgery*, **25**, 430–436.

Sachs, E. (1942) 'Hydrocephalus: an analysis of ninety-eight cases.' *Journal of the Mount Sinai Hospital*, **9**, 767–791.

Salmon, J. H. (1978) 'The collapsed ventricle: management and prevention.' *Surgical Neurology*, **9**, 349–352.

Sato, O., Bering, E. A. (1967) 'Extra-ventricular formation of cerebrospinal fluid.' *Brain and Nerve (Tokyo)*, **19**, 883–885.

Sayers, M. P., Kosnik, E. J. (1976) 'Percutaneous third ventriculostomy: experience and technique.' *Child's Brain*, **2**, 24–30.

Scarff, J. E. (1970) 'The treatment of nonobstuctive (communicating) hydrocephalus by endoscopic cauterization of the choroid plexus.' *Journal of Neurosurgery*, **33**, 1–18.

Schain, R. J. (1969) 'Carbonic anhydrase inhibitors in chronic infantile hydrocephalus.' *American Journal of Diseases of Children*, **117**, 621–625.

Schick, R. W., Matson, D. D. (1961) 'What is arrested hydrocephalus?' *Journal of Pediatrics*, **58**, 791–799.

Schwartzman, J. (1949) 'Hyaluronidase in pediatrics.' *Journal of Pediatrics*, **34**, 559–563.

Sehgal, A. D., Gardner, W. J., Dohn, D. F. (1962) 'Pantopaque arachnoiditis treatment with subarachnoid injections of corticosteroids.' *Cleveland Clinic Quarterly*, **29**, 177–188.

Selman, W. R., Spetzler, R. F., Wilson, C. B., Grollmus, J. M. (1980) 'Percutaneous lumbo-peritoneal shunt: review of 130 cases.' *Neurosurgery*, **6**, 255–257.

Shinaberger, J. H., Coburn, J. W., Clayton, L. E., Reba, R. C., Barry, K. G. (1965) 'An orally effective osmotic diuretic: effects of isosorbide on renal function in dogs.' *Clinical Research*, **13**, 314.

Shurtleff, D. B., Hayden, P. W., Weeks, R., Laurence, K. M. (1973) 'Temporary treatment of hydrocephalus and myelodysplasia with isosorbide: preliminary report.' *Journal of Pediatrics*, **83**, 651–657.

—— Kronmal, R., Foltz, E. L. (1975) 'Follow-up comparison of hydrocephalus with and without myelomeningocele.' *Journal of Neurosurgery*, **42**, 61–68.

Sonnenberg, H., Solomon, S., Frazier, D. T. (1967) 'Sodium and chloride movement into the central canal of cat spinal cord.' *Proceedings of the Society for Experimental Biology and Medicine*, **124**, 1316–1320.

Stookey, B., Scarff, J. (1936) 'Occlusion of the aqueduct of Sylvius by neoplastic and non-neoplastic processes with a rational surgical treatment for relief of the resultant obstructive hydrocephalus.' *Bulletin of the Neurological Institute, New York*, **5**, 348–377.

Swanson, H. S., Perret, G. (1950) 'Bilateral Torkildsen procedure: its application in instances of occlusion of both foramina of Monro.' *Journal of Neurosurgery*, **7**, 115–120.

Tomita, T. (1984) 'Placement of ventriculoatrial shunt using external jugular catheterization: technical note.' *Neurosurgery*, **14**, 74–75.

Torack, R. M. (1982) 'Historical aspects of normal and abnormal brain fluids. II: Hydrocephalus.' *Archives of Neurology*, **39**, 276–279.

Torkildsen, A. (1939) 'A new palliative operation in cases of inoperable occlusion of the Sylvian aqueduct.' *Acta Chirurgica Scandinavica*, **82**, 117–123.

Tromp, C. N., van den Burg, W., Jansen, A., de Vries, S. J. J. M. (1979) 'Nature and severity of hydrocephalus and its relation to later intellectual function.' *Zeitschrift für Kinderchirurgie*, **28**, 354–360.

Troncale, F. J., Shear, L., Shinaberger, J. H., Shields, C. E., Barry, K. G. (1966) 'Isosorbide: diuretic effects following oral administration to normal subjects.' *American Journal of Medical Science*, **251**, 188.

Tschirgi, R. D., Frost, R. W., Taylor, J. L. (1957) 'Inhibition of cerebrospinal fluid formation by a carbonic anhydrase inhibitor 2-acctylamino—1,2,4-thiadiazole 5-sulfonamide (Diamox).' *Proceedings of the Society for Experimental Biology and Medicine*, **87**, 373–376.

Tsingoglou, S., Forrest, D. M. (1968) 'Therapeutic and prophylactic lengthening of distal catheter of the Holter ventriculo-atrial shunt.' *Developmental Medicine and Child Neurology*, **16**, Suppl., 35–43.

—— Eckstein, H. B. (1971) 'Pericardial tamponade by Holter ventriculo-atrial shunts.' *Journal of Neurosurgery*, **35**, 695–699.

Vates, T. S. R., Bonting, S. L., Oppelt, W. W. (1964) 'Na-K. activated adenosinetriphosphatase formation of cerebrospinal fluid in the cat.' *American Journal of Physiology*, **206**, 1165–1172.

Vries, J. K. (1968) 'An endoscopic technique for third ventriculostomy.' *Surgical Neurology*, **9**, 165–168.

Weinman, D., Paul, A. T. S. (1967) 'Ventriculostomy for infantile hydrocephalus using a direct cardiac approach. Technical note.' *Journal of Neurosurgery*, **27**, 471–474.

Weiss, M. H., Nulsen, F. E., Kaufman, B. (1972) 'Control of hydrocephalus by intraventricular radioactive colloid.' *Acta Radiologica [Diagnosis]*, **13**, 615–623.

Weissenfels, E., Hemmer, R. (1981) 'Development and social status of hydrocephalic children who are now 14–20 years of age.' *Zeitschrift für Kinderchirurgie*, **34**, 100–104.

West, C. G. H. (1980) 'Ventriculovesical shunt. Technical note.' *Journal of Neurosurgery*, **53**, 858–860.

Wilkinson, H. A., Wilson, R. B., Patel, P. P., Esmaili, M. (1974) 'Corticosteroid therapy of experimental hydrocephalus after intraventricular subarachnoid hemorrhage.' *Journal of Neurology, Neurosurgery and Psychiatry*, **37**, 224–229.

Wilson, C. B., Bertan, V.(1966) 'Perforation of the bowel complicating peritoneal-shunt for hydrocephalus: report of two cases.' *American Surgeon*, **32**, 601–603.

Wise, B. L. (1974) 'A telescopic ventriculo-atrial shunt that elongates with growth.' *Journal of Neurosurgery*, **40**, 665–670.

—— Mathis, J. L., Wright, J. H. (1966) 'Experimental use of isosorbide: an oral osmotic agent to lower cerebrospinal fluid pressure and reduce brain bulk.' *Journal of Neurosurgery*, **25**, 183–188.

—— —— (1977) 'Effects of isosorbide on cerebrospinal fluid pressure and brain bulk in man.' *Cushing Society Meeting, April 1977*. (Abstract).

Wright, E. M. (1972) 'Mechanisms of ion transport across the choroid plexus.' *Journal of Physiology*, **226**, 545–571.

Yamada, H., Tajima, M. (1974) 'A method for lengthening the distal catheter of a Pudenz ventriculo-atrial shunt.' *Journal of Neurosurgery*, **40**, 663–664.

10
SURGICAL TECHNIQUES IN HYDROCEPHALUS

J. R. S. Leggate and A. J. W. Steers

From the time of Hippocrates the diagnosis and management of patients with hydrocephalus has provided the surgeon with some of the most difficult challenges in medicine. The Hippocratic approach combined medical with surgical techniques, using the administration of vegetable aperients, resorting to surgical decompression of the ventricles only when this failed. It was not until the late 19th century that the pathophysiology of CSF production and circulation led to a more logical approach to the management of hydrocephalus. The theory that CSF production occurred mainly from the choroid plexus (Dandy and Blackfan 1913) led surgical approaches to the management of hydrocephalus to be centred around the operation of choroid plexectomy. This operation persisted for almost 20 years in spite of ineffective drainage and high mortality. It was only in the late 1960s that the failure of this operation was explained by the conclusive evidence of CSF formation at the ventricular surface. Other procedures were proposed including that of third ventriculostomy (the opening of the ventricular CSF system into the subarachnoid space via the lamina terminalis), but they were of limited use because they relied on a blockage in the CSF outflow from the ventricles with the maintenance of an intact subarachnoid space and CSF absorptive pathway from the same. Ingraham and Matson (1954) first introduced the idea of polyethylene tubes to shunt the CSF into the sagittal sinus or the vena cava in experimental animals; and we still need such diversionary procedures of CSF from the ventricular system into other absorptive areas in the body. Ingraham's experiment proved, by the universal obstruction of the tubes with blood clot, that in such a system a valve was needed to ensure a one-way flow. Then Nulsen and Spitz (1952) demonstrated the practicality of incorporating a valve into a system implanted subcutaneously, thus ushering in the modern technique for the management of hydrocephalus. Since then technological advances and increasingly sophisticated valve systems have reduced the surgical mortality and morbidity, but the concept remains the same.

Techniques
The operations of choroid plexectomy and intracranial CSF diversionary procedures such as third ventriculostomy and ventriculo-cisternostomy (Torkildsen 1939) have limited application in the management of hydrocephalus. Extracranial CSF diversionary procedures can be divided into three main headings: (i) ventriculo-atrial; (ii) ventriculo-peritoneal and (iii) lumbar thecoperitoneal. Other procedures such as ventricular-pleural or arachnoid-ureterostomies are usually used in extreme circumstances when the other sites are, for clinical reasons, impossible to use.

Ventriculo-atrial shunts
This shunt, which uses the Holter valve (Nulsen and Spitz 1952, Pudenz *et al.* 1957) diverts CSF from the lateral ventricles via a valved shunt system and into the right atrium via the common facial vein which is relatively larger in children than in adults. Occasionally the external jugular vein may be used. Infection, in 10 to 30 per cent, remains the main complication of this technique. Acute infection commonly presents as septicaemia, and chronic infection may present as shunt nephritis or unexplained rashes of a vasculitic nature due to complement activation from chronic septic emboli. More recently children have been admitted and are dying in right-heart failure from pulmonary hypertension, the end result of chronic embolic phenomenon from the catheter tip lying in the right atrium. We believe that ventriculo-atrial shunting should never be used as a primary elective CSF diversionary procedure in children because of the severe consequences of infection and chronic embolic damage to the pulmonary vasculature. The ventricular peritoneal shunt must remain the primary elective CSF extracranial diversionary procedure for children presenting with hydrocephalus.

Ventriculo-peritoneal shunt
The peritoneum, as a site of absorption of CSF, was first described by Kausch (1949) although as with ventriculo-atrial shunts it was in the 1950s that the operation became clinically reliable. Initially the ventricular catheter, the valve and the peritoneal catheter were provided as separate items and the neurosurgeon assembled the shunt at the time of operation using sutures to assemble the device. It was placed along a subcutaneous tract, using one or more relieving incisions, and tunnelled from the skull and over the chest wall before being implanted via a small laparotomy into the peritoneal cavity. The main complication of ventriculo-peritoneal shunting remained infection which to the present day varies between 5 and 30 per cent. The complications of acute and chronic infection in the peritoneal cavity, however, are not severe when compared with those of ventriculo-atrial shunts.

Lumbar theco-peritoneal shunts
In certain circumstances, *e.g.* intracranial hypertension of unknown cause (benign intracranial hypertension, pseudotumour cerebri), it may be that the blockage to CSF absorption is from the subarachnoid space. In these circumstances diversion of the CSF from the lumbar CSF space into the peritoneal cavity is a safe and quick means of relieving the hydrocephalus. The risks of infection remain the same as for ventriculo-peritoneal shunting, but the technique avoids the need for a cortical puncture, and more recently the technique has been used by implanting the shunt percutaneously.

Newer technologies
With the advent of the current concept of extracranial CSF diversionary procedures, it became apparent that there would have to be an improvement in the technology of such devices. Such technological advances as have been achieved can be divided

into three main divisions: shunt tubing, valves and unitisation. These areas of improvement have been brought about by a desire to reduce the rates of infection and shunt malfunction.

Shunt tubing

In the early devices the shunt tubing was made from polyethylene. Its two main disadvantages were its tendency to become brittle and to fracture with time in the body cavities, and secondly the tube's tendency to kink and obstruct when bent beyond a certain angle. Raimondi *et al.* (1977) overcame this problem by impregnating the polysilastic tubing with a helical steel wire. Unfortunately this tended to give the shunt a degree of inflexibility and inherent stiffness which was a disadvantage in the ventricular catheter. Modern shunts are now made of kink-resistant silastic polymer which render themselves more amenable to the acute bends necessary in the placement of such devices.

Valves

The early valves of Holter and Pudenz were bulky. They relied on the principle—largely unchanged today—of elevation of a plastic membrane at a certain pressure allowing flow down the tubing. A system whereby the valve was placed at the distal end of the device in the form of a slit-valve is employed in the Raimondi catheter, Unishunt, and Pudenz-Heyer shunts and is often used for theco-peritoneal shunts. In the early 1970s the problem of over-drainage in certain groups of children was recognised with the development of overriding sutures, craniosynostosis and the slit-ventricle syndrome. This prompted the development of an anti-syphon device to be incorporated into the shunt, which certainly reduced the incidence of over-drainage in children, and reversed the situation where the slit ventricle had become established (Portnoy 1982). More recently attention has been paid to this problem by the development of a variable pressure valve (Sophy). This relies on a sapphire bevel which is spring-loaded using the variable tension of a coiled spring. This allows the adjustment of the opening pressure of the valve to range between several pre-selected opening pressures: low (2 to 5cm of CSF), medium (5 to 9cm of CSF) and high (9 to 15cm of CSF).

Unitisation

With the early devices the shunt was dispatched from the factory in separate component parts. This required the surgeon to remove the device from the sterile packaging, to cut it to the appropriate length for the patient, and then to join the component parts—usually with nylon connector tubes and silk or nylon ties. This has two main drawbacks. Firstly, the increased handling and exposure of the shunt prior to insertion into the patient increases the risk of infection; and secondly, the reliability of junctions and joins made by linking tubes tied with suture material increases the possibility of breakage and disruption of the system. Furthermore the range in requirements for the ventricular length both in children and in adults is not great (normal child ventricular catheter length 6cm, normal adult ventricular catheter length 7.5cm for parietal access to the ventricular system). With the incorporation of the valve, plus or minus the anti-syphon device at the head end of the shunt, the peritoneal catheter could be left for the surgeon to cut prior to insertion into the peritoneal cavity to the appropriate length. Pre-assembled devices, under strict sterile conditions at the factory, are dispatched with the appropriate range of valve-opening pressures and within a certain standard group of peritoneal catheter lengths for both children and adults. This minimises the exposure of the shunts to the outside environment prior to insertion into the patient and also minimises the amount of handling required.

Reservoirs
One of the major problems of shunt systems is that when they malfunction due to mechanical blockage or infection, the device fails to drain CSF from within the ventricular system, leading to development of acute hydrocephalus. This results in a rise in the ICP which may be symptomatic (*e.g.* headaches, nausea, vomiting, deteriorating conscious level) but which may be asymptomatic in up to 25 per cent of patients (Kirkpatrick *et al.* 1989). The need to gain access to the ventricles was recognised by the early shunt manufacturers who placed a reservoir in line with the ventricular catheter and the valve system. This enabled the clinician to access the device percutaneously and to establish the diagnosis of a blocked shunt, either by the presence of raised pressure in the case of a distal-end block or by the absence of CSF flow from the ventricular catheter in the case of a proximal block. However, it could only be used to relieve the pressure when the block was distally in the shunt system, and in the ventricular or proximal catheter blockage the in-line reservoir could not be used to drain and relieve the RICP. In the 1960s, Ommaya and Rickham independently developed the subcutaneous CSF reservoir devices (Rickham and Penn 1965, Ratcheson and Ommaya 1968). These devices consist of a ventricular catheter which is connected to a small chamber and placed into the frontal horn of the right lateral ventricle subcutaneously. They have been used for such practices as CSF ventricular pressure monitoring, drainage for acute hydrocephalus, external drainage of CSF in IVH in the neonatal period, and more recently for installation of chemotherapeutic agents both in bacterial infections of the CNS and also in malignancies of the CNS. Such devices have no flow in the system unless connected for external drainage of CSF, and are therefore less prone to blockage. They are also less prone to blockage when placed in the frontal horn of the right lateral ventricle which contains no choroid plexus. These devices can remain in the patient for life. They allow independent access to the shunted hydrocephalic child for the rapid diagnosis of shunt malfunction (caused by infection or blockage) and also for rapid treatment, either by external ventricular CSF drainage or by the installation of appropriate antibiotics after the diagnosis of CNS infection has been established by examination of CSF samples taken from the reservoir. It is our practice to place a separate reservoir in the right frontal region in every child who presents for investigation and management of hydrcephalus prior to insertion of a shunt.

Operative technique
This priority operation is performed by two senior surgeons. The patient is placed

on the operating table in the supine position with the head turned to the left. The head is shaved, and then the skin (of the head, neck, thorax and abdomen) is prepared in the anaesthetic room with a 4 per cent weight per volume solution of povidone iodine. This is left in contact with the skin for approximately 10 minutes prior to taking the patient into theatre. A small support is placed under the right shoulder to bring the neck, thorax and abdomen into a straight line. The patient is then prepared with another washing of povidone iodine, and after draping the patient with towels, a plastic iodine-pregnated adhesive skin-covering is applied over the whole of the operative site. The siting of the parietal burrhole is made through a 3cm curved incision placed 4cm above and behind the top of the right ear. After fashioning the burrhole, the dura is opened and at this point an iodine-soaked pledget is left in the cranial wound. A 2cm transverse abdominal incision is carried out by the second surgeon, and the peritoneal cavity is entered through a rectus-splitting approach. Using a trochar and cannula, a subcutaneous tract is established without a relieving incision between the peritoneal and cranial wounds, and a small iodine-soaked pledget is left covering the skin edges of the abdominal wound. At this stage the right lateral ventricle is cannulated and the ventricular catheter is removed, using forceps from the sterile packaging, and inserted along the tract into the right lateral ventricle. The peritoneal end of the catheter is then removed from the sterile packaging, inserted through the cannula along the subcutaneous tract, and brought out into the abdominal wound. After establishing patency of the device and collecting CSF samples for bacteriological examination, the ventricular and peritoneal ends are secured. The peritoneal catheter is inserted into the abdominal cavity and the two wounds closed by the two surgeons. At the end of the procedure, the skin wounds are covered with a small iodine-impregnated pledget via an occlusive dressing. Using this technique the entire operation from skin incision to skin closure is approximately 20 to 25 minutes.

The question of whether antibiotics should be given prophylactically for such procedures is discussed in Chapter 12: but it is our practice to give flucloxacillin in three doses, the first in the anaesthetic room, the second during the procedure and the third postoperatively.

REFERENCES

Dandy, W. E., Blackfan, K. D. (1913) 'An experimental and clinical study of internal hydrocephalus.' *Journal of the American Medical Association*, **61**, 221.
Ingraham, F. D., Matson, D. D. (1954) *Neurosurgery of Infancy and Childhood*. Springfield: C. C. Thomas.
Kausch, W. (1949) 'Shunting of cerebrospinal fluid into the peritoneal cavity.' *In* Cane, W. R., Lewis, R. D., Jackson, I. J. (Eds.) *Meeting of the American College of Physicians*. Montreal.
Kirkpatrick, M., Engleman, H., Minns, R. A. (1989) 'Symptoms and signs of progressive hydrocephalus.' *Archives of Disease in Childhood*, **64**, 124–128.
Nulsen, F. E., Spitz, E. B. (1952) 'Treatment of hydrocephalus by direct shunt from ventricle to jugular vein.' *Surgical Forum*, **2**, 399–403.

Portnoy, H. D. (1982) 'Treatment of hydrocephalus.' *In* McLaurin, R. L. (Ed.) *Pediatric Neurosurgery: Surgery of the Developing Nervous System.* New York: Grune and Stratton.

Pudenz, R. H., Russell, F. E., Hurd, A. H., Shelden, C. H. (1957) 'Ventriculo-auriculostomy: a technique for shunting cerebrospinal fluid into the right auricle. Preliminary report.' *Journal of Neurosurgery*, **14**, 171–179.

Raimondi, A. T., Robinson, J. S., Kuwamura, K. (1977) 'Complications of ventriculo-peritoneal shunting and a critical comparison of the three-piece and one-piece systems.' *Child's Brain*, **3**, 321–342.

Ratcheson, R. A., Ommaya, A. K. (1968) 'Experience with the subcutaneous cerebrospinal-fluid reservoir. Preliminary report of 60 cases.' *New England Journal of Medicine*, **279**, 1025–1031.

Rickham, P. P., Penn, I. A. (1965) 'The place of the ventriculostomy reservoir in the treatment of myelomeningoceles and hydrocephalus.' *Developmental Medicine and Child Neurology*, **7**, 296–301.

Torkildsen, A. (1939) 'A new palliative operation in cases of inoperable occlusion of the Sylvian aqueduct.' *Acta Chirurgica Scandinavica*, **82**, 117–124.

11

THE USE OF RESERVOIRS IN SHUNTED HYDROCEPHALUS AND ITS COMPLICATIONS

P.S. Baxter and R. A. Minns

Reservoirs are designed to provide access to ventricular csf. Ommaya's reservoir (Fig. 11.1), initially introduced for the intrathecal therapy of fungal meningitis, was rapidly applied to a variety of neurosurgical problems and their complications (Ratcheson and Ommaya 1968). It is characterised by a pumping chamber to allow mixing of drugs and csf. Rickham introduced a smaller version (Fig. 11.2) for the early management of infants with hydrocephalus who could not be immediately shunted because of infection or haemorrhage; the side-arm can later be connected to a shunt, thus avoiding repeat ventricular cannulation. Until then such children had either not had their raised pressure treated, or had had repeated needling of the brain, with associated morbidity (Rickham and Penn 1965). This and subsequent uses are summarised in Table 11.I, and they fall into two main categories: diagnostic (csf pressure, infection, flow) and therapeutic (decompression, intrathecal chemotherapy, and csf drug levels).

As can be seen from Table 11.I., they have been used in all age-groups. A percutaneous tap into the self-sealing rubber cap is well tolerated even in young patients (Fig. 11.3). Their widest role has been in primary and secondary cns neoplasia, to give intrathecal chemotherapy, monitor csf drug levels, drain cystic lesions and to treat hydrocephalus (Gutin *et al.* 1980, Machado *et al.* 1985): Schmid and Seiler (1986) found that their use avoids the need for a shunt in some patients. In meningitis with ventriculitis, particularly chronic forms, they have been used for antibiotic administration, with monitoring of csf drug levels and csf cellular response (Ratcheson and Ommaya 1968, Kontopolous *et al.* 1986). De Villiers *et al.* (1978) described their role in acute infective hydrocephalus, again avoiding shunts in some patients. This group concluded that early ventriculostomy wtih antibiotic therapy would salvage and improve more lives. McComb *et al.* (1983) described the use of a reservoir in acute hydrocephalus following intraventricular haemorrhage, finding it an effective and safe alternative to repeated ventricular puncture, external drainage or initial shunting. In some survivors the reservoir was later converted to a shunt (Rickham and Penn 1965). Reservoirs have also been used in neuroradiological studies (Goedhart *et al.* 1978); more recently Johnston *et al.* (1984) studied csf pathways in shunted hydrocephalus by giving isotope through a separate reservoir.

Like shunts, reservoirs have a risk of complications, particularly block and iatrogenic infections, which vary according to age and pathological condition

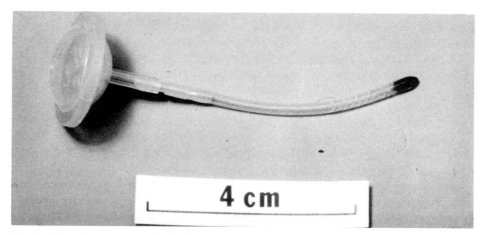

Fig. 11.1. An Ommaya reservoir showing a resealing rubber cap attached to a ventricular catheter.

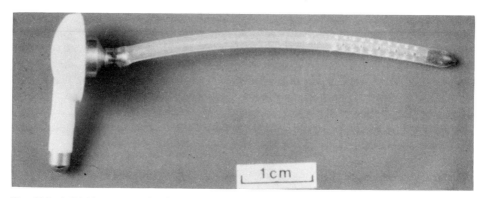

Fig. 11.2. A Rickham reservoir with a side arm.

TABLE 11.I

Experience with reservoirs

| Author | Date | Follow-up | Patients | | | | | Procedures |
			No.	Age	Path.	Block	Inf.	No.
Ratcheson	1968	1–36 months	60	A+C	All	14	9	
Diamond	1973		21		Men.	4/proc.	5/proc.	31
Galicich	1974		45	A+C	Neop.	4	4	
Lee	1977		16	N	Men.		3	
Trump	1982		31	A	Neop.		4 (21*)	
McComb	1983	0–48 days	20	N	IVH	1	0	20
Johnston	1984	5 years	27	C	Shunt		4	
Machado	1985		60	A+C	Neop.	9	3	69
Schmid	1986	1–9 years	61	A+C	Neop.		3 (3**)	

Key: *author* = first author; *date* = date of paper; *age:* A = adults, C = children, A+C = adults and children, N = neonates; *path.* = pathology; all = all types of pathology, men. = meningitis, neop. = Neoplasia, IVH = intraventricular haemorrhage, shunt = shunted hydrocephalus; *inf.* = no. of patients infected; 21* = 21 patients also had contaminants in the CSF; 3** = 3 cases had ventriculitis, and 3 more had reservoir infection or late meningitis.

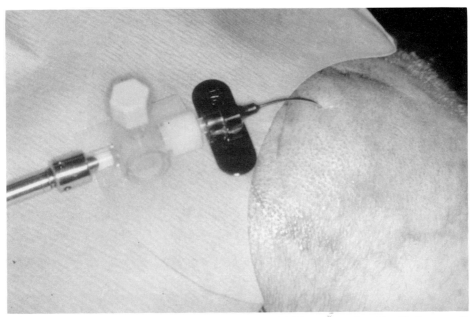

Fig. 11.3. A child with a right anterior frontal subcutaneous Rickham reservoir, with a Huebner needle *in situ*.

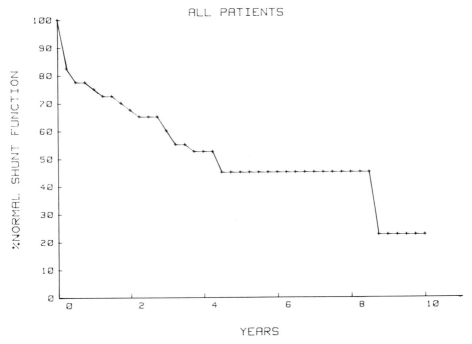

Fig. 11.4. Survival analysis (all patients) for shunt blockage showing a median survival time of 4.31 years.

(Table 11.I). However, Galicich *et al.* (1974) found no correlation between infection and the frequency of tapping the reservoir: four of the patients they described were tapped more than 40 times with no infection. The alternative procedure, ventriculostomy and external drainage without a reservoir, does seem to be associated with a higher risk of infection (Mayhall *et al.* 1984, Gardner *et al.* 1985, Stenager *et al.* 1986), although clinical circumstances differ in these series.

Most of these uses have been in patients without shunts. Before the roles of reservoirs in hydrocephalus can be discussed, it is necessary to define the problems. In spite of advances in management and shunt design, children with shunted hydrocephalus are at constant risk of block (Fig. 11.4.) (Liptak 1984, Leggate *et al.* 1988), and infection, at least for the first few years after shunt insertion or revision (Forward *et al.* 1983, Gardner *et al.* 1985). These complications are associated with an increased risk of death (Table 11.II), epilepsy (Copeland *et al.* 1982), and blindness (Gaston 1985). While a delayed diagnosis risks these problems, overdiagnosis causes unnecessary operations, usually as an emergency, with their risks of anaesthetic problems, haemorrhage and infection. The diagnosis of block or infection thus needs to be rapid, easy and accurate. Effective treatment must also be readily available.

Clinical symptoms or signs can raise the suspicion of shunt complications, but are not diagnostic (see Chapter 1) (Venes 1976, Hayden *et al.* 1983, Odio *et al.* 1984, Walters *et al.* 1984, Gardner *et al.* 1985). Unfortunately signs of an acute viral infection with fever, headache, lethargy or vomiting are common in children, as are less specific symptoms such as a rash, bad temper, waking at night or a diminished school performance, but all can indicate shunt dysfunction or ventriculitis. In addition, raised pressure may only occur when there is an increased production of CSF, as with fever or during sleep. Children can be thought to be shunt independent and some years later present suddenly with raised pressure, which can be fatal (Rekate 1982, Olsen and Frykberg 1983). The large number of proposed methods of diagnosis testifies to the importance of these problems, and suggests that none are completely satisfactory.

Indirect ways of detecting block include palpation, x-ray, CT or ultrasound scan, and methods of detecting shunt-flow. Palpation and pumping of the shunt-pumping chamber is unreliable (Hockley and Holmes 1978), and can only be applied to certain shunt types such as the Spitz-Holter. It also has the theoretical risk of sucking choroid plexus into the ventricular catheter, thus creating a block.

x-ray of the shunt shows displacement or fracture, but these are uncommon causes of block (Noetzel and Baker 1984). It does not show if there is raised pressure or not, unless there is suture separation in a young child. CT scans, or ultrasound scans if there is a sonic window, can show dilatation, and sometimes periventricular oedema or gyral flattening. In 30 CT scans of patients with blocked shunts and raised pressure, however, 10 were either normal or unchanged from previous scans, seven had equivocal and only 13 had unequivocal changes (Noetzel and Baker 1984).

Various techniques to assess flow in the shunt have been tried, particularly Doppler and direct injection of isotope or contrast. None have been particularly

TABLE 11.II
Experience with VP shunts in children

Author	Date	Follow-up	No.	Age	Path.	Procedures	Inf./Proc.	Block	Death
Little	1972	2 (2)	37	C	All	69		1/13 mths	8%
Robertson	1973	(0.1)	297	A+C	All				5%
Schoenbaum$^{\Omega}$	1975		289	0–19	All	884	13%		22% all causes
Venes	1976			C		96	9%		
George$^{\Omega}$	1979	4.2 (1–24)	410	A+C	All	840	12.7%		13% infected
Keucher	1979	5	81	C	*	266	8.6%**		11%
Mazza	1980	5.3 (1–11)	108	C	*	236			7%
McCullough	1980		257	C	All	435	5.2%		
Ajir	1981	(0.12)		C		171	6.4%		
Olsen	1983	4.8 (0–9)	104	C	All	228	11%***	58%	3% block
Odio	1984	(0–2)	297			516	11%		0
Amacher	1984	(5–12)	64	C	1°		5.6%		16% all causes
			49	C	MM		12.3%		29% all causes
Renier	1984	(0.08)	802	C	All	1174	7.9%		
Walters$^{\Omega}$	1984		1477	C		5179	5%		34% infected
Liptak	1985	4	67	C	MM	122		50%:4.8 yrs	0
Leggate	1988	4.8 (0.4–13)	56	C	1°/MM	201	14%	50%:4.8 yrs	0

Key: Ω = VA results included; *author* = first author; *date* = date of paper; *follow-up*: given as mean and (range); *age*: C = child, A+C = adults and children, 0–19 = 0–19 yrs; *path.* = pathology of hydrocephalus: all = all causes, * = all except neoplastic, 1 = primary, MM = secondary to myelomeningocoele; *inf./proc.* = infection rate per procedure: ** = infection rate for initial placements only, *** = calculated from data in text; death is given as percentage due to infection and block, unless otherwise stated.

388

useful (LaFerla *et al.* 1984), and while they may show if a shunt is patent, they cannot show whether or not there is raised pressure (Johnston *et al.* 1984). Also, neither they nor a CT scan are always readily available in all hospitals.

The diagnosis of infection causes similar difficulties (see Chapter 12). There are indirect methods such as acute-phase reactants, which will rise with bacterial infection of any part of the body, or antibody titres, which only reflect infection by the organism against which the antibody is raised, but these have not been proved to be accurate (Gardner *et al.* 1985), and may not be immediately available.

Direct methods require access to the ventricular CSF, to allow pressure measurement and sampling for analysis and culture. Even so, the criteria for diagnosing infection vary. Of the authors in Table 11.II, only Schoenbaum, Venes, George, Odio and Walters give definitions, which generally include clinical symptoms and positive cultures from CSF or the shunt. Most of the others appear to base the diagnosis on positive cultures alone. Only three (Keucher, Mazza and Odio) accepted CSF pleocytosis with negative cultures as evidence of infection. However, cultures sometimes need repeating before certain organisms (particularly *Staphylococcus epidermidis*) are isolated, and standard cultures will not detect anaerobes such as diphtheroids (Rekate *et al.* 1980). In our patients (Leggate *et al.* 1988), where infection was defined as either a postive culture and/or a CSF neutrophil count of $11/cm^3$ or more, the rate could be reduced by 35 per cent if culture-negative patients were excluded. This variation in criteria and the frequent lack of follow-up data (see Table 11.II) also renders it virtually impossible to compare published infection rates for shunt procedures.

The most popular direct method is to tap the shunt (Myers and Schoenbaum 1975, Venes 1976, Hayden *et al.* 1983, LaFerla *et al.* 1984, Noetzel and Baker 1984, Odio *et al.* 1984, Gardner *et al.* 1985, Guertin 1987). Noetzel and Baker studied 91 patients who had 209 taps: 70 of 72 episodes of block, and 12 or 13 infections, were correctly diagnosed. Distal blocks were cleared by irrigation in six cases. One child, however, died from infection and coning before surgery was possible. Hayden *et al.* (1980) reported 306 patients who had had 526 shunt taps combined with radionuclide studies. There was a low error rate, particularly in distal obstruction, but one case of distal obstruction and four cases of proximal obstruction were missed in 202 studies that were believed to be normal. This method obviously requires either a shunt chamber that can be tapped, or a reservoir in series in the shunt assembly. In distal block, decompression and the diagnosis of raised pressure and/or infection should be easy, but in proximal block, apart from the possibility of missing the diagnosis, it is also impossible to obtain CSF for analysis and culture or to decompress the ventricles, so emergency surgery would be required (Guertin 1987).

The alternative, which we prefer, is a separate reservoir cannulated through a right frontal ventriculostomy. This system has been used by Johnston *et al.* (1984) to inject isotope into the CSF and to follow its clearance by the shunt. This group report no particular complications, but give no detailed figures. In Edinburgh we have used this method for 10 years, and a recent review of 56 patients (Leggate *et al.* 1988) found, after reservoir insertion, a reduction in the number of revisions

(1/3.4 shunt years *vs* 1/2 shunt years, p < 0.01) and infections (1/10 shunt years *vs* 1/5.8 shunt years, n.s.). The risks of block, infection, epilepsy, learning difficulties, visual defect and hemiplegia were no different from published figures (Table 11.II).

The reservoir was tapped diagnostically on 210 admissions: 42 per cent were positive. 182 of these admissions were for acute symptoms and 28 were for chronic or more nonspecific symptoms such as diminished school performance.

In the latter, if the pressure was not raised on the initial tap, overnight monitoring nonetheless revealed abnormal plateau waves in patients with obstructed shunts. The reservoir failed eight times (once per 34 reservoir years). Two were due to wound infection, in two the reservoir became disconnected from the ventricular catheter, in three the catheter was blocked, and in one there was a continuous leak after tapping, with subcutaneous oedema. Apart from these situations, the only other circumstance in which the reservoir could give a false negative is that of the isolated fourth ventricle (O'Hare *et al.* 1987), which was not observed in any of these patients.

If raised pressure was found, external drainage, either intermittent or continuous, was started at once by the on-call medical staff, with antibiotics if there was a CSF pleocytosis. Surgery therefore became an elective procedure in a stable patient. The reservoir was used for drainage on 60 admissions, and for antibiotic administration and drainage on 28 admissions. In the latter it was also used during treatment to monitor CSF antibiotic levels, repeat CSF cultures and to monitor the CSF cell count (Kontopolous *et al.* 1986). With this management, none of the children died (Table 11.II).

As Ratcheson and Ommaya (1968) stated: 'In a number of central nervous system diseases it is also of value to have ease of access to the cerebral ventricles when the not altogether unexpected, and unfortunately relatively frequent, neurological crises arise. In a number of cases the subcutaneous cerebrospinal fluid reservoir has facilitated the diagnosis and institution of proper therapy and avoided the need for hastily performed emergency surgery.' In shunted hydrocephalus, a separate reservoir has these advantages, without any increase in morbidity. It can be used in an emergency in any hospital with basic facilities. We believe that the opportunity it gives for rapid diagnosis and treatment helps to prevent death from shunt complications.

REFERENCES

Ajir, E., Levin, A. B., Duff, T. A. (1981) 'Effect of prophylactic methicillin on cerebrospinal fluid shunt infections in children.' *Neurosurgery*, **9**, 6–8.
Amacher, A. L., Wellington, J. (1984) 'Infantile hydrocephalus: long term results of surgical therapy.' *Child's Brain*, **11**, 217–229.
Copeland, G. P., Foy, P. M., Shaw, M. D. M. (1982) 'The incidence of epilepsy after ventricular shunting operations.' *Surgical Neurology*, **17**, 279–281.
De Villiers, J. C., Chiver, P. F. de V., Handler, L. (1978) 'Complications following shunt operations for post-meningitic hydrocephalus.' *Advances in Neurosurgery*, **6**, 23–27.
Diamond, R. D., Bennett, J. E. (1973) 'A subcutaneous reservoir for intrathecal therapy of fungal meningitis.' *New England Journal of Medicine*, **288**, 186–188.

Forward, K. R., Fewer, H. D., Stiver, H. G. (1983) 'Cerebrospinal fluid shunt infections. A review of 35 infections in 32 patients.' *Journal of Neurosurgery*, **59**, 389–394.

Galicich, J. H., Guido, L. J., Ommaya, A. K. (1974) 'Device in carcinomatous and leukaemic meningitis. Surgical experience in forty-five cases.' *Surgical Clinics of North America*, **54**, 915–922.

Gardner, P., Leipzig, T., Phillips, P. (1985) 'Infections of central nervous system shunts.' *Medical Clinics of North America*, **69**, 297–314.

Gaston, H. (1985) 'Does the spina bifida clinic need an ophthalmologist?' *Zeitschrift für Kinderchirurgie*, **40**, Suppl. 1, 46–50.

George, R., Leibrock, L., Epstein, M. (1979) 'Long term analysis of cerebrospinal fluid shunt infections. A 25-year experience.' *Journal of Neurosurgery*, **51**, 804–811.

Goedhart, Z. D., Hekster, R. E. M., Matricali, B. (1978) 'Neurosurgical and neurological applications of the Ommaya reservoir system.' *Advances in Neurosurgery*, **6**, 45–47.

Guertin, S. R. (1987) 'Cerebrospinal fluid shunts. Evaluation, complications, and crisis management.' *Pediatric Clinics of North America*, **34**, 203–217.

Gutin, P. H., Klemme, W. M., Lagger, R. L., MacKay, A. R., Pitts, L. H., Hosobuchi, Y. (1980) 'Management of the unresectable cystic craniopharyngioma by aspiration through an Ommaya reservoir drainage system.' *Journal of Neurosurgery*, **52**, 36–40.

Hayden, P. W., Rudd, T. G., Shurtleff, D. B. (1980) 'Combined pressure-radionuclide evaluation of suspected cerebrospinal fluid shunt malfunction. A seven year clinical experience.' *Pediatrics*, **66**, 679–684.

—— Shurtleff, D. B., Stuntz, T. J. (1983) 'A longitudinal study of shunt function in 360 patients with hydrocephalus.' *Developmental Medicine and Child Neurology*, **25**, 334–337.

Hockley, A. D., Holmes, A. E. (1978) 'Computerised axial tomography and shunt dependency.' *Advances in Neurosurgery*, **6**, 48–51.

Johnston, I. H., Howman-Giles, R., Whittle, I. R. (1984) 'The arrest of treated hydrocephalus in children. A radionuclide study.' *Journal of Neurosurgery*, **61**, 752–756.

Keucher, T. R., Mealey, J. (1979) 'Long term results after ventriculoatrial and ventriculoperitoneal shunting for infantile hydrocephalus.' *Journal of Neurosurgery*, **50**, 179–186.

Kontopolous, E., Minns, R. A., O'Hare, A. E., Eden, O. B. (1986) 'Sedimentation cytomorphology of the CSF in ventriculitis.' *Developmental Medicine and Child Neurology*, **28**, 213–219.

LaFerla, G. A., Fyfe, A. H. B., Drainer, I. K. (1984) 'A simple method of assessing intracranial pressure in hydrocephalic patients with shunts.' *Developmental Medicine and Child Neurology*, **26**, 732–736.

Leggate, J. R. S., Baxter, P. S., Minns, R. A., Steers, A. J. W., Brown, J. K., Shaw, J. F., Elton, R. A. (1988) 'The role of a separate subcutaneous cerebrospinal fluid reservoir in the management of hydrocephalus.' *British Journal of Neurosurgery*, **2**, 327–337.

Lee, E. L., Robinson, M. J., Thong, M. L., Puthucheary, S. D., Ong, T. H., Ng, K. K. (1977) 'Intraventricular chemotherapy in neonatal meningitis.' *Journal of Pediatrics*, **91**, 991–995.

Liptak, G. S., Masiulis, B. S., McDonald, J. V. (1984) 'Ventricular shunt survival in children with neural tube defects.' *Acta Neurochirurgica*, **74**, 113–117.

Little, J. R., Rhoton, A. L., Mellinger, J. F. (1972) 'Comparison of ventriculoperitoneal and ventriculoatrial shunts for hydrocephalus in children.' *Mayo Clinic Proceedings*, **47**, 396–401.

Machado, M., Saleman, M., Kaplan, R. S., Montgomery, E. (1985) 'Expanded role of the cerebrospinal fluid reservoir in neurooncology: indications, causes of revision, and complications.' *Neurosurgery*, **17**, 600–603.

Mayhall, C. G., Archer, N. H., Lamb, V. A., Spadora, A. C. E., Baggett, J. W., Ward, J. D., Narayan, R. K. (1984) 'Ventriculostomy related infections. A prospective epidemiologic study.' *New England Journal of Medicine*, **310**, 553–559.

Mazza, C., Pasqualin, A., Da Pian, R. (1980) 'Results of treatment with ventriculo-atrial and ventriculoperitoneal shunts in infantile nontumoural hydrocephalus.' *Child's Brain*, **7**, 1–14.

McComb, J. G., Ramos, A. D., Platzker, A. C. G., Henderson, D. J., Segall, H. D. (1983) 'Management of hydrocephalus secondary to intraventricular haemorrhage in the preterm infant with a subcutaneous ventricular catheter reservoir.' *Neurosurgery*, **13**, 295–300.

McCullough, D. C., Kane, J. G., Presper, J. H., Wells, M. (1980) 'Antibiotic prophylaxis in ventricular shunt surgery. 1: Reduction of operative infection rate with methicillin.' *Child's Brain*, **7**, 182–189.

Myers, M. G., Schoenbaum, S. C. (1975) 'Shunt fluid aspiration. An adjunct in the diagnosis of cerebrospinal fluid shunt infection.' *American Journal of Diseases of Children*, **129**, 220–222.

Noetzel, M. J., Baker, R. P. (1984) 'Shunt fluid examination: risks and benefits in the evaluation of shunt malfunction and infection.' *Journal of Neurosurgery*, **61**, 328–332.

Odio, C., McCracken, G. H., Nelson, J. D. (1984) 'CSF shunt infections in pediatrics. A seven year experience.' *American Journal of Diseases of Children*, **138**, 1103–1108.

O'Hare, A. E., Brown, J. K., Minns, R. A. (1987) 'Specific enlargement of the fourth ventricle after ventriculo-peritoneal shunt for post haemorrhagic hydrocephalus.' *Archives of Disease in Childhood*, **62**, 1025–1029.

Olsen, L., Frykberg, T. (1983) 'Complications in the treatment of hydrocephalus in children. A comparison of ventriculoatrial and ventriculoperitoneal shunts in a 20-year material.' *Acta Paediatrica Scandinavica*, **72**, 385–390.

Ratcheson, R. A., Ommaya, A. K. (1968) 'Experience with the subcutaneous cerebrospinal-fluid reservoir. Preliminary report of 60 cases.' *New England Journal of Medicine*, **279**, 1025–1031.

Rekate, H. L., Nulsen, F. E., Mack, H. L., Morrison, G. (1982) 'Establishing the diagnosis of shunt independence.' *Monographs in Neural Sciences, Vol. 8. Shunts and Problems in Shunts*. Basel: Karger. pp. 223–226.

—— Ruch, T., Nulsen, F. E. (1980) 'Diphtheroid infections of cerebrospinal fluid shunts.The changing pattern of shunt infection in Cleveland.' *Journal of Neurosurgery*, **52**, 553–556.

Renier, D., Lacombe, J., Pierre-Kahn, A., Sainte-Rose, C., Hirsch, J.-F. (1984) 'Factors causing acute shunt infection. Computer analysis of 1,174 operations.' *Journal of Neurosurgery*, **61**, 1072–1078.

Rickham, P. P., Penn, I. A. (1965) 'The place of the ventriculostomy reservoir in the treatment of myelomeningocoeles and hydrocephalus.' *Developmental Medicine and Child Neurology*, **7**, 296–301.

Robertson, J. S., Maraqa, M. I., Jennett, B. (1973) 'Ventriculoperitoneal shunting for hydrocephalus.' *British Medical Journal*, **1**, 289–292.

Schmid, U. D., Seiler, R. W. (1986) 'Management of obstructive hydrocephalus secondary to posterior fossa tumours by steroids and subcutaneous ventricular catheter reservoir.' *Journal of Neurosurgery*, **65**, 649–653.

Schoenbaum, S. C., Gardner, P., Shillito, J. (1975) 'Infections of cerebrospinal fluid shunts: epidemiology, clinical manifestations, and therapy.' *Journal of Infectious Diseases*, **131**, 543–552.

Stenager, E., Gerner-Smidt, P., Kock Jensen, C. (1986) 'Ventriculostomy-related infections—an epidemiological study.' *Acta Neurochirurgica*, **83**, 20–23.

Trump, D. L., Grossman, S. A., Thompson, G., Murray, K. (1982) 'CSF infections complicating the management of neoplastic meningitis. Clinical features and results of therapy.' *Archives of Internal Medicine*, **142**, 583–586.

Venes, J. L. (1976) 'Control of shunt infection. Report of 150 consecutive cases.' *Journal of Neurosurgery*, **45**, 311–314.

Walters, B. C., Hoffman, H. J., Hendrick, E. B., Humphreys, R. P. (1984) 'Cerebrospinal fluid shunt infection. Influences on initial management and subsequent outcome.' *Journal of Neurosurgery*, **60**, 1014–1021.

12
SHUNT INFECTIONS AND VENTRICULITIS

Roger Bayston

Micro-organisms can colonise any implanted device, such as a hydrocephalus shunt, a Rickham or Ommaya reservoir, an external ventricular drain or an intracranially placed pressure monitor. This can give rise to a spectrum of morbidity ranging from the sub-clinical to the life-threatening.

Aetiology

A hydrocephalus shunt is inserted to circumvent the obstructed natural pathways of CSF drainage from the cerebral ventricles. The shunt consists of a ventricular catheter (usually with an integral reservoir), a valve to control rate and direction of flow, and a distal catheter leading to the drainage site. The most popular site for drainage is the peritoneal cavity, but the right cardiac atrium and the pleural space are also used. CSF can also be shunted from elsewhere in the ventricular system, or in some cases from the lumbar theca to the peritoneal cavity.

Shunt infections consist either of shunt colonisation (where organisms colonise the internal surfaces of the shunt), or of external shunt infections (which consist of wound infections around the outside of the shunt). Eventually, if no action is taken, both surfaces of the shunt will be involved in both types.

Most cases of shunt colonisation occur at the time of surgical insertion or at a subsequent revision (Bayston and Lari 1974). The organisms originate on the patient's skin despite pre-operative cleansing, and are usually present in the incisions during placement of the shunt. The most common organisms are the coagulase-negative staphylococci, though other skin organisms such as coryneforms, streptococci and *Acinetobacter* are also found. *Staphylococcus aureus* causes far fewer shunt infections than coagulase-negative staphylococci, and while again most strains are derived from the patient's skin, a few outbreaks are associated with carriers. When the internal surfaces of the shunt become colonised, the organisms are able to adhere to the shunt materials within seconds of exposure. The important factors are surface charge and hydroprobicity, both of the organism's surface and of the implanted material (Hogt *et al.* 1987). These surface properties of the organism are not expressed consistently. Soon afterwards they begin to multiply, and (in the case of some coagulase-negative staphylococci) to produce a layer of extracellular slime which serves to increase stability of microcolonies and to protect the organisms from the effects of antimicrobial drugs (Bayston and Penny 1972, Peters *et al.* 1982, Bayston 1984, Sheth *et al.* 1985).

Members of the skin flora can also gain access to the shunt lumen during tapping of the reservoir, but this is less common if proper aseptic precautions are taken. The risk is greater, however, where repeated taps are carried out in the same skin area, as with an Ommaya reservoir.

The organisms which cause external shunt infections are mainly *Staphylococcus aureus* and gram-negative rods. These must be able to resist phagocytosis for long enough to establish themselves in the tissue/shunt interface, and coagulase-negative staphylococci are not proficient at this. It should also be remembered that the skin flora of patients in hospital changes to include a higher proportion of gram-negative rods, often including *Pseudomonas aeruginosa*.

Once again, many of these organisms gain access to the external surfaces of the shunt at implantation, but they may also be secondary invaders of a slowly healing incision or of ulceration over a badly placed shunt.

Infection with mixed organisms usually follows the perforation of a hollow abdominal viscus by the lower end of the shunt. Though the actual perforation is often asymptomatic, and the protrusion of the catheter through the anus or vagina is sometimes the only presenting feature, coliforms, enterococci and *Clostridia* soon enter the ventricular system.

The valves in most shunts, and particularly the Holter, are surprisingly efficient at preventing the retrograde progress of colonisation (Bayston and Spitz 1978), but the cerebral ventricles eventually become infected in most cases. Ventriculitis can also be contracted at the operation to implant the shunt in the same way as shunt colonisation, and it is sometimes present before shunt insertion where care is not taken to exclude it. Ventriculitis can occur following closure of the back lesion in spina bifida, and here it is often due to faecal organisms such as *Escherichia coli* or enterococci.

Diagnosis
When considering the symptomatology of shunt colonisation due to skin flora, the route of drainage becomes important.

In ventriculo-atrial shunts, colonisation originates from the time of surgery, but the features of infection may be negligible for years. They consist, in insidious cases, of intermittent low-grade fevers, listlessness and anorexia, often progressing after a few months to include splenomegaly and transient rashes, sometimes with arthropathy. Later the rashes and arthropathy become more frequent and shunt nephritis often develops with hypertension, haematuria, oedema and loin pain (Black *et al.* 1965, Stauffer 1970, Bayston and Swinden 1979). This will usually become irreversible if untreated, leading to renal failure. The listlessness, anorexia and lethargy are due to increasing anaemia, an almost universal feature, and the rash, arthropathy and nephritis are due to immune-complex disease. Endocarditis is surprisingly rare.

In ventriculoperitoneal shunts, discharge of infected CSF into the peritoneal cavity gives rise to local inflammation, often with abdominal pain. Resulting adhesions and omental cyst formation lead to shunt obstruction (Bayston and Spitz 1977). Because of this, signs and symptoms of RICP are often prominent and obstruction of the shunt occurs usually between three and six months after operation. In most cases bacteraemia does not occur, but erythema and fluid collection are often found around the distal catheter where it passes over the rib-cage. The importance of recognising an infective cause for distal catheter obstruction within a few months of surgery, especially where obstruction recurs soon after revision, should be emphasised.

Ventriculitis due to coagulase-negative staphylococci, coryneforms or entero-cocci often gives rise to a very feeble inflammatory response, and symptoms can be minimal. Infection of the ventricular system by *Staphylococcus aureus* or gram-negative rods, on the other hand, usually results in a strong inflammatory response with concomitant severe generalised illness and disturbance of consciousness.

External shunt infections usually begin as local post-operative wound sepsis or infection of an erosion over a prominent part of the shunt, but often there is extension along the shunt track, causing erythema with pyrexia and bacteraemia, and eventually localised peritonitis in ventriculoperitoneal shunts. Especially if the infection involves the scalp or neck wounds, extension to the ventricular system can occur. Involvement of the interior of the shunt system can arise from the upper or lower ends, or by way of disconnections, or by tapping through infected tissue.

Blood culture is often carried out in cases of suspected shunt infection, but its drawbacks should be appreciated. The organisms commonly causing shunt in-fections are the same as those commonly found as contaminants in blood cultures, and false positives occur for this reason, necessitating repeated cultures for confirmation. Nor are positive blood cultures often found in colonised ventriculo-peritoneal shunts; even in ventriculo-atrial shunts, negative cultures can occur in the presence of proven colonisation, especially if antimicrobial drugs have been administered.

Aspiration of CSF from the shunt reservoir is a useful way of determining whether the ventricular system is infected (Myers and Schoenbaum 1975), but because of the unidirectional valve system in most shunts, one can obtain normal fluid in the presence of a colonised lower shunt. Sometimes the system can be aspirated lower down, but this is technically very difficult. Tapping also carries a risk of introducing infection, and should not be undertaken lightly.

Serological tests have been used successfully for many years in the diagnosis of shunt infection (Bayston 1975, 1979; Bayston and Swinden 1979). In ventriculo-atrial shunts which are colonised by coagulase-negative staphylococci, the circulating antibody titre to this organism rises. The rate of rise varies according to the flow-rate through the shunt, the strain of organisms involved and the use of antimicrobial drugs. The titre in uninfected individuals rises from less than 20 at about six months of age, to between 160 and 640 in adolescence. Titres of 5120 and above are not unusual in shunt colonisation. These very large amounts of antibody, with coexisting persistent antigenaemia, are instrumental in the development of immune-complex nephritis.

In colonised ventriculoperitoneal shunts the antibody titre does not usually rise, partly because events such as obstruction of the shunt lead to earlier presentation, and partly due to the way in which antigen is processed in the peritoneal cavity. However, in this group the serum c-reactive protein (CRP) concentration rises due to the intraperitoneal inflammation (Bayston 1979, Castro-Gago *et al.* 1982). CRP is one of a group of acute-phase proteins produced rapidly in the liver in response to tissue damage caused by trauma or inflammation. The CRP level will be raised for a few days following shunt surgery but should fall rapidly to normal thereafter. If the fall does not occur, or if the level continues to rise, then an active inflammatory focus is indicated. Shunt colonisation is possible if there is no local wound sepsis, infection of the respiratory or urinary tracts, or other obvious causes. The CRP level does not rise in colonised ventriculo-atrial shunts unless due to *Staphylococcus aureus* or gram-negative rods, or on development of immune-complex disease. Raised levels will be found in external shunt infections and in most cases of ventriculitis, but they will often fall to near normal with the use of antimicrobial drugs. Serological investigation should begin with a pre-operative baseline sample. Further samples can then be taken if shunt infection is suspected, though a formal surveillance system is preferable (Bayston 1975). This leads to earlier diagnosis, often before conclusive symptoms appear, and avoids complications such as peritoneal abscess, shunt nephritis and repeated revisions, as well as prolonged ill-health in those with chronic ventriculo-atrial shunt infections. I have found that with such a system, all cases will be detected either clinically or serologically within six months of operation, and that surveillance need not continue beyond this.

Treatment

The commonest organisms causing shunt infection are often resistant to a wide range of antimicrobial drugs (Christensen *et al.* 1982), which is not surprising in view of their usual role as skin commensals. The coagulase-negative staphylococci gain further protection from drugs to which they are normally susceptible by growing as slime-covered microcolonies (Sheth *et al.* 1985). Another problem is achieving therapeutic drug levels in the CSF, in the absence of a florid inflammatory response in the ventricles or the meninges.

While it may be attractive to treat shunt infection without removing the device, the success rate is very low (James *et al.* 1980), and once the shunt has been removed CSF pressure may still need to be controlled with an external ventricular drain (EVD). With a competent EVD (such as the Codman or Dow Corning), the risks of ascending secondary infection are low and the pressure control is better than that achieved by tapping. However, a few patients are best managed by reservoir insertion and tapping, and some are fortunate enough to require no further drainage.

Both the resistance of the organisms and the pharmacological problem of penetration into the CSF demand careful choice of suitable antimicrobial drugs. Chloramphenicol is one of the small number of drugs which will penetrate the uninflamed blood-brain barrier, but relapse of gram-positive infection following use of this drug is common, and it should not be used against staphylococci. Penicillins and cephalosporins do not penetrate sufficiently into the CSF except in florid inflammation and the same is true of the aminoglycosides and vancomycin.

All staphylococci and coryneforms and most streptococci are susceptible to vancomycin, however, even when resistant to most other drugs, and this has led to its administration directly into the ventricular system (Visconti and Peters 1979, Bayston *et al.* 1984, Swayne *et al.* 1987). While intravenous use of the drug can sometimes cause histamine-like reactions ('Red Man Syndrome') (Odio *et al.* 1984), and though high plasma levels are associated with renal and eighth-nerve toxicity, much higher CSF levels appear to be safe (Pav *et al.* 1986, Bayston *et al.* 1987). Indeed, experience suggests that, for intraventricular use, vancomycin is safer and more effective than aminoglycosides.

A successful treatment regimen for shunt infection consists of:

1. Shunt removal.
2. Insertion of a competent EVD to decrease the risk of secondary infection.
3. Intraventricular administration of vancomycin 20mg per day. The dose of vancomycin is related to ventricular volume, not age or body-weight. If the ventricles are very small it can be reduced to 10mg daily.
4. Intravenous administration of a suitable antimicrobial drug. The intravenous antimicrobial drug is used to eradicate infection in the shunt track and peritoneal cavity (in ventriculoperitoneal shunts) and should be chosen conventionally according to susceptibility tests. Flucloxacillin or rifampicin are commonly used, but fusidic acid, trimethoprim and netilmicin are also useful.
5. Daily examination of CSF. The CSF levels usually rise to about 100 to 300mg/l during treatment but these are not associated with toxicity, unlike high plasma levels. The success rate falls considerably if the dose is titrated so that significantly lower levels are obtained, and relapses become common.
6. Reshunting if necessary on the seventh to 10th day. There should be no waiting period between the last dose of antimicrobial drugs and reshunting.
7. The last intraventricular dose of vancomycin should be given on the operating table, when access to the ventricular system is gained during insertion of the new shunt.

While numerous other regimens are in use for shunt-associated infections due to gram-positive bacteria, their success-rate on first attempt is generally lower than the above, and treatment usually takes longer. However, occasional infections due to coagulase-negative staphylococci are eradicated after shunt removal without the need for antimicrobial drugs.

Gram-negative infections, including those involving the ventricular system, can be treated with intravenous aminoglycosides or cephalosporins after shunt removal, as these will penetrate the CSF due to the florid inflammatory response.

Patients with hydrocephalus probably have the same risk of contracting meningitis due to *Haemophilus influenzae, Neisseria meningitidis* or *Streptococcus pneumoniae* as those without, and this condition therefore occasionally presents in those with shunts. There is a temptation to remove the shunt because of the risk of colonisation and consequent complication of therapy, but a shunt appears to present no added risk and is probably beneficial as it relieves ICP, which is a feature of bacterial meningitis. Shunted patients who are treated conventionally without shunt removal respond at least as well as those without shunts (Patriarca and Laver 1980, Stern *et al.* 1988).

Prevention

In view of the known risk-period for shunt infection, any prophylactic measures should be directed towards the operation. Rigorous aseptic technique and efficient skin preparation should be the norm, but the risk can be reduced further by such measures as the use of chlorhexidine-soaked packs around the wound edges (Fitzgerald and Connelly 1984). Intravenous antimicrobial drugs will reduce the risk of wound infection and external shunt infection, but there is no evidence that they will prevent internal shunt colonisation. Numerous trials have been carried out in an attempt to determine the effectiveness of prophylactic intravenous antimicrobial drugs, but none has yielded a conclusive result, either due to poor trial design or, more usually, to insufficient patients entered. Recently the United Kingdom Hydrocephalus Group finished a multicentre trial of prophylactic intraventricular vancomycin after 30 months, but while there was no obvious benefit, again insufficient patients with shunt infections were available at the centres to achieve formal statistical validity.

A future possibility is the use of shunts which have been processed to make them antibacterial, so that if they become contaminated during insertion they will not become colonised (Bayston 1980, Bayston and Milner 1981, Bayston *et al.* 1989). Such devices are now being tested clinically, but at the moment the most effective measure seems to be excellent surgical technique based on a sound understanding of the problem.

REFERENCES

Bayston, R. (1975) 'Serological surveillance of children with CSF shunting devices.' *Developmental Medicine and Child Neurology*, Suppl. 35, 104–110.
—— (1979) 'The role of C-reactive protein test in the diagnosis of septic complications of cerebrospinal fluid shunts for hydrocephalus.' *Archives of Disease in Childhood*, **54**, 545–547.
—— (1980) 'The effect of antibiotic impregnation on the function of slit valves ,used to control hydrocephalus.' *Zeitschrift für Kinderchirurgie*, **31**, 353–359.
—— (1984) 'A model of catheter colonisation in vitro and its relationship to clinical catheter infections.' *Journal of Infection*, **9**, 271–276.
—— Barnicoat, M., Cudmore, R. E., Guiney, E. J., Gurusinghe, N., Norman, P. M. (1984) 'The use of intraventricular vancomycin in the treatment of CSF shunt-associated ventriculitis.' *Zeitschrift für Kinderchirurgie*, **39**, Suppl. II, 111–113.
—— Grove, N., Siegel, J., Lawellin, D., Barsham, S. (1989) 'Prevention of hydrocephalus shunt catheter colonisation in vitro by impregnation with antimicrobials.' *Journal of Neurology, Neurosurgery and Psychiatry*, **52**, 605–609.
—— Hart, C. A., Barnicoat, M. (1987) 'Intraventricular vancomycin in the treatment of ventriculitis associated with cerebrospinal fluid shunting and drainage.' *Journal of Neurology, Neurosurgery and Psychiatry*, **50**, 1419–1423.
—— Lari, J. (1974) 'A study of the sources of infection in colonised shunts.' *Developmental Medicine and Child Neurology*, Suppl. 32, 16–22.
—— Milner, R. D. G. (1981) 'The antimicrobial activity of silicone rubber used in hydrocephalus shunts, after impregnation with antimicrobial substances.' *Journal of Clinical Pathology*, **34**, 1057–1062.
—— Penny, S. R. (1972) 'Excessive production of mucoid substance by staphylococcus SIIA: a possible factor in colonisation of Holter shunts.' *Developmental Medicine and Child Neurology*, Suppl. 25, 25–28.
—— Spitz, L. (1977) 'Infective and cystic causes of malfunction in ventriculoperitoneal shunts for hydrocephalus.' *Zeitschrift für Kinderchirurgie*, **22**, 419–424.
—— —— (1978) 'The role of retrograde movement of bacteria in ventriculoatrial shunt colonisation.' *Zeitschrift für Kinderchirurgie*, **25**, 352–356.

—— Swinden, J. (1979) 'The aetiology and prevention of shunt nephritis.' *Zeitschrift für Kinderchirurgie*, **28**, 377–384.

Black, J. A., Challacombe, D. N., Ockenden, B. G. (1965) 'Nephrotic syndrome associated with bacteraemia after shunt operations for hydrocephalus.' *Lancet*, **2**, 921–924.

Castro-Gago, M., Sanguindeno, P., Garcia, C., Pombo, M., Ugarte, J., Cabanas, R., Pena, J. (1982) 'Valor de la proteina C-reactiva (PCR) en el diagnostico de las complicaciones infecciosas de los 'shunts' en nos niños hidrocefalos.' *Anales Españoles de Pediatria*, **16**, 47–52.

Christensen, G. D., Bisno, A. L., Parisi, J. T. (1982) 'Nosocomial septicaemia due to multiple antibiotic-resistant *Staphylococcus epidermidis*.' *Annals of Internal Medicine*, **96**, 1–10.

Fitzgerald, R., Connelly, B. (1984) 'An operative technique to reduce valve colonisation.' *Zeitschrift für Kinderchirurgie*, **39**, Suppl. 2, 107–108.

Hogt, A. H., Daakert, J., Feijen, J. (1987) 'Adhesion of coagulase negative staphylococci onto biomaterials.' *In* Pulverer, G, Quie, P., Peters, G. (Eds.) *Pathogenicity and Clinical Significance of Coagulase Negative Staphylococci. Zentralblatt für Bakteriologie, Mikrobiologie und Hygiene, Suppl. 16.* Stuttgart: Gustav Fischer.

James, H. E., Walsh, J. W., Wilson, H. D., Connor, J. D., Bean, J. R., Tipps, P. A. (1980) 'Prospective randomised study of therapy in cerebrospinal fluid shunt infections.' *Neurosurgery*, **7**, 459–463.

Myers, M. G., Schoenbaum, S. C. (1975) 'Shunt fluid aspiration; an adjunct in the diagnosis of cerebrospinal fluid shunt infection.' *American Journal of Diseases of Children*, **129**, 220–222.

Odio, C., Mohs, E., Sklar, F. H., Nelson, J. D., McCracken, G. H. (1984) 'Adverse reactions to vancomycin used as prophylaxis for CSF shunt procedures.' *American Journal of Diseases of Children*, **138**, 17–19.

Patriarca, P. A., Laver, B. A. (1980) 'Ventriculoperitoneal shunt-associated infections due to *Haemophilus influenzae*.' *Pediatrics*, **65**, 1007–1009.

Pav, A. K., Simego, R. A., Fisher, M. A. (1986) 'Intraventricular vancomycin: observations of tolerance and pharmacokinetics in two infants with ventricular shunt infections.' *Pediatric Infectious Diseases*, **5**, 93–96.

Peters, G., Locci, R., Pulverer, G. (1982) 'Adherence and growth of coagulase negative staphylococci on surfaces of intravenous catheters.' *Journal of Infectious Diseases*, **146**, 479–482.

Sheth, N. K., Franson, T. R., Sohnle, P. G. (1985) 'Influence of bacterial adherence to intravascular catheters on in vitro antibiotic susceptibility.' *Lancet*, **2**, 1266–1268.

Stauffer, U. G. (1970) 'Shunt nephritis: diffuse glomerulo-nephritis complicating ventriculoatrial shunts.' *Developmental Medicine and Child Neurology*, Suppl. 22, 161–164.

Stern, S., Bayston, R., Hayward, R. J. (1988) '*Haemophilus influenzae* meningitis in the presence of cerebrospinal fluid shunts.' *Child's Nervous System*, **4**, 164–165.

Swayne, R., Rampling, A., Newsom, S. W. B. (1987) 'Intraventricular vancomycin for treatment of shunt-associated ventriculitis.' *Journal of Antimicrobial Chemotherapy*, **19**, 249–253.

Visconti, E. B., Peters., G. (1979) 'Vancomycin treatment of cerebrospinal fluid infections. Report of two cases.' *Journal of Neurosurgery*, **51**, 245–246.

13

'BENIGN' INTRACRANIAL HYPERTENSION (PSEUDOTUMOUR CEREBRI)

R.A. Minns and A. H. Hamilton

Benign intracranial hypertension (BIHT) is a clinical syndrome consisting of symptomatic RICP, usually with papilloedema but without focal neurological signs, in a neurologically stable patient with normal CSF composition.

The entity was first recognised by Quincke (1897) and has been known variously since then as pseudotumour (Warrington 1914), pseudo-abscess (Adson 1924), otitic hydrocephalus (Symonds 1931), intracranial pressure without brain tumour (Dandy 1937), hypertensive meningeal hydrops (Davidoff and Dyke 1937), toxic hydrocephalus (McAlpine 1937), brain-swelling of unknown cause (Sahs and Hyndman 1939, Sahs and Joynt 1956), papilloedema of indeterminate aetiology (Yaskin *et al.* 1949), and benign intracranial hypertension (Foley 1955).

Aetiology
There are half a dozen causes of pseudotumour cerebri:

Endocrine
(1) Addison's disease
(2) Pregnancy
(3) Menstrual abnormalities
(4) Gross obesity. The CSF pressure in some neurologically normal obese patients is increased and overlaps with the levels of CSF pressure measured in patients with BIHT (Corbett and Mehta 1983)
(5) Oral progestational agents
(6) Congenital adrenal hyperplasia (while on steroid therapy)
(7) Prolonged steroid therapy (especially triamcinolone, either oral or topical) used in patients with nephrotic syndrome, leukaemia, ulcerative colitis, and collagen diseases. Nine years of continuous steroids were reported in one case of BIHT
(8) Sudden steroid withdrawal
(9) Hyperthyroidism and thyroid hormone treatment
(10) Hyper- and hypoparathyroidism.

For all these endocrine abnormalities, laboratory estimates of steroids and oestrogens have been measured and found to be normal.

Drugs
(1) Psychotherapeutic drugs
(2) Tetracyclines (especially during the long-term treatment of acne with normal-dose regimes of oral tetracyclines of any group, *e.g.* minocycline, demeclocycline

and oxytetracycline. The syndrome may occur after weeks or months of therapy
(3) Other antibiotics (amoxycillin, co-trimoxazole, sulphamethoxazole, penicillin, gentamicin)
(4) Vitamin A in large doses
(5) Vasopressin
(6) Nalidixic acid
(7) Indomethacin
(8) Lithium carbonate.

Haematological
(1) Iron-deficiency anaemia
(2) Polycythaemia and hypercoagulation states
(3) Other blood dyscrasias
(4) Histiocytosis x
(5) Ataxia telangiectasia
(6) Cryofibrinogenaemia
(7) Sickle cell anaemia
(8) Pernicious anaemia
(9) Wiskott-Aldrich syndrome
(10) Gastrointestinal haemorrhage
(11) Haemophilia.

Injury/neurological
(1) Postoperative (unilateral or bilateral, radical neck dissection)
(2) Minor head injury
(3) Neck injury (jugular-vein injury?)
(4) Guillain-Barré syndrome
(5) Recurrent polyneuritis
(6) Dural sinus thrombosis.

Infectious
(1) Ear disease is the most common aetiological factor, *e.g.* chronic otitis media or mastoiditis in children and adults, with or without lateral sinus thrombosis (if there is lateral sinus thrombosis, then this has been designated otitic hydrocephalus)
(2) Thrombosis of superior sagittal sinus
(3) Upper respiratory infections (influenza, sinusitis, bronchitis)
(4) Gastro-enteritis
(5) Chicken pox
(6) Post-infectious states (parotitis, tuberculosis, urinary tract infection).
(7) Infectious mononucleosis
(8) Lyme disease.

Other associations
(1) Systemic lupus erythematosus and connective tissue disorders
(2) Monoclonal gammopathy (Gilman *et al.* 1983)

(3) Familial metabolic defect (Rothner and Brust 1974)

(4) Familial or acquired deficiency of functioning villi (Donaldson 1981)

(5) Chronic hypoxia

(6) Sarcoidosis

(7) Paget's disease

(8) Pulmonary hypoventilation

(9) Serum sickness

(10) Cryoglobulinaemia

(11) 'Catch-up' growth

(12) Nephrotic syndrome

(13) Allergic conditions

(14) Galactosaemia.

In a review of 23 cases at the War Memorial Children's Hospital in London, Ontario, a cause could be found for all but six patients (Amacher and Spence 1985). But in a retrospective review, Johnston and Paterson (1974a) found 56.3 per cent of cases with no apparent cause.

Clinical features

Symptoms

HEADACHE

While headache is almost invariably present in adults, in children it is less frequent and is present in 57 per cent of cases (Grant 1971). It tends to be generalised, aggravated by coughing and sneezing and manoeuvres that increase the intra-cerebral venous pressure.

NAUSEA AND VOMITING

This occurs in 20 to 40 per cent of cases (Weisberg 1975, Rush 1980).

VISUAL SYMPTOMS

These occur in 35 to 68 per cent of cases (Weisberg 1975, Rush 1980): (i) blurring of vision in one or both eyes, which may be of short duration or continuous; (ii) transient visual obscurations (photopsias, which are the classic visual symptoms of raised pressure from any cause, lasting a few seconds and consisting of pulsating halos, black spots or psychedelic lights made worse by changes in posture; and (iii) diplopia, which occurs in 35 per cent of cases, due to a sixth-nerve palsy (Rush 1980).

OTHER SYMPTOMS

Dizziness occurs in 50 per cent of cases (Weisberg 1975). Other symptoms, such as facial pain, tinnitus, paraesthesiae, may also occur. Asymptomatic cases account for about 5 per cent (Rush 1980).

Clinical signs

PAPILLOEDEMA

While this is almost always present, cases have been reported where it has been absent (Lipton and Michelson 1972, Scanarini *et al.* 1979). Papilloedema was absent in 12 out of 23 cases reviewed in Ontario (Amacher and Spence 1985). It was unilateral in four out of the 57 cases of Corbett *et al.* (1982). The papilloedema is generally of moderate degree, 4 dioptres or less in most cases.

SIXTH-NERVE PALSY
This may be unilateral or bilateral, and is a non-localising sign of RICP. The frequency has been variously reported as 9 per cent (Boddie *et al.* 1974*a*), 16 per cent (Rush 1980) and 31 per cent (Smith 1958). A unilateral third-nerve lesion may also occur as a false localising sign (McCammon *et al.* 1981).

VISUAL ACUITY
This is better than 6/9 in most patients. Early visual loss usually indicates a worse prognosis, but the visual loss accompanying chronic papilloedema takes two to four months to develop (Rush 1980, Corbett *et al.* 1982).

VISUAL FIELDS
The common feature is of an asymptomatic, enlarged blind-spot. Others have reported the contraction of the infero-nasal quadrant (Dersh and Schlezinger 1959). There is also a generalised constriction of the periphery of the visual fields and occasionally paracentral scotoma or homonymous hemianopia.

SUDDEN VISUAL LOSS
This rare complication is due to ischaemic optic neuropathy, *i.e.* vascular occlusion (Green *et al.* 1980). Sudden monocular visual loss is rarely due to sub-retinal neovascular membrane which may produce haemorrhage and a picture similar to macular degeneration (Troost *et al.* 1979). Permanent visual loss may occur in patients with pseudotumour cerebri.

COGNITIVE DYSFUNCTION
Cognitive dysfunction with asthenia and memory disturbance (Klein 1978, Klosterkotter 1982), together with persistent headache, may occur within three years of onset of BIHT, despite medical treatment. This is therefore a symptom of chronic BIHT, and drainage of CSF offers the best chance of relief for these patients (Foley 1977).

Diagnostic criteria
(1) Papilloedema and enlarged blind spot
(2) Exclusion of other conditions known to cause papilloedema, in particular venous sinus thrombosis
(3) No focal neurological signs
(4) A CT scan showing normal or small ventricles and no mass lesion or hydrocephalus
(5) A high CSF pressure, with normal composition of the CSF in terms of protein and cellular content.

CT scan

CT scans of patients with dural sinus thrombosis are easily recognisable and clearly these patients require different treatment, *e.g.* with heparin. Rarely, a frontal-lobe tumour and midbrain glioma has been found on repeated CT scans in patients initially thought to have pseudotumour cerebri. Normally, however, the CT scan shows small ventricles; and Reid *et al.* (1980) studied the volume of the lateral and third ventricle by CT scan in 18 patients with BIHT, and compared these with normals matched for age and sex. They found the ventricles significantly smaller (at the 0.1 per cent level) than in the normal patients. The ventricular volume was a mean of 4.9ml in the BIHT patients, whereas in control patients the mean volume was 11.7ml. They postulated that the mechanism for BIHT was therefore not due to impaired CSF absorption, or a problem at the arachnoid villi, because this would have resulted in dilatation of the CSF pathways. These smaller-than-normal ventricles indicated cerebral swelling resulting from oedema or engorgement. In a fascinating follow-up study, Reid *et al.* (1981) showed that their patients who responded to treatment subsequently had increased ventricular volume on later scans, while those who remained symptomatic did not.

CSF pressure

RICP is the usual finding, and this may be extreme with plateau waves and B waves, despite the minor subjective symptoms. Continuous ICP monitoring confirms that normal levels of ICP are occasionally found. Rabinowicz *et al.* (1968) monitored ICP by *lumbar puncture* in eight patients prospectively, and found a fluctuating range of normal and high values. The intracranial pressure in BIHT, therefore, is intermittently normal. The pressure range varies between 100mm and 500mm of water.

Long-term ICP monitoring using an *implantable epidural sensor* was done in four patients by Gucer and Viernstein (1978), who unequivocally demonstrated occasional normal ICP levels. Pressures ranged from 100mm to 500mm of water over a 24-hour period before any treatment had been started. In patients with a symptomatic clinical picture of BIHT, where normal pressure is initially found at lumbar puncture, the lumbar pressure measurement should be repeated.

Apart from the lumbar and epidural recordings, other methods of pressure-recording have been employed. In one patient under local anaesthetic, Amacher and Spence (1985) inserted a sterile plastic *catheter into the lumbar theca* via a number 14 Toohy needle. This was connected to a strain gauge, and a 10-hour tracing obtained. Sorenson *et al.* (1988) used epidural transducers and lumbar cannulas to obtain 30-minute and one-hour recordings.

Johnston and Paterson (1974b) did continuous monitoring and studies of CSF dynamics on 21 patients. Twenty patients had continuous *intracranial ventricular pressure monitoring*, lasting from six to 68 hours. They showed that the mean ICP ranged from 1 to 33mmHg. This confirmed that there are long periods when the pressure is low or normal, between short periods when there is marked intracranial hypertension. There were 13 patients with unequivocally raised CSF pressure (*i.e.* >15mmHg), and seven with doubtful pressure-levels (<15mmHg). The latter group had predominantly flat and featureless ICP records, with only occasional atypical plateau waves. The ICP waveform characteristics of those patients with unequivocally raised CSF pressure were: (i) low-amplitude (10 to 20mmHg) waves at 1 per minute, with no associated clinical concomitants; (ii) plateau waves (50 to 80mmHg) lasting from five to 20 minutes, again with no clinical associations, although in one patient this seemed to be precipitated by drinking; and (iii) 'plateau-like' waves (30 to 40mmHg) of shorter duration (five to 10 minutes), which occurred in clusters.

Simultaneous ventricular and lumbar recordings show a close association between these two pressure measurements, and the lumbar route can safely be used to drain CSF in order to bring the pressure back to less than 10mmHg. Calculations, derived from the average time for the pressure to return to its pre-drainage levels, have indicated average CSF production rates of 0.26ml/min, the normal rate of production being 0.3 to 0.5cc/min. Simultaneous blood-pressure and ICP measurements, in three patients over several hours, showed that the blood pressure changed little with increasing ICP even during moderately high plateau waves. High-amplitude sharp waves, however, could be associated with a transient increase in blood-pressure (Johnston and Paterson 1974*b*). This absence of a Cushing response with plateau waves means that there is a potential for ischaemic damage from a low CPP during an acute rise in ICP. Langfitt *et al*. (1965) showed that an acute rise in ICP was associated with a fall in CBF, but chronic ICP resulted in no appreciable effect on CBF. In BIHT, therefore, the damage to vision may be brought about by the rapid increases in ICP without a significant Cushing response. This results in a low perfusion with acute intermittent ischaemia to the optic nerve-head and calcarine cortex.

Illustrative cases
This patient, a previously well six-year-old boy, presented with a three-week history of fever, early-morning headache, photophobia, vomiting and general malaise for which he had been treated with antibiotics. Intermittent double vision developed, with a squint, one week prior to admission. On initial examination, he was found to be hyporeflexic with bilateral papilloedema and a right sixth-nerve palsy. **CASE 1**

An urgent CT scan showed a low-density area in the medial part of the left temporal lobe, probably an arachnoid cyst, or perhaps an area of focal encephalitis or a partially treated pyogenic meningitis.

A lumbar puncture was performed and the CSF pressure measured as previously described. The initial pressure was markedly elevated at 40mmHg with a wide pulse pressure (Fig. 13.1). 7ml/kg of 20 per cent solution of mannitol was infused without appreciable effect, but the removal of aliquots of CSF to a total of 25ml resulted in a fall to normal levels (10mmHg). The PVI in the acute state on several calculations was high but variable, like the estimated CSF production rate.

A subarachnoid screw was inserted and the ICP continuously monitored overnight. A gradual increase, to between 20 and 30mmHg was satisfactorily managed by removal of further aliquots of CSF.

Meanwhile, he was treated with penicillin, chloramphenicol, metronidazole and acyclovir. When the initial CSF examination proved to be normal and the culture clear, dexamethasone (2mg four-hourly initially) was added, with rapid resolution of ICP within 48 hours of admission. Subsequently, all viral and bacterial investigations proved negative and a repeat CT scan was unchanged, tending to support the view that the abnormality in the temporal lobe was of long standing and an incidental finding. He was discharged well, 20 days after admission, on a reducing dose of dexamethasone. Recovery of his sixth-nerve palsy took 30 days but the papilloedema took three months to be fully resolved.

CASE 2 This five-year-old boy was already having neurological follow-up on account of ataxia, developmental delay and plagiocephaly secondary to a chromosomal abnormality (4p+). He presented with a four-week history of malaise and vomiting. Two weeks prior to admission he was found to have a left otitis media which was treated successively with ampicillin and co-trimoxazole. During these courses of antibiotics he developed a purulent discharge from the left ear followed two days before admission by a left convergent squint with continued vomiting and increasing drowsiness.

On admission, he complained of left-sided otalgia and headache and was found to have a left sixth-nerve palsy (the right optic disc was thought abnormally pale) with early papilloedematous changes on the left. A CT scan was normal apart from opacification in the left mastoid sinus. A lumbar puncture was performed with CSF pressure-monitoring by transducer. Initial CSF pressure measurements reached 80mmHg, although he was struggling at this time. This settled to 20mmHg after infusion of 20 per cent mannitol, and went down further to normal pressure levels with the removal of 2ml of CSF (Fig. 13.2).

Subsequently an unsuccessful attempt was made to insert an in-dwelling spinal catheter, then a ventricular catheter was inserted and continuous use of drainage commenced. Penicillin, cefotaxime and metronidazole were started and dexamethasone added once examination of the CSF had proven normal.

Ventricular drainage was continued for two days until surgery for exploration of the mastoid (cortical mastoidectomy) and removal of a cholesteatoma was performed. Twenty-four hours later the need for continuous drainage was well demonstrated when the ICP rose suddenly after clipping off the drainage, indicating poor intracranial compliance (Fig. 13.3). The patient remained on ventricular pressure-monitoring and drainage for a total of six days. Thereafter the ICP was normal. All microbiological parameters on the CSF subsequently proved normal and the pressure level remained normal after weaning from the dexamethasone. His sixth-nerve palsy resolved after 16 days, but there remained residual fundal changes 3½ months later. He has subsequently required further surgery for recurrent cholesteatoma.

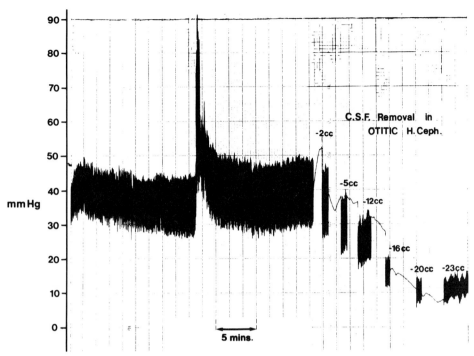

Fig. 13.1. CSF pressure in a six-year-old boy with BIHT, showing the grossly widened pulse pressure and the beneficial effect of removal of CSF.

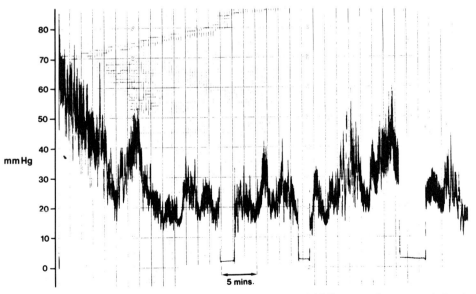

Fig. 13.2. Lumbar CSF pressure in a five-year-old boy with BIHT, initially responding to mannitol and the removal of 3 aliquots of CSF. The fluctuating baseline pressure was especially noticeable.

CASE
3

This seven-year-old girl had no relevant past medical history. She suffered a minor blow to the head from a child's swing two weeks prior to admission. She was seen in the Accident and Emergency Department at the time, but no abnormality was found. Subsequently she complained of frequent headaches and finally two days of double vision. At that time she was seen by a clinical medical officer at school who found a squint and referred her urgently to hospital.

On examination, she was found to have marked bilateral papilloedema with bilateral sixth-nerve palsy and some dilatation of the scalp veins. Her visual acuity was normal and no other abnormal neurological signs were present.

The CT scan was normal apart from small ventricles. Subsequently, at lumbar puncture, CSF pressure was found to be markedly elevated at 40 to 50mmHg. CSF was removed in 1ml aliquots until normal pressure levels were reached after a total of 16ml of CSF were removed (Fig. 13.4.)

She was thereafter managed with twice-daily lumbar punctures for removal of sufficient CSF to maintain a normal ICP. This course of management was chosen because she tolerated each lumbar puncture exceptionally well.

After three days it proved possible to reduce the lumbar punctures to one per day, and after a further four days to alternate-day lumbar punctures, decreasing in frequency to weekly and then fortnightly, finally discontinuing altogether with the last lumbar puncture two months from the onset. At this time the ICP was persistently normal, but over the two months a mean of 9.6ml of CSF was required to be removed at each lumbar puncture in order to establish normal pressure levels.

When the CSF had proved to be normal she was also treated with a reducing dose of dexamethasone and long-term acetazolamide. The papilloedema resolved in one month and the squint improved within two weeks of treatment. She subsequently returned to normal health.

CASE
4

This boy presented at age 13 with a left-sided headache which he had had for the previous two weeks. It was occasionally severe, occasionally associated with vomiting, and would sometimes wake him at night. The family practitioner diagnosed otitis media, and he was treated with co-trimoxazole for 11 days without effect. He had no significant past medical history. No abnormality was noted on admission, other than his excessive weight; he weighed more than 90kg, i.e. well over the 97th centile for age. Skull x-ray and full blood-count, urea and electrolytes were normal. He was observed and discharged with anti-migraine therapy.

He was next admitted seven weeks later, again with frontal headaches for the previous two weeks, pain in his forearms, swelling and tenderness which he localised to the back of his neck and the lumbo-sacral region of his spine. He had vomited twice, was lethargic, and also complained of paraesthesia in his left index finger. There was no improvement with an

408

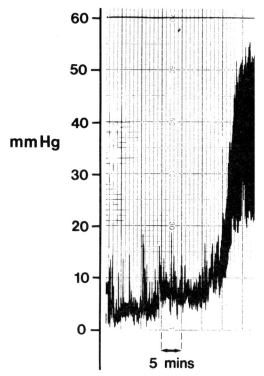

5 mins

Fig. 13.3. Closed ventricular drainage kept the ICP at normal levels until the ventricular drainage was clamped with a resultant plateau of pressure.

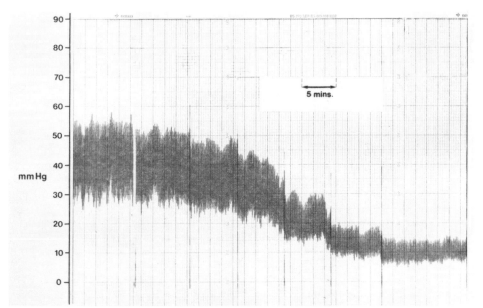

5 mins.

Fig. 13.4. Lumbar CSF pressure in a seven-year-old girl with BIHT showing the opening pressure of almost 40mmHg, and the effect of removal of small volumes of CSF. There is a corresponding decrease in the pulse pressure, but at 10mmHg it is still abnormally enlarged.

409

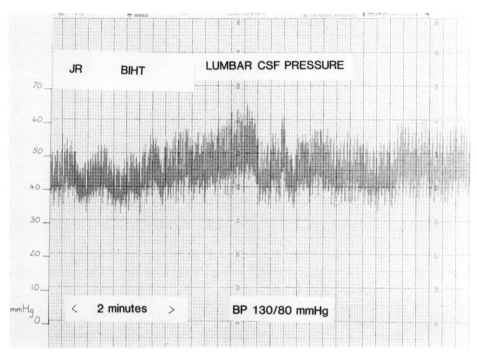

Fig. 13.5. Lumbar pressure of a grossly obese 13-year-old boy with BIHT, which did not respond to mannitol.

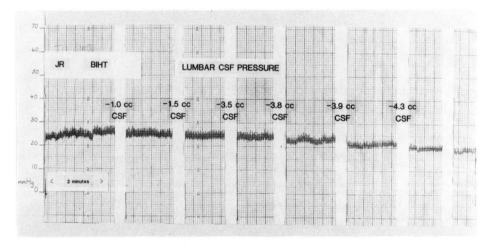

Fig. 13.6. The same patient (Case 4) responded poorly to removal of CSF, but dramatically to strict dieting measures.

analgesic/anti-emetic preparation. Examination at that time showed obese striae, papilloedema (more marked on the right), and diplopia on upward and lateral gaze. He also complained of hyperacusis. He had normal visual acuity, the CT scan proved normal, and subsequently CSF-pressure measurement at lumbar puncture showed an opening pressure of 40mmHg (Fig. 13.5). He was immediately given 20 per cent mannitol, 3 to 4ml/kg, without effect. Removal of 1ml aliquots of CSF (total of 16.5ml) resulted in slow decompression to an eventual CSF pressure of 17mmHg. His blood pressure remained at 130/80mmHg, before and after the procedure. That is, his CPP at the beginning of the recording was 57mmHg and after removal of the CSF was 80mmHg. He was commenced on dexamethasone, 2mg t.d.s., once the CSF had been examined and was found to be clear. On this admission his weight was 92.5kg. A dietician was introduced. A skull x-ray revealed no abnormalities in his mastoids, his visual evoked potentials were normal, and all subsequent virology was negative. While there was an increase in the size of his blind spot, the papilloedema showed signs of resolving within one week. The osmolality of the CSF from the first lumbar puncture was 282mmol/kg. A second lumbar puncture six days later showed an opening pressure of 25mmHg; a total of 18cc was removed on this occasion with a closing pressure of 19mmHg, and again his blood-pressure was 120/70mmHg (Fig. 13.6). The osmolality was now 269mmol/kg. His weight had not decreased and was still approximately 92kg.

Eight days after admission he had a mean transit-time estimation which showed hemispheric transit times of 13.6 and 14.3 seconds (Fig. 13.7)—symmetrically and substantially prolonged compared to the normal range of two to eight seconds. This is a sign that the cerebral perfusion reserve is reduced, but it is not known whether this reduction in cerebral perfusion reserve is due to an increase in the blood volume or a diminution in bloodflow. $PaCO_2$ at the time was 4.97 and 5.57kPa.

Re-lumbar puncture on the 10th day after admission showed pressure of 8mmHg. Dexamethasone was further reduced to 1mg on alternate days. The patient's weight had declined to 89.5kg (a decrease of 2.5kg), coinciding with this decrease in CSF pressure. An MRI scan was performed, together with T1 and T2 measurements through the corona radiata level: these were not significantly elevated (*i.e.* there was no substantial increase in brain water at this time). His blood pressure was now 110/65mmHg and $PaCO_2$ measured 5.57kPa.

Seventeen days after admission, after he had been previously discharged, he was reviewed and an opening pressure on this occasion was 12.5mmHg; 15cc of CSF was removed and his closing pressure was 10.5mmHg. Dexamethasone was stopped altogether on that day. Two days later, however, he was admitted again. He was lethargic with orbital pain, and a swollen face; his eyes were watery, he had been momementarily disoriented during the night, and was complaining of very severe

411

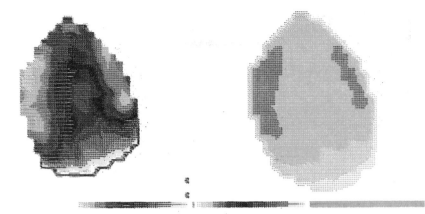

L   NETT TRANSIT TIME   R   L   FRACTIONAL FLOW   R
L 13.6+-2.2   N=157   L .07 +-.01   N=168
R 14.3+-2.2   N=122   R .07 +-.02   N=138

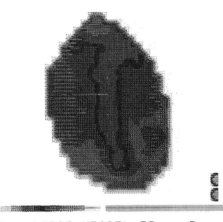

L   LARGE VESSEL TT   R
L 4.0 +-.6   N=168
R 3.9 +-.6   N=133

INPUT FUNCTION
ARRIVAL TIME 8.8 SEC.
TRANSIT TIME 8 SEC.

Fig. 13.7. Colour-coded map of same patient as in Figures 13.5 and 13.6, showing grossly prolonged hemispheric transit times.

412

headache. He also had diarrhoea, which was considered the cause for his new symptoms.

He was reviewed 29 days after the initial admission. The dexamethasone had been stopped 10 days previously. He was asymptomatic, and only the nasal margins of his optic discs were slightly blurred. His opening pressure was 21mmHg and his closing pressure was 14mmHg following removal of 22cc of CSF.

One week later (*i.e.* 36 days after the initial admission) he was again admitted because his opening pressure at lumbar puncture was 28mmHg. There was still slight blurring of his discs, but he was otherwise asymptomatic.

25cc of CSF was removed and the closing pressure was 18mmHg. CSF osmolality was 286mmol/kg, and blood pressure was 120/70mmHg. This increase in his CSF pressure appeared to be parallelled by an increase in his weight, which had again increased to 90.5kg.

Strict dieting was enforced, and he was re-started on dexamethasone 8mg/day. Seven days later his CSF pressure was 17.5mmHg and he required 7cc of CSF to be removed for the pressure to drop to 14mmHg. His blood pressure was now 115/55mmHg, but his weight had again decreased to 88.5kg. He was again discharged, asymptomatic and with a reducing steroid dosage for the next five weeks. There had been recurrence of his headaches occasionally and his weight fluctuated up to a maximum of 93.25kg, but six months after the initial admission his weight had dropped to 86kg, he was exercising, he was normotensive and had had no headaches for the preceding month. Calculation of PVI and CSF production rate (I_f) on two separate occasions in the course of this boy's acute illness with high pressure, produced variable but high values for PVI and estimated production rate above the normal range.

A 12½-year-old girl began suffering from headaches three years previously, was diagnosed as myopic, and was prescribed spectacles which she wore for one year, with apparent correction of her visual defect. She was admitted with a two-week history of headache, nausea, vomiting and abdominal pain; she had also complained of double vision for one week prior to admission. Her medical diagnostic background was non-contributory other than sub-acute asthma on exertion, for which she used a salbutamol inhaler. Examination showed her to be afebrile and not ill-looking with left occipital lymphadenopathy. She was alert and oriented, with equal, normally reacting pupils. There was mild diplopia on extreme lateral gaze and bilateral papilloedema. A CT scan was normal. **CASE 5**

There had been an additional history of trauma two weeks previously when she fell off her bike and banged her head, but retained consciousness. She had had no unusual bruising. She was overweight and pubertal in development. Her blood pressure was 120/96mmHg.

A lumbar puncture revealed an ICP of 60mmHg, although two days

413

later the lumbar CSF pressure was 12mmHg. CSF bacteriology and bio-chemistry were normal and she was treated with prednisolone. A third lumbar puncture, three weeks after the initial admission, showed a pressure of 15mmHg, and prednisolone was continued in reducing doses. The only symptom persisting was lethargy. The headache and blurred vision had abated, and the papilloedema was resolving in both eyes. There were no focal neurological signs. It was decided to treat her with steroids and therapeutic lumbar punctures when necessary.

CASE 6   This was a seven-year-old boy with a medical background of asthma, for which he had been treated for two years with salbutamol syrup (prn), beclomethasone dipropionate inhalation (200mg, four times a day) and salbutamol powder inhalation (four times a day). Three weeks before admission he developed vomiting and diarrhoea, which was managed at home with clear fluids. Following that, he had been increasingly lethargic and had complained of severe frontal headaches which sometimes woke him from sleep. He also complained of blurring of vision and 'spots' before his eyes. On the day of admission he was bright and chatty, with a normal blood pressure and pulse, and no neck stiffness. He had a full range of extra-ocular movements and full visual fields, although bilateral papil-loedema. A CT scan, done urgently, was found to be normal, and on lumbar puncture the CSF pressure was 17mmHg. He had evidence of a truncal ataxia and, following removal of CSF, there was a dramatic improvement in his general level of activity and symptoms.

One week later he had a further lumbar pressure recording, at which the opening pressure was 10mmHg, and closing pressure was 5mmHg after removal of 5cc of CSF. The papilloedema was resolving by this time and he continued on salbutamol aerosol inhalation for slight wheeze. The prolonged inhalational steroids for two years in this boy, and cessation of the steroids 19 days before admission, almost certainly contributed to precipitating his pseudotumour cerebri. All his CSF biochemistry and bacteriology were normal, including oligoclonal band studies and IgG index. His CSF showed no evidence of recent viral infection.

Few reports in the literature comment on continuous recordings of CSF pressure in benign intracranial hypertension. It may be necessary, for example with otitic hydrocephalus. On other occasions, if equivocal or normal CSF pressure levels are found, then it may be necessary to repeat the lumbar puncture.

Our cases illustrate the use of a pressure transducer: firstly at diagnosis, and at the time of lumbar puncture. It is a safe, objective method of measurement of the CSF pressure before removal of CSF. The continuous measurement of the pressure via a strain gauge transducer attached to the end of the lumbar puncture needle means that withdrawal of small amounts of CSF can be undertaken and titrated against the falling CSF pressure until normal values are reached.

In one case in our series we attempted lumbar cannulation, a procedure which has been reported previously, giving recordings for up to 24 hours. Another two cases were associated with measurement of the pressure at the cranial end, one via a ventricular catheter in a child who was treated with closed ventricular drainage, and the other by means of measurement in the cortical subarachnoid space with a subarachnoid screw. Unfortunately, this method does not allow removal of CSF at the time of intermittent abrupt elevations of pressure which are likely to occur.

The lumbar pressure method is a routine treatment-room method for measuring CSF pressure. The graphs illustrate the increase in the CSF pulse pressure as the ICP rises, indicating decreasing compliance as autoregulation fails. What is noticeable is the persistence of the increased pulse pressure after the ICP has returned to normal following removal of CSF. This suggests that poor compliance persists immediately after CSF removal. This is occasionally seen in children with malfunctioning CSF shunts, in whom the baseline pressure often returns to normal soon after CSF evacuation: but the pulse pressure remains increased in cases where there has been substantial periventricular oedema. The ventricular drainage clearly drains the ventricles first and then (because the intraventricular pressure is reduced) the brain. Our methods of measurement included the subarachnoid screw, ventricular catheter, and repeated lumbar punctures, depending upon individual cases. Repeated lumbar punctures, which permit spells of continuous monitoring, are not always acceptable even to the most co-operative patients. Insertion of a spinal catheter after the first diagnostic lumbar puncture is technically difficult, but would be an ideal method for observation of the CSF pressure measurement over a prolonged period, and calculation of CSF dynamics. Once the diagnosis has been made, and knowing that there is good communication between the ventricular and spinal compartment, CSF can be removed from either compartment safely.

The cases discussed here have been managed differently, but each illustrates the value of an immediate and, if necessary, continuous read-out of ICP. Case 1 illustrates the wide pulse pressure and the ineffectiveness of mannitol in reducing the pressure, whereas the removal of aliquots of CSF was very effective. In Case 2 the pressures were extremely high, at 80mmHg. Some of the highest intracranial pressures ever measured in adults or children have been in BIHT. It seems that the more severe and pathogenic the organism responsible for chronic otitis media and mastoiditis, the worse will be the pressure problems encountered in BIHT. The pressure problems continued in Case 2 until surgical removal of the cholesteatoma and adequate drainage. Case 3 was included to illustrate the acceptability of twice-daily lumbar punctures followed by daily, then alternate day, then weekly lumbar punctures in a seven-year-old girl. Case 4 similarly showed little effect from mannitol. The CSF removal was effective transiently, and while steroids began to resolve the papilloedema within one week, the pressure level fluctuated repeatedly for some time. At eight days into this child's treatment, a mean transit time study was excessively prolonged indicating a decreased flow reserve. That is an increase in the cerebral blood volume/cerebral bloodflow ratio. The most significant therapeutic measure reducing this child's CSF pressure was strict dieting. Case 5 showed a quick reduction of the CSF pressure from 60mmHg to normal levels within

TABLE 13.I

Summary of BIHT cases

	Case	Age (years)	Sex	Duration of symptoms	Presentation	Method of ICP measurement	Opening pressure	Management
1.	GF	6	M	3 weeks	Early-morning headache, photophobia, vomiting, malaise, intermittent diplopia, squint for 1 week, right 6th-nerve palsy, bilateral papilloedema	LP pressure and subarachnoid space measurement	40mmHg	CSF removal in aliquots
2.	KM	5	M	4 weeks	Clinical background: ataxia, developmental delay, plagiocephaly, chromosome 4P+ abnormality. Presentation: malaise, vomiting, purulent otorrhoea, squint, vomiting and drowsiness for 2 weeks, left 6th-nerve palsy, papilloedema with abnormal pallor of discs	LP pressure and ventricular catheter	80mmHg	Closed ventricular drainage and steroids
3.	VK	7	F	2 weeks	Minor blow to the head, 2 days diplopia and squint, bilateral papilloedema, bilateral 6th-nerve palsy, scalp veins distended	LP	45mmHg	Daily lumbar punctures, steroids, and acetazolamide
4.	JR	13	M	7 weeks	Headache, vomiting, otitis media, obesity, pains in the arm, neck and back, lethargy, paraesthesia, hyperacusis, bilateral papilloedema and diplopia	LP pressure	40mmHg	CSF removal, steroids and dieting
5.	LF	12.5	F	2 weeks	Minor blow to the head, headache, vomiting, diplopia, drowsiness, photophobia, pyrexia, occipital lymphadenopathy, bilateral papilloedema, diplopia to the right	LP pressure	60mmHg	CSF removal via LPs and steroids
6.	GW	7	M	3 weeks	Diarrhoea and vomiting 3 weeks prior to admission, previous asthmatic, on inhalational steroids for 2 years, stopped 3 weeks prior to admission, bilateral papilloedema	LP pressure	17mmHg	CSF removal, steroids

48 hours following the initial CSF removal. Case 6 developed his BIHT following inhalational steroids, which had been withdrawn after a two-year period. It is known from the literature that cases of BIHT have been reported following withdrawal of topical steroid, but to my knowledge not from inhalational steroid withdrawal (see Table 13.I for a summary of the cases).

Pathogenesis
There is no totally satisfactory explanation for RICP in benign intracranial hypertension, nor for the relationship between the RICP and the aetiological agents which have so far been recognised. The absence of ventricular dilatation has been a particularly difficult feature to explain. It is possible that some of the studies on the pathogenesis of BIHT may well have been conducted while the patients were on treatment (such as steroids) and the finding of abnormalities (such as an increased size of the subarachnoid space or decreased CSF absorption) may well have been confirming the known effects of the steroids. Some of the theories of pathogenesis are outlined below in brief, and this is followed by a new hypothesis based on the known experimental findings so far reported.

Endocrine factors have long been suggested in the pathogenesis in view of the female preponderance in this condition. However, the studies measuring plasma steroid and oestrogen have not confirmed any abnormalities of a primary endocrinological nature.

Several investigators have found evidence of increased CBV. Raichle *et al.* (1978) found a 33 per cent rise in the CBV and they suggested this was in the venules and smaller capillaries which were not seen on CT scan. There was no suggestion why the CBV should be increased, and a 33 per cent rise of CBV would account for a 1 per cent rise in intracranial volume, and probably insufficient to be responsible for the substantially raised ICP. The authors also considered that a *diffuse brain-swelling* in the form of parenchymal water also occurred. Since then, PET scan evidence of an increased CBV and brain water content has been confirmed, and intra- and extracellular brain oedema found at biopsy of 10 patients with BIHT (Sahs and Joynt 1956). The ventricular volume is significantly reduced on CT scan in patients with BIHT compared to controls (Reid *et al.* 1980).

Boeri *et al.* (1981) speculated that the increased CBV was due to an *increase in venous pressure* from one cause or another, and that this increased venous pressure prevented normal absorption of CSF through the arachnoid villi.

Donaldson (1981) believed that there was an *increased CSF secretion* and that this was the prime abnormality in obese young females. His finding of increased CSF oestrone in fat cells and in the CSF led to this belief, although the precise effects of oestrone on the CSF production rate is not known. Because of the presence of large amounts of retinol-binding prealbumin in the choroid plexus and in the ventricular fluid, it has been speculated that vitamin A overdosage causes BIHT by increasing CSF production.

A *disturbance of the venous pulse valve* between the intracranial sinuses and the jugular venous bulb has been postulated. In these cases, the CT scan may show a large sinus rectus confluens and venous congestion. Disturbance of this valve by stenosis may occur after chronic otitis media because of the close anatomical contact between the inner ear and the jugular bulb.

Perhaps the most popular of the various theories has been that of *decreased CSF absorption* (Bercaw and Greer 1970, Johnston and Paterson 1974*b*). At first it was thought that the decreased CSF absorption was due to unrecognised dural sinus thrombosis resulting in decreased CSF production and absorption; later it became obvious that there were far too many cases of BIHT without obvious dural sinus thrombosis for this to be the reason in all patients. Johnston and Paterson (1974*b*), following their study with isotope cisternograms and ventriculograms, showed a delay in the CSF circulation with holdup of isotope in the subarachnoid space, and postulated that the cause of the RICP was due to an increased CSF volume from delayed CSF absorption, which in turn could have been due to one of two mechanisms: either an increased *resistance to flow across the arachnoid villi* or a *reduction in the pressure gradient* from an increase in the pressure in the superior sagittal sinus (P_{SSS}) between the subarachnoid space and the superior sagittal sinus. Such a delayed absorption would result, they felt, in CSF production rate at less than the normal rate, but still an increased CSF volume and distensibility of the subarachnoid space, which is often claimed to occur. Approximately half were noted to have a markedly distended subarachnoid space.

Their theory was supported by (i) the decreased CSF absorption which they measured; (ii) the seeming ease with which CSF is removed in this condition, indicating increased CSF volume; (iii) periods of normal ICP followed by a build-up of pressure; (iv) the free communication between lumbar and cerebral CSF; (v) their estimated CSF production rate being below the normal range; and (vi) the increased resistance to CSF absorption with a decreased CSF bulk flow, which had been previously reported with intra-thecal infusion tests. Evidence against this theory of decreased CSF absorption is the brain oedema which has been found, and the well-being of the patient with very high levels of RICP, together with the increase in CBV which has been unequivocally demonstrated.

In trying to explain the absence of ventricular dilatation they claim that CSF, added to a freely communicating cistern, would be accommodated within the subarachnoid space (SAS) and not result in ventricular dilatation. Their view of BIHT as a CSF-absorption syndrome was formulated as follows:

$$\text{Flow across villi} \propto \frac{P_{SAS} - P_{SSS}}{R_{AV}}$$

Decreased absorption, therefore, might be due to an increased pressure within the sagittal sinus, *e.g.* from middle-ear disease, extracranial venous obstruction, or an increase in resistance across the villi due to altered vitamin A levels, steroid function and tetracyclines (Sklar *et al.* 1979, Janny *et al.* 1981).

RICP from other causes will result in an increase in the P_{SSS}, but removal of CSF can cause the CSF pressure to fall to zero although the P_{SSS} will not fall below the JVP (about 5mmHg), *i.e.* there is a reversible collapse of the sigmoid sinus due to RICP. Sainte-Rose *et al.* (1984) found that in achondroplasia or craniosynostosis removal of the CSF will cause the CSF pressure to fall, but the P_{SSS} remains elevated above the JVP. They postulated, therefore, that a *fixed obstructive lesion in or about the sinuses* could be repsonsible, and this may be one of the mechanisms in BIHT where there is associated venous sinus malformation.

Haar and Miller (1975) reviewed the literature of cases of dural sinus hypertension. Some of these cases were associated with hydrocephalus and others with a BIHT picture. Those that were associated with hydrocephalus had a generalised increase in the venous sinus pressure and they postulated that there was absent venous cushioning of the choroid plexus arterial pulse wave with consequent hydrocephalus. By contrast those with a BIHT syndrome had *normal pressure in some of the intracranial venous structures.* Bering (1955) had noted earlier that the arterial pulse wave is normally transmitted to the CSF, but is cushioned by the intracranial venous system. In a later study on experimental animals subjected to bilateral jugular/vertebral obliteration, he found dural sinus hypertension and hydrocephalus in 75 per cent of the cases (Bering and Salibi 1959).

Junck (1985) advanced the theory of *abnormal collapsibility of the dural venous sinuses* operating under a pressure gradient. Normally the P_{CSF} is $< P_{SSS}$. Partial collapse of the sinuses increases resistance which increases the P_{SSS} and further increases the P_{CSF}, with collapse of the venous sinuses. Apart from the well recognised cases of lateral sinus thrombosis, no site of obstruction is regularly found in the dural sinuses in most cases of BIHT and one therefore still needs a hypothesis to explain the increased P_{SSS}. He considered that an increase in the CSF flow or an increase in the resistance across the arachnoid villi might precipitate BIHT in susceptible patients with an underlying weakness in the sinus walls.

Hypothesis

We postulate that the defect in BIHT is on the venous side of the circuit, and that it is essentially a vasoparalysis. This hypothesis is supported by the known anatomical and experimentally confirmed findings of:

(1) An increase in the venous sinus pressure ($P_{SSS} = P_{CSF}$)

(2) A decreased CSF absorption

(3) An increase in the CBV

(4) Small volume compressed ventricles and an increase in brain water

(5) Sluggish CSF circulation and poor CSF bulk flow

(6) Diminished or increased CSF production

(7) An absence of muscles or valves in the sinuses

(8) The presence of dilatations of sinusoidal plexuses at the junction of the great cerebral vein and the straight sinus (and other sites) which exert a ball-valve control over the outflow from the great cerebral vein (and hence the internal cerebral, choroidal, and thalamostriate veins)

(9) Achondroplasia or craniosynostosis (fixed obstructive lesion of the sinuses) results in hydrocephalus

(10) Ligation or obliteration of bilateral jugular and vertebral veins results in dural sinus hypertension and hydrocephalus in 75 per cent of the cases.

If there is a vasoparalysis then it is possible to fit these observations to a holistic theory of BIHT which incorporates an explanation for the two most difficult questions: the cause for the dural sinus hypertension, and the absence of ventricular dilatation in BIHT.

In BIHT vasoparalysis of the cerebral veins (because there is no muscle in the sinuses) results in pooling of venous blood, until the capacitance is exhausted, when an increase in the cerebral venous and venous sinus pressure, and cerebral venous blood volume will result. The sinusoidal projections into the great cerebral vein become engorged and exert a ball-valve protection over the drainage from the internal cerebral and choroidal veins. The pressures in these deep internal venous structures are normal. The P_{SSS} will equal the P_{CSF} and there will be a secondary decrease in CSF absorption with a consequent increase in CSF pressure. The arterial pulsation in CSF will be buffeted by the normal venous pressure in the choroidal veins and ventricular dilatation will not occur. This increase in CSF volume and decreased CSF absorption and decreased bulk flow will result in transependymal migration of CSF into the brain white matter with resultant hydrostatic brain oedema. Other cerebral venous congestions result in small compressed ventricles on CT scan, *e.g.* cyanotic congenital heart disease and fibrocystic disease.

In obstructive conditions of the venous sinuses without vasoparalysis then the more *proximal obstructions* (superior sagittal sinus or lateral sinus) are likely to result in a BIHT picture. The venous sinus pressure will increase proximally and there will be the same secondary decrease of CSF absorption, increase in CSF pressure and volume, and decreased CSF flow. The drainage from the deep venous sinuses will be protected from the retrograde pressure and will thus be able to cushion subsequent increases in the arterial pulse of the CSF.

Obstructive conditions more distal without vasoparalysis (superior vena cava or jugular) will result in such a massive increase in venous sinus pressure that the ball-valve operation will be overcome with a build-up of pressure in the internal cerebral veins and a lack of buffering of the arterial CSF pulse wave and consequent ventricular dilatation. The obstruction will result in a massive retrograde pressure to the arterial side of the circuit with an increase in CSF production and no impediment to the ventricular dilatation.

Exactly how the known aetiologies affect the venous circuit is more conjectural. In otherwise normal individuals, treatment with prolonged steroids would interfere with absorption of villi and increase capacitance (venous), the gradient across the villi will be only slightly reduced and a secondary brain atrophy will occur with ventricular dilatation. Children taking prolonged steroids for leukaemia invariably show atrophy on their CT scan (Fig. 13.8). Steroid withdrawal, however, would have the opposite effect and, because of the decreased elastance within the venous system, be responsible for BIHT. Chronic otitis media and mastoiditis may well have an associated phlebothrombosis in the great veins adjacent to the jugular bulb, and certainly lateral sinus thrombosis or obstruction is one unequivocal mechanism for BIHT. Head injury and jugular vein injury may act in the same way (Fig. 13.9).

Treatment

Because BIHT is largely a self-limiting condition, the effectiveness of therapy is

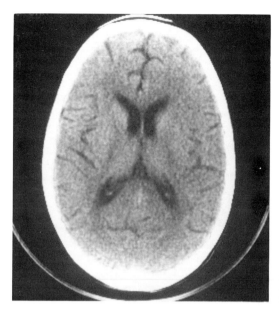

Fig. 13.8. CT scan of child being treated with long-term steroids on account of leukemia, showing significant cerebral atrophy.

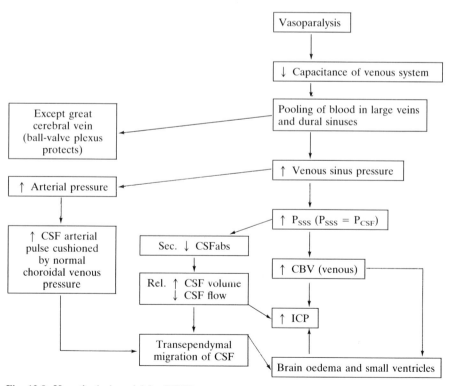

Fig. 13.9. Hypothetical model for BIHT.

difficult to evaluate and there have not been any controlled studies on the various treatments available.

REPEATED LUMBAR PUNCTURES WITH CSF REMOVAL
In the Weisberg (1975) series, 25 per cent of patients remitted after the first diagnostic lumbar puncture. Initially the lumbar puncture may have to be done daily, and thereafter at increasing intervals. About a third of all patients respond to this method of treatment alone.

STEROIDS
These were used first by Paterson *et al.* (1961) and Weisberg (1975), but again there has been no properly controlled evaluation of them. It is claimed that the pressure drops to normal within 24 hours of institution of steroids in most cases.

ORAL ACETAZOLAMIDE
Acetazolamide in a dose of 500mg b.d. is frequently reserved for patients who fail to have an adequate response to steroids. The effect is to block carbonic anhydrase in the choroidal villi and cause a decreased CSF production. But it is only effective in far greater doses than those required to suppress aqueous formation in the eye. The failure to use large doses may explain why so many cases do not respond to acetazolamide; alternatively, over-secretion may not play any part in the aetiology (see above).

DIURETIC AND ACETAZOLAMIDE
Sorenson *et al.* (1988) had success in controlling symptoms with this combination in most patients. In a prospective study of 24 patients, they found that steroids were ineffective where this combination had failed. Long-term diuretics will mean that hypokalaemia is a distinct possibility.

LUMBO-PERITONEAL OR VENTRICULO-PERITONEAL SHUNT
Most people use a theco- or lumbo-peritoneal shunt for patients with failed medical treatment. This treatment bypasses the fundamental problem, but reduces intraventricular pressure and relieves symptoms and the papilloedema. In our study, six out of 23 children required surgical treatment (Amacher and Spence 1985). The later development of low-pressure headache prompted the removal of the shunt in three patients, without recurrence of symptoms, and presumably their low-pressure headaches signalled the disappearance of benign intracranial hypertension. Gucer and Viernstein (1978), in three patients who had lumbo-peritoneal shunts, found that all three developed shunt malfunctions with a slow progressive increase in the measured ICP when the shunts malfunctioned. Apart from shunt malfunction with blockage, and spinal meningitis, other complications of lumbo-peritoneal shunts may also occur: hyperlordosis of spine, over-drainage with possible spinal stenosis, and acute non-communication from an intercurrent illness such as mumps meningitis (or aqueductitis) with serious compartmental pressure differences.

OPTIC NERVE DECOMPRESSION

Kaye *et al.* (1981) decompressed the optic nerve and found symptomatic relief and reversal of visual loss, without any effect on the RICP. The rationale here is to treat the target organ which is most at risk in this condition.

SYSTEMIC BLOOD-PRESSURE REDUCTION

In a series by Corbett *et al.* (1982) the single most important risk factor for visual loss in patients with pseudotumour cerebri was systemic hypertension. Judicious use of systemic blood-pressure reduction may be required.

ORAL GLYCEROL

In a dose of 15 to 60g, four to six times a day, this has been used by some investigators as an adjunct to steroid therapy, although its side-effects would preclude its use from most cases.

DIETARY CONTROL

Strict dietary control and weight reduction may be advised in obese patients.

In monitoring the effectiveness of treatment one should serially measure the blind-spot enlargement (Jefferson and Clark 1976), as well as visual evoked potential latencies and lumbar punctures if there is recurrence of symptoms.

Recurrence and prognosis

BIHT is nearly always self-limiting and has good long-term prognosis for most patients. The recurrence rate has been suggested at between 1 and 37 per cent (Lysak and Svien 1966, Guidetti *et al.* 1968, Boddie *et al.* 1974, Johnston and Paterson 1974*a*, Weisberg 1975, Rush 1980, Rousseaux *et al.* 1985). The incidence of permanent visual loss has been variously reported in different series from 2 to 50 per cent (Symonds 1956, Boddie *et al.* 1974, Weisberg 1975, Bulens *et al.* 1979, Rush 1980, Corbett *et al.* 1982). Of 124 patients retrospectively analysed, 24 developed some other related illness after the signs and symptoms of BIHT had resolved, *e.g.* fits, cerebrovascular disease, meningitis, diabetes mellitus, Simmonds' disease and other conditions (Johnston and Paterson 1974*a*).

REFERENCES

Adson, A. W. (1924) 'Pseudobrain abscess.' *Surgical Clinics of North America*, **4**, 503–512.
Amacher, A. L., Spence, J. D. (1985) 'Spectrum of benign intracranial hypertension in children and adolescents.' *Child's Nervous System*, **1**, 81–86.
Bercaw, B. L., Greer, M. (1970) 'Transport of intrathecal ^{131}I RISA in benign intracranial hypertension.' *Neurology*, **20**, 787–790.
Bering, E. A. Jr. (1955) 'Choroid plexus and arterial pulsation of cerebrospinal fluid. Demonstration of the choroid plexuses as a cerebrospinal fluid pump.' *Archives of Neurology and Psychiatry*, **73**, 165–172.
—— Salibi, B. (1959) 'Production of hydrocephalus by increased cephalic-venous pressure.' *Archives of Neurology and Psychiatry*, **81**, 693–698.
Boddie, H. G., Banna, M., Bradley, W. G. (1974) '"Benign" intracranial hypertension: a survey of the

clinical and radiological features and long-term prognosis.' *Brain*, **97**, 313–326.

Boeri, R., Grottaglie, G. D., Tagliabue, G. (1981) 'Pathogenesis of cerebral pseudotumors: report of 54 cases'. *Neuro-ophthalmologie*, **1**, 199–202.

Bulens, C., De Vries, W. A. E. J., Van Crevel, H. (1979) 'Benign intracranial hypertension. A retrospective and follow-up study.' *Journal of the Neurological Sciences*, **40**, 147–157.

Corbett, J. J., Savino, P. J., Thompson, H. S., Kansu, T., Schatz, M. J., Orr, L. S., Hopson, D. (1982) 'Visual loss in pseudotumor cerebri: follow-up of 57 patients from 5 to 41 years and a profile of 14 patients with severe visual loss.' *Archives of Neurology*, **39**, 461–474.

—— Mehta, M. P. (1983) 'Cerebrospinal fluid pressure in normal obese subjects and patients with pseudotumour cerebri.' *Neurology*, **33**, 1386–1388.

Dandy, W. E. (1937) 'Intracranial pressure without brain tumour, diagnosis and treatment.' *American Surgeon*, **106**, 492–513.

Davidoff, L. M., Dyke, C. G. (1937) 'Hypertensive meningeal hydrops: syndrome frequently following infection in middle ear or elsewhere in the body.' *American Journal of Ophthalmology*, **20**, 908–927.

Dersh, J., Schlezinger, N. S. (1959) 'Inferior nasal quadrantanopia in pseudotumour cerebri.' *Transactions of the American Neurological Association*, **84**, 116–118.

Donaldson, J. O. (1981) 'Pathogenesis of pseudotumour cerebri syndromes.' *Neurology*, **31**, 877–880.

Foley, J. (1955) 'Benign forms of intracranial hypertension—"toxic" and "otitic" hydrocephalus.' *Brain*, **78**, 1–41.

Foley, K. M. (1977) 'Is benign intracranial hypertension a chronic disease?' *Neurology*, **27**, 388. *(Abstract.)*

Gilman, J. K., Smith, C. G., Davis, C. E., Hibri, N. (1983) 'Benign intracranial hypertension, monoclonal gammopathy, and superior sagittal sinus thrombosis.' *Southern Medical Journal*, **76**, 658–660.

Grant, D. N. (1971) 'Benign intracranial hypertension. A review of 79 cases in infancy and childhood.' *Archives of Disease in Childhood*, **46**, 651–655.

Green, G. J., Lessell, S., Lowenstein, J. I. (1980) 'Ischemic optic neuropathy in chronic papilledema.' *Archives of Ophthalmology*, **98**, 502–504.

Gucer, G., Viernstein, L. (1978) 'Long-term intracranial pressure recording in the management of pseudotumour cerebri.' *Journal of Neurosurgery*, **49**, 256–263.

Guidetti, B., Giuffre, R., Gambascosta, D. (1968) 'Follow-up study of 100 cases of pseudotumour cerebri.' *Acta Neurochirurgica*, **18**, 256–267.

Haar, F. L., Miller, C. A. (1975) 'Hydrocephalus resulting from superior vena cava thrombosis in an infant: case report.' *Journal of Neurosurgery*, **42**, 597–601.

Janny, P., Chazal, J., Colnet, G., Irthum, B., Georget, A.–M. (1981) 'Benign intracranial hypertension and disorders of CSF absorption.' *Surgical Neurology*, **15**, 168–174.

Jefferson, A., Clark, J. (1976) 'Treatment of benign intracranial hypertension by dehydrating agents with particular reference to the measurement of the blind spot area as a means of recording improvement.' *Journal of Neurology, Neurosurgery and Psychiatry*, **39**, 627–639.

Johnston, I., Paterson, A. (1974) 'Benign intracranial hypertension. I: Diagnosis and prognosis.' *Brain*, **97**, 289–300.

—— —— (1974*b*) 'Benign intracranial hypertension. II: CSF pressure and circulation.' *Brain*, **97**, 301–312.

Junck, L. (1985) 'Benign intracranial hypertension and normal pressure hydrocephalus: theoretical considerations.' *In* Miller, J. D., Teasdale, G. M., Rowan, J. O., Galbraith, S. L., Mendelow, A. D. (Eds.) *Intracranial Pressure, Vol VI*. Berlin: Springer. pp. 447–450.

Kaye, A. H., Galbraith, J. E. K., King, J. (1981) 'Intracranial pressure following optic nerve decompression for benign intracranial hypertension.' *Journal of Neurosurgery*, **55**, 453–456.

Klein, D. (1978) 'Pseudotumor cerebri. Untersuchung zu Krankheitbild und Krankheitsverlauf sowie zur Frage nach verschiedenen Erscheinungsformen.' *Medical Faculty, Dissertation*, University of Köln.

Klosterkotter, J. (1982) 'Pseudotumour cerebri mit psychischen Störungen und ungünstiger Prognose.' *Nervenarzt*, **53**, 411–413.

Langfitt, T. W., Kassell, N. F., Weinstein, J. D. (1965) 'Cerebral blood flow with intracranial hypertension.' *Neurology*, **15**, 761–773.

Lipton, H. L., Michelson, P. E. (1972) 'Pseudotumor cerebri syndrome without papilledema.' *Journal of the American Medical Association*, **220**, 1591–1592.

Lysak, W. R., Svien, H. J. (1966) 'Long-term follow-up on patients with diagnosis of pseudotumor cerebri.' *Journal of Neurosurgery*, **25**, 284–287.

McAlpine, D. (1937) 'Toxic hydrocephalus.' *Brain*, **60**, 180–203.

McCammon, A., Kaufman, H. H., Sears, E. S. (1981) 'Transient oculomotor paralysis in pseudotumor cerebri.' *Neurology*, **31**, 182–184.

Paterson, R., DePasquale, N., Mann, S. (1961) 'Pseudotumour cerebri.' *Medicine*, **40**, 85–99.

Quincke, H. (1897) 'Ueber meningitis serosa und verwandte Zustände.' *Deutsche Zeitschrift für Nervenheilkunde*, **9**, 149–168.

Rabinowicz, I. M., Ben-Sira, I., Zauberman, H. (1968) 'Preservation of visual function in papilloedema: observed for 3 to 6 years in cases of benign intracranial hypertension.' *British Journal of Ophthalmology*, **52**, 236–241.

Raichle, M. E., Grubb, R. L., Phelps, M. E., Gado, M. H., Caronna, J. J. (1978) 'Cerebral hemodynamics and metabolism in pseudotumor cerebri.' *Annals of Neurology*, **4**, 104–111.

Reid, A. C., Matheson, M. S., Teasdale, G. (1980) 'Volume of the ventricules in benign intracranial hypertension.' *Lancet*, **2**, 7–8.

—— Teasdale, G. M., Matheson, M. S., Teasdale, E. M. (1981) 'Serial ventricular volume measurements: further insights into the etiology and pathogenesis of benign intracranial hypertension.' *Journal of Neurology, Neurosurgery and Psychiatry*, **44**, 636–640.

Rothner, A. D., Brust, J. C. (1974) 'Pseudotumour cerebri: report of a familial occurrence.' *Archives of Neurology*, **30**, 110–111.

Rousseaux, P., Vieillart, A., Scherpereel, B., Bernard, M. H., Motte, J., Guyot, J. F. (1985) 'Hypertension intracranienne benigne (17 cas) et thromboses veineuses cérébrales (49 cas).' *Neurochirurgie*, **31**, 381–389.

Rush, J. A. (1980) 'Pseudotumour cerebri: clinical profile and visual outcome in 63 patients.' *Mayo Clinic Proceedings*, **55**, 541–546.

—— (1983) 'Pseudo problems, pseudotumour cerebri.' *British Journal of Hospital Medicine*, **29**, 320–325.

Sahs, A. L., Hyndman, O. R. (1939) 'Intracranial hypertension of unknown cause: cerebral edema.' *Archives of Surgery*, **38**, 429–434.

—— Joynt, R. J. (1956) 'Brain swelling of unknown cause.' *Neurology*, **6**, 791–803.

Sainte-Rose, C., La Combe, J., Pierre-Kahn, A., Renier, D., Hirsch, J. F. (1984) 'Intracranial venous sinus hypertension: cause or consequence of hydrocephalus in infants.' *Journal of Neurosurgery*, **60**, 727–736.

Scanarini, M., Mingrino, S., d'Avella, D., Della Corte, V. (1979) 'Benign intracranial hypertension without papilledema: case report.' *Neurosurgery*, **5**, 376–377.

Sklar, F. H., Beyer, C. W., Ramanathan, M., Cooper, P. R., Clark, W. K. (1979) 'Cerebrospinal fluid dynamics in patients with pseudotumor cerebri.' *Neurosurgery*, **5**, 208–215.

Smith, J. L. (1958) 'Pseudotumor cerebri.' *Transactions of the American Academy of Ophthalmology and Otolaryngology*, **62**, 432–440.

Sorenson, P. S., Krogsaa, F., Gjerris, F. (1988) 'Clinical course and prognosis of pseudotumour cerebri. A prospective study of 24 patients.' *Acta Neurologica Scandinavica*, **77**, 164–172.

Symonds, C. P. (1931) 'Otitic hydrocephalus.' *Brain*, **54**, 55–71.

—— (1956) 'Otitic hydrocephalus.' *Neurology*, **6**, 681–685.

Troost, B. T., Sufit, R. L., Grand, M. G. (1979) 'Sudden monocular visual loss in pseudotumor cerebri.' *Archives of Neurology*, **36**, 440–442.

Warrington, W. B. (1914) 'Intracranial serous effusions of inflammatory origin: meningitis or ependymitis serosa-meningism with a note on "pseudo-tumours" of brain.' *Quarterly Journal of Medicine*, **7**, 93–116.

Weisberg, L. A. (1975) 'Benign intracranial hypertension.' *Medicine*, **54**, 197–207.

Yaskin, J. C., Groff, R. A., Shenkin, H. A. (1949) 'Severe bilateral papilledema of indeterminate etiology with report of 12 cases.' *Confinia Neurologia*, **9**, 108–112.

425

14

BRAIN DAMAGE AND RAISED INTRACRANIAL PRESSURE— BIOCHEMICAL AND NEUROPHYSIOLOGICAL PARAMETERS

Neville R. Belton

Chemical analysis of CSF constituents has been undertaken primarily to learn more about brain metabolism, and in the hope that it will help in the diagnosis and treatment of neurological disorders. There are, however, few studies in which ICP has been related to changes in CSF constituents. In part this is probably because the measurement of ICP has not been routine, although clinical signs have been used for much longer to diagnose the presence of raised ICP. With recent improvements in equipment design and electronics, enabling continuous monitoring of ICP in children, it is likely that biochemical changes in the CSF may be related directly to alterations in ICP. Mann and Punt (1986) indicated some of the conditions in which ICP monitoring may be beneficial (Table 14.I). All these conditions are either metabolic in origin, or involve profound metabolic changes in the brain: and these changes may be reflected in the CSF. Chapters 1 and 2 of this volume indicate more fully the causes and mechanisms of RICP.

Loss of homeostasis is caused by such important events as changes in CBF, metabolic acidosis in the brain, extracellular acidosis, decreased CSF pH secondary to hypoxia or hypercapnia, and accumulation of intracellular sodium and water leading to tissue oedema, and these changes may be reflected in concentrations of various constituents of the CSF. Some of the differences already measured in CSF constituents have been related to hypoxia or asphyxia, and these events may be secondary to existing RICP or may be part of the pathogenesis of subsequent increases in ICP.

This chapter will examine evidence of brain damage in a variety of clinical conditions, as the results may have implications for the development and therapy of RICP, even though increased pressure may not have been measured and RICP may not have been identified as a clinical symptom.

Sampling

Accurate clinical evaluations of CSF data require close attention to sampling methodology and appropriate storage to ensure stability of the sample constituents. Sampling times may be important, as circadian rhythms have been identified in the CSF concentrations of catecholamines, monoamine metabolites, cyclic adenosine monophosphate (CAMP) and gamma-aminobutyric acid (GABA) (Ziegler *et al.* 1976,

426

TABLE 14.I

Conditions in which ICP monitoring may be beneficial

Severe head injury
Reye's syndrome
Acute encephalopathies (viral/idiopathic)
Lead encephalopathy
Burns encephalopathy
Severe perinatal asphyxia
Hepatic coma
Cerebral oedema in diabetes — following profound hypoglycaemia
                                      — as a complication of ketoacidosis
Near drowning
Post-craniotomy
Hydrocephalus

Perlow and Lake 1980), ventriculo-spinal gradients for CSF neurotransmitters and their metabolites, ions and some peptides (Luerssen and Robertson 1980, Wood 1980); and several studies have shown considerable variations in total protein along the neuraxis showing the lowest values in the ventricles, intermediate concentrations in the cisterna magna, and the highest figures for lumbar fluid (Hill *et al.* 1958, Hunter and Smith 1960, Weisner and Bernhardt 1978). CSF composition and gradients are changed by obstruction of CSF circulation, as in hydrocephalus (Anderson and Roos 1969), and by spinal canal blockage, *i.e.* by tumour (Post *et al.* 1973).

pH, organic acids, electrolytes and other ions

CSF acid-base parameters were reviewed by Rossandra and Sganzerla (1976), who considered that CSF pH is normally less than arterial plasma by 0.06 to 0.1 units, and that this difference is caused by greater PCO_2 in the CSF, with the bicarbonate concentration being approximately the same in CSF and plasma. In lumbar CSF, the pH is less by 0.02 to 0.04 units, and the PCO_2 greater by 3 to 4mmHg than in the cisternal fluid (Van Heist *et al.* 1966, Plum and Price 1973). Similar observations have been made in infants (Krauss *et al.* 1972). These relationships may be lost in critically ill patients (Plum and Price 1973, Kalin *et al.* 1975). In studies on infants with gastroenteritis, dehydration and resulting metabolic acidosis, Horovitz *et al.* (1985) found five out of 21 infants with neurological signs and symptoms (coma, convulsions or both) associated with CSF acid-base disequilibrium (mean CSF pH 7.24, PCO_2 30.8mmHg and bicarbonate 13.8mmol/l). Kalin *et al.* (1975) found that during acute anoxia of the CNS, the lumbar-cisternal pH difference was reversed with a more profound respiratory and metabolic acidosis in the cisternal CSF. They also found, however, that the normal milieu was rapidly established after resuscitation. Lumbar CSF should not be used as a reliable index of cerebral acid-base state, especially in patients with acute circulatory imbalance (Plum and Price 1973).

Organic acids

Lactate production in the CSF has been shown by Kjallquist *et al.* (1969) to be increased at very low arterial PCO_2, *i.e.* at alkaline blood pH, indicating that lactic acid can contribute some 4 to 5mmol/l to the buffer-base of the CSF. However,

427

because lactate and pyruvate are freely diffusible through most cell membranes, their measurement in the CSF and the calculation of lactate/pyruvate ratios has been widely used as an index of cerebral hypoxia. High lactate concentrations or an increased lactate/pyruvate ratio were proposed by Siesjo and Plum (1971) as indicative of impairment of cerebral oxidative metabolism, and to reflect the cytoplasmic NADH/NAD$^+$ system in brain cells.

Early studies tended to confirm this hypothesis (Svenningsen and Siesjo 1972). Simpson et al. (1977) suggested that on the basis of observations of high CSF lactate concentrations and high lactate/pyruvate ratios, cerebral hypoxia and possible brain damage might be a hazard of prolonged or rapidly recurring short convulsions in children. It may be inferred from the experimental work of Wasterlain and Plum (1973) and Wasterlain (1976) in immature rats, and of Myers et al. (1969) in monkeys, that the immature brain is particularly vulnerable to convulsive hypoxia and early asphyxia. Certainly McGuinness et al. (1983) have shown higher CSF lactate concentrations in normal neonates than in older children and adults. Similarly Mathew et al. (1980) showed elevated lactate concentrations in non-asphyxiated newborns, particularly in the first eight hours of life, and even higher values in asphyxiated neonates. Vannucci et al. (1980) found ventricular fluid lactate concentrations were increased almost twofold in infants with post-haemorrhagic obstructive hydrocephalus compared with those with congenital (non-haemorrhagic) obstructive hydrocephalus. However, there was no significant correlation between the lactate concentrations and ICP measured at the time of sampling.

In adults, Edgren et al. (1987) showed a good negative correlation between CSF lactate at 24 hours following cardiac arrest, with subsequent hypoxic ischaemic coma and a good outcome. CSF lactate has been proposed as a diagnostic and prognostic indicator for bacterial meningitis ever since Levinson (1917) observed low pH values in the CSF of patients with bacterial meningitis, believing that this was due to lactic acid; Killion (1925) showed that CSF lactate was elevated in bacterial meningitis. Eross et al. (1981), in their review of the literature, suggested that CSF lactate concentrations below 3.0mmol/l may be considered neurologically safe, while values above 4.0mmol/l are found in life-threatening states in which survival may lead to permanent neurological damage.

Pyruvate estimated on its own does not appear to be a valuable CSF investigation, and it is doubtful whether measurement of the lactate/pyruvate ratio is any more useful than that of the CSF lactate itself. Studies on CSF citrate (Martensson and Thunberg 1951) and acetate have not shown such estimates to have any pathological significance or therapeutic benefit.

Sodium, osmolality and water
Persistent disturbance of homeostasis in the extracellular fluid, evidenced by alterations in the plasma concentration of sodium in the CSF or by abnormal osmolality results, has long been recognised as deleterious to brain metabolism and function. The sodium-potassium pump, which is modulated by sodium-potassium-adenosine triphosphatase (NA-K-ATPase) within the choroid plexus epithelial cell,

moves sodium across the cell into the CSF. Water appears to migrate via the osmotic gradient established by the active sodium secretion. This process is dependent on the supply of protons from the hydration of carbon dioxide, as sodium enters the epithelial cell in exchange for hydrogen ions. This is illustrated by the reduction of CSF secretion by carbonic anhydrase inhibitors.

In humans, following an acute increase in plasma osmolality, it may take approximately four hours for a similar change to be seen in the CSF (Belton and Brown 1979).

Mannery and Bale (1941) and Forbes and Perley (1951) showed that there was a delay in the equilibration of ^{22}Na between serum and CSF, although the concentration of sodium in the CSF approaches that in serum water more rapidly. Thus migration of water from CSF occurs more quickly than entry of sodium, and osmotic equilibrium is achieved before equilibrium of sodium has occurred. This is confirmed by experimental studies by Finberg et al. (1959). Kravath et al. (1970) showed experimentally in cats that the rapid intravenous injection of hypertonic solutions caused rapid changes in CSF pressure and could cause intracranial haemorrhage.

Simmons et al. (1974) suggested that excessive sodium bicarbonate administration to newborns (>8mmol/kg/day) could increase the likelihood of intracranial haemorrhage. Anderson et al. (1976) did not agree that sodium bicarbonate therapy played a major role in the pathogenesis of IVH.

Hypernatraemic dehydration due to high solute load in young infants has been widely observed and documented, but there are no data on whether there were changes in CSF pressure or composition.

RICP may occur in the asphyxiated neonate for a variety of reasons, including a space-occupying blood clot, cerebral congestion due to high PCO_2, excess CSF production and oedema of the brain (Brown 1976).

Cerebral oedema, e.g. from water intoxication (Brown and Habel 1975), increases brain volume and this may or may not increase ICP. A study by Anderson and Belton (1974) confirmed that many infants who were severely asphyxiated at birth and subsequently showed clinical signs of cerebral irritation, had at autopsy marked electrolyte disturbances including decreased potassium and increased sodium in the brain. The syndrome of inappropriate antidiuretic hormone secretion (SIADH) with hyponatraemia, low plasma osmolality and high urine osmolality, has been described in neonates and young infants (Feldman et al. 1970, Nolph and Schrier 1970, David et al. 1981). The definitive mechanism of SIADH and its relevance to water intoxication remains unclear.

Both hypernatraemia and hyponatraemia have been extensively seen in children suffering from dehydration. There is evidence that the extracellular changes in osmolality will be reflected in the CSF. When marked hypernatraemia and hyperosmolality are present, rehydration usually takes between six and 24 hours. This will protect the brain and CSF from rapid fluid and electrolyte shifts. The dangers of rapid correction of hyponatraemia have also been highlighted. Central pontine myelinolysis (CPM), originally described by Adams et al. (1959), and extra-pontine myelinolysis, are considered by Laureno and Karp (1988) to be caused by the rapid correction of hyponatraemia. They consider that CPM and hypoxic brain damage are distinct clinically, aetiologically and pathologically, and that correction of hyponatraemia should not cause the serum sodium to rise more than 12mmol/l in the first 24 hours and even less in each subsequent 24-hour period if the danger of myelinolysis is to be avoided. Arieff (1987), however, listed the major causes of permanent brain damage in CPM as: an episode of hypoxia or coma, a change of serum sodium of more than 20 to 25mmol/l in the initial 24 hours of therapy of hyponatraemia, the presence of associated medical conditions known to result in abnormalities of the blood-brain barrier, (*i.e.* hepatic cirrhosis), and delay in initiation of therapy for symptomatic hyponatraemia. CSF analysis is likely to show marked electrolyte disturbance in CPM, and osmotic pressure changes may well be central in the pathogenesis of CPM.

Other ions
While the CSF concentration of sodium is similar to that of plasma (140 to 150mmol/l) the CSF potassium concentration is normally only approximately two-thirds that of plasma values. Few modifications are seen in pathological syndromes, although Kalin *et al.* (1975) found that after acute anoxia, CSF potassium tended to rise, particularly in cisternal fluid, suggesting that potassium (and hydrogen) ions flow from brain cells into brain extracellular fluid, following anoxia, and that these changes are more accurately reflected by cisternal rather than lumbar fluid. Stutchfield and Cooke (1989) found that six out of 29 (21 per cent) of neonates with IVH had raised potassium concentrations in the CSF (3.7 to 30mmol/l); five developed cerebral infarctions. They consider that raised concentrations of potassium in the CSF occur with IVH and may contribute to the development of cerebral infarction.

While CSF concentrations of magnesium are about 30 per cent higher than those in serum, those of calcium and zinc are 50 per cent lower (Woodbury *et al.* 1968). Virtual independence of the CSF calcium concentration from fluctuations in the plasma has been demonstrated (Bradbury 1965), although passage of ^{45}ca from blood into CSF certainly occurs (Davson *et al.* 1987). The main cause of the discrepancy is the high degree of protein-binding of calcium. Studies have shown, however, that when sera of different calcium concentrations are studied, the proportion of ionised calcium remains the same. Venkataraman *et al.* (1987) confirmed that, in children, CSF calcium (and phosphorus) is lower and CSF magnesium higher than that of serum. In a study of trace elements in the CSF, Mitchell *et al.* (1984) found a lower concentration of cobalt in patients with motor neuron disease. In general, however, there is little evidence of any significant modifications in pathological states of any of these ions.

Proteins
CSF contains protein in a concentration very much less than that in plasma (neonates 400 to 1200, infants 200 to 800, children and adults 150 to 450mg/1). This is because formation of CSF in the choroid plexuses largely excludes these large molecular-weight substances. Leakage of serum protein, through membranes

whose main function is to exclude them, probably accounts for most of the proteins in the CSF—principally fibrinogen, albumin and globulin—but protein also comes from nervous tissue, through brain-tissue leakage.

The increase in protein content along the neuraxis previously mentioned (Hill *et al.* 1958, Weisner and Bernhardt 1978) presumably reflects additions of protein from adjacent nervous tissue. In particular, additional IgG may be added to the CSF independently of plasma along the neuraxis (Weisner and Bernhardt 1978). Beta$_2$-microglobulin has a concentration higher in human CSF than in plasma, and is even higher in meningitis and encephalitis (Tenhunen *et al.* 1978), and prealbumin represents a high percentage of proteins in the CSF compared with serum. Bock (1978) identified a number of proteins specific to nervous tissue.

Opinions about the nature and timing of the development of the blood-brain and blood-CSF barrier remain controversial (Adinolfi 1985, Saunders 1986), but it is clear that newborns and young infants have much higher CSF protein concentrations than do older infants, children and adults (Arnhold and Zetterstrom 1958, Widell 1958, Pilliero and Lending 1959).

Increases in total protein concentration, with significant increases in albumin, transferrin, and gammaglobulin, were demonstrated in infants with hydrocephalus (Pepe and Hochwald 1967). Cerda and Basauri (1980) defined three different CSF protein patterns found in children with hydrocephalus: a barrier-damage pattern, an obstructive pattern and a degenerative pattern. In a later paper (1985) they found that CSF calcium was increased in all three groups of patients when they were classified according to the CSF protein pattern. Those with a barrier-damage pattern had increased CSF phosphorus and magnesium, and those with a degenerative pattern had increased magnesium. The degenerative protein pattern was significantly associated with severe intracranial hypertension, and the obstructive pattern with mild intracranial hypertension. The authors suggest that measurement of these protein and ionic parameters may be of prognostic value in hydrocephalus.

Myelin basic protein (MBP)
MBP appears to be specific to myelin, and its presence in CSF is an index of active demyelination (Cohen *et al.* 1980). Although its measurement in the CSF has been used primarily in diagnosis and monitoring of multiple sclerosis, it is considered that it may also be beneficial in acute traumatic demyelination and leucoencephalopathy. Kohlschütter (1978) suggested that in newborns and older children, the presence of MBP in the CSF may be associated with severe brain-tissue destruction. Palfreyman *et al.* (1978, 1979) found that MBP in serum and CSF is high following head injury, and also that MBP assay may be valuable in the assessment of severity of brain damage and prediction of outcome in such patients (Thomas *et al.* 1978). CSF-MBP has been shown to be high in the leukodystrophies (Cohen *et al.* 1980) and in children with necrotising leukoencephalopathy associated with acute lymphoblastic leukaemia (Gangji *et al.* 1980). Many of this latter group had received intracranial irradiation and/or intrathecal methotrexate.

Because RICP may cause acute demyelination, high MBP in the CSF may be associated with RICP.

Enzymes

Measurements of enzymes and isoenzymes in both CSF and serum have been made for many years in an attempt to find reliable indicators of brain damage which may be used for diagnosis and prognosis of neurological disorders. Creatine kinase, lactic dehydrogenase and their isoenzymes have been widely studied for this purpose. The creatine kinase isoenzyme (CF-BB) was found by Pfeiffer *et al.* (1983) and by Worley *et al.* (1985) in both neurons and astrocytes, although Thompson *et al.* (1980) found it only in astrocytes. Studies by Herschkowitz and Cumings (1964) and Nathan (1967) found elevations of total CSF creatine kinase (CK) in patients with progressive hydrocephalus, and Sherwin *et al.* (1969) demonstrated that the source of CK in the CSF was the brain isoenzyme BB. Katz and Liebman (1970) considered that CK activity in the CSF was associated with CNS damage, Belton (1970) suggested that high concentrations of CK in the CSF in newborn infants were indicative of brain damage and indicated a poor prognosis, while Drummond and Belton (1972) indicated that CSF-CK measurements could be of value in the management of blocked or malfunctioning shunts in children with myelomeningocele and hydrocephalus. More recently two studies have looked at the relationship of the creatine kinase isoenzyme BB or CPK_1 and clinical status using the Glasgow coma scale devised by Teasdale and Jennett (1974) in patients with neurological injury, particularly head injury. Bakay and Ward (1983) found that CSF CPK_1 correlated with the degree of trauma and outcome in that the isoenzyme appeared in the acute phase, disappeared within three days and returned only if there was secondary injury to the brain causing additional neurological damage. Their studies on increased ICP demonstrated the presence of CPK_1 only in the presence of plateau waves and clinically significant deteriorations associated with the elevated ICP. They considered that the isoenzyme presence was not due to ICP itself, but that the imbalancing of pressure gradients with secondary brain injury results in the destruction of tissue and is the enzyme source. Hans *et al.* (1983) found CK-BB isoenzyme in ventricular CSF (and serum) within 13 hours following severe head injury, and noticed a good correlation between total CK and CK-BB in the CSF (but not in serum). They considered that the CK enzyme concentrations correlate well with both the Glasgow and Liège coma scales, are a quantitative index of primary brain damage, and that high enzyme values at admission correlate well with a poor outcome at six months. However, they did not find a correlation between CK-BB activity in the CSF and CK-BB.

CK in CSF is maximal 24 to 48 hours after resuscitation following cardiac arrest, according to Bøhmer *et al.* (1983), who considered that CK and hypoxanthine were more specific indicators of anoxic cerebral damage than lactate, pyruvate and potassium.

Elevation of CK-BB in serum following perinatal asphyxia is a sensitive indicator of brain damage in preterm infants (Cuestas 1980) and in term infants (Becker and Menzel 1978, Warburton *et al.* 1981, Walsh *et al.* 1982, Amato *et al.* 1986, Fernandez *et al.* 1987). Shields and Feldman (1982) and Speer *et al.* (1983) also found that increased serum CK-BB occurs after IVH. Walsh *et al.* (1982) thought that the measurements correlated well with neurologic outcome and with computerised

432

tomographic and radionuclide scanning as a method of prediction following asphyxia, but Fernandez *et al.* (1987) felt that the serum CK-BB results were of limited prognostic value. Lactic dehydrogenase (LDH) and its isoenzymes have also been extensively studied in the CSF in infants and children with intracranial pathology and neurological disease. Lending *et al.*(1959, 1964) found that LDH was increased in children with hydrocephalus prior to operative correction, whereas only minimal elevation was seen after shunt procedures. Bakay and Ward (1983) also studied serum and CSF LDH isoenzymes and found CSF LDH elevated following neurological trauma but thought LDH isoenzymes of less value in detecting secondary injuries than CK isoenzyme measurements. Conversely Dalens *et al.* (1981) thought LDH (and hydroxybutyrate dehydrogenase) measurements in CSF more closely related to psychomotor events at one year. Nelson *et al.* (1975) reported that increased concentrations of LDH were present in CSF in children with hydrocephalus and RICP, and Fernandez *et al.* (1986) concluded that LDH isoenzyme patterns in CSF may be of value in the assessment of anoxic brain damage. 2',3' cyclic nucleotide 3'-phosphohydrolase (CNP) has been shown to be associated with myelin (Kurihara and Tsukada 1967), probably with oligodendroglial membranes, and is considered a glial marker enzyme (Schousboe 1982). Its development in the CNS parallels that of myelination, including the accumulation of cholesterol (Belton and Anderson 1973, Toews and Horrocks 1976). Although its activity has been measured in the CSF by several workers, however, its measurement as an indicator of tissue damage and active demyelination has been considered to be less reliable than that of myelin basic protein (Sprinkle and McKhann 1978, Banik *et al.* 1979, Raes *et al.* 1981).

Other enzymes measured in the CSF include aspartate transaminase (formerly glutamic oxalacetic transaminase) (Lending *et al.* 1959, 1964; Dalens *et al.* 1981), enolase, aldolase, beta-hexosaminidase, beta-galactosidase, adenylate kinase, pyruvate kinase, cholinesterase and pseudo-cholinesterase (Royds *et al.* 1981, Simpson *et al.* 1984, Davson *et al.* 1987), but none of these appears to be of as much value as the studies which have shown a possible benefit for the measurement of CK, LDH and their isoenzymes in the assessment of brain damage in neurological disorders, and these enzymes would appear to be the best available for any prognostic studies regarding the effects of RICP.

Neuropeptides
We do not know the origin or fate of peptides found in the CSF (Krieger and Martin 1981). Table 14.II gives some peptides detected in human CSF (Jackson 1980). However, almost all the peptides with putative neurotransmitter modulation roles in the CNS have been measured in the CSF (Post *et al.* 1982). Since neural peptides occur not only in the hypothalamus and brain but also in the spinal cord, caution must be exercised in the interpretation of measured concentrations of peptides in the CSF. Increased concentrations of somatostatin have been found in various destructive and degenerative disorders of the CNS (Patel *et al.* 1977).

Measurements of beta-endorphins in the CSF have been made in newborns and in adults. Newborn concentrations appear to be higher than adult values, and to be

TABLE 14.II

Some peptides detected in human cerebrospinal fluid

Thyrotrophin-releasing hormone (TRH)
Luteinising-hormone-release hormone (LH-RH)
Somatostatin
Corticotrophin-releasing factor (CRF)
Growth hormone-releasing factor (GH-RF)
Gastrin
Cholecystokinin (CCK)
Vasoactive intestinal peptide (VIP)
Angiotensin II
Substance P
Sleep factor
Antimelanotropic protein
Adenohypophyseal hormones (growth hormone, adrenocorticotrophin, prolactin)
Neurohypophyseal hormones (vasopressin, oxytocin)
Opioid peptides (beta-endorphin)

increased in prolonged infant apnoea (Burnard *et al.* 1982, Orlowski 1986) and in near-miss sudden infant death syndrome (Sankaran *et al.* 1986). Laungani *et al.* (1985) found highly significant inverse correlation between one-minute Apgar scores and CSF beta-endorphin-like activity. Sankaran *et al.* (1986) showed that beta-endorphin concentrations in the CSF of infants did not correlate with plasma measurements. This confirmed a previous report in adults by Jeffcoate *et al.* (1978), who found that CSF values were always higher than plasma values.

Further studies on the role of neural peptides in the CSF are needed but their unique distribution raises the possibility that their measurements may provide a sensitive marker for the anatomical diagnosis of specific areas of CNS damage (Jackson 1980, Luerssen and Robertson 1980).

Neurotransmitters, their precursors and metabolites and cyclic nucleotides
Study of CSF precursors and metabolites of neurotransmitters has for some time been carried out as a biochemical approach to pathological changes in the brain. Moir *et al.* (1970) considered that interpretation of such analyses required the absence of CSF contamination by peripheral transmitters and their metabolites, and that increased concentrations of CSF amine metabolites could be a consequence of decreased elimination of metabolites from the CSF and/or a greater turnover of brain amines.

Amino acids in the CSF are present in general at a concentration of only 5 to 25 per cent of plasma. CSF glutamine, however, is present in approximately equal concentration to that in plasma, while cystine and proline are present in extremely low concentrations. Concentrations of CSF tryptophan, the precursor of serotonin, were 80 per cent higher in patients with an ICP greater than 25mmHg compared with controls (Hyyppä *et al.* 1977).

Gamma-aminobutyric acid (GABA) is a putative inhibitory neurotransmitter and lumbar CSF concentrations are considered to reflect brain GABA metabolism (Wood *et al.* 1978, 1979). Enna *et al.* (1977) observed an increasing GABA concentration during continuous lumbar CSF drainage. Bala Manyam *et al*. (1980) showed that patients with acute hypoxic encephalopathy had a higher mean GABA concentration than that of controls. Gamma-hydroxybutyric acid (GHB), a metabolite of GABA which itself has potent neuropharmacological and neurophysiological effects (Snead 1977), has been found in higher concentration in the CSF of young infants than in older children, in higher concentration in ventricular fluid than in lumbar CSF and in high concentration in the CSF of children with seizures (Snead *et al*. 1981).

Acetylcholine, its metabolism and concentration in CSF were reviewed by Haber and Grossman (1980). Although they consider that CSF obtained from intracranial sites rather than lumbar CSF would more accurately reflect biochemical processes in specific brain areas, they suggest that head injury and patients with ischaemic-anoxic brain damage may have the highest acetylcholine concentrations in CSF.

Monoamine metabolites. Shaywitz *et al*. (1980) reviewed the data on CSF monoamine metabolites in neurological disorders of childhood.

They monitored ventricular CSF serially in children with coma after cardiac arrest, in whom a ventricular catheter had been placed to monitor ICP. They found 5-hydroxyindoleacetic acid (5-HIAA) slightly above that observed in hydrocephalic children, their 'contrast' group, and homovanillic acid (HVA) more clearly elevated in concentration, reflecting what they believe to be the effects of cerebral oedema. Hyyppa *et al*. (1977), however, found the concentrations of HVA and 5-HIAA to be reduced in patients with high ICP compared to those with normal CSF pressures, while Porta and co-workers noted reduced HVA and no alteration in 5-HIAA in lumbar CSF in 10 patients (ages four to 28, mean 14.1 years) with chronic brain post-traumatic syndromes following head injury (Bareggi *et al*. 1975) but increased concentrations of HVA and 5-HIAA in ventricular CSF in acute brain post-traumatic syndromes (Porta *et al*. 1975). Shaywitz *et al*. (1979) found increased HVA but no changes in CSF concentrations of 5-HIAA in children with Reye's syndrome. Maira *et al*. (1975) studied adults with normal pressure hydrocephalus.The CSF HVA concentration was low and remained low after shunt procedure, although values increased if shunt obstruction occurred. No significant changes were found in lumbar and ventricular concentrations of 5-HIAA. 5-HIAA concentrations in the CSF were also studied by Massarotti *et al*. (1978) in children with hypertensive hydrocephalus before and after ventricular shunting. Some decrease in 5-HIAA occurred after shunting. In summary, lumbar monoamine metabolites appear to be elevated in traumatic coma and in ventricular CSF of children with Reye's syndrome and post-anoxic coma, as well as hydrocephalus (Shaywitz *et al*. 1980).

Ebert *et al*. (1980) pointed out that HVA, the major metabolite of dopamine, is present in high concentrations in the lateral ventricle because of its proximity to the caudate nucleus, and that there is a twofold decrease as CSF flows into the fourth ventricle and an additional decrease as CSF is sampled from the cisterna magna. Thus the lumbar concentration of HVA is 2 per cent of that found in the lateral ventricle. Similarly the concentration of 5-HIAA, the major metabolite of serotonin, also declines considerably as CSF moves from the ventricles to the lumbar space, but the gradient is not as steep as for HVA.

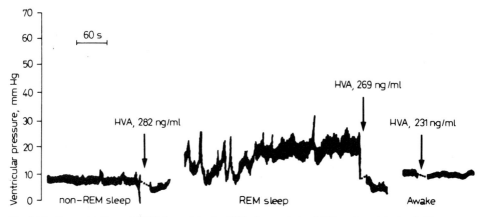

Fig. 14.1. Concentrations of HVA in ventricular CSF after periods of different ventricular fluid pressure in a 13-month-old boy, taken at 50-minute intervals. (Yates and Minns 1981).

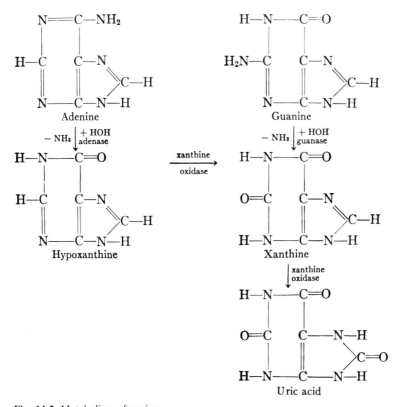

Fig. 14.2. Metabolism of purines.

The major metabolites of noradrenaline are vanillylmandelic acid (VMA) and 3-methoxy-4-hydroxyphenyl glycol (MHPG). Their concentrations are significantly higher in the third and fourth ventricles compared with the lateral ventricle (Gordon *et al.* 1975). This may reflect the increased concentration of noradrenaline in hypothalamic and brainstem structures. In contrast to HVA and 5-HIAA, no decrease in gradient from ventricles to lumbar space has been demonstrated. Yates and Minns (1981) found that concentrations in ventricular CSF of 5-HIAA, HVA and MHPG were not related to ventricular fluid pressure (Fig. 14.1), but noted that the mean concentration of MHPG was negatively correlated with age, being significantly higher in children up to six months of age than in older children. Habel *et al.* (1981) also found that CSF concentrations of 5-HIAA and HVA in children of mean age 2.5 years (range six months to six years) were about twice those found in adults. Langlais *et al.* (1985) confirmed this significant inverse correlation with age of MHPG, 5-HIAA and HVA in CSF in children aged one day to 10 years.

Nevertheless, Anderson *et al.* (1985) thought it unlikely that measurement of neurotransmitter precursors and metabolites in the CSF in neonates would be of much use in the diagnosis and treatment of conditions such as seizures, hydrocephalus and apnoea. The role of brain neurotransmitters and neuromodulators, and their measurement in paediatrics, was reviewed by Johnston and Singer (1982).

Nucleotides and cyclic nucleotides. Linking energy-production and energy-consuming processes are the nucleotides, especially adenosine and guanosine di- and tri-phosphates and also phosphocreatine. Cessation of energy production and the non-availability of energy stores occurs rapidly in total ischaemia (Siesjo and Wieloch 1985). Depletion of ATP and phosphocreatine are seen following birth asphyxia (Hope *et al.* 1984), Hope and Reynolds 1985) and the failure to maintain energy stores is a major factor in neuronal damage and death. ATP and to a lesser extent ADP are among the most labile constituents of brain. Hence their measurement in CSF is unlikely to be of value and so is rarely undertaken. Studies on their metabolites (particularly the cyclic nucleotides and oxypurines) have been more beneficial, and evidence suggests that measuring CSF cyclic adenosine 3′,5′-monophosphate (cyclic AMP or CAMP) and cyclic guanosine 3′,5′-monophosphate (CGMP) is more useful in studying alterations of these brain nucleotides than assaying plasma or urine concentrations (Heikkinen *et al.* 1975, Fleischer and Tindall 1980). Sebens and Korf (1975) suggest that cisternal CSF cyclic AMP concentrations reflect brain cyclic AMP content. Rudman *et al.* (1976a) showed the same concentration of CAMP (15 to 30nM/l) in ventricular and lumbar CSF from patients with normal ICP, although ventricular CSF CAMP was found to be higher than lumbar by other workers (Tsang *et al.* 1976), who also considered that cyclic AMP in lumbar CSF may not be totally dependent on the brain as the major source of this nucleotide but may also reflect spinal nucleotide metabolism. A significant correlation has been reported between the level of consciousness and ventricular CAMP in patients comatose following head trauma or intracranial haemorrhage. Improvement to normal sensorium was associated with CAMP concentrations returning towards normal values, whereas patients who remained comatose had persistent, markedly diminished ventricular CSF cAMP values, emphasising that prolonged traumatic coma is associated with a disturbance of cAMP metabolism within the CNS (Rudman *et al*. 1976*b*, Fleischer *et al*. 1977, Fleischer and Tindall 1980). Acute cerebral trauma has, however, been reported as increasing CSF cAMP (Brooks *et al*. 1980). CSF cGMP concentrations have been shown to be increased in patients with RICP (Goldberg *et al*. 1970, Rudman *et al*. 1976*b*, Fleischer *et al*. 1977). Metabolism of cyclic nucleotides in the CNS and their measurement in CSF have been reviewed by Brooks *et al*. (1980).

Oxypurines (hypoxanthine and xanthine). Xanthine, hypoxanthine and uric acid are produced by the catabolism of adenine and guanine (Fig. 14.2). Increased catabolism of adenine nucleotides occurs during tissue hypoxia, and accumulation of metabolites such as hypoxanthine occurs in the tissues. Concentration of hypoxanthine in the plasma (Saugstad 1975) and in CSF (Saugstad *et al*. 1976, Saugstad 1977) was proposed as a good indicator of tissue hypoxia. Manzke and Staemmler (1981) showed that extremely high concentrations of hypoxanthine, xanthine and uric acid were present in the CSF of children with various diseases of the nervous system. Levin *et al*. (1984) demonstrated a highly significant correlation between ICP and CSF hypoxanthine and xanthine concentrations in children with hydrocephalus. Harkness and Lund (1983) had shown that large rises in CSF hypoxanthine and to a lesser extent xanthine occurred about 24 hours after hypoxia in newborns, children and adults and that high concentrations were associated with later evidence of brain damage or subsequent death. Bejar *et al*. (1983) found high CSF concentrations of hypoxanthine in preterm infants with post-haemorrhagic hydrocephalus and that following successful treatment of the ventriculomegaly by lumbar puncture or by ventriculoperitoneal shunt the values decreased. They considered that the brain hypoxia was probably a consequence of the ventriculomegaly and not of the haemorrhagic insult. Harkness and his colleagues also showed that oxypurine excretion in the urine is raised after intrapartum hypoxia and perinatal asphyxia and that the excretion of hypoxanthine may be used either to exclude the possibility of post-asphyxial damage or to select asphyxiated infants who require further investigation (Harkness *et al*. 1982, 1983; Laing *et al*. 1988).

Lipids

The origin of lipids in the CSF has long been discussed. Lipids enter CSF with their carrier proteins, and although Tourtelotte (1959) concluded that CSF could be regarded as diluted serum with respect to lipids, there is clearly some modification by brain metabolism. For instance the percentage of cholesterol (33 per cent) in CSF is higher than in serum (20 per cent), while the concentration of linoleic acid is much lower in CSF. Seidel *et al*. (1980), however, showed a positive correlation between albumin and linoleic acid in the CSF. Illingworth and Glover (1971) compared the lipid composition in CSF in children and adults, and Sastry and Stancer (1968) measured the relative composition of phospholipids of CSF in children from infancy to 14 years. Phospholipids and cholesterol are the predominant lipids and lecithin is the major phospholipid. Despite this knowledge of lipid composition in controls, little diagnostic or prognostic use has been made of the estimation of CSF lipids. Even in multiple sclerosis, where Seidel *et al.* (1980) showed changes in CSF lipid profile, such estimations do not appear to be a better diagnostic tool than the usual routine procedures. Ondera and Ito (1977) showed increased total fatty acid concentrations in the CSF of 40 children aged one month to two years with congenital hydrocephalus who were studied prior to insertion of a shunt. In addition, in those whose ventricular pressure was above 150mm H_2O, the fatty-acid concentration was greater than in those with a pressure below 150mm. Furthermore, post-operatively those who showed a bad prognosis had higher concentrations than those with a good prognosis. The proportion of macrophages in CSF which are positive for sudanophilic lipid has been shown by Chester *et al.* (1971) to indicate the state of brain tissue in contact with CSF, and the proportion of fat-laden macrophages was correlated with evidence of brain damage and RICP. Furthermore, relief of the RICP resulted in a rapid diminution of the number of these fat-containing cells. Apart from this, there is little evidence that assay of lipids will contribute much to the clinical management of RICP.

Spectrophotometry

CSF in healthy individuals is optically clear. For nearly a century, however, it has been recognised that certain cerebrovascular accidents may cause the CSF to become coloured or xanthochromic. Oxyhaemoglobin, bilirubin and methaemoglobin are the three substances mainly responsible for the xanthochromia. Spectrophotometric scanning has been used to examine CSF to establish the nature of the substances in a specimen and thus to clarify the cause of the xanthochromia (Kunnas and Leppänen 1967, Kjellin 1979, Hellström and Kjellin 1971). Oxyhaemoglobin has an absorbance peak at 415λ (nm), methaemoglobin at 406, free bilirubin is represented by a flattened peak with a maximum at about 455, and conjugated bilirubin (bilirubin glucuronides) has a maximum peak at 422 (Fig. 14.3). Haemoglobin in the CSF is broken down to bile pigments which after about eight hours impart the yellow xanthochromic colour to the CSF. This reaches a maximum at 48 hours and disappears in 10 to 20 days (Brown 1974). Figure 14.4 shows sequential spectrophotometric scans over 14 days of CSF samples from a child following IVH. Oxyhaemoglobin alone indicates either a traumatic lumbar puncture or a recent intracranial haemorrhage. The presence of methaemoglobin with or without bilirubin in the presence of bilirubin in increased amounts is indicative of an earlier intracranial haemorrhage. Stroes and Van Rijn (1987) used derivative spectrophotometry to measure quantitatively very small quantities of oxyhaemoglobin, methaemoglobin and bilirubin in CSF. Spectrophotometric scanning has proved to be a useful diagnostic tool, but ultrasound can now provide good evidence of intracranial haemorrhage and is thus of increasing value in the investigation of RICP.

Nuclear magnetic resonance spectroscopy (NMRS)

The application of NMRS to *in vivo* studies of intracellular metabolism in the human brain is likely to provide important evidence on the pathophysiology and metabolism in cerebral hypoxia-ischaemia (Cox 1988). This non-invasive, non-

439

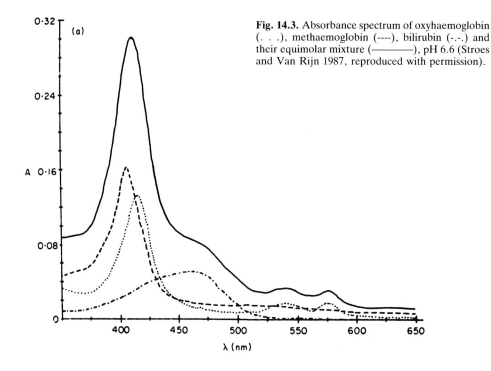

Fig. 14.3. Absorbance spectrum of oxyhaemoglobin (. . .), methaemoglobin (----), bilirubin (-.-.) and their equimolar mixture (————), pH 6.6 (Stroes and Van Rijn 1987, reproduced with permission).

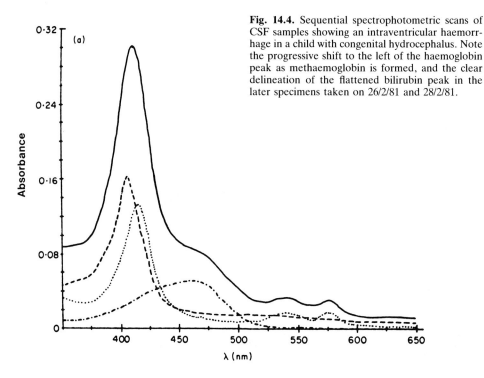

Fig. 14.4. Sequential spectrophotometric scans of CSF samples showing an intraventricular haemorrhage in a child with congenital hydrocephalus. Note the progressive shift to the left of the haemoglobin peak as methaemoglobin is formed, and the clear delineation of the flattened bilirubin peak in the later specimens taken on 26/2/81 and 28/2/81.

440

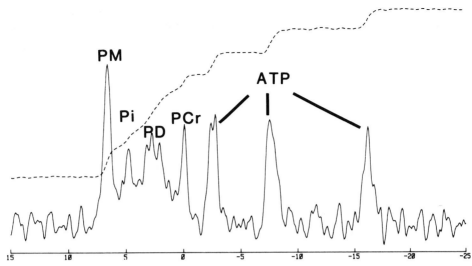

Fig. 14.5. ^{31}p NMR spectrum recorded from a normal full-term infant aged 16 hours. The x axis is chemical shift in parts per million and y axis is signal intensity. ATP = adenosine triphosphate (β, α and γ from r to l); PCr = phosphocreatine; PD = phosphodiester and phospholipids; Pi = inorganic orthophosphate; PM = phosphomonoester, mainly phosphoethanolamine. The interrupted line is the integral of the spectrum (Hope *et al*. 1984, Hope and Reynolds 1985, reproduced with permission).

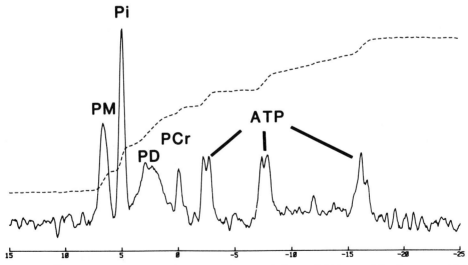

Fig. 14.6. ^{31}p NMR spectrum recorded from a full-term baby aged 48 hours, following severe birth asphyxia. Compare with Figure 10.5; note small PCr and large Pi peaks (Hope *et al*. 1984, Hope and Reynolds 1985, reproduced with permission).

441

destructive technique is being used increasingly to study the mechanism of changes in brain tissue that may lead to irreversible structural damage. Such studies should help our understanding of the importance of RICP. Already phosphorus ^{31}P has been used to study asphyxiated infants (Figs. 14.5, 14.6) (Hope *et al.* 1984), those with intraventricular haemorrhage (Younkin *et al.* 1988), and to follow changes in intracellular metabolism and the effect of therapy with mannitol (Cady *et al.* 1983). Using ^{31}P-MRS, signals can be detected from high-energy phosphates such as ATP and phosphocreatine, from inorganic phosphate and from compounds involved in membrane synthesis and breakdown (phosphomonoesters and phosphodiesters). ^{1}H-MRS may also be used in following changes in lactate concentration that may be a more sensitive marker of ischaemia and metabolic disease than variations in ^{31}P-MRS (Crockard *et al.* 1987). ^{13}C-MRS may prove to be useful in studying carbohydrate metabolism. Clearly studies in animals (Hope *et al.* 1987) will provide evidence on the mechanisms of asphyxial and hypoxial changes in the brain, but ultimately it is hoped that *in vivo* NMRS studies on body fluids such as CSF will provide important data which will enable better management of clinical problems such as RICP. Similarly, near infra-red spectrophotometry may provide valuable quantitative data at the cotside for the management of sick infants and for studying the pathophysiology of damage to the brain (Wyatt *et al.* 1986).

REFERENCES

Adams, R. D., Victor, M., Mancall, E. L. (1959) 'Central pontine myelinolysis. A hitherto undescribed disease occurring in alcoholic and malnourished patients.' *Archives of Neurology*, **81**, 154–172.

Adinolfi, M. (1985) 'Development of human blood-CSF-brain barrier.' *Developmental Medicine and Child Neurology*, **27**, 532–537.

Amato, M., Gambon, R. C., Von Muralt, G. (1986) 'Accuracy of Apgar score and arterial cord-blood pH in diagnosis of perinatal brain damage assessed by CK-BB isoenzyme measurement.' *Journal of Perinatal Medicine*, **14**, 335–338.

Anderson, G. M., Hoder, E. L., Shaywitz, B. A., Cohen, D. J. (1985) 'Neurotransmitter precursors and metabolites in CSF of human neonates.' *Developmental Medicine and Child Neurology*, **27**, 207–214.

Anderson, H., Roos, B. E. (1969) '5-hydroxyindoleacetic acid in cerebrospinal fluid of hydrocephalic children.' *Acta Paediatrica Scandinavica*, **58**, 601–608.

Anderson, J. M., Bain, A. D., Brown, J. K., Cockburn, F., Forfar, J. O., Machin, G. A., Turner, T. L. (1976) 'Hyaline-membrane disease, alkaline buffer treatment, and cerebral intraventricular haemorrhage.' *Lancet*, **1**, 117–119.

—— Belton, N. R. (1974) 'Water and electrolyte abnormalities in the human brain after severe intrapartum asphyxia.' *Journal of Neurology, Neurosurgery and Psychiatry*, **37**, 514–520.

Arieff, A. I. (1987) 'Hyponatremia associated with permanent brain damage.' *Advances in Internal Medicine*, **32**, 325–344.

Arnhold, R. G., Zetterstrom, R. (1958) 'Proteins in the cerebrospinal fluid in the newborn.' *Pediatrics*, **21**, 279–289.

Bakay, R. A. E., Ward, A. A. Jr. (1983) 'Enzymatic changes in serum and cerebrospinal fluid in neurological injury.' *Journal of Neurosurgery*, **58**, 27–37.

Bala Manyam, N. V., Katz, L., Hare, T. A., Gerber, J. C. III, Grossman, M. H. (1980) 'Levels of gamma-aminobutyric acid in cerebrospinal fluid in various neurologic disorders.' *Archives of Neurology*, **37**, 352–355.

Banik, N. L., Mauldin, L. B., Hogan, E. L. (1979) 'Activity of 2',3'-cyclic nucleotide 3'-phosphohydrolase in human cerebrospinal fluid.' *Annals of Neurology*, **5**, 539–541.

Bareggi, S. R., Porta, M., Selenati, A., Assael, B. M., Calderini, G., Collice, M., Rossandra, M., Morselli, P. L. (1975) 'Humovanillic acid and 5-hydroxyindoleacetic acid in the CSF of patients after a severe head injury. I. Lumbar CSF concentration in chronic brain post-traumatic syndromes.' *European Neurology*, **13**, 528–544.

Becker, M., Menzel, K. (1978) 'Brain-typical creatine kinase in the serum of newborn infants with perinatal brain damage.' *Acta Paediatrica Scandinavica*, **67**, 177–180.

Bejar, R., Saugstad, O. D., James, H., Gluck, L. (1983) 'Increased hypoxanthine concentrations in cerebrospinal fluid of infants with hydrocephalus.' *Journal of Pediatrics*, **103**, 44–48.

Belton, N. R. (1970) 'Creatine phosphokinase (CPK); blood and CSF levels in newborn infants and children.' *Archives of Disease in Childhood*, **45**, 600.

—— Anderson, J. M. (1973) '2',3'-cyclic nucleotide 3'-phosphohydrolase in the developing brain.' *Archives of Disease in Childhood*, **48**, 325.

—— Brown, J. K. (1979) *Unpublished observations.*

Bock, E. (1978) 'Nervous system specific proteins.' *Journal of Neurochemistry*, **30**, 7–14.

Bøhmer, T., Kjekshus, J., Vaagenes, P. (1983) 'Biochemical indices of cerebral ischemic injury.' *Scandinavian Journal of Clinical and Laboratory Investigation*, **43**, 261–265.

Bradbury, M. W. B. (1965) 'Magnesium and calcium in cerebrospinal fluid and in the extracellular fluid of brain.' *Journal of Physiology*, **179**, 67–68P.

Brooks, B. R., Wood, J. H., Diaz, M., Czerwinski, C., Georges, L. P., Sode, J., Ebert, M. H., Engel, W. K. (1980) 'Extracellular cyclic nucleotide metabolism in the human central nervous system.' *In* Wood, J. H. (Ed.) *Neurobiology of Cerebrospinal Fluid: I.* New York: Plenum. pp. 113–139.

Brown, J. K. (1974) 'Systematic neurology.' *In* Cockburn, F., Drillien, C. M. (Eds.) *Neonatal Medicine.* Oxford: Blackwell. pp. 556–626.

—— (1976) 'Infants damaged during birth. Pathology.' *In* Hull, D. (Ed.) *Recent Advances in Paediatrics. Vol. 5.* Edinburgh: Churchill Livingstone. pp. 35–56.

—— Habel, A. H. (1975) 'Toxic encephalopathy and brain swelling in children.' *Developmental Medicine and Child Neurology*, **17**, 659–679.

Burnard, E. D., Todd, D. A., John, E., Hindmarsh, K. W. (1982) 'Beta-endorphin levels in newborn cerebrospinal fluid.' *Australian Paediatric Journal*, **18**, 258–263.

Cady, E. B., Costello, A. M. de L., Dawson, M. J., Delpy, D. T., Hope, P. L., Reynolds, E. O. R., Tofts, P. S., Wilkie, D. R. (1983) 'Non-invasive investigation of cerebral metabolism in newborn infants by phosphorus nuclear magnetic resonance spectroscopy.' *Lancet*, **1**, 1059–1062.

Cerda, M., Basauri, L. (1980) 'Isoelectric focusing of CSF proteins in children with non-tumoral hydrocephalus.' *Child's Brain*, **7**, 169–181.

—— (1985) 'Cerebrospinal fluid protein patterns in children with hydrocephalus: relation to clinical parameters and electrolyte levels.' *Journal of Pediatric Neurosciences*, **1**, 245–253.

Chester, D. C., Penny, S. R., Emery, J. L. (1971) 'Fat-containing macrophages in the cerebrospinal fluid of children with hydrocephalus.' *Developmental Medicine and Child Neurology*, **25**, 33–38.

Cohen, S. R., Brooks, B. R., Jubelt, B., Herndon, R. M., McKhann, G. M. (1980) 'Myelin basic protein in cerebrospinal fluid. Index of active demyelination.' *In* Wood, J. H. (Ed.) *Neurobiology of Cerebrospinal Fluid: I.* New York: Plenum. pp. 487–494.

Cox, I. J. (1988) 'Nuclear magnetic resonance spectroscopy.' *British Journal of Hospital Medicine*, **40**, 165.

Crockard, H. A., Gadian, D. G., Frackowiak, R. S. J., Procter, E., Allen, K., Williams, S. R., Russell, R. W. (1987) 'Acute cerebral ischaemia: concurrent changes in cerebral blood flow, energy metabolites, pH and lactate measured with hydrogen clearance and ^{31}p, and ^{1}H nuclear magnetic resonance spectroscopy. II. Changes during ischaemia.' *Journal of Cerebral Blood Flow and Metabolism*, **7**, 394–402.

Cuestas, R. A. (1980) 'Creatine kinase isoenzymes in high-risk infants.' *Pediatric Research*, **14**, 935–938.

Dalens, B., Viallard, J. L., Raynaud, E. J. Dastugue, B. (1981) 'Enzyme studies and neonatal brain damage.' *Acta Paediatrica Scandinavica*, **70**, 743–749.

David, R., Ellis, D., Gartner, J. C. (1981) 'Water intoxication in normal infants: rôle of antidiuretic hormone in pathogenesis.' *Pediatrics*, **68**, 349–353.

Davson, H., Welch, K., Segal, M. B. (1987) *The Physiology and Pathophysiology of the Cerebrospinal Fluid.* Edinburgh: Churchill Livingstone.

Drummond, M. B., Belton, N. R. (1972) 'Creatine phosphokinase (CPK) in the CSF; its value in the management of children with myelomeningocele and hydrocephalus.' *Archives of Disease in Childhood*, **47**, 672.

Ebert, M. H., Kartzinel, R., Cowdry, R. W., Goodwin, F. K. (1980) 'Cerebrospinal fluid amine metabolites and the probenecid test.' *In* Wood, J. H. (Ed.) *Neurobiology of Cerebrospinal Fluid: I.*

New York: Plenum. pp. 97–112.

Edgren, E., Hedstrand, U., Nordin, M., Rydin, E., Ronquist, G. (1987) 'Prediction of outcome after cardiac arrest.' *Critical Care Medicine*, **15**, 820–825.

Enna, S. J., Wood, J. H., Synder, S. H. (1977) 'Gamma-aminobutyric acid in human cerebrospinal fluid: radioreceptor assay.' *Journal of Neurochemistry*, **28**, 1121–1124.

Eross, J., Silink, M., Dorman, D. (1981) 'Cerebrospinal fluid lactic acidosis in bacterial meningitis.' *Archives of Disease in Childhood*, **56**, 692–698.

Feldman, W., Drummond, K. N., Klein, M. (1970) 'Hyponatraemia following asphyxia neonatorum.' *Acta Paediatrica Scandinavica*, **59**, 52–57.

Fernandez F., Ouero, J., Verdu, A., Ferreiros, M. C., Daimiel, E., Roche, M. C. (1986) 'LDH isoenzymes in CSF in the diagnosis of neonatal brain damage.' *Acta Neurologica Scandinavica*, **74**, 30–33.

—— Verdu, A., Ouero, J., Perez-Higueras, A. (1987) 'Serum CPK-BB isoenzyme in the assessment of brain damage in asphyctic term infants.' *Acta Paediatrica Scandinavica*, **76**, 914–918.

Finberg, L., Luttrell, C., Redd, H. (1959) 'Pathogenesis of lesions in the nervous system in hypernatraemic states. II. Experimental studies of gross anatomic changes and alterations of chemical composition of the tissues.' *Pediatrics*, **23**, 46–53.

Fleischer, A. S., Rudman, D. R., Fresh, C. B., Tindall, G. T. (1977) 'Concentration of 3',5' cyclic adenosine monophosphate in ventricular CSF of patients following severe head trauma.' *Journal of Neurosurgery*, **47**, 517–524.

—— Tindall, G. T., (1980) 'Cerebrospinal fluid cyclic nucleotide alterations in traumatic coma.' *In* Wood, J. H. (Ed.) *Neurobiology of Cerebrospinal Fluid: I.* New York: Plenum. pp. 337–344.

Forbes, G. B., Perley, A. (1951) 'Estimation of total body sodium by isotopic dilution I. Studies on young adults.' *Journal of Clinical Investigation*, **30**, 558–565.

Gangji, D., Reaman, G. H., Cohen, S. R., Bleyer, W. A., Poplack, D. G. (1980) 'Leukoencephalopathy and elevated levels of myelin basic protein in the cerebrospinal fluid of patients with acute lymphoblastic leukemia.' *New England Journal of Medicine*, **303**, 19–21.

Goldberg, N. D., Lust, W. D., O'Dea, R. F., Wei, S., O'Toole, A. G. (1970) 'A rôle of cyclic nucleotides in brain metabolism.' *Advances in Biochemical Psychopharmacology*, **3**, 67–87.

Gordon, E., Perlow, M., Oliver, J., Ebert, M., Kopin, I. (1975) 'Origins of catecholamine metabolites in monkey cerebrospinal fluid.' *Journal of Neurochemistry*, **25**, 347–349.

Habel, A., Yates, C. M., McQueen, J. K., Blackwood, D., Elton, R. A. (1981) 'Homovanillic acid and 5-hydroxyindoleacetic acid in lumbar cerebrospinal fluid in children with afebrile and febrile convulsions.' *Neurology*, **31**, 488–491.

Haber, B., Grossman, R. G., (1980) 'Acetylcholine metabolism in intracranial and lumbar cerebrospinal fluid and in blood.' *In* Wood, J. H. (Ed.) *Neurobiology of Cerebrospinal Fluid: I.* New York: Plenum. pp. 345–350.

Hans, P., Born, J. D., Chapelle, J. P., Milbouw, G. (1983) 'Creatine kinase isoenzymes in severe head injury.' *Journal of Neurosurgery*, **58**, 689–692.

Harkness, R. A., Lund, R. J. (1983) 'Cerebrospinal fluid concentrations of hypoxanthine, xanthine, uridine and inosine: high concentrations of the ATP metabolite, hypoxanthine, after hypoxia.' *Journal of Clinical Pathology*, **36**, 1–8.

—— Simmonds, R. J., Coade, S. B., Lawrence, C. R. (1983) 'Ratio of the concentration of hypoxanthine to creatinine in urine from newborn infants: a possible indicator for the metabolic damage due to hypoxia.' *British Journal of Obstetrics and Gynaecology*, **90**, 447–452.

—— Whitelaw, A. G. L., Simmonds, R. J. (1982) 'Intrapartum hypoxia: the association between neurological assessment of damage and abnormal excretion of ATP metabolites.' *Journal of Clinical Pathology*, **35**, 999–1007.

Heikkinen, E. R., Simila, S. Myllyla, V. V., Hokkanen, E. (1975) 'Cyclic adenosine-3',5'-monophosphate concentration and enzyme activities of cerebrospinal fluid in meningitis in children.' *Zeitschrift für Kinderheilkunde*, **20**, 243–250.

Hellström, B., Kjellin, K. G. (1971) 'The diagnostic value of spectrophotometry of CSF in the newborn period.' *Developmental Medicine and Child Neurology*, **13**, 789–797.

Herschkowitz, N., Cumings, J. N. (1964) 'Creatine kinase in cerebrospinal fluid.' *Journal of Neurology, Neurosurgery and Psychiatry*, **27**, 247–250.

Hill, N. C., McKenzie, B. F., McGuckin, W. F., Goldstein, N. P., Svien, H. J. (1958) 'Proteins, glycoproteins and lipoproteins in the serum and cerebrospinal fluid of healthy subjects.' *Proceedings of the Mayo Clinic*, **33**, 686–698.

Hope, P. L., Cady, E. B., Chu, A., Delpy, D. T., Gardner, R. M., Reynolds, E. O. R. (1987) 'Brain metabolism and intracellular pH during ischaemia and hypoxia: an in vivo ^{31}p and ^{1}H magnetic resonance study in the lamb.' *Journal of Neurochemistry*, **49**, 75–82.

—— Costello, A. M. de L., Cady, E. B., Delpy, D. T., Tofts, P. S., Chu, A., Hamilton, P. A., Reynolds, E. O. R., Wilkie, D. R. (1984) 'Cerebral energy metabolism studied with phosphorus NMR spectroscopy in normal and birth-asphyxiated infants.' *Lancet*, **2**, 366–370.

—— Reynolds, E. O. R. (1985) 'Investigation of cerebral energy metabolism in newborn infants by phosphorus nuclear magnetic resonance spectroscopy.' *Clinics in Perinatology*, **12**, 261–275.

Horovitz, Y., Tal, I., Keynan, A. (1985) 'Acid base balance in blood and cerebrospinal fluid.' *Archives of Disease in Childhood*, **60**, 579–581.

Hunter, G., Smith, H. V. (1960) 'Calcium and magnesium in human cerebrospinal fluid.' *Nature*, **186**, 161–162.

Hyyppa, M. T., Langvik, V. A., Nieminen, V., Vapalahti, M. (1977) 'Tryptophan and monoamine metabolites in ventricular cerebrospinal fluid after severe cerebral trauma.' *Lancet*, **1**, 1367–1368.

Illingworth, D. R., Glover, J. (1971) 'The composition of lipids in cerebrospinal fluid of children and adults.' *Journal of Neurochemistry*, **18**, 769–776.

Jackson, I. M. D. (1980) 'Significance and function of neuropeptides in cerebrospinal fluid.' *In* Wood, J. H. (Ed.) *Neurobiology of Cerebrospinal Fluid.* New York: Plenum. pp. 625–650.

Jeffcoate, W. J., McLoughlin, L., Hope, J., Rees, L. H., Ratter, S. J., Lowry, P. J., Besser, G. M. (1978) 'Beta-endorphin in human cerebrospinal fluid.' *Lancet*, **2**, 119–121.

Johnston, M. V., Singer, H. S. (1982) 'Brain neurotransmitters and neuromodulators in pediatrics.' *Pediatrics*, **70**, 57–68.

Kalin, E. M., Tweed, W. A., Lee, J., Mackeen, W. L. (1975) 'Cerebrospinal fluid acid-base and electrolyte changes resulting from cerebral anoxia in man.' *New England Journal of Medicine*, **293**, 1013–1016.

Katz, R. M., Liebman, W. (1970) 'Creatine phosphokinase in central nervous system disorders and infections.' *American Journal of Diseases of Children*, **120**, 543–546.

Killian, J. A. (1925) 'Lactic acid of normal and pathological spinal fluids.' *Proceedings of the Society for Experimental Biology and Medicine*, **23**, 255–257.

Kjallquist, A., Nardini, M., Siesjo, B. K. (1969) 'The CSF/blood potential in sustained acidosis and alkalosis in the rat.' *Acta Physiologica Scandinavica*, **71**, 255–256.

Kjellin, K. G. (1970) 'Bilirubin compounds in the CSF.' *Journal of the Neurological Sciences*, **13**, 161–173.

Kohlschütter, A. (1978) 'Myelin basic protein in cerebrospinal fluid from children.' *European Journal of Pediatrics*, **127**, 155–161.

Krauss, A. N., Thibeault, D. W., Auld, P. A. (1972) 'Acid-base balance in cerebrospinal fluid of newborn infants.' *Biology of the Neonate*, **21**, 25–34.

Kravath, R. E., Aharon, A. S., Abal, G., Finberg, L. (1970) 'Clinically significant physiologic changes from rapidly administered hypertonic solutions: acute osmol poisoning.' *Pediatrics*, **46**, 267–275.

Krieger, D. T., Martin, J. B. (1981) 'Brain peptides.' *New England Journal of Medicine*, **304**, 876–884; 944–951.

Kunnas, M., Leppänen, V. V. (1967) 'Spectrophotometric studies in the cerebrospinal fluid in the newborn, especially for the demonstration of blood.' *Annales Paediatriae Fenniae*, **13**, 89–95.

Kurihara, T., Tsukada, Y. (1967) 'The regional and subcellular distribution of 2′,3′-cyclic nucleotide 3′-phosphohydrolase in the central nervous system.' *Journal of Neurochemistry*, **14**, 1167–1174.

Laing, I., Brown, J. K., Harkness, R. A. (1988) 'Clinical and biochemical assessments of damage due to perinatal asphyxia: a double blind trial of a quantitative method.' *Journal of Clinical Pathology*, **41**, 247–252.

Langlais, P. J., Walsh, F. X., Bird, E. D., Levy, H. L. (1985) 'Cerebrospinal fluid neurotransmitter metabolites in neurologically normal infants and children.' *Pediatrics*, **75**, 580–586.

Laungani, S. G., Delivoria, B., Gintzler, A., Wong, S., Glass, L. (1985) 'Apgar scores and cerebrospinal fluid beta-endorphin-like immunoreactivity during the first day of life.' *American Journal of Diseases of Children*, **139**, 403–404.

Laureno, R., Karp, B. A. (1988) 'Pontine and extrapontine myelinolysis following rapid correction of hyponatraemia.' *Lancet*, **1**, 1439–1441.

Lending, M., Slobody, L. B., Stone, M. L., Hosbach, R. E., Mestern, J. (1959) 'Activity of glutamic-oxalacetic transaminase and lactic dehydrogenase in cerebrospinal fluid and plasma of normal and abnormal infants.' *Pediatrics*, **24**, 378–388.

—— —— Mestern, J. (1964) 'Cerebrospinal fluid glutamic oxalacetic transaminase and lactic dehydrogenase activities in children with neurologic disorders.' *Journal of Pediatrics*, **65**, 415–421.

Levin, S. D., Brown, J. K., Harkness, R. A. (1984) 'Cerebrospinal fluid hypoxanthine and xanthine concentrations as indicators of metabolic damage due to raised intracranial pressure in hydrocephalic children.' *Journal of Neurology, Neurosurgery and Psychiatry*, **47**, 730–733.

Levinson, A. (1917) 'The hydrogen ion concentration of cerebrospinal fluid: studies in meningitis.' *Journal of Infectious Diseases*, **21**, 556–570.

Luerssen, T. G., Robertson, G. L. (1980) 'Cerebrospinal fluid vasopressin and vasotocin in health and disease.' *In* Wood, J. H. (Ed.) *Neurobiology of the Cerebrospinal Fluid: I.* New York: Plenum.

Maira, G., Bareggi, S. R., Di Rocco, C., Calderini, G., Marselli, P. L. (1975) 'Monoamine acid metabolites and cerebrospinal fluid dynamics in normal pressure hydrocephalus: preliminary results.' *Journal of Neurology, Neurosurgery and Psychiatry*, **38**, 123–128.

Mann, N., Punt, J. (1986) 'Intracranial pressure monitoring in children.' *Care of the Critically Ill*, **2**, 143–146.

Mannery, J. F., Bale, W. F. (1941) 'The penetration of radioactive sodium and phosphorus into the extra and intracellular phases of tissues.' *American Journal of Physiology*, **132**, 215–231.

Manzke, H., Staemmler, W. (1981) 'Oxypurine concentration in the CSF in children with different diseases of the nervous system.' *Neuropediatrics*, **12**, 209–214.

Martensson, J., Thunberg, T. (1951) 'Studies on the citric acid in the cerebrospinal fluid.' *Acta Medica Scandinavica*, **140**, 454–463.

Massarotti, M., Migliore, A., Roccella, P., Tegos, S., Toffano, G. (1978) '5-hydroxy-indoleacetic acid (5-HIAA) levels in the cerebrospinal fluid of hydrocephalic children before and after ventricular shunting procedure.' *Child's Brain*, **4**, 195–204.

Mathew, O. P., Bland, H., Boxerman, S. B., James, E. (1980) 'CSF lactate levels in high risk neonates with and without asphyxia.' *Pediatrics*, **66**, 224–227.

McGuinness, G. A., Weisz, S. C., Bell, W. E. (1983) 'CSF lactate levels in neonates. Effect of asphyxia, gestational age and postnatal age.' *American Journal of Diseases of Children*, **137**, 48–50.

Mitchell, J. D., Harris, I. A., East, B. W., Pentland, B. (1984) 'Trace elements in cerebrospinal fluid in motor neurone disease.' *British Medical Journal*, **288**, 1791–1792.

Moir, A. T. B., Ashcroft, G. W., Crawford, T. B. B., Eccleston, D., Guldberg, H. C. (1970) 'Cerebral metabolites in cerebrospinal fluid as a biochemical approach to the brain.' *Brain*, **93**, 357–368.

Myers, R. E., Beard, R., Adamsons, K. (1969) 'Brain swelling in the newborn rhesus monkey following prolonged partial asphyxia.' *Neurology*, **19**, 1012–1018.

Nathan, M. (1967) 'Creatine phosphokinase in the cerebrospinal fluid.' *Journal of Neurology, Neurosurgery and Psychiatry*, **30**, 52–55.

Nelson, P. V., Carey, W. F., Pollard, A. C. (1975) 'Diagnostic significance and source of lactate dehydrogenase and its isoenzymes in cerebrospinal fluid of children with a variety of neurological disorders.' *Journal of Clinical Pathology*, **28**, 828–833.

Nolph, K. D., Schrier, R. W. (1970) 'Sodium, potassium and water metabolism in the syndrome of inappropriate antidiuretic hormone secretion.' *American Journal of Medicine*, **49**, 534–545.

Onodera, Y., Ito, H. (1977) 'Fatty acid in cerebrospinal fluid of congenital hydrocephalus.' *Child's Brain*, **3**, 101–108.

Orlowski, J. P. (1986) 'Cerebrospinal fluid endorphins and the infant apnea syndrome.' *Pediatrics*, **78**, 233–237.

Palfreyman, J. W., Thomas, D. G. T., Ratcliffe, J. G. (1978) 'Radioimmunoassay of human myelin basic protein in tissue extract, cerebrospinal fluid, serum and its clinical application to patients with head injury.' *Clinica Chimica Acta*, **82**, 259–270.

—— Johnston, R. V., Ratcliffe, J. G., Thomas, D. G. T., Forbes, C. D. (1979) 'Radio-immuno-assay of serum basic protein and its application to patients with cerebrovascular accident.' *Clinica Chimica Acta*, **92**, 403–409.

Patel, Y. C., Rao, K., Reichlin, S. (1977) 'Somatostatin in human cerebrospinal fluid.' *New England Journal of Medicine*, **296**, 529–533.

Pepe, A. J., Hochwald, G. M. (1967) 'Trace proteins in biological fluids III.' *Proceedings of the Society of Experimental Biological Medicine*, **126**, 630–633.

Perlow, M. J., Lake, C. R. (1980) 'Daily fluctuations in cerebrospinal fluid concentrations of catecholamines, monoamine metabolites, cyclic AMP and γ aminobutyric acid in rhesus monkeys.' *In* Wood, J. H. (Ed.) *Neurobiology of Cerebrospinal Fluid: I.* New York: Plenum.

Pfeiffer, F. E., Homburger, H. A., Yanagihara, T. (1983) 'Creatine kinase BB isoenzyme in CSF in neurological diseases: measurement by radioimmunoassay.' *Archives of Neurology*, **40**, 169–172.

Pilliero, S. J., Lending, M. (1959) 'Protein studies in normal newborn infants.' *Journal of Diseases of Children*, **97**, 785–789.

Plum, F., Price, R. W. (1973) 'Acid-base balance of cisternal and lumbar cerebrospinal fluid in hospital patients.' *New England Journal of Medicine*, **289**, 1346–1351.

Porta, M., Bareggi, S. R., Collice, M., Assael, B. M., Selanati, A., Calderini, G., Rossanda, M.,

446

Morselli, P. L. (1975) 'Homovanillic acid and 5-hydroxyindoleacetic acid in the CSF of patients after a severe head injury. II. Ventricular CSF concentrations in acute brain post-traumatic syndromes.' *European Neurology*, **13**, 545–554.

Post, R. M., Goodwin, F. K., Gordon, E. (1973) 'Amine metabolites in human cerebrospinal fluid: effects of cord transection and spinal fluid block.' *Science*, **179**, 879–899.

—— Gold, P., Rubinow, D. R., Ballenger, J. C., Bunney, W. E. Jr., Goodwin, F. K. (1982) 'Peptides in the cerebrospinal fluid of neuropsychiatric patients: an approach to central nervous system peptide function.' *Life Sciences*, **31**, 1–15.

Raes, I., Weissbarth, S., Maker, H. S., Lehrer, G. M. (1981) 2'3'-cyclic nucleotide 3'-phosphodiesterase in cerebrospinal fluid.' *Neurology*, **31**, 1361–1363.

Rossanda, M., Sganzerla, E. P. (1976) 'Acid-base and gas tension measurements in cerebrospinal fluid.' *British Journal of Anaesthesia*, **48**, 753–760.

Royds, J. A., Timperley, W. R., Taylor, C. B. (1981) 'Levels of enolase and other enzymes in the cerebrospinal fluid as indices of pathological change.' *Journal of Neurology, Neurosurgery and Psychiatry*, **44**, 1129–1135.

Rudman, D., O'Brien, M. S., McKinney, A. S., Hoffman, J. C., Patterson, J. H. (1976a) 'Observations on the cyclic nucleotide concentrations in human cerebrospinal fluid.' *Journal of Clinical Endocrinology and Metabolism*, **42**, 1088–1097.

—— Fleischer, A. S., Jutner, M. S. (1976b) 'Concentration of 3',5' cyclic adenosine monophosphate in ventricular cerebrospinal fluid of patients with prolonged coma after head trauma or intracranial hemorrhage.' *New England Journal of Medicine*, **295**, 635–638.

Sankaran, K., Hindmarsh, K. W., Wallace, S. M., McKay, R. J., O'Donnell, M. (1986) 'Cerebrospinal fluid and plasma beta-endorphin concentrations in prolonged infant apnea (near-miss sudden infant death syndrome).' *Developmental Pharmacology and Therapeutics*, **9**, 224–230.

Sastry, P. S., Stancer, R. C. (1968) 'Quantitative analysis and fatty acid composition of phospholipid constituents in cerebrospinal fluid of various age groups.' *Clinica Chimica Acta*, **22**, 301–307.

Saugstad, O. D. (1975) 'Hypoxanthine as a measurement of hypoxia.' *Pediatric Research*, **9**, 158–161.

—— (1977) 'Hypoxanthine as an indicator of tissue hypoxia: a study of plasma, cerebrospinal fluid and brain tissue concentrations.' *Journal of Oslo City Hospital*, **27**, 29–40.

—— Schrader, H., Aasen, A. O. (1976) 'Alteration of the hypoxanthine level in cerebrospinal fluid as an indicator of tissue hypoxia.' *Brain Research*, **112**, 188–189.

Saunders, N. R. (1986) 'Development of human blood-CSF-brain barrier.' *Developmental Medicine and Child Neurology*, **28**, 261–262.

Schousboe, A. (1982) 'Glial marker enzymes.' *Scandinavian Journal of Immunology*, **15**, Suppl. 9, 339–356.

Sebens, J. B., Korf, J. (1975) 'Cyclic AMP in cerebrospinal fluid: accumulation following probenecid and biogenic amines.' *Experimental Neurology*, **46**, 333–344.

Seidel, D., Heipertz, R., Weisner, B. (1980) 'Cerebrospinal fluid lipids in demyelinating disease. II. Linoleic acid as an index of impaired blood-CSF barrier.' *Journal of Neurology*, **222**, 177–182.

Shaywitz, B. A., Cohen, D. J., Bowers, M. B. Jr. (1980) 'Cerebrospinal fluid monoamine metabolites in neurological disorders of childhood.' *In* Wood, J. H. (Ed.) *Neurobiology of Cerebrospinal Fluid I.* New York: Plenum. pp. 219–236.

—— Venes, J., Cohen, D. J., Bowers, M.B. Jr. (1979) 'Monoamine metabolites in ventricular fluid.' *Neurology*, **29**, 467–472.

Sherwin, A. L., Norris, J. W., Bulcke, J. A. (1969) 'Spinal fluid creatine kinase in neurologic disease.' *Neurology*, **19**, 993–999.

Shields, W. D., Feldman, R. C. (1982) 'Serum CPK-BB isoenzyme in preterm infants with periventricular hemorrhage.' *Journal of Pediatrics*, **100**, 464–468.

Siesjo, B. K., Plum, F. (1971) 'Cerebral energy metabolism in normoxia and hypoxia.' *Acta Anaesthesiologica Scandinavica*, Suppl. **45**, 81–101.

—— Wieloch, T. (1985) 'Cerebral metabolism in ischaemia: neurochemical basis for therapy.' *British Journal of Anaesthesia*, **57**, 47–62.

Simmons, M. A., Adcock, E. W., Bard, H., Battaglia, F. C. (1974) 'Hypernatraemia and intracranial hemorrhage in neonates.' *New England Journal of Medicine*, **291**, 6–9.

Simpson, H., Habel, A. H., George, E. L. (1977) 'Cerebrospinal fluid acid-base status and lactate and pyruvate concentrations after convulsions of varied duration and aetiology in children.' *Archives of Disease in Childhood*, **52**, 844–849.

Simpson, R. M., Besley, G. T. N., Moss, S. E., Eden, O. B. (1984) 'CSF lysosomal enzyme activities in children treated for acute leukaemia.' *European Paediatric Haematology and Oncology*, **1**, 183–186.

Snead, O. C. (1977) 'Gamma hydroxybutyrate.' *Life Sciences*, **20**, 1935–1943.
—— Brown, G. B., Morawetz, R. B. (1981) 'Concentration of gamma-hydroxybutyric acid in ventricular and lumbar cerebrospinal fluid.' *New England Journal of Medicine*, **304**, 93–95.
Speer, M. E., Ou, C. N., Buffone, G. J., Frawley, V. L. (1983) 'Creatine phosphokinase BB isoenzyme in very-low-birth-weight infants: relationship with mortality and intraventricular hemorrhage.' *Journal of Pediatrics*, **103**, 790–793.
Sprinkle, T. J., McKhann, G. M. (1978) 'Activity of 2',3'-cyclic-nucleotide 3'-phospho-diesterase in cerebrospinal fluid of patients with demyelinating disorders.' *Neuroscience Letters*, **7**, 203–206.
Stroes, J. W., Van Rijn, H. J. M. (1987) 'Quantitative measurement of blood pigments in cerebrospinal fluid by derivative spectrophotometry.' *Annals of Clinical Biochemistry*, **24**, 189–197.
Stutchfield, P. R., Cooke, R. W. I. (1989) 'Electrolytes and glucose in cerebrospinal fluid of premature infants with intraventricular haemorrhage: rôle of potassium in cerebral infarction.' *Archives of Disease in Childhood*, **64**, 470–475.
Svenningsen, N. W., Siesjo, B. K. (1972) 'Cerebrospinal fluid lactate/pyruvate ratio in normal and asphyxiated neonates.' *Acta Paediatrica Scandinavica*, **61**, 117–124.
Teasdale, G., Jennett, B. (1974) 'Assessment of coma and impaired consciousness. A practical scale.' *Lancet*, **2**, 81–83.
Tenhunen, R., Iivanainen, M., Kovanen, J. (1978) 'Cerebrospinal fluid beta$_2$-micro-globulin in neurological disorders.' *Acta Neurologica Scandinavica*, **57**, 366–373.
Thomas, D. G. T., Palfreyman, J. W., Ratcliffe, J. G. (1978) 'Serum myelin basic protein assay in diagnosis and prognosis in patients with head injury.' *Lancet*, **1**, 113–115.
Thompson, R. J., Kynoch, P. A. M., Sarjant, J. (1980) 'Immunohistochemical localization of creatine kinase BB isoenzyme to astrocytes in human brain. *Brain Research*, **201**, 423–426.
Toews, A. D., Horrocks, L. A. (1976) 'Developmental and aging changes in protein concentration and 2',3'-cyclic nucleosidemonophosphate phosphodiesterase activity (EC 3.1.4.16) in human cerebral white and gray matter and spinal cord.' *Journal of Neurochemistry*, **27**, 545–550.
Tourtelotte, W. W. (1959) 'Study of lipids in the cerebrospinal fluid. VI.' *Neurology*, **9**, 375–383.
Tsang, D., Lal, S., Sourkes, T. L., Ford, R. M., Aronoff, A. (1976) 'Studies on cyclic AMP in different compartments of cerebrospinal fluid.' *Journal of Neurology, Neurosurgery and Psychiatry*, **39**, 1186–1190.
Van Heist, A. N. P., Maas, A. H. J., Visser, B. F. (1966) 'Comparison of the acid-base balance in cisternal and lumbar cerebrospinal fluid.' *Pflugers Archives*, **287**, 242–246.
Vannucci, R. B., Hellmann, J., Dubynsky, O., Page, R. B., Maisels, M. J. (1980) 'Cerebral oxidative metabolism in perinatal post-haemorrhagic hydrocephalus.' *Developmental Medicine and Child Neurology*, **22**, 308–316.
Venkataraman, P. S., Kirk, M. R., Tsang, R. C., Chen, I. W. (1987) 'Calcium, phosphorus, magnesium and calcitonin concentrations in the serum and cerebrospinal fluid of children.' *American Journal of Diseases of Children*, **141**, 751–753.
Walsh, P., Jedeikin, R., Ellis, G., Primhak, R., Makela, S. K. (1982) 'Assessment of neurologic outcome in asphyxiated term infants by use of serial CK-BB isoenzyme measurement.' *Journal of Pediatrics*, **101**, 988–992.
Warburton, D., Singer, D., Oh, W. (1981) 'Effects of acidosis on the activity of creatine phosphokinase and its isoenzymes in the serum of newborn infants.' *Pediatrics*, **68**, 195–197.
Wasterlain, C. G. (1976) 'Effects of neonatal status epilepticus on rat brain development.' *Neurology*, **26**, 975–986.
—— Plum, F. (1973) 'Vulnerability of developing rat brain to electro-convulsive seizures.' *Archives of Neurology*, **29**, 38–45.
Weisner, B., Bernhardt, W. (1978) 'Protein fractions of lumbar, cisternal and ventricular cerebrospinal fluid.' *Journal of Neurological Science*, **37**, 205–214.
Widell, S. (1958) *On the Cerebrospinal Fluid in Normal Children and in Patients with Acute Bacterial Meningo-encephalitis*. Lund, Berlingska Boktryckeriet.
Wood J. H. (1980) 'Sites of origin and concentration gradients of neurotransmitters, their metabolites and cyclic nucleotides in cerebrospinal fluid.' *In* Wood, J. H. (Ed.) *Neurobiology of Cerebrospinal Fluid: I*. New York: Plenum.
—— Glaeser, B. S., Enna, S. J., Hare, T. A. (1978) 'Verification and quantification of GABA in human cerebrospinal fluid.' *Journal of Neurochemistry*, **30**, 291–293.
—— Hare, T. A., Glaeser, S. B., Ballenger, J. C., Post, R. M. (1979) 'Low cerebrospinal fluid gamma-aminobutyric acid content in seizure patients.' *Neurology*, **29**, 1203–1208.
Woodbury, J., Lyons, K., Carretta, R., Hahn, A., Sullivan, J. F. (1968) 'Cerebrospinal fluid and serum levels of magnesium, zinc and calcium in man.' *Neurology*, **18**, 700–705.

Worley, G., Lipman, B., Gewolb, I. H., Green, J. A., Schmechel, D. E., Roe, C. R., Gross, S. J. (1985) 'Creatine kinase brain isoenzyme: relationship of cerebrospinal fluid concentration to the neurological condition of newborns and cellular localization in the human brain.' *Pediatrics*, **76**, 15–21.

Wyatt, J. S., Cope, M., Delpy, D. T., Wray, S., Reynolds, E. O. R. (1986) 'Quantification of cerebral oxygenation and haemodynamics in sick newborn infants by near infrared spectro-photometry.' *Lancet*, **1**, 1063–1066.

Yates, C. M., Minns, R. A. (1981) 'Monamine metabolites and ventricular fluid pressure in children.' *Child's Brain*, **8**, 138–144.

Younkin, D., Medoff-Cooper, B., Guillet, R., Sinwell, T., Chance, B., Delivoria-Papadopoulos, M. (1988) 'In vivo ^{31}p nuclear magnetic resonance measurement of chronic changes in cerebral metabolites following neonatal intraventricular hemorrhage.' *Pediatrics*, **82**, 331–336.

Ziegler, M. G., Lake, C. R., Wood, J. H. (1976) 'Circadian rhythm in cerebrospinal fluid noradrenaline of man and monkey.' *Nature*, **264**. 656–658.

INDEX

tumours, 26
volume, 14
see also Cerebral
Brain death, 309–311
Brainstem (vegetative) failure, 43, 69 (table)
  progressive, 69–70
Bromide partition test, 217
Bulk extracellular flow, 27
Burns, 286–287

C

Calcium, 297
Calcium channel blockers, 160–161
Carbon dioxide, 21–22, 56–57
  apnoea unresponsive to, 73
  cerebrovascular response, 9–10, 42, 44
    localised loss, 10
  changes in cerebral bloodflow, 292
  reactivity in coma, 292, 296–297
Carbonic anhydrase, 16
Cardiac arrest, 287–288
Carotid artery development, 38–39
Carotid sinus, 43
Ceftasidine, 328
Ceftriaxone, 328, 332
Cella media index, 222
Central nervous system infections, intracranial
  hypertension, 284–285
Central neurotransmitter labels, 106 (table)
Cerebellar astrocytoma, 19
Cerebral abscess, 202–203
  tuberculous, 220
Cerebral bloodflow (circulation), 6–7, 38–73,
  77–113
  autoregulation, 10–11, 21, 41 (table), 41–44,
    295–296
    impairment in head injury, 187
    in non-traumatic coma, 295
    paralysis by anoxic ischaemic damage, 25
  changes on reperfusion after ischaemia, 293
  clinical conditions affecting, 55 (fig.)
  control, 40–41
    local biochemical, 44
  definition, 77
  development, 38–39
  measurements, 7–8, 46–56, 77–113
    autoradiography, 78 (table), 80
    diffusible tracers, 87–88
    Doppler velocitometry, 47–49, 82–86
    electrical impedance, 78 (table)
    experimental/reference techniques, 77–82
    first pass methods *see* First pass methods
    flow meters, 77
    impedance plethysmography, 47
    inert gas wash-out *see* Inert gas wash-out
    inert tracer wash-out, 78 (table), 81–82
    magnetic resonance, 78 (table), 86–87
    mercury strain gauge plethysmography, 47
    microspheres, 78 (table), 79–80
    nitrous oxide method, 42

PET scan, 49, 78 (table), 97
radio-isotope methods, 46–47
SPECT, 52, 95 (table)
ultrasound, 78 (table), 182
wash-in, 78 (table)
  post-cerebral insult, 294
  venous, 39
Cerebral congestion, 21–22
Cerebral diabetes, 43
Cerebral gliosis, 23
Cerebral herniation, early signs, 289 (table)
Cerebral infarction, impaired perfusion-
  induced, 58–59
Cerebral oedema, 4, 22–24, 429
  biochemical estimation, 34–35
  classification, 24–30
  clinical diagnosis, 30–35
    neurosurgical, 34
  CT scan, 31–32
  cytotoxic, 22
  focal, 26
  generalised inflammatory, 203–204
  hydrostatic, 27, 42
  intracellular, 27–28
  intracranial pressure measurement, 33–35
  magnetic resonance imaging, 34
  myelinoclastic, 22, 30
  necrotic, 30, 204
  neuropathological confirmation, 34
  osmotic, 28–30
    diabetic ketoacidosis as cause, 29, 30
    fatal, 29
    hyperosmolar brain to plasma, 28–29
    hyperosmolar plasma to brain, 28
  osmotic imbalance-induced, 203
  pathophysiology, 23
  raised intracranial pressure signs, 31
  situational causation, 31
  status epilepticus-induced, 31
  types, 22 (table)
  vasogenic, 22, 25–27
    causes, 25 (table)
  white-matter, 204
Cerebral perfusion pressure, 6, 44–45, 157
Cerebral protection, 160–162
Cerebral tumours, vasoactive substances secretion, 26
Cerebral vascular disease, 112
  intracranial hypertension, 285
Cerebral vasomotor paralysis, 4
Cerebral veins, 39
  blood obtaining, 7
  infarction, 147
  pressure, 6
Cerebritis, 203
Cerebrospinal fluid
  absorption, 19–20
  amino acids, 434
  bilirubin, 439
  calcium, 430

453

Phospholipids, 438
Pinocytosis, 24, 25
Plasma, osmolality, 29
Platybasia, 18
Pontine glioma, 19
Positron emission tomography, 97–99
Post-asphyxial encephalopathy, 143–144,
  159–160
Posterior fossa tumours, 19
Post-haemorrhagic ventricular dilatation,
  157–158
Post-hypoxic rigidity, 175
Pressure-volume index, 5, 230
Primitive neuroectodermal tumour, 19
Prolactin, 434
Prolonged infant apnoea, 434
Propranolol, 16, 42
Prostacyclin, 161–162, 329
Prostaglandin(s)
  PG$_{12}$, 24
  PGE$_2$, 24
Prostaglandin inhibitors, 161–162
Proteus mirabilis
  cerebral abscess, 202
Pseudo-cholinesterase, 433
Pseudo-phaeochromocytoma syndrome, 43
Pseudotumour cerebri *see* Benign intracranial
  hypertension
Pulmonary oedema, 71–72
Purine metabolism, 436 (fig.)
Pyogenic meningitis, 189–216
  cerebral abscess, 202–203
  cerebral congestion, 205
  cerebral oedema, 203–205
  choroid plexitis, 197–198
  clinical features, 191–192
  CSF pressure measurement, 194 (fig.)
  ependymitis, 201
  imaging, 192–193
  intracranial pressure measurement, 193–195
  lumbar puncture
    contraindications, 190
    repeat, 190
  Luschka/Magendie foramina obstruction, 201
  neurosurgery, 210–215
  perfusion defects, 205
  pressure cones, 189–191
  raised intracranial pressure, 195–209
  subdural effusion, 201
  subdural empyema, 201
  therapeutic failure, 215–216
  ventriculomegaly, 192
Pyruvate, 428
Pyruvate kinase, 433

Q
Queckenstedt test, 22

R
Raised intracranial pressure

birth asphyxia infant, 156–157
brainstem failure, 69 (table), 69–70
causes, 3–5
cerebral perfusion loss, 68–69
cerebral perfusion pressure, 6
cerebral venous pressure, 6
conscious level, 64–67
eye signs, 62–63
homeostasis disorders, 67–73
  biochemical/endocrine, 73 (table)
  cardiovascular, 72 (table)
  gut, 71 (table)
  respiratory, 71 (table)
local pressure necrosis, 69
midbrain compression, 67
motor signs, 63–64
neck retraction, 64 (fig.)
production mechanisms, 13–35
  hydrocephalus *see* Hydrocephalus
  space occupation, 13–14
shifts/cones, 60
symptoms, 3
vascular compression, specific, 69
Renal disease, 286
Respiratory arrhythmias, 71
Respiratory centre, 43
Re-uptake blockers, 106 (table)
Reye's syndrome, 28, 31, 32, 259–274, 330 (fig.)
  aetiology, 259
  arterial blood pressure monitoring, 271–272
  biochemical defects, 262–263
  clinical features, 259–262
  incidence, 259
  management, 263–274
    antibiotics, 270
    arteriovenous oxygen difference (AVDO$_2$),
      268
    blood gases, 273
    calcium, 274
    cerebral bloodflow, 269
    chest therapy, 274
    clinical status at presentation, 263
    CPP monitoring, 265–268
    CT scan, 263
    CVP continuous monitoring, 271
    Dextrostix, 274
    drugs/substances to be avoided, 273
    ECG, 273
      monitoring, 272
    elective paralysis/ventilation, 264
    electrolytes, 270, 273–274
    end of monitoring, 274
    fluids, 270
    glucose chain, 263–264, 274
    head elevation, 265
    ICP monitoring, 265–268
    initial coagulation study, 274
    jugular venous oxygen saturation, 268–269
    neomycin ± lactulose, 273
    non-steroidal anti-inflammatory drugs, 271